ESSENTIALS OF COMMUNITY-BASED NURSING

Karen Saucier Lundy, PhD, RN, FAAN

PROFESSOR
COLLEGE OF NURSING
UNIVERSITY OF SOUTHERN MISSISSIPPI
HATTIESBURG, MISSISSIPPI

Sharyn Janes, PhD, RN, ACRN

PROFESSOR
COLLEGE OF NURSING
UNIVERSITY OF SOUTHERN MISSISSIPPI
HATTIESBURG, MISSISSIPPI

JONES AND BARTLETT PUBLISHERS
Sudbury, Massachusetts
BOSTON   TORONTO   LONDON   SINGAPORE

World Headquarters
Jones and Bartlett Publishers
40 Tall Pine Drive
Sudbury, MA 01776
978-443-5000
info@jbpub.com
www.jbpub.com

Jones and Bartlett Publishers Canada
2406 Nikanna Road
Mississauga, ON L5C 2W6
CANADA

Jones and Bartlett Publishers International
Barb House, Barb Mews
London W6 7PA
UK

Library of Congress Cataloging-in-Publication Data

Lundy, Karen Saucier.
    Essentials of community health nursing / Karen Saucier Lundy, Sharyn Janes.
        p. ; cm.
    Includes bibliographical references and index.
    ISBN 0-7637-2348-7 (alk. paper)
    1. Community health nursing. I. Janes, Sharyn. II. Title.
    [DNLM: 1. Community Health Nursing—United States. WY 106 L962e 2003]
RT98 .L863 2003
610.73'43—dc21   2002044438

Chief Executive Officer: Clayton Jones
Chief Operating Officer: Don W. Jones, Jr.
Executive V.P. & Publisher: Robert W. Holland, Jr.
V.P., Design and Production: Anne Spencer
V.P., Sales and Marketing: William Kane
V.P., Manufacturing and Inventory Control: Therese Bräuer
Acquisitions Editor: Penny M. Glynn
Production Manager: Amy Rose
Associate Editor: Karen Zuck
Associate Production Editor: Karen C. Ferreira
Production Assistant: Jenny L. McIsaac
Senior Marketing Manager: Alisha Weisman
Associate Marketing Manager: Joy Stark-Vancs
Marketing Associate: Jennifer Killam-Zambrano
Manufacturing and Inventory Coordinator: Amy Bacus
Composition: Northeast Compositors
Text Design: PageMasters and Company
Cover Design: Kristin E. Ohlin
Printing and Binding: DB Hess
Cover Printing: DB Hess

Printed in the United States of America
07 06 05 04 03   10 9 8 7 6 5 4 3 2 1

Contents

A - W

PART ONE   Community-Focused Nursing Care

PART TWO   Diversity in Community-Based Nursing Roles

PART THREE   Community-Based Nursing Care

Dedication

I am honored to dedicate this book to my family and friends who make up my life community and who provided me with the love and commitment needed to see this book come to life. To bring a text of this size and breadth to print consumes time, energy, and focus from many. Special recognition to my husband, Dr. Chris Lundy, who acted as gentle critic and editor and gave me time and space when I needed it. Thank you for staying the distance with me and making my dream, your dream. For my son, Parker Lundy, who still believes that anything is possible; you are the joy of my existence and my connection to the faculty of wonder. For my father, Marshall Saucier, from whom I learned the value of intellectual curiosity and the importance of the circle of community that gives life meaning. You have always been my inspiration. I am eternally grateful for your love and intellectual presence in my life. And I am most grateful to Marcelle Saucier Stinson, Wayne Saucier, and John Lundy for the encouragement needed to see this to the end. And for being a part of this book in so many ways, I thank Judy Barton and Ann Lanier for their belief in me and being with me through the years, sharing your hearts and your wisdom. A special thanks to Tom Lochhaas, for giving me my first publishing opportunity when I had little to say or to offer in publishing; I am grateful that you had faith in me and that I benefited from your extraordinary editing talents on this text as well. It was a fitting completion of our publishing journey together over the past decade. I am thankful for the good fortune, in the face of extraordinary personal challenges, to benefit from the healing gifts of Nagan Bellare, MD. You helped me find my way back to health, which made it possible for me to complete this text. For the healing environment created by Charlotte McDonnell, RN, BSN, OCN, and your nursing staff, to Dolly Mathis, RN, BSN, Brad Archer, RN, BSN, and Spencer, you all have been critical to my healing and embody the essence of good nursing care. And to my friend and co-author, Dr. Sharyn Janes, without whom this book would not have happened. Thank you for helping me to believe that anything was possible, even when the rest of the world seemed to suggest otherwise. For your friendship and shared vision of this text, I remain eternally grateful.

Karen Saucier Lundy

This dedication is for all of my family and friends who have encouraged and supported me along the way and who gave me the strength to complete the journey that was the creation of this book. A very special thanks to my mother, Joan Janes, for always believing in me and helping me to believe in myself and to my daughter, Heather Rakauskas Sherry, for always making me proud of her in every way and for her special contributions to this book. To my son-in-law Cliff Sherry, my sisters Diane Janes and Joan Kilvitis, and my brother and sister-in-law Harry and Lana Janes—thanks for being an endless source of love and encouragement. My siblings are nurses who have provided constant "feedback" and support for this project. Special thanks to Justin, Holly, and Oscee just for being them and loving me. There are three very special friends deserving of mention: First, Dr. Gale Spencer, professor and director of my master's program at SUNY Binghamton, who introduced me to the world of public health. Her friendship and guidance helped shape the early stages of my career. For Evelyn Jenkins, who has been a nurse for more than 50 years and is truly a role model for professional nursing. She taught me that to be a "good" nurse you must care about your clients, your profession, and yourself. Finally Dr. Kay Lundy, my friend and colleague, who has given me both professional and personal opportunities that I could only have imagined in my dreams. We have shared laughter, tears, and most of all the belief in a common dream. She is much more than a friend. She is family.

Sharyn Janes

About the Authors

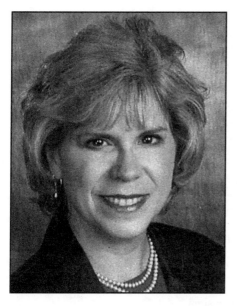

Karen Saucier Lundy, PhD, RN, FAAN, is currently a Professor at the University of Southern Mississippi College of Nursing in Hattiesburg, Mississippi. She has practiced in community and public health in diverse settings, such as state health departments, migrant health programs, the U.S. Public Health Service, school health, and high-risk maternity and child health. She has also functioned in neonatal intensive care as a staff nurse, clinical instructor, and transport nurse in regional referral medical centers. Dr. Lundy has taught community health at the baccalaureate and master's levels. In addition, Dr. Lundy has taught holistic health, research, maternal child health, and philosophy of science in the doctoral program. She has been responsible for undergraduate and graduate courses in community health nursing and doctoral courses in philosophy of science and qualitative research. Dr. Lundy served as Dean at Delta State University School of Nursing in Cleveland, Mississippi, and was on faculty at the University of Mississippi, Loretta Heights College in Denver, Colorado, and the University of Colorado School of Nursing in Denver. Dr. Lundy has also taught sociology at the University of Colorado in Boulder, including courses in family, gender roles, deviance, and social theory. Her scholarly presentations and publications have been in the areas of community health, philosophy of science, gender role and the family, historical research, media, and international health and education in Great Britain, Germany, Jamaica, and Cuba. She holds a BS in nursing from the University of Southern Mississippi College of Nursing, an MS in community health nursing from the University of Colorado School of Nursing in Denver and an MA and PhD in sociology from the University of Colorado in Boulder. Dr. Lundy is the author of *Perspectives in Family and Community Health,* which was named an American Journal of Nursing Book of the Year in 1990.

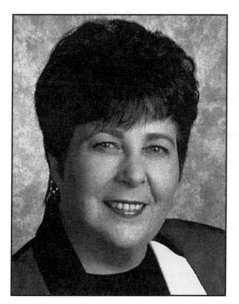

Sharyn Janes, PhD, RN, ACRN, is currently a Professor at the University of Southern Mississippi College of Nursing in Hattiesburg, Mississippi, where she teaches community health nursing at the baccalaureate and master's levels. She also teaches health care policy at the doctoral level, international health courses in Cuba and Jamaica, and graduate and undergraduate courses in transcultural nursing. Dr. Janes is the Director of the University of Souther Mississippi's Center for International Health. Prior to her tenure at the University of Southern Mississippi, Dr. Janes was an associate professor in the School of Nursing at Florida Agricultural and Mechanical University in Tallahassee, Florida. She earned her BSN at Marywood College, Scranton, Pennsylvania; her MS in community health nursing at the State University of New York at Binghamton; and her PhD in Higher Education at Florida State University, Tallahassee. Dr. Janes has practiced nursing in a variety of community settings, including home health, hospice, and school health and in several acute care settings, including medical-surgical units and emergency departments. She holds certification in HIV/AIDS nursing. Her scholarly presentations and publications are predominantly in the areas of HIV/AIDS education and prevention; cultural issues in nursing education, practice, and research; and international health and education.

Contributors

A. Serdar Atav, PhD
Associate Professor
Decker School of Nursing
Binghamton University
Binghamton, New York

Joan H. Baldwin, DNSc, RN
Professor
College of Nursing
Brigham Young University
Provo, Utah

Lucy Bradley-Springer, PhD, RN, ACRN
Associate Professor and Director
Mountain Plains AIDS Education and Training Center
School of Medicine
University of Colorado Health Sciences Center
Denver, Colorado

Margaret A. Burkhardt, PhD, RN, CS, HNC
Director
Healing Matters
Beckley, West Virginia

Patricia Butterfield, PhD, RN
Associate Professor
College of Nursing
Montana State University–Bozeman
Bozeman, Montana

Janie B. Butts, DSN, RN
Assistant Professor
College of Nursing
The University of Southern Mississippi
Hattiesburg, Mississippi

Venus Callahan, RNC, MSN, FNP, WHNP
Family Nurse Practitioner
Mississippi State Department of Health
Mississippi Family Health Care Center
Pascagoula, Mississippi

Cynthia O'Neill Conger, PhD, RN
Assistant Clinical Professor
School of Nursing
University of Texas at Austin
Austin, Texas

Virginia Lee Cora, DSN, RN, CS
Adult/Geriatric Nurse Practitioner
Assistant Professor
Division of Geriatrics
School of Medicine
University of Mississippi Medical Center
Jackson, Mississippi

Norma G. Cuellar, DSN, RN
Assistant Professor
College of Nursing
The University of Southern Mississippi
Hattiesburg, Mississippi

Susan Oliver Dodds, MSN, RN, CRNP
Family Nurse Practitioner
Private Practice
Marlton, New Jersey

Joseph E. Farmer, RN, MSN
Instructor
College of Nursing
The University of Southern Mississippi–Gulf Park
Long Beach, Mississippi

Barbara Foster, RN, MSN
Division of Associate Degree Nursing
Copiah-Lincoln Community College
Wesson, Mississippi

Gail A. Harkness, DrPH, RN, FAAN
Professor and Chair
Department of Nursing
School of Health and Human Services
University of New Hampshire
Durham, New Hampshire

Sherry Hartman, DrPH, RN
Associate Professor
College of Nursing
The University of Southern Mississippi
Hattiesburg, Mississippi

Loretta Sweet Jermott, PhD, RN, FAAN
Associate Professor and Director, Center for Urban
    Health Research
School of Nursing
University of Pennsylvania
Philadelphia, Pennsylvania

Harriet J. Kitzman, PhD, RN
Loretta C. Ford Professor of Nursing
School of Nursing
University of Rochester
Rochester, New York

Anne C. Klijanowicz, MS, PNP, CS
Senior Advanced Practice Nurse, Pediatrics
University of Rochester Medical Center
Rochester, New York

Debra K. Lance, RN, MSN
St. Luke's Home Care
Boga Chitta, Mississippi

Sarah Steen Lauterbach, MSPH, EdD, RN
Associate Professor
Florida State University
School of Nursing
Tallahassee, Florida

Russell C. McGuire, RN, PhD
Director
Clinical Services
Appalachian Regional Healthcare, Inc.
Hazard, Kentucky

Michelle Cousins Mott, RN, MSN, CRNP
Family Nurse Practitioner
Penn Nursing Network Practices
School of Nursing Center for Urban Health Research
University of Pennsylvania
Philadelphia, Pennsylvania

Bonita R. Reinert, PhD, RN
Professor
College of Nursing
University of Southern Mississippi
Hattiesburg, Mississippi

Heather Rakauskas Sherry, MS, PhD
Student Services Policy Specialist
Florida State Board of Community Colleges
Former Legislative Analyst
Florida House of Representatives
Tallahassee, Florida

Jean Shreffler, PhD, RN
Assistant Professor
College of Nursing
Montana State University–Bozeman
Missoula, Montana

Gale A. Spencer, PhD, RN
Associate Professor and Director
Kresge Center for Nursing Research
Decker School of Nursing
Binghamton University
Binghamton, New York

Mary E. Stainton, MS, RN-C, FAAN
Retired President
South Mississippi Home Health, Inc.
Hattiesburg, Mississippi

Vicki Sutton, RN, MSN
Division of Associate Degree Nursing
Copiah-Lincoln Community College
Wesson, Mississippi

Linda Beth Tiedje, PhD, RN, MA, FAAN
Adjunct Associate Professor
College of Human Medicine
Department of Epidemiology
Michigan State University
East Lansing, Michigan

Karen B. Utterback, RN, MSN
Vice President of Operations
Adult Nursing Division
Deaconess HomeCare, Inc.
Hattiesburg, Mississippi

H. Lorrie Yoos, PhD, CPNP
Associate Professor of Clinical Nursing
School of Nursing
University of Rochester Medical Center
Rochester, New York

Contributors to Chapter Special Features

Margaret M. Aiken, PhD, RN
Sexual Assault Nurse Examiner (SANE)
Memphis Sexual Assault Resource Center
Memphis, Tennessee

Ruth D. Berry, RN, MSN
Associate Professor
Community Health Nursing/Administration
College of Nursing
University of Kentucky
Parish Nurse, Second Presbyterian Church
Lexington, Kentucky

Ilene Purvis Bloxsom, BSN, RN
Director
Dale Medical Center Home Health
Ozark, Alabama

Ann Elizabeth Kaiser Brown, MSN, RN
School Nurse Consultant
Natchez, Mississippi

Miriam Cabana, MSN, RN
Coordinator of Learning Center
College of Nursing
The University of Southern Mississippi
Hattiesburg, Mississippi
Former Nursing Supervisor
Mississippi State Penitentiary
Parchman, Mississippi

Lynne Cameron, ANP
Skagway Medical Center
Skagway, Alaska

Alvara Leonard Castillo
Assistant Professor of Nursing
Instituto Superior de Ciencias Médicas
President of Havana Chapter of Cuban Nurses Society
Havana, Cuba

Emily Chandler, MS, MDIV, PhD, RN
Coordinator of Psychiatric/Mental Health Nursing Track
Graduate Program in Nursing
MGH Institute of Health Professions
Boston, Massachusetts

Betty Dickson
Executive Director and Lobbyist
Mississippi Nurses Association
Jackson, Mississippi

Mary Fisher
Author and AIDS Activist
Washington, DC

Marjaneh Fooladi, PhD, RN
Assistant Professor
College of Nursing
The University of Southern Mississippi
Hattiesburg, Mississippi

Jim Jones, BEd, RN
Case Manager and Home Health Nurse
South Mississippi Home Health
Hattiesburg, Mississippi

Deborah Konkle-Parker, MSN, RN, FNP, ACRN
Family Nurse Practitioner
Department of Medicine
Division of Infectious Diseases
The University of Mississippi Medical Center
Jackson, Mississippi

Ann Thedford Lanier, PhD
National Science Foundation
Washington, DC

Judith K. Leavitt, MEd, RN, FAAN
Professor of Nursing
School of Nursing
The University of Mississippi Medical Center
Jackson, Mississippi

Debendra Manandhar, MPA
Community Development Consultant with NGOs
Kathmandu, Nepal

Frances R. Martin, PhD, CFNP
Family Nurse Practitioner and Associate Director
Student Health Services
Hattiesburg, Mississippi

Lic. Juana Daisy Berdayes Martinez
Associate Dean for Graduate Studies and Research
Julio Trigo School of Nursing
Instituto Superior de Ciencias Médicas
Havana, Cuba

Arlene McFarland, DNS, RN
Family Therapist and Author
Fort Payne, Alabama

Anayda Fernandez Naranjo, MD
Dean
Julio Trigo School of Medical Sciences
Instituto Superior de Ciencias Médicas
Havana, Cuba

Sharon L. Oswald, PhD
Associate Professor of Management
Director of Graduate Management Programs
College of Business
Auburn University
Auburn, Alabama

Regina Hood Posey, MSN, RN
Instructor
The University of Southern Mississippi
College of Nursing
Hattiesburg, Mississippi

Bonnie Rogers, DrPH, COHN-S, RN, FAAN
Associate Professor and Director
Occupational Health Nursing Program
School of Public Health
University of North Carolina at Chapel Hill
Chapel Hill, North Carolina

Elizabeth A. Simnons
Graduate Student
Auburn University
Auburn, Alabama

Connie Thompson, BSN, RN, ACRN
HIV Case Manager
Delta Region AIDS Education and Training Center
The University of Mississippi Medical Center
Department of Medicine
Division of Infectious Diseases
Jackson, Mississippi

Ntombodidi Muzzen-Sherra (Zodidi) Tshotsho, MCur, DCur
Deputy Director
Child Youth, Women and Mental Health in the National
Directorate: Mental Health and Substance Abuse
Pretoria, South Africa

Jean Watson, PhD, RN, FAAN, HNC
Distinguished Professor of Nursing
Endowed Chair in Caring Science
University of Colorado Health Sciences Center
Denver, Colorado

Anna Frances Z. Wenger, PhD, RN, FAAN
Affiliate Faculty, Neil Hodgson Woodruff School of Nursing
Faith and Health Consortium Coordinator
Interfaith Health Program
Rollins School of Public Health
Emory University
Atlanta, Georgia

Reviewers

Kathleen Masters, DNS, RN
Assistant Professor
The University of Southern Mississippi
College of Nursing
Hattiesburg, Mississippi

Janette S. McCrory, MSN, RN
Instructor
Delta State University
School of Nursing
Cleveland, Mississippi

Marjorie McCullagh, RN, PhD
North Dakota State University
Department of Nursing
Fargo, North Dakota

Carol O'Neil, RN, PhD
University of Maryland-Baltimore
School of Nursing
Baltimore, Maryland

Lisa Paine, CNM, DrPH, FAAN, FACNM
Boston University
School of Public Health
Boston, Massachusetts

Heather R. Sherry, BA, MS, PhD(c)
Student Services Policy Specialist
Florida State Board of Community Colleges
Former Legislative Analyst
Florida House of Representatives
Tallahassee, Florida

Nancy A. Sowan, RN, PhD
University of Vermont
School of Nursing
Burlington, Vermont

Mary Stewart, MSN, RN, PhD(c)
Assistant Professor
William Carey College
Hattiesburg, Mississippi

Pat Torsella, RN, DNSc
Bloomsburg University
Department of Nursing
Bloomsburg, Pennsylvania

Foreword

The health of people is a reflection of the communities in which they live, play, work, and learn. Communities shape the lifestyles that people adopt and their likelihood of living safe, fulfilling, and productive lives. For those who seek to understand human health, the community is an important force to understand. For those who wish to improve the health of others, the community is an essential factor in the equation of people's health and well-being.

The relationship between the health of people and their communities lies at the core of nursing's work. As a profession whose hallmark is concern for human health, nursing has had a long history of engagement in the community. Nurses have practiced in this context, have exercised social activism and advocacy for community causes, and are themselves active members of their communities. Many of nursing's greatest leaders have come from the ranks of nurses working in community and public health.

Despite the close relationship between nurses and the community, the advancement of medical technology, the rise of institutions in which people receive care, and the financial systems supporting services have overshadowed the roles that nurses play in the community context. The public perception of nurses is frequently one in which the nurse is seen as a provider of services to people in hospitals. This view, coupled with the fact that the majority of nurses do work in institutional settings, has had a negative impact on the development of specialties within the community—and the education that prepares them for these roles. One indication of this is the relatively small number of outstanding texts available for teaching community-based nursing.

Fortunately, community health nursing is now moving into its renaissance. The fastest growing context for nursing services is now the community. And, there is widespread recognition that the challenges facing health care today can only be addressed if early interventions are delivered in the community context. In short, the day of community health nursing has arrived.

This text heralds the arrival of this new era for community health nursing. It does so in a manner that sets it apart from previous works of this type. It is an exciting and innovative collection of important information, ideas, and perspectives that promise to meet the challenge of educating nurses for ef-fective, community-based nursing practice. It is also a text that makes significant connections between theory, practice, and learning, in ways that are grounded in the emerging reality of community health nursing.

There are many important and useful features to this text. First, it has value as a text specifically designed for undergraduate ADN nursing programs. Second, the text is designed to support education that integrates community health nursing across content and specialty practice areas. It can also support individual specialty course work in community health nursing. This is a text that has widespread applicability across types of education and curricular designs.

The contributors to this book are also noteworthy in that they represent some of the very best thinkers in the field. They are practitioners, researchers, educators, policy makers, and innovators in the field. They bring important viewpoints, challenging readers to think beyond conventional views of community health.

Perhaps most important is that this book is a significant and timely contribution to the advancement of the public's health. The theme that ties this work together is one that focuses on the real goal of nursing education and practice: meeting the health needs of people everywhere. This theme is one that recurs throughout the text with great clarity.

The editors of this book are really its architects—they have conceptualized and brought to fruition a wonderfully designed project that serves its mission very well. They had the foresight to see the movement of community health nursing into new importance in the health of people and to help move the field forward through enhancing the education of those practicing in its specialties.

Marla E. Salmon, ScD, RN, FAAN
Associate Vice President for Nursing Science
Woodruff Health Sciences Center
Dean and Professor
Nell Hodgson Woodruff School of Nursing
Emory University
Former Director, The Division of Nursing
U.S. Department of Health and
    Human Services

Preface

Community health nursing has historically responded to changes in health care needs of the population and met those needs in a variety of diverse roles and settings. As we enter the 21st century, the health care needs of the public can seem overwhelming to the beginning nurse. The health care system in the United States has produced technological advancements never thought possible at the beginning of the last century. Public health, along with scientific and technological progress, has resulted in an ever-increasing average life span for Americans while other parts of the world struggle to meet basic health care needs. Greater life expectancy of individuals with chronic and acute conditions has continued to challenge the health care system's ability to provide efficient and quality care for its population. As the population of the United States has become increasingly more diverse, the need for change in community health nursing is imperative; practice must now reflect an awareness of these diverse values and beliefs of populations from the homeless to children with AIDS. Morbidity and mortality statistics reveal significant disparities among population groups, while socioeconomic and cultural factors have led to increased violence and substance abuse. Health care must be provided within the client population's cultural context, whether influenced by age, gender, race, or ethnicity. In this text, we have attempted to represent diversity among our authors, in the selection of chapter content, and in the general visual presentation of the text. By doing so, we hope to have produced a textbook that is more representative of what communities are in the United States—a unified society made up of many different populations and unique health perspectives.

This text is intended to serve as a primary text for ADN nursing students throughout the curriculum with an *emphasis on community-based nursing practice* directed toward health promotion and primary prevention in the community. National League for Nursing's *Educational Competencies for Graduates of Associate Degree Nursing Programs* guided the conceptual development of chapter selection, structure, and content of the book.

Rising costs and an aging population have both contributed to the shift to a community-based health care system. As Baby Boomers move into their aging years, their rising expectations for a healthy life span have resulted in a shift from episodic, acute care management to a more chronic focus. Such a change has contributed to population-based outcomes. The community has largely become the setting for chronic disease management and prevention. ADN nurses must have the additional skills and knowledge in such areas as epidemiology and environmental sciences in order to care for patients in community-based settings. Nurses will need to demonstrate skills in managed care at the individual level, keeping an ever-vigilant eye on population influenced variables, such as age, gender, and cultural factors.

During the last 30 years of the 20th century, the cost of health care in the United States approached 15% of the gross national product (GNP). No longer just the interests of economists and policy makers, everyone has joined the debate about how to pay for the public's increasing expectations of quality health care at every life stage. More than 40 million U.S. citizens lack adequate health insurance while certain health indicators lag behind those of other comparable advanced countries who are spending far less for health care. The growing economic and health disparity between competing segments of the population has taken on national political significance, as all political parties struggle to find acceptable solutions. The impact of federal and state policy on the delivery of community health services cannot be ignored if nurses in the community expect to influence the delivery of appropriate services to the population. This text provides chapters on culture, politics, and the health care system by prominent nurse scholars who help beginning nurses understand how the knowledge of these often abstract forces can be used in everyday clinical practice.

With the *technological explosion* of the past decade, advances in digital technology have increased applications in telehealth, bringing together health providers and clients without regard to geographical proximity. The community health nurse of the 21st century must use computer technology as the public health nurse of the 18th century used quill and ink. With faster and more current data access in community and acute care settings, new dimensions are emerging in client assessment and intervention. This text is the first community health nursing text to include a chapter on nursing informatics in the community.

With advances in information technology and global travel, global health issues create challenges for all nurses, not just those who work in international settings. With the global community becoming smaller with every passing day, the spread of disease as well as health information occurs in *hours* rather than the *years* of the past. These dramatic risks have created the need for different approaches for the community health nurse. Opportunities are vast for nurses in global health, and inaccessible populations throughout the world can now be reached through the advent of telehealth and telecommunications.

The passive health consumer of yesterday has given way to the well-informed, fully participating client of today. With almost total access to information, which until recently has been available only to health professionals and scientists, individuals can participate as full partners in their care decisions and in the management of their health, which has raised expectations of care outcomes for clients and nurses. Through the almost phenomenal proliferation of the World Wide Web, most individuals can access unlimited information about health and health choices. This has greatly increased the power of consumer groups in health and has resulted in greater demands for services and access. The nurse in the community setting will have even greater responsibilities in the educator role as community populations demand the most current information and become more assertive about securing services.

The increased interest in the use of complementary and alternative, non-Western health practices among Americans to enhance health, healing, and a more holistic sense of well-being continues to influence the health care system. Nurses in the community are often confronted with unfamiliar health practices that may or may not have a research basis for use. Attempts to legitimatize many unconventional approaches are occurring at research medical centers and through the federal government. A greater interest in the spiritual aspects of health is part of the movement among health care consumers for more emphasis on the subjective experience of health. With greater awareness of health information and greater participation in alternative health practices, community health nurses must be more prepared to understand these revolutionary changes. Nurses in the community are in an ideal position to help clients navigate through these uncharted and unfamiliar areas, making ethically sound and informed decisions. This text includes a chapter on complementary holistic health to prepare the nurse for these challenges, *breaking new ground for community health nursing textbooks.*

With the extension of life through technology and improved living conditions, *end-of-life issues have changed dramatically as well.* The traditional approaches to caring for the dying are no longer as acceptable to clients accustomed to having more control in health care decisions. More clients and families are electing to die at home with hospice services and nurses as part of this team approach to a more dignified and humane end of life. In recognition of these needs, this text includes an *extended section on hospice* in the chapter on home health nursing.

This text features a unique collaborative model of chapter authorship. Nursing education is moving to integrate a more collaborative and interdisciplinary practice in the curriculum at the undergraduate level. The ADN nurse will be called on to coordinate care in an increasingly complex health care system. Although most of our authors are community health nurse special-

ists, we also use other specialists in chapters that benefit from diverse perspectives. We believe that by securing well-known authors from nursing and other community health–related fields, we present a strong text and support our ideology of a more integrated approach to community health nursing. The inclusion of clinical practitioners as authors further provides a clinical authenticity that is often missing from nursing textbooks. A further strength of this text was in our review process. In addition to the traditional review process by community health nurse authors and faculty, we included nurses in other specialties; student nurses; and beginning practicing nurses and experienced nurses in community health practice. These reviews were extremely enlightening, and we believe that through such an extensive and diverse group of reviewers, the text is more accessible for a broader section of nursing students and the final version of the text is more grounded in current practice.

Change has always been a certainty in the U.S. health care system. These changes present community health nurses with unlimited opportunities to influence the public's health. It is up to the student nurses of today to fully realize such possibilities. Nurses of the future must be in partnership with the health care system, which requires a broad understanding of community structure and process. The need for a commitment to lifelong learning and critical thinking skills emerges as critical for the nurse who will be successful in the challenging nursing roles of the future. We challenge faculty and students to use this text as the basis for their future professional practice, whatever the setting or role.

Organization

The book is organized into six units with 23 chapters and is designed to be used throughout the ADN curriculum. **Unit I** provides an overview of community-based nursing which includes the history of public and community health nursing, the major features of community-based nursing practice, an overview of the health care delivery system, and an introduction to epidemiology.

Unit II addresses the major influences on the health of a community. Health care and nursing are viewed from cultural and international perspectives. Environmental influences on community health are explored and discussed. The influence of politics on health care delivery is described and examined and communicable disease is examined as a community health problem.

Unit III addresses the various approaches to community health nursing practice including informatics, health education, health promotion and wellness, and holistic and complementary health.

Unit IV provides a view of the diversity in community health nursing roles and functions. The chapters in this unit describe the rapidly changing and constantly evolving functions of nurses in many community settings including ambulatory care, home health, and hospice. The home visiting process is outlined and described. A chapter on disasters in the community is also included.

Unit V focuses on the foundations of family care and nursing interventions for both healthy and unhealthy families, and **Unit VI** presents an overview of health issues specific to men, women, pregnant adolescents, children, and elders. Finally, mental health nursing from a community perspective is described and discussed.

Pedagogy

The chapters are organized to facilitate faculty use and enhance student learning. Most chapters contain the following:

- *An outline of chapter content and a list of questions to be considered in the chapter*
- *Key terms*
- *Research briefs*
- *Case studies*
- *Short original essays, interviews, or quotes from well-known persons representing diverse views relevant to the chapter focus*
- *Poems, quotes, and other featured boxed material which enhance learning of chapter content*
- *Healthy People 2010 Objectives*
- *FYI boxes containing interesting facts*
- *A web icon at the end of every chapter, directing the reader to the accompanying web site (http://communitynursing.jbpub.com) for more information about topics covered in the chapter*
- *Critical thinking activities*
- *Carefully selected photographs and graphics to enhance reading and understanding of chapter content*
- *A reference list*

Teaching Support

An Instructor's Manual is available to supplement the teaching aids already provided by the chapter features in the text. The Instructor's Manual is an integrated package of teaching and learning tools that enhances teaching effectiveness. The Instructor's Manual also provides noncommunity health instructors with specific directions and ample clinical examples of how to make the community-based portion of the text in Part 3 relevant to their content areas in the curriculum. In addition, there is a web site that provides regular updates, student and faculty resources, web links, in-depth and current material for further inquiry for each chapter, a sample course syllabus, a testbank, and PowerPoint™ presentation outlines for each chapter and communication with text authors.

Available to accompany this text is *Hospital to Home: A Pocket Guide.* The pocket guide serves as a convenient reference for nurses assisting clients with the transition from hospital to home.

Acknowledgments

Many people have contributed to the development and completion of this book. The contributing chapter authors have honored us with their contributions to this text and have enriched our lives through our interactions with them. We thank them for making this book come to life. The ideas and eventual structure of this text have evolved over many conversations and interactions with faculty, colleagues, and students over many years. We thank those who have inspired us and given us the hope and confidence that the time was right for such a text. We remain in debt to the following people for their encouragement and belief in seeing us through this project with their professional support: Lenell Ford, Dr. Marie Farrell, and the University of Southern Mississippi College of Nursing faculty and students. And for Jones and Bartlett Publishers who believed in the importance of this project, especially Tom Lochhaas, for his insights, which go far beyond the critical eye of a manuscript editor—you saved us in so many ways, our debt is immeasurable; Karen Zuck for her management of the manuscript; Dr. Penny Glynn, for her insights and valuable critical evaluation of the entire manuscript; and Karen Ferreira, for her remarkable ability in managing the production of what seemed an impossible task. For those who participated in the critical review of this text, we thank them for their interest, enthusiasm, and courage to produce candid, detailed evaluations of this text throughout the many stages of development: Dr. Kaye Bender; Dr. Joan Baldwin; Brigham Young University faculty and students; University of Southern Mississippi undergraduate and graduate students in community health nursing; Juanita Mikell and John Hodnett, for their extraordinary reviews and constructive suggestions; Barbara Foster; Vicki Sutton; Dr. Judith A. Barton; Dr. Chris Lundy; Dr. Arlene McFarland; and Dr. Jerri Laube for the extra attention to context and detail.

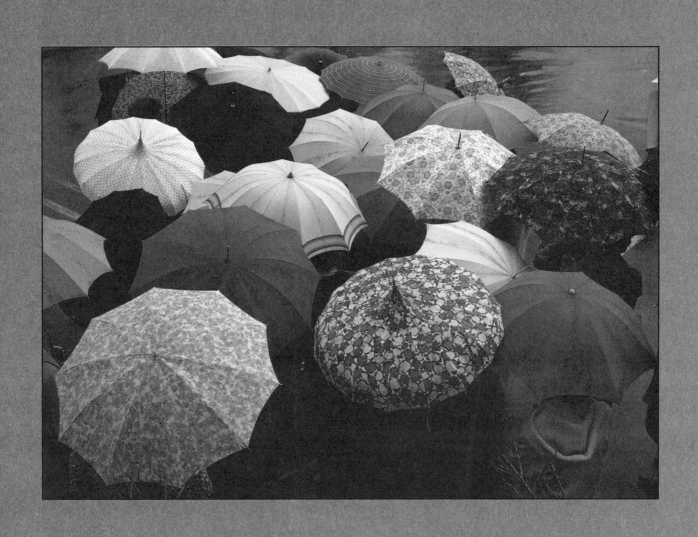

PART ONE

Community-Focused Nursing Care

What does it mean to take care of a community? Community-focused nursing care is often difficult to define and even more difficult to practice. Baccalaureate nurses are educated to practice nursing in all health care settings. Community health nurses care for populations. Since the late 1800s, professional public health nurses have cared for communities. Those communities have changed over time, and the practice of community health nursing has changed as well. Community health nursing has evolved into a complex, multifaceted nursing specialty that is constantly challenged by rapidly changing delivery systems. While reading about the history of community and public health nursing, both similarities and differences in today's community health nursing practice will emerge. Community health nursing, which evolved from public health nursing and is accountable to the public for meeting the population's health care needs, has responded to changes in society to include the care of such diverse populations as school children, women with HIV/AIDS (human immunodeficiency virus/acquired immunodeficiency syndrome), and the homeless. Part One introduces the student to the world of the community health nurse: the focus, the settings, and the historical issues relevant to today's community health practice. As a broadly based specialty, community health nursing practice is more affected by structural changes in society than are other nursing specialties. The community health nurse must be aware of the health care system, social trends, economics, and culture to deliver effective care to the public. Part One assists the student in understanding the uniqueness of community health nursing and the structural influences that must be considered when delivering effective care for an entire community.

Unit I

The Context of Community Health Nursing

Chapter 1

Opening the Door to Health Care in the Community

Karen Saucier Lundy, Sharyn Janes, and Shery Hartman

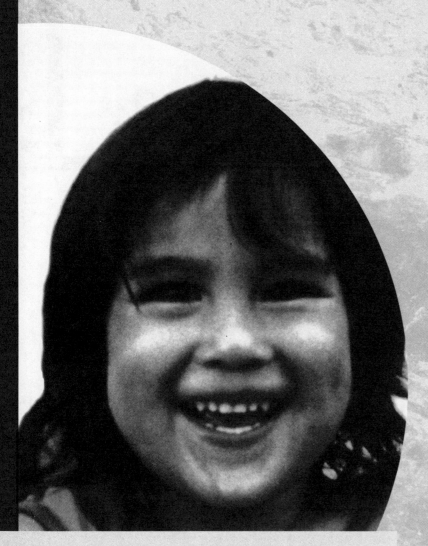

Money would be better spent in maintaining health in infancy and childhood than in building hospitals to cure diseases.

Florence Nightingale, 1894

CHAPTER FOCUS

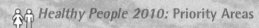
QUESTIONS TO CONSIDER

After reading this chapter, answer the following questions:

1. How does the definition of health affect the way we care for populations?
2. How have settings for health care changed in recent decades?
3. What implications does managed care have for nurses?
4. What is health care reform and prevention and how has it influenced the U.S. health care system?
5. What is the significance of *Nursing's Agenda for Health Care Reform?*
6. What is the role of the National League for Nursing Educational Competencies for Graduates of Associate Degree Nursing Programs?
7. What is *Healthy People 2010* and how does it influence the health care system related to a policy of prevention?
8. What are the distinctions of the concepts of community health, population-focused care, and acute care?
9. What is a community and a population?
10. What are the three major influences on community health?
11. What is *epidemiology?*
12. What is the relationship between the natural history of disease and the three levels of prevention?
13. How is a population's health measured?

KEY TERMS

Care management
Community
Community-based nursing
Culture
Environment
Epidemiology
Ethics
Florence Nightingale
Health care reform
Healthy People 2010
Home health care
Managed care

National League for Nursing (NLN)
National League for Nursing Educational Competencies for Graduates of Associate Degree Nursing Programs
Natural history of disease
Nursing's Agenda for Health Care Reform
Population
Population-focused nursing
Primary prevention
Public health nursing
Secondary prevention
Tertiary prevention
World Health Organization (WHO)

....

It is cheaper to promote health than to maintain people in sickness.
                                    Florence Nightingale, 1894

....

The world of nursing and the nurse's role are always changing, but it is probably safe to say that those who choose nursing at the new millennium are caught in unprecedented currents of change: change in health care, change in nursing, and change in setting of care. These forces for change have been developing for some time now, engulfing all health care professionals in "shifting sands" in their practice. In response to new demands, new opportunities, new possibilities, and a complex health care environment, current nursing students are in a curriculum that their predecessors might not recognize. The nurse's place in the health care system is at the client's side, not just in the hospital, but in any setting where people work, play, learn, worship, shop, surf on the World Wide Web or call a hot line; the nurse has an opportunity to promote health for people in communities. The *National League for Nursing (NLN)*, which nationally accredits nursing programs that meet the highest standards of excellence, has developed its "Vision for Nursing Education" (Box 1-1) based on these dramatic changes

A Conversation With...

Nursing's story is a magnificent epic of service to mankind. It is about people: how they are born, and live and die; in health and in sickness; in joy and in sorrow. Its mission is the translation of knowledge into human service.

Nursing is compassionate concern for human beings. It is the heart that understands and the hand that soothes. It is the intellect that synthesizes many learnings into meaningful administrations.

For students of nursing the future is a rich repository of far-flung opportunities around this planet and toward the further reaches of man's explorations of new worlds and new ideas. Theirs is the promise of deep satisfaction in a field long dedicated to serving the health needs of people.

—Professor Martha Rogers, PhD
The Education Violet, June 1966,
New York University.

BOX 1-1 A VISION FOR NURSING EDUCATION

Nursing's vision for a health care system that ensures access, quality, and cost containment through a new approach to the delivery of care is within reach. The nursing education system required by that new approach must move quickly to provide adequate numbers of appropriately prepared nurses.

Successful implementation of nursing's approach to health care delivery requires the following:

- Significant increases in the numbers of advanced nurse practitioners prepared to provide primary health care to communities and primary care services in group and interdisciplinary practice

- A shift in emphasis for all nursing education programs to ensure that all nurses—whatever their basic and graduate education and wherever their basic and graduate education and wherever they choose to practice—are prepared to function in a community-based, community-focused health care system

- An increase in the numbers of community health nursing centers and their increased utilization as model clinical sites for nursing students

- A shift in emphasis for nursing research and an increase in the numbers of studies concerned with health promotion and disease prevention at the aggregate and community levels

- Targeted national initiatives to recruit and retain nurse providers, faculty, administrators, and researchers from diverse racial, cultural, and ethnic backgrounds

Source: A vision for nursing education. New York: National League for Nursing, 1993.

to a community-based environment. Even if the world around us appears to remain chaotic and complex, as some suggest, the nursing ideals and commitments will fulfill the promise of the dreams that bring most nurses to the profession.

With the headlines often heralding hospital closures, mergers, and downsizing, where does that leave the nurse? What is the story behind where we are today? What kind of job will there be for you after graduation? When you graduate from nursing school, you will join more than 2.2 million registered nurses (RNs) in the United States. The good news is that the federal government predicts that RN will be one of the top 10 careers, with the most job openings in the year 2006 (Bureau of Labor Statistics, 1998).

The Division of Nursing of the Bureau of Health Professions in the Health Resources and Services Administration (HRSA), a division of the Department of Health and Human Services, released its national survey of registered nurses in the United States in 2000. Although nearly 60% of RNs still work in hospitals, that percentage has dropped more than 6 points since 1992. The greatest changes have been an increase in the percentage of nurses who work in community-ambulatory care, home health, public health, and other community-based settings (National Sample Survey of Registered Nurses, 2000). Dramatic changes in the way health care is delivered have led to the discharge of sicker clients to their homes. As managed care continues to result in fewer hospitalizations, nurses in acute care settings are facing assignments on a daily basis to different units and in diverse settings, including outpatient, home health, and other community-based agencies housed in or associated with their own facility. As the client census (the number of occupied beds in a hospital on a daily basis) fluctuates, nurses must be flexible, willing, and competent in multiple settings. So no matter where you ultimately choose to work as a nurse, community health will be an influence on you and on your clients' lives.

According to Gebbie (1997), the U.S. vision of public health is that of healthy people *in healthy communities* because individual health can be fully realized only if the community itself is in good shape as well. For a closer look at how much our health is influenced by public health measures, see "A Personal Look at Public Health" on the following page.

In this chapter the history, context, and setting for nursing practice are discussed, as well as some of the current controversies and confusions specific to the "new" move to "the client's side" in the community. So many things influence health: In this century we continue to find out through research how much in the environment, in our own behavior, and in the kind of health care we deliver affects whether we are healthy or ill. Why some people get sick and some people don't has intrigued health care providers for centuries. This chapter introduces health as a concept, presents the historical insights we have learned, and reveals what we can expect nursing and health care to look like in the new millennium. Sometimes, the ways in which we use terms can confuse and obscure the focus of community and public health nursing. In this chapter the terms related to community, population, and nursing roles are discussed in the context of health care delivery. The ways in which a population's health is determined are introduced as well as concepts related to disease and illness prevention and health promotion.

A Closer Look at Health

We hear much of "contagion and infection" in disease. May we not also come to make health contagious and infectious?
Florence Nightingale, 1890

Before we can talk in more detail about the U.S. health care system and nursing roles in today's health care arena, we need an understanding of what "health" is. That seems simple; after all, everyone knows what health is. However, there are many definitions and descriptions of health depending on one's perspective and purpose. The most well-known and widely cited description of health is the World Health Organization's (WHO) definition of health as "a state of complete physical, mental, and social well-being and not merely the absence of disease or infirmity" (WHO, 1958). When this definition was drafted in 1948, it began a trend that has persisted for more than 50 years to define health more broadly, including social terms in addition to medical terms. In 1986, the WHO definition of health was expanded to include a community concept of health. WHO now defines health as "the extent to which an individual or group is able, on the one hand, to realize aspirations and satisfy needs; and on the other hand, to change or cope with the environment. Health is, therefore, seen as a resource for everyday life, not the objective of living; it is a positive concept emphasizing social and personal resources, as well as physical capacities" (WHO, 1986). An individual or community then must be able to attain and use resources effectively and exhibit a resilience when facing change.

Although WHO's definition of health is the most common, many other definitions also imply a social or community focus. Health has been defined as "a purposeful and integrated method of functioning within an environment" (Hall & Weaver, 1977, p. 7), and "the common attainment of the highest level of physical, mental, and social well-being consistent with available knowledge and resources at a given time and place" (Hanlon & Pickett, 1984). Even Florence Nightingale's definition of health as "not only to be well, but to use well every power that we have" can be used to describe health for both individuals and communities (Nightingale, 1860).

Many social issues surround the concept of health, making it difficult to limit it to only one definition and perspective. Health is defined by the society and culture in which we live. How individuals, families, and communities perceive what health means is often determined by social, cultural, and economic conditions that limit health choices (Kuss, Proulx-Girouard, Lovitt, Katz, & Kennelly, 1997). To put this another way: Health is highly dependent on where and how we live. A 20-year-old man may consider himself healthy only if he can run up the stairs at work. For an 80-year-old woman, retrieving her own mail at the mailbox may be her idea of health.

FYI

A Personal Look at Public Health

The first rays of sunlight peek through your bedroom curtains, accompanied by the fresh air of a new day. You breathe deeply and enjoy the clean air that public health protects by monitoring radiation levels and developing strategies to keep them low.

Rousing the children, you usher them into the bathroom for their showers. You brush your teeth, knowing the water won't make you sick because safe drinking water is the responsibility of public health.

You check your smile in the mirror. You can't remember your last cavity, thanks in part to the fluoride public health helps add to the water. Through similar programs, public health has always sought to promote good health by preventing disease altogether.

The family clambers to the table just as you finish pouring the milk, which is safe to drink because the State Department of Health checks and monitors it from the dairy to the grocery store.

After breakfast, you call your sister—who is pregnant with her first child—and find out her routine doctor's visit went perfectly. Even in the small town where she lives, your sister can visit a local doctor. Public health recognized the need for doctors in rural areas and helped place one there.

Your sister tells you her doctor suggested she visit the county health department and enroll in the Women, Infants, and Children Program, another public health service that ensures children get the proper nutrition to prevent sickness later in life.

You walk outside and guide the children into the car. You buckle their seatbelts without realizing it. Seatbelts have become a habit now, because public health has explained how proper seatbelt use has greatly reduced automobile-related deaths nationwide.

Playmates greet your children at the child care center with yelps of youthful joy. As you watch the children run inside to play, you know they'll stay safe while you're away at work. Public health has licensed the center and made certain the staff knows the proper ways to avoid infectious disease outbreaks that can occur among young children.

And thanks to the immunizations your children have gotten, you know they'll be safe from life-threatening diseases like polio and whooping cough.

In fact, public health has eliminated the deadly smallpox virus worldwide, so your children will never catch it. Maybe your children's children won't have to worry about polio or whooping cough.

You arrive at work and find a flyer for a new exercise program tacked to the bulletin board. You decide to sign up, remembering the public health studies that show you can reduce the risks of chronic disease by staying physically active.

The morning goes well, and you feel good because your company became a smoke-free work place this month. Science shows that tobacco can cause cancer and other ailments in those who use tobacco and among those who breathe second-hand smoke. Public health encourages people and organizations to quit smoking so that all people can live more healthful lives.

Walking to a nearby fast food restaurant for lunch, you pass a bike rider with a sleek, colorful helmet, another example of a public health message that can influence healthy behaviors. Inside, you order a hamburger and fries.

You notice the food service license signed by the State Health Officer on the wall, and you know the food is sanitary and free of disease-causing organisms. Still, a State Department of Health public service announcement from TV rings in your head, and you make a mental note to order something with a little less cholesterol next time.

You finish your day at work, pick up the kids, and head to the community park to let the children play. You watch the neighborhood children launch a toy sailboat into the park pond, knowing public health protects lakes and streams from dangerous sewage runoff.

At home, your spouse greets you at the door. You sort the mail and discover a letter from your uncle. He's doing fine after his surgery in the hospital and will head back to the nursing home in 2 days. You know he's getting quality care at both facilities because public health monitors and licenses them to ensure a commitment to quality standards.

Even the ambulance that transported him to the hospital met public health standards for emergency medical services.

After dinner, you put the children to bed and sit to watch the evening news. The anchor details a new coalition dedicated to preventing breast and cervical cancer. A representative of the State Department of Health issues an open invitation for members from all walks of life. You jot down the telephone number and promise yourself you'll call first thing tomorrow.

As you settle into bed, you decide that public health is more than a point-in-time recognition. Without even realizing it, you'll rely on public health every day for an entire lifetime.

Source: Mississippi State Department of Health Annual Report (1997), pp. 2–3.

....

[Health is] a way of life, an attitude, an outlook, a history, a context with socio-cultural norms, a belief, and a tradition. Being healthy is managing, negotiating, achieving, growing, becoming, and helping others grow and become. Being and becoming healthy may be parts of a whole perception of health. Becoming healthy is hopefulness, transcending worries, realizing options, advocating, and accessing resources.

A. L. Meleis, 1996

....

....

Health [is rather] a modus vivendi enabling imperfect men to achieve a rewarding and not too painful existence while they cope with an imperfect world.

Rene Dubos, 1968

....

Nurses differ in their perception of health and are influenced by their own background, age, and experiences. In a study that explored the perceptions of community health nurses about health, the nurses interviewed described health as an "interactive vision" between nurses and client (Leipert, 1996). This vision of health varies with each nurse-client relationship, depending on the values and characteristics of the nurse, the client, and the setting where the interaction occurs. Some of the characteristics that can greatly affect the vision of health are age, culture, social environment, and economic status. Clients in this context include individuals, families, groups, and communities.

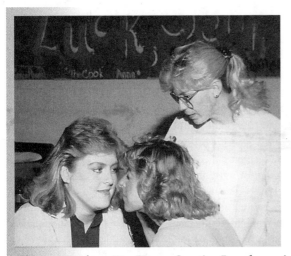

Chapter author, Dr. Karen Saucier Lundy, assists nursing students learning individual assessment skills. Community health nursing skills often involve additional data collection, such as morbidity and mortality statistics.

Historical Insights

Sickness and suffering have always been a part of human existence. As a result, from the beginning there have been men and women who served as caregivers to the sick and injured. Early on, most care was provided by family members. As human society evolved, moral consciousness became formalized into religious codes, and religious groups assumed more responsibility for the ill. Although efforts were commendable, they were limited because so little was known about disease management or prevention.

Florence Nightingale is recognized as the founder of modern professional nursing, as well as for developing the first school of nursing at London's St. Thomas' Hospital in 1860. Although her initial efforts focused on preparing nurses to care for the sick in hospitals and infirmaries, she continued throughout her life to promote "well" nursing in the community. Nightingale's directive was to manipulate the patient's environment to allow "nature" to take its course in the healing process.

Through scientific inquiry during the 19th century, causes of the devastating communicable diseases of these earlier centuries began to emerge and professional intervention became possible. During the mid to late 1800s, public health measures were established as the process of contagion between human hosts and their environment became better understood.

Throughout the 20th century medical science grew in leaps and bounds, and the manipulation of "nature" became the drive that resulted in significant medical discoveries and inventions. The United States experienced unprecedented growth in technology and medical science in the 20th century. We learned more about the causes of diseases and generated a broad knowledge base about disease and injury detection, treatment, and prevention. The resulting health care system, which early on was divided into public and private sectors, focused on the diagnosis and treatment of disease in the highly specialized and centralized setting of the hospital. For most individuals, health care was synonymous with the local hospital. During the 20th century, most nurses were employed in hospital settings as skilled caregivers for the acutely ill; nursing education was mostly focused on care of the sick. Nursing students gained experience almost exclusively in hospitals. But even as we were credited worldwide with having the most advanced health technology for treating disease, and while health care spending vastly increased during the 1960s and 1970s, health professionals expressed a growing concern that the health care needs of all citizens were not being met.

In the 1990s, we came to realize that as a society our obligation is to provide an environment in which achievement of good health for all is not only possible but expected. Yet there are population groups, such as the homeless, the elderly, and the poor, whose illnesses and death rates exceed those of the general population and may require additional resources to achieve good health. Health care costs in the United States already amount to more than 14% of the gross domestic product (GDP), more than twice that of other countries that can boast better health statistics.

FYI

Health Care Spending Projected to Double in Decade

Spending for health care in the United States will double over the next decade, reaching $2.1 trillion by the year 2007, according to U.S. government projections. Spending per person will jump from $3,759 in 1996 to $7,100 in 2007. Hospitals will account for only 30% of all health care expenditures by 2007, compared with 35% in 1996, as the trend continues toward more community-based care.

Source: The Wall Street Journal, *September 14, 1998.*

Americans would probably be willing to live with the high price tag of health care if it made us all healthier than people in other countries (*Consumer Reports*, 1990). However, that is not the case. In the United States, where the health care system is heralded as the most sophisticated in the world, when compared with similar countries such as Great Britain, Germany, or France, we are lagging behind:

- *We have high infant mortality rates relative to other highly developed industrialized nations.*

- *We rank 12th in the world in life expectancy, behind Japan, Italy, France, and the Scandinavian countries.*

- *At least one third of our population has limited access to basic health services and one third of the uninsured are children.*

- *We are the only industrialized nation in the world without guaranteed access to basic health care services.*

Much must be done in this country for many to achieve levels of health that are acceptable and equitable. Many deaths and disabilities could be reduced by environmental improvements and lifestyle changes. A hundred years ago, most deaths were caused by infectious diseases; today the leading causes of death are related to societal influences, lifestyle, and behavioral choices. Progress in technology has created environmental threats to our air, water, and food. Health problems such as addiction and violence have emerged as serious threats to our well-being. "Good health cannot be achieved without a social concern for ethical, humane decision-making . . . a just and caring society does not withhold health care from its citizens; sickness after all is never something people deserve" (Keck, 1994, pp. 4–5).

Beyond looking at our own country's struggle with internal decisions about health care delivery and connecting it with the broader determinants of health, there has been a concurrent recognition of the global connectedness and importance of concerns for health. As the millennium dawns, the achievement of world health has increasingly become a global expectation. Although nurses are still needed as skilled caregivers who improve the health of the individual, a broader perspective has evolved as population health interventions are realized to be at least equally if not more significant in the attainment of health for all. Solutions to the health problems of populations worldwide now exceed the resources and control of any one individual (McKenzie & Pinger, 1997).

Nursing in the New Millennium

Trossman (1998, p. 1), in *American Nurse*, stated that "in the early part of the next century, hospitals will still be a major place of employment for nurses. The type of work will slowly change, though, as these hospitals become the care zones for the nation's oldest and sickest individuals. At the same time, other settings, such as home health and community based care, will provide increased opportunities for R.N.s." Hospitals are relinquishing their role as the recognized hub of care delivery while health care services continue to increase at home, at work, at play, in schools and churches, online with the World Wide Web through the Internet, and on the telephone. *Who* delivers health care, *what* is provided, and *when* and *where* clients are seen have changed. Cost containment, managed care systems, technology, societal expectations, and politics have all influenced these changes. Clients stay less often in the hospital, and when they do, they stay fewer days. Clients are generally sicker when they are admitted and when they are discharged than they have been in the past. There has not been a significant decrease in client numbers, but rather the settings for care have changed; with this shift, population health issues have become more of a focus. There are greater demands on the health care system than ever before, and nurses are needed more than ever. Nurses, as always, continue to meet the needs of clients; we move to care for populations in whatever setting they are found.

In a study conducted by the American Nurses Associations' (ANA) Department of Labor Relations and Workplace Advocacy, nurse executives from acute, home health, extended, and managed care settings reported on the skills seen as most important for the next generation of nurses. Nurses should possess skills of self-reliance, independence, flexibility, and decision making, as well as a "systems-thinking" approach to health care, client education and critical thinking skills, and computer skills. The conclusion of the study was that nurses need to be prepared to provide the four rights of nursing practice: give the right care, in the right setting, at the right time, and at the right cost (Canavan, 1996).

Educating Nurses for Community Health Nursing Practice

Educational Competencies for Graduates of Associate Degree Nursing Programs (NLN, 2000), provides recommendations regarding the ADN educational content essential for entry level in community health nursing practice. To survive as a profession, NLN recognizes that nursing must evolve along with the health care system. Nurses of the future will practice in a more complex health care system that involves both care of individuals outside of hospital settings (community-based care) and care of whole populations (community-focused care). Details of the competencies can be found in the Appendix. This book uses the NLN document as the basis for its content and organization (NLN, 2000).

One of the most intriguing and challenging aspects of the health problems that we face in the new millennium is that we already know effective interventions for many diseases and conditions in our society. According to Salmon and Vanderbush (1990), "Never before have we known as much about health as we do now; what we don't know is how to put this knowledge into action" (p. 192).

BOX 1-2 TERMS TO KNOW . . .

A community *is a group of people who share something in common and interact with one another, who may exhibit a commitment with one another and may share a geographic boundary.*

A population *is a group of people who have at least one thing in common and who may or may not interact with each other.*

Community-Based, Population-Focused, and Community-Focused Care

Community-based, population- and community-focused, and *personal client care*—what do these phrases actually mean? What does it mean that health care is "moving out" to the community? **Community-based nursing** refers to both the *setting* and the *practice* of the nursing role. The *setting* usually means any kind of health care *other than acute care settings*. The nurse who practices community-based nursing is referred to as a *community health nurse* (CHN) and ADN nurses are prepared for these settings. To further complicate our use of terms, a hospital may have both acute care (labor and delivery, coronary care units, emergency

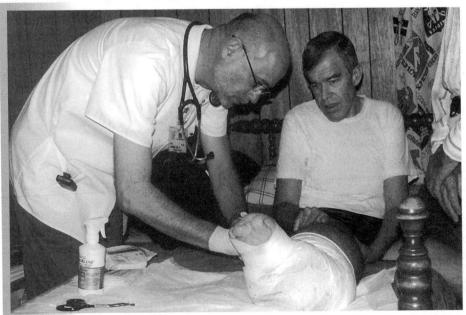

Home health nursing practice is the fastest growing community health nursing role.

care) and community-based health care (outpatient surgery, day care for children and elders in home health) within its scope.

Communities and Populations

When we think of the word *community*, we may have many pictures in our mind, because the word has a variety of meanings. Andy Griffith lived in the community of Mayberry, and Mr. Rogers' neighborhood is also a community. Most television situation comedies revolve around a community, such as the shows *Seinfeld* or *Friends*. In this text the word **community** is defined as *a group of people who share something in common and interact with one another, who may exhibit a commitment with one another and may share a geographic boundary*. A **population** is defined as *a group of people who have at least one thing in common and who may or may not interact with each other*.

Examples of communities include the following:

* *Lesbians in a communal living setting*
* *The town of Nederland, Colorado*
* *The nursing faculty at the University of West Virginia*
* *The "Devil's Own" neighborhood urban gang*

Examples of populations include the following:

* *People who drink alcohol and drive*
* *Parents with preterm infants*
* *Sexually active teenagers*
* *Nurses who work the night shift*
* *Professional athletes*
* *Foreign-educated RNs*
* *Teenagers with diabetes*

According to Schultz (1994), interaction is essential in a community, whereas members of a population may or may not interact with one another. To put it another way, communities are usually aware of their "communityness," which binds them into a collective entity and "to which they give a name" (Cottrell, 1976, pp. 114–115). Some populations evolve into communities over time; elderly persons who participate in a water aerobics class, for example, may develop into a cohesive community of older women who share other common activities and interests.

The average life span of Americans increased from 45 years to 75 years during the 20th century, but it is interesting to note that only five of those years are attributable to individual preventive or curative interventions such as cardiac surgery. Twenty-five of the additional years of life have resulted from public health efforts to provide for safe water, effective waste disposal, adequate housing, and other improvements in the overall health of communities (Bunker, Frazier, & Mosteller, 1994).

There are many ways in which nurses are moving into new settings and expanding their application of community-based nursing skills. Although these nurses are bringing expertise of acute care and technology to community settings, they are often

RESEARCH BRIEF

Seldes, R., Grisso, J., Pavell, J., Berlin, J., Tan, V., Bowman, B., Kinman, J., Fitzgerald, R. (1999). Predictors of injury among adult recreational in-line skaters: A multicity study. American Journal of Public Health, 89(2), 238–242.

The rising number of injuries caused by in-line skating has resulted from the increased popularity of this sport. An estimated 105,000 in-line skating injuries occurred in 1996, representing a 191% increase from 1993. This research study focused on the population of adults who participate in recreational skating. The researchers interviewed 964 skaters and administered a questionnaire about skating activities, use of safety equipment, procedures, and frequency of skating. In addition, interviewers made observations about the presence of safety equipment. Use of safety gear was generally low. Helmets and elbow, wrist, and knee guards were reportedly used sometimes or nearly never by 96% of those sampled. Eleven percent of those sampled reported injuries, including injuries to the wrist and knee, fractures, and contusions; 65% of the injuries required medical treatment. Only 7% of the injured skaters reported wearing safety gear at the time of the accident. The study concluded that safe skating education programs should recognize this at-risk population and consider specifically targeting more advanced skaters in their campaigns.

lacking in their knowledge of community dynamics and public health concepts (Gebbie, 1996). If nurses are to continue to be a dynamic part of health care in the future, we must be able to understand the complex and community-based nature of health promotion, illness prevention, recovery from illness and injury, and health restoration (Kurtzman et al., 1980). We need to expand our knowledge and expertise in the care of individuals and our skills in hospital-based clinical management of illness and injury to include care of individuals in community settings (Hall & Stevens, 1995). By using our knowledge and experience in medical-surgical, maternal-child, and psychiatric nursing, we can assist individuals, families, and groups to make choices that promote health and wellness (Smith, 1995).

Acute Care Versus Community-Based Nursing

Let's compare acute care and community-based nursing to more fully understand how these nursing roles differ both in setting and practice focus. In the acute care setting, there is the issue of

FYI

Common Definitions in Community Health Nursing

Community-based nursing refers to both the setting and the practice of the nursing role. Nursing care that occurs in a setting other than acute care is also referred to as *community health nursing* (CHN). ADN educated nurses are prepared to practice community-based nursing.

Population- and community-focused care refers to interventions aimed at health promotion and disease prevention that shape a community's overall health status and is generally practiced at the BSN level.

Public health nursing is a population-focused, community-oriented nursing practice and the dominant responsibility is to the care of the larger community. A BSN is often the preferred preparation.

provider control. Clients are well aware of who is in control in the hospital setting—the health care professional. The client is in a subordinate position to the nurse, who remains the ultimate authority regarding when to go to sleep, what to wear, when and how much to urinate, what kind of diet to eat and when, and

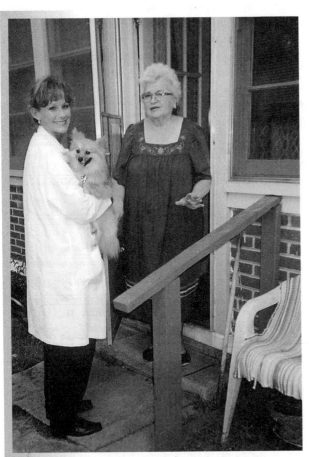

Community nurses work with clients in their homes to improve health. For many elders, pets are considered "family."

whether visitors are allowed. Treatments and interventions are done "to" the client and scheduled at staff and hospital convenience. Clients, who are often identified by their "condition" (e.g., the gallbladder in room 214), are isolated from friends, family, and pets, who are excluded from the "health" care setting. Little individualized care that takes into consideration the client's lifestyle and preferences is given. When a person changes into a hospital gown, the role of client is assumed. Personal items such as medications, glasses, and false teeth are often relinquished, and self-care is limited, with permission often required from nurses for activities taken for granted at home. Many questions are asked, sometimes over and over by different health professionals, and most often these questions are of a very personal and intimate nature. Rarely does the client receive any explanation for why information is needed, for to question is to risk being labeled a "difficult" client—and we know what that means (Armentrout, 1998)! (Refer to Table 1-1 for differences in nursing interventions by setting.) The controlled environment of the acute care setting, however, has many benefits for the nurse:

- *Predictable routine*
- *Maintenance of hospital policy*
- *Predictability of nursing and medical goals*
- *Resource availability, both human and material*
- *Collegial collaboration and consultation*
- *Controlled client compliance with plan of care: the client takes correct medicine and treatment on time*
- *Standardization of care*

The community-based setting is completely different from acute care, especially in home care. Nurses tend to be dependent on clients' willingness to adhere to the plan of care, and clients on their own "turf" act very differently than in the acute care setting. A significant advantage is that the nurse is able to assess environmental conditions, food and other critical resources, lifestyle influences, and social support system, such as friends, family, and pets. Transportation issues, which impact

| | TABLE 1-1 | DIFFERENCES IN NURSING INTERVENTIONS BY SETTING | |

HEALTH PROBLEM	ACUTE CARE SETTING: HOSPITAL	COMMUNITY-BASED SETTING: HOME HEALTH
Osteoporosis resulting in degenerative hip disease	Treatment Surgery and recovery (total hip replacement)	Teach client how to walk after surgery. Involve family with encouraging activity and flexibility exercises.

the ability to adhere to medical and nursing goals, often become overriding concerns that are not even considered in the hospital setting. The lack of colleagues to consult about problems and challenges encountered in community settings is a cause of stress among new graduates and nurses who have never worked outside the controlled environment of the hospital (Armentrout, 1998). Benefits for the community client include the following:

- *Familiar and comfortable environment*
- *Routine that is less determined by the nurse or health professional*
- *Diverse resources, including friends, family, pets, available for support and comfort*
- *Autonomy and choice in health decisions*

Reform and the Reinvention of Systems of Care

Our health care system is but one of the many overlapping and interacting systems created by society. Societies create systems that reflect the commonly held values of that society. This is the realm of policy, politics, and power. Health care reform initiatives arise in this realm of competing and conflicting values. Groups who advocate values related to well-being, sustenance, quality of life, equity, fairness, and justice often compete with other values related to economic self-interest. Even when values do not seem to be in conflict, the methods recommended to act on those values often cannot be agreed upon. The capitalistic values of the health care delivery system in the United States have been questioned by health care leaders and policy makers in other countries (Moon, 1993). They often do not understand how we can consider ourselves a highly industrialized and civilized country and not provide basic, essential health care for all. A caring society would not allow individuals (especially children) to be deprived of health care. Many find our "nonsystems" approach to health care confusing.

Indeed, among Americans as well, there are few who would not argue that, although the health-illness system has changed, it still needs improvement. Many of the authors throughout this text make reference to **health care reform**. Enacted reforms, proposed

reforms, and preferred reforms all have actual and possible effects on the populations for which nurses provide care and the conditions under which they provide it. Reform is not new, nor is it controlled; rather it is *episodic*, responding to multiple forces for change. *Reform* implies some major change in the process of the delivery of health care. We often refer to reform as change that originates at the national level but is implemented by the states, by payers, or by provider systems. When change is not a "broad" and "sweeping" reform, it is considered an "incremental change," meaning smaller adjustments occur over time. This is the type of health care reform that occurred during the 1990s.

Historically, there have been numerous reform proposals. Major health care reform was attempted following World War II, in 1948, when President Harry Truman proposed national health insurance. What many thought were the beginnings of broad health coverage were introduced in the 1960s as Medicaid and Medicare. In the 1970s, Senator Edward Kennedy (D-Massachusetts) was one of the major supporters of nationwide reform. Most recently, the presidential campaigns of the early 1990s were marked by health reform issues. Despite various proposals from both political parties, no reform initiatives were passed. Even though there was initial support from diverse stakeholders, many of these stakeholders, such as businesses, physicians, and insurance companies, eventually opposed the reform approaches. In addition, the public was confused and did not recognize the cost and choice consequences to individuals (Starr, 1993).

Nursing's Agenda for Health Care Reform

The failed effort of the 1990s to redesign the American health care system had at least one positive consequence for nursing. In an unprecedented collaboration, more than 75 nursing associations endorsed the document jointly developed by the ANA and the NLN, *Nursing's Agenda for Health Care Reform*. This document was significant in terms of its expression of nursing's values and in furthering an understanding of the profession itself. Values such as health services for all, illness prevention, and wellness were prominent. Many nurses played influential and visible roles during the health care reform attempts. Nursing supported the need for cost containment but wanted assurance of quality of care, reduced barriers to advanced practice nursing, and promotion of nursing care as the link between consumers and the health care system. According to the document, "the cornerstone of nursing's plan for reform is the delivery of primary health care services to households and individuals in convenient, familiar places" (ANA, 1991, p. 9).

Managed Care and the Future of Nursing

Although major health care reform proposals are still debated, significant change at the national level is unlikely in the near future. The controversial issues most debated are expanding federal coverage (access) and controlling costs. Many policy and regulation changes, however, have had significant impact on health care delivery systems and providers. "**Managed care**" and a market approach based on "managed competition" have emerged as our major strategies to control costs. These connected strategies have together transformed the organization and methods of care delivery. **Care management** is a growing practice arena for nurses. Within the managed care environment, there is a focus on care management, which is the attempt to provide more timely and coordinated care for individuals. Individuals move among the following possible states: being well and promoting that state, having acute care needs, needing outpatient surgery, needing follow-up home care, and so on (ANA, 1994).

Health care organizations now see the economic and quality outcome benefits of caring for clients and managing client care over a continuum of possible settings and needs. Traditional health care was episodic, with individuals moving with little connection from one episode of need to the next (often waiting until the need for care was acute) and one facility to another. When care is managed, the term *discharge planning* is now more accurately referred to as *transition planning*. The client does not "leave" the system but merely requires another type of care, including wellness care or health promotion. Clients are followed much more closely both during illness care and with follow-up when well. Care managers can practice from a base in many settings, including the offices of a payer. To more clearly conceptualize this change in thinking, instead of a client being "discharged" from the hospital, more importantly, he or she is being "admitted" back to the community.

When the health care providers in a system have the responsibility for all types of care for the plan's "enrolled population," they have an incentive to coordinate or "manage" that care efficiently. The goal is to provide the best value in the most efficient way to be competitive in the health care market. A market economy for health care delivery dramatically changes health care services and incentives. For nurses who are historically committed to "doing whatever it takes" for their clients, cost consciousness is an unfamiliar and often resisted viewpoint. Nurses in today's health care system must remain informed about the complexities of managed care to sustain professional identity and to assist clients in the navigation through the market systems. The continued growth of managed care as a system for health financing and delivery provides unique challenges and opportunities for nurses, especially those prepared in community health. Nurses remain the only health care professionals who are specifically educated to assess health status and risks, unhealthful lifestyles, and health education needs for clients and families; who provide support and reassurance while caring for present and potential health problems; and who act as advocates for primary and preventive care services. Managed care organizations, as well as all agencies that provide health care services in a managed care environment, have come to value quality and recognize the importance of prevention, wellness, and early intervention. The community health nurse is especially well prepared to provide managed care with the direction needed to focus on providing a full range of quality, cost-effective services in the promotion of a population's health (ANA, 1994). Health care delivery in the context of managed care will be discussed in Chapter 2.

Money would be better spent in maintaining health in infancy and childhood than in building hospitals to cure diseases.
Florence Nightingale, 1894

Back to the Future: From Hospital to Community, from Cure to Prevention

As we have learned from the history of health care, early attempts to improve health, treat disease, and prevent disability occurred primarily in the home. The primary characteristic of the emerging system has been the move back to the community practice setting. Perhaps the major force behind much of the change has been economic, with efforts to contain what many see as the exploding costs of our health care system. One cost-related factor encouraging a community focus has been the movement of clients out of expensive acute care facilities into community settings, where many of their illness needs can be adequately met at a much lower cost. This movement has encouraged the growth of home care, hospice care, outpatient clinics, and outpatient surgeries. Another among the many results of cost-containment efforts has been the recognition of the connection between prevention and keeping populations healthy. Healthy populations have lower morbidity (disease rates) and mortality (death rates) statistics.

My view, you know, is that the ultimate destination of all nursing is the nursing of the sick in their own homes. . . . I look to the abolition of all hospitals and workhouse infirmaries. But no use to talk about the year 2000.
Florence Nightingale, 1867

Home Health Care

Home health care is the fastest growing community-based nursing role outside of the acute care setting. This is just one of many roles

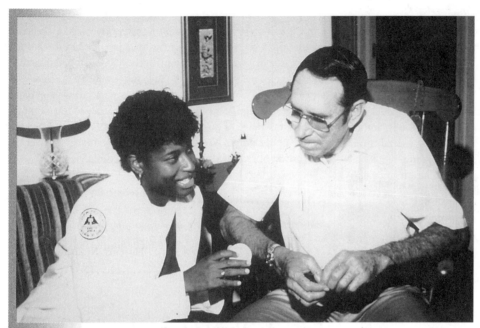

Home health nurses deliver care in the client's home. A goal of home care is to teach clients and their families self-care.

available in community health and is covered in various chapters in the text. Home health nursing is discussed briefly here as an example of an emerging role that has resulted from changes in the way health care is delivered and paid for. One attempt at major health care cost containment in the early 1980s was the shift from cost reimbursement to prospective payment for hospital care, which means that payment was based on standard disease categories. Because of this change, hospitals could make money if they were efficient in taking care of the clients' problems and could discharge them quicker. Home health boomed as clients were discharged while still needing nursing care in their homes. Even with recent government attempts to regulate the growth of home health by changing reimbursement patterns, home health continues to grow and present new and challenging opportunities for nursing (Trossman, 1998).

Cure and Prevention: Can We Really Do It All?

Most people spend little time thinking about or planning for their own good health or the community's health. Research tells us that our health is influenced more by our social and biological environment, lifestyle choices, and self-care initiatives than by our inherited traits, yet we continue to pour money into newer and better treatments rather than into learning about what we can do to promote health and prevent illness from the beginning. We are discovering that we have overemphasized cure with a disease-based medical model for health care. As early as 1977, the Centers for Disease Control and Prevention (CDC) reported an analysis of the proportional contributions to mortality in the United States of four "health field elements": lifestyle, human bi-

ology, environment, and health care. Their conclusions were that approximately 50% of premature mortality in the United States is due to lifestyle, 20% to human biology, 20% to environment, and only 10% to inadequacies in health care. Seventy percent of the potential for reducing premature mortality lies in the areas of health promotion and disease prevention, but only about 3.5% of the health care dollar is spent in those areas. Therefore, although the health status of a population is related more to the determinants of health than it is to the causes of disease, we have developed a system that pays for illness care rather than a system designed to create the healthiest population possible.

Certainly, people having access to competent and skilled health practitioners and technologies related to the diagnosis and treatment of disease is important, but no more so than having clean water to drink, safe food to eat, meaningful employment with an adequate wage, adequate housing and childcare, a good education, a life free of discrimination, and a safe environment. Such insights are leading to a "reinvention" of health services organizations at all levels—from single facilities organized to serve sick clients to complex networks organized to serve populations of mostly well people (Shortell & Gilles 1995).

Prevention activities and population-focused care are often contrasted with the more immediately "gratifying" and "exciting" acute care. Community-focused care is long term, often behind the scenes, taken for granted, and largely unseen unless something goes amiss. Nurses have always promoted the welfare and health of those in their care. Wolf (1989) contends that nursing has difficulty being visible because much of the work of nursing goes unnoticed. Health care reform and the move to health promotion and illness prevention may provide the opportunity for nursing to shine as a profession.

Despite the "excitement" of acute care, there are many economic, social, and political factors that suggest that the future focus of health care should be on health promotion and disease prevention in a health-based model with a "community orientation" (Proenca, 1998). These areas and such networking have traditionally been the domain of the less visible and less financially supported practice of public health. Mechanic (1998) has pointed out that an alignment of public health with the growing managed care health plans would be a logical and potential benefit to the mission of our public health system. The vision of public health for more than a century has been one of health promotion and disease prevention that depends on a community perspective to activate identification of risks and protective and restorative interventions.

Health care providers in managed care plans are increasingly subject to competition and are evaluated on their successes in improving outcomes for their plan's enrollees. They have become more interested in the population activities and methods long carried out by public health. Acknowledging the economic value of population health promotion and disease prevention activities within the health care marketplace encourages the adoption of these approaches. Thus, for many nurses caring for individuals, the focus on community health nursing roles represents a transition to the community in practice setting.

Nurses have been optimistic about the trends in health care practice and reform. With the increasing impetus for health promotion, nurses seem well poised as a result of their longstanding commitment to and expertise in keeping people healthy. In the past, when nurses have made claims about the benefits of health promotion and disease prevention strategies, the thoughts have been on benefits to the individual, not on any financial benefit or loss. Now we as nurses are beginning to embrace the possibilities of teaming up with a market-driven business world to also realize financial benefits and improved health for populations.

Benefits Versus Costs

Anderson (1997) cautions against a naive understanding of what we take for granted. Indeed, she describes the case of smoking cessation programs, proven to have economic benefits. However, a potential financial loss scenario is possible for preventing cardiopulmonary diseases in middle-aged clients. Prevention may actually increase managed care costs by prolonging a person's life and thus incurring greater costs for the complex medical problems of old age. Similarly, early detection of HIV in at-risk populations should permit early drug treatment to prevent costly AIDS-related illnesses. For a managed care organization, early detection would imply costly antiviral treatment at thousands of dollars yearly. Nondetection and an early death would actually save money for a private health care provider and increase its

> ## A Conversation With...
>
> *I am more convinced than ever that the major health problems in this and future decades—chronicity, aging, the personal and public health problems generated by social and economic dislocations, the prevention of illness, and the promotion of healthy communities—are all within the nursing genius to address and ameliorate. These are the very things that we are known for. They are the things we do best and we are the best to do them. . . . I truly believe that we are at a place in nursing that we will never see again. This is our big chance. . . . We cannot wait for anybody to let us do anything. . . . We have more capacity to play in the health care game, we have the obligation to take charge, to endorse professional values and improve health outcomes.*
>
> **—Melanie C. Dreher, PhD, RN, FAAN**
> Past President of Sigma Theta Tau International.
> December 6, 1997, Indianapolis, Indiana, cited
> in *Reflections* (1998), first quarter, pp. 36–37.

profits. Nurses are socialized to value life. Health care companies are in business to make a profit first.

With those warnings, nurses must realize the competing values often at work in the health care arena. Community-focused health promotion strategies also can face ideological, political, and religious differences that cause conflict. Needed sex education to prevent teenage pregnancy has long met with resistance from some groups. Strategies must be developed at the individual and societal levels to bring about change that aligns with all interested parties' goals and needs. In the case of smoking cessation, other community groups could be approached to encourage health promotion interventions and policies. Employers could be motivated to realize the financial gain of less employee illness and fewer work days lost. They would then negotiate for managed care plans that cover health promotion activities.

Healthy People 2010: Goals for the Nation

Even before the more recent reform efforts and regulations encouraged increased use of prevention practices, it became obvious in the 1970s, based on the CDC's study of premature deaths, that health promotion and disease prevention could save lives

HEALTHY PEOPLE 2010

PRIORITY AREAS

Promote Healthy Behaviors

1. Physical activity and fitness

2. Nutrition

3. Tobacco use

Promote Healthy and Safe Communities

4. Educational and community-based programs

5. Environmental health

6. Food safety

7. Injury/violence prevention

8. Occupational safety and health

9. Oral health

Improve Systems for Personal and Public Health

10. Access to quality health care services

   1. Preventive care

   2. Primary care

   3. Emergency services

   4. Long-term care and rehabilitative services

11. Family planning

12. Maternal, infant, and child health

13. Medical product safety

14. Public health infrastructure

15. Health communication

Prevent and Reduce Diseases and Disorders

16. Arthritis, osteoporosis, and chronic back conditions

17. Cancer

18. Diabetes

19. Disability and secondary conditions

20. Heart disease and stroke

21. HIV

22. Immunization and infectious diseases

23. Mental health and mental disorders

24. Respiratory diseases

25. Sexually transmitted diseases

26. Substance abuse

Source: DHHS, 2000.

---

and perhaps reduce health care costs. In 1980, the federal government issued a set of national health objectives that were evaluated to measure progress in the nation's health goals and health care services. The process proved valuable and was repeated with the issuing of a new set of objectives to guide the 1990s. That plan was titled Healthy People 2000: National Health Promotion and Disease Prevention Objectives.

The process was again repeated, culminating in the release of a ***Healthy People 2010*** document in October 2000. Two overarching goals, "increase years of healthy life" and "eliminate health disparities," are proposed. Four enabling goals provide support. They are concerned with promoting healthful behaviors, protecting health, achieving access to quality health care, and strengthening community prevention. These objectives provide a tool that the creators envision for public health policy makers and all policy makers at both state and local levels as well. Meeting these ob-

jectives requires that all health care providers move toward a community-based practice or focus. They must move from illness and cure to health promotion and illness prevention.

....

Of all the forms of inequality, injustice in health care is the most shocking and inhumane.

Martin Luther King

....

....

Preventable disease should be looked on as a social crime.

Florence Nightingale, 1894

....

Influences on a Community's Health: Culture, Environment, and Ethics

There are so many different things that influence health care that it is difficult to decide which are the most important. For the nurse to isolate any one factor for assessment and intervention with both individuals and communities is like the captain of a ship seeing only the tip of the iceberg and not looking for the real threat to the ship's safety that lies underneath. However, there are three major components of health care that are addressed in this first chapter because they have a profound affect on all aspects of client care. The influence of **culture**, **environment**, and **ethics** are discussed in greater detail in later chapters.

Culture

The numerous global, social, demographic, economic, and political changes in recent years have alerted health care professionals to the need to provide attention to increasing diversity in our society and the affect of that diversity on people's health (Meleis, 1996). International travel and advances in communication through the Internet and satellite television make it essential for today's nurses to have the skills needed to provide care that recognizes complexities and differences among clients (Janes & Hobson, 1998).

The United States is the most culturally diverse nation in the world. In fact, in 1994, *Time Magazine* designated the United States "the first universal nation" (Grossman, 1994). The 1990 census reported that almost 25% of Americans were members of ethnic minority groups, including 12% African Americans, 9% Hispanics, and 2.9% Asian Americans. It is predicted that by the year 2050, the African American population will increase to 16%, Hispanics to 21%, and Asian Americans to 11% (Norbeck, 1995).

So what exactly do we mean by the term *culture*? According to Madeleine Leininger (1995), culture refers to the "learned and shared beliefs, values, and life ways, of a designated or particular group which are generally transmitted intergenerationally and influence one's thinking and action modes." Giger and Davidhizar (1995) say the culture is "a patterned behavioral response that develops over time as a result of imprinting the mind through social and religious structures and intellectual and artistic manifestations." Purnell and Paulanka (1998) define culture as "the totality of socially transmitted behavioral patterns, art, beliefs, values, customs, life ways, and all other products of human work and thought characteristics of a population of people that guide their world view and decision making." Obviously, culture is more than just ethnicity. Culture is language, religion, food, traditions, customs, clothing, and everything that makes one group of people unique from another. Cultural values, beliefs, and behaviors can also be related to age, gender, sexual orientation, socioeconomic status, and profession. There is a "culture of nursing" that all nurses belong to, with its own language, values, and traditions, that often clashes with clients whose cultural beliefs about health care differ from those of their nurses.

When considering cultural issues, we need to look beyond the borders of our own country. Those who hold privileged and recognized positions in societies by virtue of specialized expertise, such as nursing, have an obligation to give back to those societies. To make such contributions, nurses should become "global citizens" holding a broad vision of international health. In today's connected world, no profession can be truly effective without interactions and viewpoints that include international perspectives. Community health nurses especially, who by definition practice within a broad systems perspective, must incorporate understandings from international health efforts in their own interventions. Comparing and drawing insights from methods and successes of nurses delivering care in other countries holds the promise of improving the care to U.S. clients. In addition, there is a need to understand and support collaborating agencies at the international level. Principles of pluralism, consultation, coherence, consensus, compassion, partnership, and cooperation are the hallmarks of nurses who practice and embrace global citizenship (Neufield, 1992). For example, control measures for effectively reducing AIDS infections have involved the active cooperation of most countries worldwide.

Environment

The environment has been a concern for nursing since the days of Florence Nightingale. In *Notes on Nursing* (1860), Nightingale emphasizes the fact that recovery from illness can occur only in a bright, clean, well-ventilated environment. She states:

> The very first canon of nursing, the first and the last thing upon which a nurse's attention must be fixed, the first essential to a client, without which all the rest you can do for him is nothing, with which I had almost said you may leave all the rest alone, is this: TO KEEP THE AIR HE BREATHES AS PURE AS THE EXTERNAL AIR, WITHOUT CHILLING HIM.

When Nightingale spoke of the patient's environment, she meant the room in the hospital or home in which the patient stayed during the course of his or her illness. In more recent years, the public health definition of environment has come to mean all the surroundings and conditions that affect the health of individuals, families, and communities. The environment has many different components, including social, cultural, political, economic, and ecological factors.

• •

The work we are speaking of has nothing to do with nursing disease, but with maintaining health by removing the things which disturb it . . . dirt, drink, diet, damp, draughts, and drains.
Florence Nightingale, 1860

• •

Environmental issues have been in the forefront of many political campaigns during the last few years and seem to be gaining momentum, with many governmental and private community groups supporting legislation to protect the environment. Most of this activity has been focused on the ecological component of environmental health—primarily clean air and water and a safe food supply.

Nurses are beginning to take a more active role in promoting environmental health, reducing environmental health risks, and protecting the earth's resources. In fact, several nursing organizations, such as the American Holistic Nurses Association and the International Council of Nurses, have developed position statements to delineate the nurse's role in promoting environmental health. A specialty organization called Nurses for Environmental and Social Responsibility has been formed specifically to educate nurses and the public about environmental health hazards.

Ethics

Since the time of Florence Nightingale, the nursing profession has been addressing ethical concerns related to patient care issues. The ANA's *Code for Nurses with Interpretive Statements* (2001) provides guidance for ethical decisions made by nurses in the clinical setting.

Ethical dilemmas have traditionally included such things as informed consent and individual freedom of choice, autonomy, truth telling, protection of privacy and confidentiality, and discrimination. In addition, public health nurses have also had to make ethical decisions related to the dual obligation to protect the public's welfare while respecting the rights of individual clients (Folmar, Coughlin, Bessinger, & Sacknoff, 1997). However, today's changing health care delivery system brings with it additional ethical dilemmas for nurses. We are now concerned with problems related to equity in health care delivery, environmental safety, politicization of health care interventions, euthanasia, elder abuse in nursing homes, provider-client relationships, and community partnerships (Graham, 1997). Recent advancements in science and technology are presenting ethical dilemmas that Florence Nightingale could not have envisioned in even her wildest fantasies. These include such issues as physician-assisted suicide, living wills, gene therapy, in vitro fertilization, and human cloning. All nurses would do well to follow Spicer's advice to nursing students in an editorial in *Imprint* (1998). She says, "As you prepare for your careers, remember your professional commitment to place your patient first in all decisions. Take time to establish your ethical boundaries. . . . Base your decisions from your head and your heart."

Epidemiology: The Science of Public Health

Whether a person is healthy or ill results from numerous constantly changing interacting forces. The actual occurrence of disease results from a triad of factors, referred to as the *epidemiological model* or *triangle*. The triad is composed of the host, the agent, and the environment. The host is the human body influenced by such variables as gender, age, race, and behavior. The agent is a physical, chemical, or biological element that can cause illness or injury. Examples might include a tuberculosis bacilli or nicotine. The environment is perhaps the most complex component. As we learn more about health and its determinants, the environment holds more and more keys to explaining health risks to our human hosts. The environment not only includes the physical environment, such as climate and terrain, but also the sociocultural-political environment, such as poverty, racism, and other stressors that influence health.

Prevention strategies are made up of measures that protect people from disease and take the form of efforts that we use to protect ourselves and others from specific diseases and conditions and their resulting consequences. There are three levels of prevention: primary, secondary, and tertiary. Nurses in all settings use all three levels of prevention as a basis for practice. The nurse caring for clients in an acute care setting may primarily use secondary and tertiary interventions, and the occupational health nurse may use primary and secondary interventions in his or her role. These levels of prevention were originally conceptualized by Leavell and Clark in 1953 and were tied to what these authors described as the **natural history of disease**. Their assumption is that disease in humans is a process: The conditions that promote either health or disease are present in the human's biological, physical, emotional, and social environments as well as in the human host itself.

The relationship between levels of prevention and the natural history of any given disease condition or health state is the basis for community health interventions. Disease occurs in two stages: prepathogenesis and pathogenesis. The intervention strategies or levels of prevention must coincide with predictable events within the stages of prepathogenesis (predisease) and pathogenesis (disease, condition, or injury). One can readily see that applying the levels of prevention requires that the nurse know the natural history of a given disease or condition. The less known about the disease or condition, the greater the likelihood of interventions occurring in secondary or tertiary prevention levels. In other words, the more we learn about disease, disability, and injury, the earlier we can intervene to prevent the illness from occurring. The goal of preventive health then is to intervene at the earliest possible stage in the natural history of disease in order to prevent complications, limit disability, and halt irreversible changes in health status (Leavell & Clark, 1979).

Primary prevention refers to those measures that focus on prevention of health problems *before* they occur. Primary prevention is *not* therapeutic, which means that it does *not* consist of symptom identification and use of the typical therapeutic skills of the nurse (Shamansky & Clausen, 1980). This level includes both generalized health promotion and specific protection against certain identified diseases or conditions. The purpose is to reduce the person's vulnerability to the illness by strengthening the human host's capacity to withstand physical, emotional, and environmental stressors. An example would be teaching a person about adequate nutrition, exercise, and hygiene. Specific protection includes numerous interventions associated with public health nursing: immunizations, bicycle helmets, auto seatbelts, safety caps on electrical outlets, handrails on bathtubs, and drug education for children.

Secondary prevention begins when pathology is involved and is aimed at early detection through diagnosis and prompt treatment. This level of prevention is aimed at halting the pathological process, thus shortening its duration and severity and getting the client back to a normal state of functioning. All screening tests, such as breast self-examinations, hypertensive assessments, and Pap smears, are included in this level of prevention. The goal of this level is to identify groups of individuals who have early symptoms of disease so that they may be treated as soon as possible in the natural history of the disease, condition, or injury. If the disease, condition, or injury cannot be cured, further complications and disability move the level of prevention to that of tertiary prevention.

Tertiary prevention consists of activities designed around rehabilitation of a person with a permanent, irreversible condition. The goal of tertiary prevention goes beyond halting the disease process to restoring the client to an optimal level of functioning *within the constraints of the disability*. Nursing strategies at this level might include teaching a stroke patient how to ambulate with assistance or assisting a child with cystic fibrosis to reduce risks of respiratory infection while maintaining an active lifestyle.

The boundaries between secondary and tertiary prevention are often fuzzy and more difficult to identify as either one or the other. One feature that helps in this identification is that tertiary intervention takes place *only if the condition results in a permanent disability* (Shamansky & Clausen, 1980). This may be influenced by the age or development of the patient rather than by the condition itself. For example, if a 15-year-old high school athlete suffers a simple broken femur during a soccer game, intervention would occur at the secondary prevention level. Although the athlete may require extensive physical rehabilitation after the cast is removed, unless there are serious complications, she should eventually be able to return to her normal state of health. Compare this with a 75-year-old man who falls from a roof and suffers the identical injury. Most likely, this client would need both secondary and tertiary intervention strategies because of the aging process, recovery, and the likelihood of permanent disability resulting from this fall.

Shamansky and Clausen (1980) use the following example to illustrate how all levels of prevention are often used with the same client and family:

> A nurse is conducting a group session with young parents and uses values clarification as a method to discuss issues of parental responsibility for providing a safe yet stimulating environment for the young, curious child. This is primary prevention; health promotion occurs, since the discussion is general and directed toward nonspecific efforts to ensure the well-being of the young child. Later, on a home visit, the nurse encourages a mother to use screens on a second story window, since she perceives the window is dangerously accessible to the active three year old. This, too, is primary prevention, an example of specific protection, because one is attempting to remove a risk factor from the environment of a vulnerable child. If the screen is not used and the child falls out of the window onto a cement driveway below, the mother's and emergency personnel's use of appropriate emergency first aid would be secondary prevention through the use of prompt treatment. If the child sustained a severe head injury, was hospitalized (and secondary measures were used in the hospital), and later released to home care, teaching the mother to turn, feed, and give range of motion exercises would represent the disability limitation aspect of secondary prevention. Several months later if the child is found to have some permanent brain damage, tertiary prevention would take the form of referrals to special education classes, or physical or speech therapy to increase the child's maximum potential level of functioning, although the damage itself is irreversible. (pp. 106–107)

Measuring a Community's Health: How Do We Know When We Get There?

Outcomes and measurements of community health interventions take the form of health statistics such as birth rates, infant mortality rates, and incidence and prevalence rates for various diseases and age groups. Most threats to health do not occur at random (i.e., by chance). Natural forces influence health threats, but by no means do they dictate the outcome. In this century we have learned through epidemiological research that most threats or risks to our health and well-being are associated with *patterns* of human activity and behavior. It is those patterns that we use to evaluate health interventions and the multitude of influences on people's health (Cohen, 1989). For example, breast cancer rates in the United States are high compared with other countries such as Japan and China. In other words, breast cancer is not universal among all females, nor is it randomly distributed in the female population (Cohen, 1989).

We can see from epidemiological research that individual behavior has a significant effect on a person's "chance" of developing breast cancer. Breast cancer may be associated with a high-fat, high-protein, high-calorie diet, and with high levels of estrogen (either produced by the woman's own body or ingested in diet and medication). Women who do not have or nurse children or have them later in life have higher rates of breast cancer. These lifestyle factors clearly influence the chances of a woman's contracting breast cancer

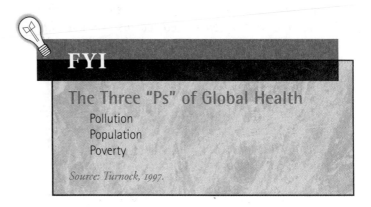

FYI

The Three "Ps" of Global Health

Pollution
Population
Poverty

Source: Turnock, 1997.

| TABLE 1-2 | A COMPARISON OF INDIVIDUAL, FAMILY, COMMUNITY, AND GLOBAL POPULATION-FOCUSED CARE |

INDIVIDUAL CARE	FAMILY	COMMUNITY	GLOBAL
Injuries suffered by woman in violent spousal domestic relationship	Family dysfunctions, such as inability to provide appropriate behavioral roles for conflict resolution Children exhibiting early and inappropriate use of firearms	Child unable to function in school setting because of disruptive behavior in classroom Gang violence resulting in neighborhood isolation, decreased population, diminished economic base because of business closure and decreased funds available for education and family assistance	Woman and children refugees in war-torn Pakistan and Afghanistan suffering from injuries as a result of acts of war violence

in her lifetime. The availability of cutting-edge technology and diagnostic interventions cannot prevent women from contracting breast cancer; they can improve chances of survival only once cancer is detected (Kolata, 1987; Marx, 1986; Winick, 1980). In another example, maternal death risk in childbirth plummeted during the 20th century in developed countries as a result of research application of prenatal care, use of antibiotics, and infectious disease control. In the United States, a woman has only a 1 in 3,700 chance of dying in childbirth, yet in Latin America, a woman's mortality risk is 1 in 130 and women in parts of Africa have an alarming *1 in 16 chance* of dying as a result of childbearing (Whaley & Hashim, 1995). Table 1-2 provides an illustration of the links among all levels of care. You will learn in this text how these group rates of disease, health, injury, and disability reflect more accurately the values of a society and how health professionals measure not only their interventions but the influences of many variables on health.

CASE STUDY

Community-Based Care: An Example from Practice

A 3-year-old child is brought to a public health department for her first set of immunizations. As the nurse assesses the child, she finds that the child has a generalized red rash all over her body. The mother complains that the child scratches and cries about the rash and that she has been using a cortisone skin cream for three days. The nurse attends to the immediate concerns of the mother about home care comfort measures and possible causes. The nurse then delivers direct client care to the child and to her family, while considering the following community implications:

- Does anyone else in the family exhibit those symptoms?
- Does the child go to day care?
- Have there been any other children in the clinic recently with similar symptoms? If so, how does this case compare with cases in recent months?
- What is the likely pathogen that is causing the rash?
- Are there any pregnant women in the clinic or in the home setting?

1. What are possible conclusions that the nurse can make that have individual implications?
2. Are there community and public health issues that may be present that the nurse must address?

CONCLUSION

In community-based care, community clients are the focus wherever they live, work, or reside. The *focus* of the nurses' practice may be on the individual client but various influences on a community's health and how the health care system has organized services around societal needs and expectations must be considered. Nurses will play a critical role in the future of managed care, which is organized around prevention and a healthy population. Epidemiology is the science that provides community and public health with a framework for addressing the primary, secondary, and tertiary health needs for a population and directs community health nursing practice. The personal well-being of individuals is more than an individual matter. Humankind does not live in isolation, unaffected by others. Community health is a dynamic of the community and is influenced by the context of where and how the population lives, works, and addresses health care needs.

CRITICAL THINKING ACTIVITIES

1. After reading "A Personal Look at Public Health" on p. 10, respond to the following questions:
   - What three risks described in the essay were unknown a century ago?
   - What is the responsibility of the individual in creating a safe environment?
   - What three public safety measures mentioned in the essay do not exist in underdeveloped countries?

2. How can heart disease be both a personal health problem and a community health problem?

3. For several decades now, nurses have worked primarily in hospitals using a medical model approach to health and illness. Does nursing have a vision of the profession with community at the center or has nursing become so institutionalized into hospital-based practice over the past decades that we will resist the tremendous opportunities to care for people in a myriad of settings and situations?

4. After reading this chapter, watch an episode of *ER, Chicago Hope,* or any program on television that features a trauma setting. Identify the kinds of problems that are presented on the program. Which ones could have been prevented? How?

5. Could a community health nurse work in such an environment? If so, what would the role be?

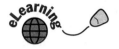

Explore Community Health Nursing on the web! To learn more about the topics in this chapter, use the passcode provided to access your exclusive web site: http://communitynursing.jbpub.com
If you do not have a passcode, you can obtain one at this site.

REFERENCES

American Nurses Association (ANA). (1980). *ANA social policy statement.* Kansas City, MO: Author.

American Nurses Association. (2001). *Code for nurses with interpretive statements.* Kansas City: Author.

American Nurses Association. (1986). *Standards of community health nursing practice.* Kansas City: Author.

American Nurses Association. (1991). *Nursing's agenda for health care reform: Executive summary.* Washington, DC: Author.

American Nurses Association. (1994). *Managed care: challenges and opportunities for nursing.* Washington, DC: Author.

Anderson, C. (1997). The economics of health promotion. *Nursing Outlook, 45*(3), 105–106.

Armentrout, G. (1998). *Community-based nursing. Foundation for practice.* Stamford, CT: Appleton & Lange.

Bunker, J. P., Frazier, H. S., & Mosteller, F. (1994). Improving health: Measuring effects of medical care. *Milbank Quarterly, 72,* 225–258.

Bureau of Labor Statistics. (1998). *Statistics of employment 1996–2006: A summary of BLS projection* (Bulletin No. 2502). Washington, DC: U.S. Government Printing Office.

Canavan, K. (1996). Nursing education on cusp of shift in focus: Faculty grapple with preparing students for changing health care delivery. *American Nurse, 28*(6), 1, 11.

Cohen, M. (1989). *Health and the rise of civilization.* New Haven, CT: Yale University Press.

Consumer Reports. (1992, July). Wasted health care dollars, 435–448.

Consumer Reports. (1990, September). The crisis in health insurance part 2, 608–617.

Cottrell, K. (1976). The competent community. In B. H. Kaplan, R. N. Wilson, & A. H. Leighton (Eds.), *Further explorations in social psychology.* New York: Basic Books.

Dubos, R. (1968). *Man, medicine and environment.* New York: Mentor.

Flynn, B. C. (1997). Are we ready to collaborate for community-based health services? *Public Health Nursing, 14*(3), 135–136.

Folmar, J., Coughlin, S. S., Bessinger, R., & Sacknoff, D. (1997). Ethics in public health practice: A survey of public health nurses in southern Louisiana. *Public Health Nursing, 14*(3), 156–160.

Gebbie, K. M. (1996, November 18). *Preparing currently employed public health nurses for changes in the health care system: Meeting report and suggested action steps.* New York: Columbia University School of Nursing Center for Health Policy and Health Sciences Research. (Report based on meeting in Atlanta, GA, July 11, 1996.)

Giger, J. N., & Davidhizar, R. E. (1995). *Transcultural nursing. Assessment and intervention* (2nd ed.). St. Louis: Mosby.

Graham, K. Y. (1997). Ethics: Do we really care? *Public Health Nursing, 14*(1), 1–2.

Grossman, D. (1994). Enhancing your cultural competence. *American Journal of Nursing, 94*(7), 58–62.

Hall, J. M., & Stevens, P. E. (1995). The future of graduate education in nursing: Scholarship, the health communities, and health care reform. *Journal of Professional Nursing, 11*(6), 332–338.

Hall, J. E., & Weaver, B. R. (1977). *Distributive nursing practice: A systems approach to community health.* Philadelphia: Lippincott.

Hanlon, J. J., & Pickett, G. E. (1984). *Public health: Administration and practice* (8th ed.). St. Louis: Mosby.

Heinrich, J. (1983). Historical perspectives on public health nursing. *Nursing Outlook, 32*(6), 317–320.

http://odphp.osophs.dhhs.gov/pubs/hp2000/newsbit.html.

Institute of Medicine. (1988). *The future of public health.* Washington, DC: National Academy Press.

Keck, E. W. (1994). Community health: Our common challenge. *Family and Community Health, 17*(2), 1–9.

Kolata, G. B. (1987). !Kung hunter-gatherers: Feminism, diet, and birth control. *Science, 185,* 932–934.

Kurtzman, C., Ibgui, D., Pogrund, R., & Monin, S. (1980, December). Nursing process at the aggregate level. *Nursing Outlook, 28*(12), 737–739.

Kuss, T., Proulx-Girouard, L., Lovitt, S., Katz, C. B., & Kennelly, P. (1997). A public health nursing model. *Public Health Nursing, 14*(2), 81–91.

Lancaster, J. (1984). History of community health and community health nursing. In M. Stanhope & J. Lancaster (Eds.), *Community health nursing. Process and practice for promoting health* (pp. 3–31). St. Louis: Mosby.

Leininger, M. (1995). *Transcultural nursing. Concepts, theories, research, & practices* (2nd ed.). New York: McGraw-Hill.

Leipert, B. D. (1996). The value of community health nursing: A phenomenological study of the perceptions of community health nurses. *Public Health Nursing, 13*(1), 50–57.

Janes, S., & Hobson, K. (1998). An innovative approach for affirming cultural diversity among baccalaureate nursing students and faculty. *Journal of Cultural Diversity,* Winter Issue.

Leavell, H. R., Clark, E. G. (1953). *Preventive medicine for the doctor in his community.* New York: McGraw-Hill.

Leavell, H. R., Clark, E. G. (1979). *Preventive medicine for the doctor in his community: An epidemiological approach* (3rd ed.). Huntington, NY: RE Dreges.

Marx, J. (1986). Viruses and cancer briefing. *Science, 241,* 1039–1040.

McKenzie, J. F., & Pinger, R. R. (1997). *An introduction to community health.* Boston: Jones and Bartlett.

Mechanic, D. (1998). Topics of our times: Managed care and public health. *American Journal of Public Health, 88*(6), 84–85.

Meleis, A. I. (1990). Being and becoming healthy: The core of nursing knowledge. *Nursing Science Quarterly, 3,* 107–114.

Meleis, A. L. (1996). Culturally competent scholarship: Substance and rigor. *Advances in Nursing Science, 19*(2), 1–16.

Moon, M. (1993). Health care reform. *The Future of Children, 3*(2), 21–36.

Division of Nursing, Bureau of Health Professions, Health Resources and Services Administration, Health and Human Services. (2000). *National Sample Survey of Registered Nurses.* Washington, DC: U.S. Government Printing Office.

National League for Nursing (NLN). (2000). *Educational Competencies for Graduates of Associate Degree Nursing Programs.* Sudbury, MA: Jones and Bartlett Publishers and National League for Nursing.

Neufeldt, V., & Guralnik, D. B. (Eds.). (1994). *Webster's new world dictionary* (3rd college ed.). New York: Prentice Hall.

Neufield, V. (1992). Training: a Canadian perspective. In Pan American Health Organization (Ed.), *International health: North south debate.* (Human Resource Development Series, pp. 95, 193–203). Washington, DC: Pan American Health Organization.

Nightingale, F. (1860). *Notes on nursing: What it is and what it is not.* London: Harrison.

Norbeck, J. S. (1995). Who is our consumer? Shaping nursing programs to meet consumer needs. *Journal of Professional Nursing, 11*(6), 325–331.

Proenca, E. J. (1998). Community orientation in health services organizations: the concept and its implementation. *Health Care Management Review, 23*(2), 28–38 (51 ref.).

Purnell, L. D., & Paulanka, B. J. (1998). *Transcultural health care. A culturally competent approach.* Philadelphia: F. A. Davis.

Salmon, M., & Vanderbush, P. (1990). Leadership and change in public and community health nursing today: The essential intervention. In J. C. McCloskey, & H. K. Grace (Eds.), *Current issues in nursing* (3rd ed., pp. 187–193). St. Louis: Mosby.

Schultz, P. R. (1987). When client means more than one: Extending the foundational concept of person. *Advances in Nursing Science, 10*(1), 71–86.

Schultz, P. R. (1994). *On the matter of populations, aggregates, and communities.* Unpublished manuscript, University of Washington, Seattle.

Shamansky, S. L., & Clausen, C. L. (1980, February). Levels of prevention: Examination of the concept. *Nursing Outlook, 28*(2), 104–108.

Shortell, S. M., & Gilles, R. R. (1995). Reinventing the American hospital. *Milbank Quarterly, 73*(2), 131.

Smith, C. M. (1995). Responsibilities for care in community health nursing. In C. M. Smith & F. A. Maurer (Eds.), *Community health nursing. Principles and practice* (pp. 3–29). Philadelphia: Saunders.

Spicer, G. (1998). Learning right from wrong. *Imprint, 45*(3), 4.

Starr, P. (1993). The framework of health care reform. *New England Journal of Medicine, 329,* 1666–1672.

Trossman, S. (1998, March/April). Self-determination: The name of the game in the next century. *The American Nurse,* 1.

Turnock, B. (1997). *Public health: What it is and how it works.* Baltimore: Aspen.

Whaley, R. F., & Hashim, T. J. (1995). *A textbook of world health.* New York: Parthenon.

Whelan, E. M. (1995). The health corner: A community-based nursing model to maximize access to primary care. *Public Health Reports, 110*(2), 184–188.

Winick, M. (1980). *Nutrition in health and disease.* New York: John Wiley.

Wolf, Z. R. (1989, October). Uncovering the hidden work of nursing. *Nursing and Health Care, 10*(8), 462–467.

World Health Organization. (1958). *The first ten years of the World Health Organization.* New York: Author.

World Health Organization. (1986). Health promotion. A discussion document on the concept and principles. *Public Health Reviews, 14*(3–4), 245–254.

Chapter 2
Health Care Systems in Transition

Bonita R. Reinert

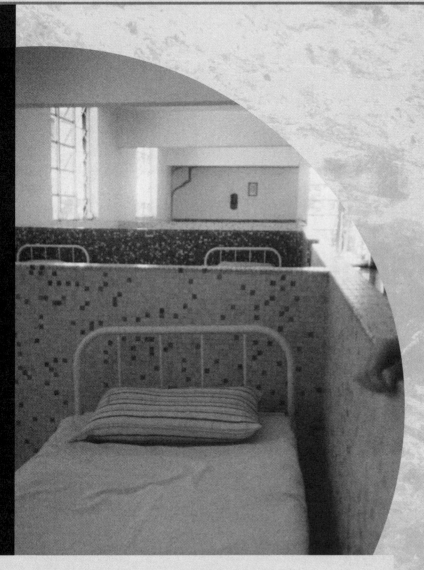

Health care is one of the largest industries in the United States, employing an estimated 10 million workers. The health care system in the United States includes the most technology-rich facilities and the most advanced practices in the world. The most well-educated physicians, nurses, and other health care workers use sophisticated treatments on a daily basis to prolong life and restore function.

CHAPTER FOCUS

Evolution of the U.S. Health Care Delivery System
Private Health Care
Public Health Care
Military Health Care
Health Care Reform

Current U.S. Health Care Delivery System
Levels of Care
Health Care Providers
Health Care Settings
Issues Affecting Delivery of Health Care Services

Managed Care
Managed Care Delivery Systems

Managed Care Organizations
Patient Care Outcomes

Health Politics and Policy
Government Policy
Public Opinion and Special Interest Groups
Nursing and Health Care Policy

New Nursing Opportunities
Advanced Practice Nurses
Entrepreneurs
Data Management
Research

QUESTIONS TO CONSIDER

After reading this chapter, answer the following questions:

1. How did the current U.S. health care system evolve to its present form?
2. What is the difference between private and public health care?
3. What are some of the current issues affecting health care delivery in the United States?

4. How do politics and policy influence the health care delivery system?
5. What are some of the current and evolving health care settings?
6. What impact is managed care having on health care delivery?
7. What are some potential roles for nurses within the changing health care system?

KEY TERMS

Capitation
Diagnosis-related groups (DRGs)
Fee-for-service
Health care delivery system
Health maintenance organizations (HMOs)
Integrated health care systems
Managed care

Managed competition
Point-of-service (POS) plans
Preferred provider organization (PPO)
Preventive care
Primary care
Prospective payment system (PPS)
Third-party payer

As a result of its cutting-edge nature, the U.S. health care system is the most costly, in terms of resources, in the world. Current patterns of health care delivery have resulted in an annual cost that exceeds $9.8 billion (HCFA, 1998), a figure that is significantly higher than that of any other industrialized nation. By the year 2011, it has been projected that health care costs in the United States could exceed $2.8 trillion, a figure that will represent more than 17% of the country's gross domestic product (HCFA, 2002).

Despite technological advances and high health care costs, clinical outcomes are not always significantly better in the United States when compared with other industrialized nations. For example, among the industrialized countries, the United States ranks 1st in health care technology but 17th in rates of low-birth-weight babies and 12th in life expectancy (Children's Defense Fund, 1998). Access to health care is believed to be one of the determinants of our less-than-auspicious health indicators.

A lack of access to quality health care services can take several forms. For example, needed services may simply not be available in an accessible location or during hours when individuals are able to use them. The health care site may not be organized in a user-friendly manner so that individuals can obtain timely and acceptable services. For example, providers may not be as culturally sensitive or as multilingual as is needed in certain locations of this country.

Routine health care may also not be accessible because of a lack of personal funds and/or insurance coverage. Medications and special treatments may be beyond the financial resources of the individual despite a provider's carefully developed plan of care. Finally, individuals may not have a regular provider and may have to receive care from a variety of providers in a number of unconnected facilities. Thus, care may not be comprehensive or timely.

Although leaders in government, health care, and consumer groups continue to express concern over access issues, inequities in the current system are readily apparent. By most accounts, more than 45 million (16%) Americans are uninsured. In addition, many more U.S. citizens are underinsured, and the figure is growing. Individuals working at part-time and minimum wage jobs make up a large part of the uninsured and underinsured in this country.

A lack of insurance often results in a lack of prevention services and early interventions. Lack of adequate prenatal care and infant immunizations, especially for the poor and minority populations, has led to illness, disability, and ultimately, increased financial demands on the public health care system. Statistically, African Americans fair worse in virtually every condition that affects health (U.S. National Center for Health Statistics, 1998). The rates of infectious disease such as tuberculosis, sexually transmitted diseases, and acquired immunodeficiency syndrome (AIDS) continue to rise, especially within at-risk populations. A lack of accessible community mental health services has resulted in a number of tragedies and untold stress for families.

Attempts to contain spiraling costs, deal with the dissatisfaction of consumers and providers, and address issues of uneven access and poor clinical outcomes have resulted in cost containment legislation, new configurations of providers, and new ways of providing care. Because nursing care holds the answer to many of the current dilemmas, the nursing profession appears to be poised at the edge of an exciting and challenging future.

Evolution of the U.S. Health Care Delivery System

The term **health care delivery system** refers to a multilevel industry that transforms various resources into essential services designed to meet the health care needs of a population. This transformation occurs through a complex set of interactions among consumers, providers, payers, employers, and the government. Resources include things such as physical structures, personnel, technology, supplies, and financing. The system is both guided and, in some instances, undermined by competition, demands for profit, technological innovation, standards, and government regulations.

Many critics suggest that the health care system in the United States is not actually a system at all because it is not a coordinated whole with interrelated parts. Instead, health care in this country often occurs as a series of fragmented episodes that may be isolated, unrelated, confusing, or even competing. Furthermore, in the United States, there is no single source of oversight, policies, or goals, nor is there a set of shared values and concerns among the various entities in the delivery system.

Services may be provided in traditional settings, such as hospitals or physicians' offices, and in less traditional settings, such as shelters, specially equipped vans, or shopping malls. Client care information may or may not be shared among the providers in the subsystems or even between providers at separate sites in a single subsystem. Furthermore, follow-up contact between providers and clients is rare.

Reimbursement may come from one or more of the following sources: private insurance companies, managed care organizations, government agencies, foundations, and the client. The client is often the one who has to decide who to bill, what to do when reimbursement is denied, or who to talk to when the bill is only partially reimbursed.

Finally, services may need to be accessed in private, public, and/or military health care systems. Each system has a unique set of rules and requirements. Coverage may be overlapping, costs of care are different, and reimbursement occurs in different ways.

Private Health Care

Our complicated private health care system has changed dramatically in the last 200 years. In the 19th century, family, servants, or close friends cared for clients in the home with physicians making visits as needed. Treatment involved medicinal herbs and comfort measures. Medical knowledge was limited, and most medical practitioners in the United States lacked a standardized education. Medical treatments were based on common sense, and physicians often lacked acceptance as professionals. Care was purchased out of private funds or provided on a charity basis. The few hospitals that existed basically served indigent clients, without family or support, who found themselves at death's door. Medical treatments performed in these early hospitals were often crude and seldom very effective.

After the middle of the 19th century, large jumps in medical knowledge occurred that paved the way for significant gains in surgical interventions and the treatment of disease. The new, more sophisticated procedures required centralized facilities to house the new technology and train the personnel needed to provide client care. This resulted in an era of extensive hospital construction, the institutionalization of health care, and the establishment of the hospital as the center of health care delivery (see Box 2-1).

After World War I, the medical profession in this country grew in prestige and power. This transformation was based on trends such as the following: movement to cities away from family and friends, advances in medical science and technology, organization of medicine and adoption of state licensing requirements, establishment of worker's compensation and growth of health insurance, and educational requirements for providers (Shi & Singh, 1998).

To ensure that hospital bills would be paid, insurance companies such as Blue Cross were formed. With the establishment of broader health insurance coverage, providers were at less financial risk, and insurance policies provided for the reimbursement of increasing numbers of clients. Clients selected the provider. Providers simply decided on the appropriate course of care for the client, implemented that care, and then submitted bills at the end of the illness episode. This form of payment was known as fee-for-service.

Fee-for-service is a form of retrospective payment for health care in which a facility or provider submits a bill for services rendered at the completion of the health care episode. An advantage of this type of billing is that care is reimbursed according to the acuity of the client based on the services required. However, some health care experts now believe that paying a fee for each service performed encourages unnecessary services and frequent return visits, which increases health care costs.

The Hill-Burton Act was passed in 1946 to help communities build hospitals. The National Institutes of Health became a major funding source for health care research in the 1950s. The Medicare Act was passed in 1965 to provide hospital insurance for the elderly. Each of these efforts increased the organizational strength of the health care system.

Two acts passed by Congress have significantly affected the methods by which hospitals are reimbursed for care. The Tax Equity and Fiscal Responsibility Act of 1982 (TEFRA) established

a cost-per-case basis for Medicare-reimbursed inpatient services. The 1983 amendments to the Social Security Act established a prospective payment method of paying for inpatient services for Medicare clients based on a system of admitting diagnoses known as **diagnosis-related groups (DRGs)**.

Under the **prospective payment system (PPS)**, an annual fixed (prospective) rate was established for reimbursing providers for care based on 467 diagnoses or procedures. The prototype for the prospective payment system was developed at Yale University. Under the Yale program, reimbursement amounts bore "little or no relationship to length of stay, services rendered, or costs of care" (Williams & Torrens, 1999, p. 137). Rules stated that costs above the established amount for a given DRG would be absorbed by the hospital, but if the care was delivered for less than the established amount, the hospital could keep the difference and make a profit.

Third-party payers are agencies or organizations like insurance companies or health maintenance organizations that are responsible for all or part of an insured individual's health care costs. Third-party payers also adopted the DRG system as a part of their cost-saving measures. It has been suggested that prospective payment legislation introduced a new era of fiscal constraints, demands for accountability, and pressure to provide services in innovative ways. This new era involved the constant evaluation of practices, policies, and procedures to limit costs whenever possible and has resulted in concerns about access, equitable treatment decisions, and quality of care (Box 2-1).

As a result of the need to control costs, provide quality care, and meet the needs of increasing numbers of individuals, a variety of creative and innovative health care organizations have developed. Often called *alphabet health care*, acronyms such as

---

BOX 2-1 PHASES OF HEALTH CARE SYSTEM DEVELOPMENT

Development of the private health care delivery system occurred in four phases:

1. Prior to the 1850s: Illness and disability were handled at home. Few hospitals and clinics existed, and they provided mostly indigent care.

2. 1850–1930: Significant gains in medical knowledge occurred. Technological advances necessitated an increase in the number of hospitals and nurses.

3. 1930–1980: Health care became more organized. Insurance became available, so people were more likely to go to hospitals for care.

4. 1980 to present: Soaring costs resulted in reorganization, restructuring, reallocation of scarce resources, and difficult ethical decisions.

HMOs (health management organizations), PPOs (preferred provider organizations), POS (point-of-service plans), and MCOs (managed care organizations) have become part of our new health care vocabulary (Feldstein, 1999). With these new health care models have come some difficult ethical questions. Is health care a right? If a treatment or procedure is available and I want it, should my insurance pay for it? Who should decide on the appropriateness of medical treatment plans, the doctor or the insurance company? These questions are probably going to be with us for some time because there are no easy answers.

Public Health Care

"Public health can be defined as an effort organized by society to protect, promote, and restore people's health" (Fairbanks & Wiese, 1998). The U.S. public health system is an interwoven local, state, and national governmental agency designed to look at broad community-based health issues and protect the general public from the hazards that result from living in populated urban areas.

Massachusetts was the first state to establish a state department of health, modeled, in part, after the British General Board of Health. Lemuel Shattuck, from Massachusetts, produced a visionary report in 1850 titled *Report of the Sanitary Commission of Massachusetts*. In that report, he outlined the health needs of the state and offered recommendations related to the need for sanitary engineers, accurate vital statistics, inspectors, food and drug regulations, public health education, and routine preventive health care for all citizens. Despite its carefully written and documented recommendations, it was virtually ignored for almost 20 years.

In 1872, the Public Health Association was formed. Its membership focused on interdisciplinary efforts to improve health, and it developed a number of health promotion and illness prevention materials for the public. In the 1880s, based on work by Pasteur and Koch, public health moved from a narrow emphasis on environmental sanitation to a broader view that included bacteriology and immunology.

During the first decades of the 20th century, public health services began to expand. The Social Security Act of 1935 provided federal funding for support of local health departments and marked the first step toward the development of a nationwide network of public health agencies. Public health agencies were responsible for providing health care services to special populations such as urban poor, mothers, babies, Native Americans, and so on (Fairbanks & Wiese, 1998).

Today, public health agencies range in size and scope from local health departments to the Centers for Disease Control and Prevention (CDC) in Atlanta and focus on ensuring that the public health of the community is protected, promoted, and restored. To meet that goal, public health departments currently have a wide range of population-based goals (Box 2-2). To meet the goal of healthy communities, public health agencies have expanded their core functions to include community assessment, policy development, limited medical services (e.g., immunizations, well

---

BOX 2-2 PUBLIC HEALTH GOALS

The public health system is responsible for the following:

- Preventing epidemics and the spread of disease
- Reducing environmental hazards
- Preventing injuries
- Promoting healthy behaviors
- Providing disaster services
- Ensuring the quality and accessibility of health services

Source: Fairbanks & Wiese, 1998.

---

baby checkups, sexually transmitted disease treatment and surveillance), and program evaluation (Keck & Scutchfield, 1997).

Military Health Care

One of the most important fringe benefits of military life is a system of well-organized, comprehensive health care services provided at little or no extra cost (Williams & Torrens, 1999). Military personnel are also covered for service-connected problems for life. Health care is always available when needed, although personnel may have little choice of provider. Finally, the military health care system emphasizes prevention in addition to illness care.

Ambulatory care is provided in base and regional clinics. Simple hospital services, including short-term stays, are available through base dispensaries or sick bays on-board ships. More advanced care is available in regional hospitals. Well-trained medics, nurses, and physicians, in facilities owned by the U.S. government, provide most of the care. The system of care is well organized, integrated, and sophisticated.

Dependents and families of active duty personnel are covered by an extensive health insurance plan known as the Civilian Health and Medical Program of the Uniformed Services (CHAMPUS). This program allows dependents and families to obtain health care from private clinics and practitioners, local hospitals, and HMOs when similar services are not available from a nearby military base.

A second program, the Veterans Administration (VA) health care system, is a hospital and long-term care system that exists to care for retired and disabled military personnel. A hospital clinic system is available for complicated ambulatory services, but most simple ambulatory services are obtained through other systems of care. The VA health care system is probably the largest long-term care provider in the United States and is funded through an annual appropriation from Congress.

Health Care Reform

The current health care delivery system is undergoing dramatic changes. Advances in research and technology have resulted in the most sophisticated care in the world, and the most costly. At the same time, millions of Americans have limited or no access to health care services. When the uninsured do receive care, it is often in costly emergency rooms and after the condition has become unnecessarily complex. Uncompensated care is on the rise, and many providers are limiting their numbers or refusing to care for uninsured or underinsured clients. Clients without a regular provider are often forced to seek care in emergency rooms, where care is often fragmented, after conditions have become serious. Consequently, it is not surprising that health care reform draws many supporters.

Health care reform is not a new issue. Major legislative initiatives directed at health care reform were proposed seven times during the 20th century. The administrations of Roosevelt, Truman, Kennedy, Nixon, Ford, Carter, and Clinton all attempted to design some type of health care reform. Only the Social Security Act, supported by President Kennedy before his death, passed successfully.

Each time, the need for health care reform was based on the need to control health care costs while providing access to quality health care services to increasing numbers of people. Before 1993, the prototypes for Clinton's health care reform bill had been debated through three elections and defeated by two legislatures because of concerns about increased costs and governmental control.

A massive reorganization attempt was started during the first year of President Clinton's administration under the direction of Hillary Clinton. The plan, based on the concept of **managed** competition, would have guaranteed all individuals access to a basic benefit package of selected primary and preventive services while ensuring cost containment and quality care. The benefits would have been financed by employers, individuals, or (in the case of unemployed, indigent individuals) the government.

The failure of the Clinton plan is generally attributed to a number of structural, strategic, and tactical mistakes (Shi & Singh, 1998). The opposition was well organized, the President had differences within his own party, the plan was too complex, the drafters of the plans were politically naive, and the President's political base of support was narrow. The arguments that were most often heard were that the plan was too expensive and too confusing and taxpayers did not want to pay for health care for poor people. The failure of the plan left the United States and South Africa as the only major industrialized nations in the world without some form of universal insurance coverage. Although the reform package was never passed, health care changes did occur.

Current U.S. Health Care Delivery System

In response to a need for change, a number of new and innovative organizations are emerging, and many traditional components of

THE NATION'S HEALTH DOLLAR: 2000

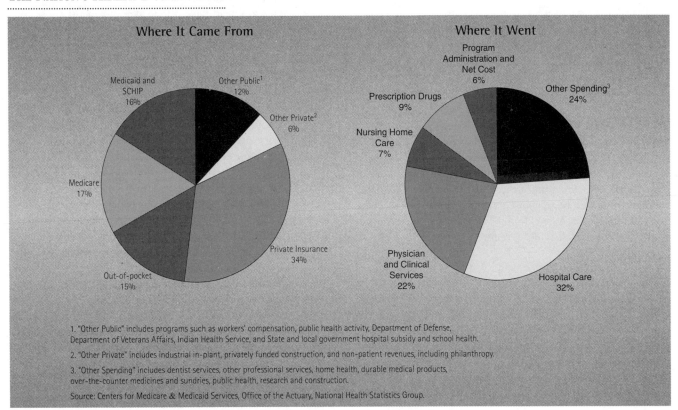

1. "Other Public" includes programs such as workers' compensation, public health activity, Department of Defense, Department of Veterans Affairs, Indian Health Service, and State and local government hospital subsidy and school health.

2. "Other Private" includes industrial in-plant, privately funded construction, and non-patient revenues, including philanthropy.

3. "Other Spending" includes dentist services, other professional services, home health, durable medical products, over-the-counter medicines and sundries, public health, research and construction.

Source: Centers for Medicare & Medicaid Services, Office of the Actuary, National Health Statistics Group.

the system are in transition. A single hospital operating independently or a physician in an individual practice is becoming unusual. Hospitals, physicians, clinics, and other providers have been forced into a variety of interrelated systems. Growth and consolidation of smaller providers into larger organizations, horizontal and vertical integration of services within organizations, changes from government-owned facilities to private nonprofit and for-profit facilities, and diversification of traditional health care services are occurring at an amazing rate (Lee & Estes, 1997). Large purchasers of medical services are demanding wholesale prices for services and even dictating terms. Insurance coverage is constantly changing and client choices have been reduced.

Levels of Care

Our health care delivery system provides six basic levels of care: preventive, primary, secondary, tertiary, restorative, and continuing or long-term health care. Preventive care includes education and screening programs. Primary care includes services directed at reducing the potential for a disease through continuous, coordinated, and comprehensive care. **Preventive care** and **primary care** generally take place in the primary care provider's office. Secondary care is concerned with early detection and treatment of acute illness and injury to prevent disability and mortality. Secondary care usually occurs in the primary care provider's office or in a community hospital. Tertiary care is concerned with slowing the progression of established disease, preventing further disability, and improving the individual's degree of functioning. Tertiary care sometimes occurs in community hospitals and sometimes in large medical referral centers.

Restorative care includes hospice and chronic care and occurs in hospitals or special rehabilitation facilities. Long-term care occurs in long-term care facilities such as nursing homes and hospice facilities. Historically, this country has focused most of its resources on tertiary care provided in large medical care institutions.

Health Care Providers

Registered nurses and physicians are the two largest groups of health-care professionals, but as health care has become more complex, the number and variety of providers has increased proportionately. The American Medical Association identified 29 allied health training occupations accredited through the association's Committee on Allied Health Education and Accreditation, as described in the following sections.

Physicians

Physicians make up the second largest group of health care professionals. A total of 463,870 physicians are currently practicing in the United States (U.S. Department of Labor, 1998). They diagnose and treat clients in an attempt to cure or improve their clients' conditions. Physicians may be allopathic (MDs) or osteopathic (DOs). In the past, most physicians were in solo practice. Today, many physicians are joining group practices or con-

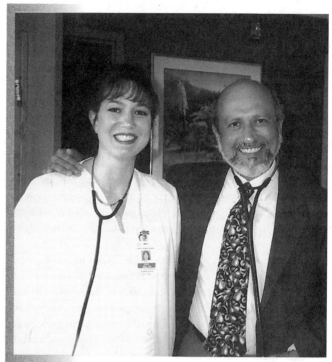

Physicians and nurses work in acute care settings in collaboration to improve health of clients.

tracting with health care corporations. By joining groups, physicians are able to spread their workload and their risks.

Nurses

Nurses make up the largest group of health care providers. There are 2,007,030 nurses employed in the United States (U.S. Department of Labor, 1998). Approximately 66% of all nurses work in hospitals, 10% work in community/public health, 8% in ambulatory care, and 7% in nursing homes and extended care (ANA, 1998). Nurses both deliver and coordinate health care for clients within settings and across sites, collaborate with physicians, and carry out day-to-day treatments and care.

More than 140,000 registered nurses have the education and credentials to call themselves advanced practice nurses (ANA, 1998). The category "advanced practice nurse" contains several different specialty areas, including clinical nurse specialists, nurse practitioners, nurse midwives, and nurse anesthetists. These advanced roles have grown over the years, usually in response to a physician shortage or a physician maldistribution. Each role has its own certification, rules and regulations, and state recognition process. Nurses are at an important juncture in the development of the profession. They currently have the opportunity to show their value in providing quality care at a reasonable cost while obtaining positive client outcomes.

Physician Assistants

The physician assistant (PA) role is new to the health care delivery system. The first training program for PAs was started at Duke University in 1965. In 1995, there were 80 PA programs in the United States (Fowkes & Mentink, 1997). Approximately 52,716 PAs are currently practicing in the United States (AAPA, 2002). The PA training program is typically the last 2 years of an undergraduate degree program and focuses on medical science and clinical skills. PAs work directly under the supervision and license of physicians, who are responsible for their performance. PAs can provide various medical services, such as history taking and physical examinations, minor medical diagnosis and care, follow-up care for acute and chronically ill clients, hospital rounds, surgical assistance, and so on.

Specialized Care Providers

Within the health care delivery system, certain groups of professionals provide focused care services. Examples are clinical psychologists, dentists, podiatrists, and optometrists. These professionals are licensed, although standards vary from state to state. They are usually addressed as "doctor," and in some areas, they may have prescriptive authority and hospital privileges (i.e., they can admit and treat clients in a hospital setting). Their education is in depth in their specialty areas at a master's level or higher.

Technicians/Therapists

Many people who provide ancillary health care services are called *technicians* or *technologists*; examples include the medical laboratory technician or medical technologist, the medical record technician, the x-ray technician, and the dietary technician. Other ancillary health care professionals are called *therapists*; examples are respiratory, occupational, physical, mental health, and speech therapists. Each is educated and licensed to provide a specific service and are educated at a bachelor's level or higher.

Other Providers

Other providers include professionals such as pharmacists and social workers. Pharmacists are specialists in the science of drugs and can make recommendations about drug therapy. Most programs preparing pharmacists are 5 years long and include an internship. Pharmacists make up the third largest group of health care providers.

Social workers are assuming increasingly important roles in today's health care delivery system. These professionals counsel clients and families, often directing them to various health care resources, and may also be involved in discharge planning.

Chaplains address the spiritual and emotional needs of clients and families from a nondenominational perspective.

Health Care Settings

Services may be provided in traditional settings, such as hospitals, nursing homes, physicians' offices, ambulatory clinics, and homes. Today, services may also be provided in less traditional settings such as shelters, shopping malls, pharmacies, schools, and job sites.

Acute Care Facilities

Hospitals, or acute care facilities, make up the largest component of the U.S. health care delivery system and account for 40% of the total personal health expenditures in 1991 (U.S. Department of Commerce, 1997). Hospitals include federal, state, and local government facilities and those owned by private organizations. Privately owned hospitals include voluntary (not for profit) or proprietary (for-profit) hospitals. Religious or charitable groups operate voluntary hospitals and may be independent or represent health maintenance organizations or cooperatives. Individuals, partnerships, or corporations own proprietary hospitals. The last decade has seen an increase in investor-owned hospital corporations; the stock of these large corporations is traded on the stock exchange.

In the current health care market, many hospitals have established home health agencies to help clients as they transition from the hospital to the home environment. Community health nurses can provide a critical link between hospital care and home care.

Short-Term Specialized Care Facilities

Some facilities, such as mental health centers, substance abuse facilities, and rehabilitation centers, offer very specialized services, and clients are admitted for a short-term stay to learn how to function with their disability(ies). Another example of a short-term facility is a respite care facility that provides temporary inpatient services for individuals who are usually cared for at home. The purpose of respite care is to offer relief to the informal caregiver, usually a family member.

Short-term facilities may be part of a network of coordinated services or a single independent entity. Centers may be staffed with a variety of health care providers, including physicians, nurses, and social workers.

Short-term specialized care facilities discharge clients into the community after short stays. Community health nurses could provide family and home assessments to determine the client's needs upon discharge and serve as a resource to clients once they are at home.

Long-Term Facilities

Long-term care may be defined as a wide range of social, personal, and health care services in addition to medical care. These services may include arranging social functions, exercise classes, and shopping trips to improve mental and physical function. The services might also include assistance with eating and bathing, arranging for therapy sessions, dental treatments, and visits by health care providers. These services may be needed by older individuals or individuals who have lost their ability to care for themselves through disease or injury. Long-term care focuses on maintaining as much function as possible and emphasizes activities of daily living (basic needs such as eating, dressing, bathing, and ambulating).

Most long-term care occurs in nursing homes but may also take place in a variety of other ways, such as assisted living facilities, hospice organizations, and home health care agencies. Community health nurses have excellent skills at assessing community resources and individualized client needs in each of these long-term care modalities.

Ambulatory Care Sites

Clients can receive care for conditions not requiring hospitalization at ambulatory care sites. Clinics and physicians' offices are the most common types of ambulatory sites, but this category would also include specially equipped trucks and buses that make scheduled stops in underserved areas. Many ambulatory care sites are affiliated with hospitals, but others operate independently. Traditional "walk-in" clinics have existed for many years and are often supported by government funding or charitable organizations. People often use the clinics in lieu of a personal physician. Centers may operate on an appointment or drop-in basis. Some clinics are specialized, such as family-planning clinics or those offering only women's health care services, and nurse practitioners or PAs often provide the care. Community health nurses can provide essential services in assisting clients while they try to meet their health care needs and stay at home.

Rural Health Centers

Rural health centers were developed as a result of federal funding and the need to provide care in rural, impoverished areas with few or no local physicians. Teams of residents and physicians from medical centers, along with nurse practitioners and PAs, often provide much of the care in rural health centers. These providers may cover several clinics on a rotating basis. Community health nurses play an important role in providing continuity in the care of clients who are often seen by many different providers.

Day-Care Centers

Day-care centers target specific client populations; for instance, many day-care centers serve elderly clients who cannot be left alone for long periods but who can carry out activities of daily living. Other day-care centers serve clients who are physically or mentally challenged, such as those with cerebral palsy or Down syndrome, or those who have chemical dependencies. These centers care for clients when family members are working and offer services such as meals, rehabilitation, and occupational therapy. Because the primary needs of these clients are in the area of personal care needs, nurses play an important role in these facilities.

Hospice

A hospice, run by public or private agencies, is designed to care for terminally ill clients and their families by providing noncuring, supportive, and palliative services. Many clients receiving these services have cancer, although conditions such as AIDS, multiple sclerosis, or end-stage renal disease may also require hospice care. Although nurses play the major role, a team approach, including physicians, therapists, volunteers, and clergy, is often used. Nursing activities focus on managing pain, treating symptoms, and preparing the client and family for death and bereavement.

Retirement Communities

In the last 20 years, the number of retirement communities in the United States has increased significantly. These communities take many forms, such as entire small towns, retirement subdivisions, apartments or condominiums, and continuing-care communities. Although the services vary, retirement communities usually provide a number of levels of care. In an arrangement known as assisted living, older people live independently but have care nearby if needed. A convalescent center may be associated with the facility, and services such as physical and occupational therapy may be provided. Other health care services such as dental care may also be available. Residents are guaranteed access to various health care services, and the financial responsibilities are spread over the entire community. Some of the fees, such as entry fees, must be prepaid and may be very expensive. Entry fees and monthly maintenance fees are often high, thus limiting access to some of these facilities to more affluent retirees.

Home Health Care

As prospective payment has forced clients to be discharged from hospitals earlier, home health care has become an essential part of the health care delivery system. Care is provided by registered nurses skilled in assessment and practical nurses and aides trained to provide safe client care. Agencies receiving Medicare reimbursement must be certified and must meet certain conditions and federal standards.

Technology, previously found only in hospitals, is now provided by home care agencies. Treatments may include such things as intravenous feedings and medications, ventilators, portable dialysis machines, and cardiac monitoring. Although home health care has changed dramatically, it is still the traditional practice area for community health nurses. In addition to skilled nursing care, home health care may include services such as physical, occupational, or speech therapy, homemaker services, and home-delivered meals.

Alternative Health Care

Alternative health care involves nontraditional treatments such as acupressure, acupuncture, therapeutic touch, herbal treatments, hypnosis and imagery, and homeopathy. Alternative health care treatments are now being studied to see how they can be used to support more traditional medical plans of care. Congress established the Office of Alternative Medicine in 1992 to sponsor research in this field to attempt to determine the value of nontraditional treatments on client outcomes. Nurses have often been supportive of and practiced alternative health care. Current research has recently focused more attention on some of

BOX 2-3 FACTORS AFFECTING HEALTH CARE DELIVERY

- Failure of competition as a strategy following deregulation of health care
- Emphasis on secondary and tertiary health care instead of prevention
- Increasing consumerism
- Escalating cost of technology
- Aging of the population
- Cost of defensive medicine
- Government regulation and administrative costs

these modalities and made them more acceptable in mainstream health care.

Issues Affecting Delivery of Health Care Services

Many issues have contributed to the growth, complexity, and expense of our health care delivery system such as deregulation, consumerism, technology, the graying of America, and our litigious society (Box 2-3). Local, state, and federal governments have attempted to address these issues at one time or another. However, short-term fixes for any one factor have had little impact on the overall problem.

Deregulation

In the last few years, the United States has experienced deregulation of health care. The result has been a proliferation of facilities and technology (e.g., computed tomography [CT] scans and magnetic resonance imaging [MRI]) in some urban areas, which has resulted in excess capacity and, in turn, increased expensive competition. This expense is passed along to the clients, and maldistribution of essential services is seen in underserved areas. Competition as a price control strategy has not helped control health care costs. Americans still want the specialist, the newest technology, the cutting edge treatment, and the hospital that looks like a four-star hotel. They simply hope their insurance will pay for it.

Focus on Secondary and Tertiary Health Care Services

Historically, we have allocated the majority of our resources to the care that occurs after the client has become critically ill. Vast amounts of money are spent on critical care units, technical procedures, and sophisticated surgical techniques, but little money has been spent preventing the illness in the first place. Education and screening services are often not reimbursed by third-party payers and are undervalued by busy providers. Although MCOs

often say they value what these preventive services can accomplish, the cost is often more than they wish to pay. As a result, managed care often makes decisions about which preventive services are the most valuable and ignore the rest.

Increasing Consumerism

Health care consumerism is the public's involvement in determining the type, quality, and cost of their health care. Today, consumers are reading, looking up information, subscribing to newsletters specializing in their health care problem, and attending support groups. They are better informed and are asserting their right to have an active part in decisions related to their care.

In the past, the poor often either went without health care or had to be satisfied with a lesser quality of care. However, values are changing, and equal access to health care is now viewed by many as a right.

Technological Advances

Advances made in technology have drastically changed health care and altered how physicians treat hospitalized clients. For example, the life expectancy of a client with diabetes has increased considerably. New chemotherapy treatments have extended cancer clients' lives and, in some cases, greatly increased the quality of their lives. Heart, lung, and liver transplants, unheard of three decades ago, have become commonplace. The latest antibiotic therapies ward off deadly diseases. All these advances have reduced hospital stays and allowed people to live longer.

The new technology is expensive, and some advances have raised formidable ethical questions. If you can extend the life of an 80-year-old man for a short time by putting him on a ventilator, should you do it? If you can keep a premature baby alive on life support but you know that the child has multiple irreparable problems that will result in incredible future costs, should you do it? For the cost of the care of one elderly man on a ventilator for several weeks, you could provide prenatal care to a large group of pregnant women.

Increasing Longevity of Americans

Americans born in 1995 can expect to live an average of 76 years (men 73, women 80), compared with 47.3 years for those born in 1900 (U.S. Department of Commerce, 1997). The fastest-growing age group is people 85 and older. Because the heaviest users of health services are the elderly, more emphasis is being placed on their needs, the need for services has increased, and gerontology has become a significant branch of medicine and nursing. Topics such as living wills and powers of attorney are becoming more widely discussed as people become concerned about their ability to maintain life, as well as the quality of that life.

Defensive Medicine and Government Regulation

The cost of defensive medicine and government regulations has been a major factor affecting the delivery of health care in this country. Physicians are often forced to pay extremely high costs for malpractice insurance and attorney fees when they are sued. As a result, some physicians have simply stopped offering high-risk services such as obstetrics or they have stopped providing care to indigent clients as a way to increase their profits.

Physicians also tend to practice defensive medicine by ordering more tests or more expensive treatments. In addition, increased government regulation has caused many physicians to increase their office staff, reduce their client load, or join health care systems where billing services are provided. The results of the increased costs are that the physician must become much more cost conscious and health care has become a business rather than a service.

Managed Care

Total integration of services is expected to be the future economic structure of the health care delivery system. Networks are expected to compete for clients by becoming more efficient, charging lower prices, offering a wider range of services, and ensuring quality care for a fixed cost for the individual. They will maintain a central database to ensure comprehensive care as the client moves from provider to provider within the system. These networks are called managed care.

Managed Care Delivery Systems

The concept of **managed care** encompasses a wide variety of organizational structures and is quickly becoming the dominant management strategy of our health care delivery system. By definition, *managed care* refers to a system that, for a set fee, assumes responsibility and accountability for the health of a population through the use of effective, responsible, and cost-efficient care.

> Managed care integrates the financing and delivery of health care services to covered individuals, most often by arrangements with providers. These systems offer packages of health care benefits, explicit standards for the selection of health care providers, formal programs for ongoing quality assurance and utilization review, significant financial incentives for its members to use providers, and procedures associated with the plan (ANA, 1998).

MCOs made their appearance in the 1970s and 1980s as the insurance industry was faced with employers starting to self-insure and health care costs that were soaring. The huge reserves of money that insurance companies had previously invested were being depleted. Strategically thinking insurance companies redefined their market and began developing managed care organizations. Today, managed care involves some 70 million Americans (Herzlinger, 1997).

The goals of managed care are achieved by keeping clients healthy and treating them in the lowest-cost setting using providers that have also agreed to provide services at a reduced rate. Under this system, primary care replaces the hospital as the center of care. The goal is to keep people out of the hospital, not to keep the hospital beds full. More treatments and care are provided in clinics and physicians' offices. Ambulatory clients go home to recover from surgery rather than upstairs for a leisurely recovery in a private room.

Managed care has transformed health care from a service industry into a competitive, market-driven business. The question now is whether health care decisions are made based on the client's needs or the need to show a profit for the organization and its stakeholders. Who is making the decisions about treatment options, and who is caring for the client with complex, multisystem problems? Is the cheapest treatment the best treatment? All of these questions are currently without answers.

If managed care looks at the long-term answer to client care questions, the answer lies in the premise that a healthy client is cheaper to care for that an unhealthy one. Therefore, preventive care is the only answer. If managed care looks at the short-term answer, then cheaper is better.

....

Nursing is managed care . . . Since the beginning of the century, expert nurses have been shepherding the care of acute and chronic patients in homes, clinics, and hospitals. Much has changed since those early days, but much has stayed the same. It's our job as nurses to develop a strong enough understanding of the needs of the system, of our own skills and strengths and those of our communities, that we can—collectively and individually—actively help craft the emerging system.

B. B Gray in Turner, 1999a, p. xii

....

Managed Care Organizations

The majority of MCOs can be categorized into three basic types: HMOs, PPOs, and POSs. **Capitation** refers to the amount of money that is paid to an HMO to cover the cost of health care for a group of clients. An agency or organization representing a group of individuals seeking health care contracts with a group of providers and pays a predetermined fee periodically, usually quarterly.

Health Maintenance Organizations

Federally recognized **health maintenance organizations (HMOs)** are prepaid health management plans that offer an organized system for providing a predetermined set of health care services in a geographic area to a voluntarily enrolled group of people for an established fee. This system combines traditional insurance and health care delivery in one organization and provides a wide range of services, including inpatient and outpatient hospital care, infertility and mental health services, therapeutic x-ray treatments, alcohol and drug addiction treatment, and physical therapy.

HMOs were first established in 1973 under a federal program. The number of HMOs in existence grew from 175 in 1976 to 556 in 1992 (U.S. Department of Commerce, 1997). Enrollment is voluntary; members have the option to select another plan. Because the fee paid by members is fixed annually, the organization tries to minimize costs. To do this, HMOs must place greater emphasis on health promotion and disease prevention. Some HMOs hire providers as employees and some contract with providers for services.

Preferred Provider Organizations

A **preferred provider organization (PPO)** is a type of managed care plan composed of a group of physicians, and possibly one or more hospitals, that get together and offer a prepaid health care plan to employers. In preferred provider arrangements, clients select their health care providers from the list of preferred providers and receive services at a discounted cost. If a consumer chooses to seek services from a provider who has not contracted with the plan, a substantial deductible fee is assessed or the service is not covered. In the future, PPOs are likely to grow larger with a wider range of providers.

Point-of-Service Plans

Point-of-service (POS) plans are also known as open-ended HMOs. POS plans provide a set of services that are covered under the established fee, but members are also given the choice of going out of the network for services. Members share in costs with the HMO if they decide to go out of the network for care.

Multilevel Integrated Systems

Integrated health care systems consist of a mix of many types of health care facilities and providers connected through different types of contractual arrangements. These complex systems will be able to supply a broad range of services, from in-house care to outpatient and from traditional to nontraditional care, within their own system (vertically integrated) or will arrange for the services to be provided by other systems (horizontally integrated). Primary care providers, hospitals, retirement communities, wellness centers, pharmacies, health food outlets, rehabilitation centers, counseling centers, and many other types of providers from a large geographical area will be connected and accessible to members.

The process of changing traditional systems into new, multilevel integrated systems is often complicated and emotionally difficult. The literature is full of words designed to make the transformation process sound less cold and calculating. The first term to appear was *downsizing*, which immediately was changed to *rightsizing*. This term simply refers to cutting the number of funded positions to decrease costs. *Redesigning* was the next term to make an appearance. Redesigning referred to the process of examining all job descriptions for equitable distribution of activities, role overlap, excess specialization, and waste. The next term to appear was *restructuring*. Restructuring refers to an assessment of the overall organizational structure in an attempt to improve productivity. Finally, *reengineering* refers to a comprehensive and often radical process to look at jobs and organizational structure

as a way to form new relationships, new visions, and improved functioning and productivity. Future integrated health care systems will be larger and more comprehensive. The opportunities for nurses will be many and varied (Box 2-4).

Patient Care Outcomes

The term *patient care outcomes* refers to the consequences of care that the client receives or does not receive. Outcome studies are becoming very popular in MCOs as a way to predict and provide effective client care. Outcome studies look for trends over time in client status and adverse events. Adverse patient care outcomes are occurrences that are not expected as a result of the client's disease process or treatment. Data obtained from client care studies are used as a basis for decisions, the development of policies and procedures, and changes in health care practice.

Improved patient care outcomes involve assessing individual clients' care and recovery as well as large data sets from across the country and world. Large national databases will be used in the future to provide predictive information on which to base treatments, types of care, lengths of care, and level of provider needed to achieve positive outcomes.

Health Politics and Policy

How did our health care delivery system become so expensive? Who should pay for the ever-increasing costs of health care and hospitalization? These questions have become the basis for untold numbers of legislative reports, articles, studies, and documentaries. The astronomical cost of some forms of treatment has made it impossible for the average client to pay personally for needed medical, surgical, and nursing services. Single illness episode bills well above $10,000 are no longer the exception. Many people rely on government interventions to help with soaring costs and inaccessible services.

Government Policy

Health insurance provides protection against the high cost of medical care and hospitalization arising from illness or injury. Most Americans look to their jobs for health insurance, but increasingly, insurance benefits are not available at work sites. The number of Americans who are uninsured or underinsured is increasing at an alarming rate. Americans have appealed to their legislators for help.

Government policy focuses on health care on several levels. Legislation establishes boards to govern the practice of health care professionals and health care agencies, establishes commissions to examine health care delivery and make recommendations, and sets guidelines for the payment of Medicare benefits. Medicare guidelines affect the entire health care industry because the government is the third-party payer for more than 45% of all expenditures in health care (HFCA, 2002).

The publication of *Healthy People 2010*, based on the progress made under *Healthy People 2000* goals, again moves forward the agenda of disease prevention and health promotion for all citizens (APHA, 1998). The goals for the year 2010 fall into two categories: increasing the years of healthy life and reducing health disparities. Before the publication of *Healthy People 2000* and *2010*, these goals were not central in health legislation. However, in a time of escalating fiscal austerity, these goals make increasing sense. Keeping people well is much less costly than trying to cure or rehabilitate them.

Finally, there have been many debates about whether the United States should adopt a national health insurance plan or support market competition. Under a national plan, taxpayers would pay the government for the coverage, much as insurance companies currently collect funds from subscribers, and everyone would be covered at a predetermined basic level of services. The disadvantage is that government plans rarely operate very efficiently, and many people believe that it is inappropriate for government to meddle in individuals' health care decisions.

Market competition has been promoted as another way to keep health care costs at a reasonable level while ensuring quality care. Under this system, the government would allow a rivalry between health care providers for the purpose of attracting clients. However, an unequal distribution of the most ill clients might keep corporations from wanting to insure the very clients who need care the most.

Public Opinion and Special Interest Groups

Public opinion expressed through special interest groups is very influential in the development of public policy. Many special interest groups, such as the American Hospital Association, the American Medical Association, and the American Insurance Association, spend huge amounts of time and money providing legislators with information on which to base health care decisions. Many legislators lack an in-depth understanding of health care issues. As a result, information provided by special interest groups often serves as a basis for health care decisions. When that happens, decisions may fail to reflect the best interests of the majority.

Nursing and Health Care Policy

As the largest health care provider group, it is important for nurses to be both a visible and vocal advocate for quality health care. To meet that important goal, the American Nurses Association (ANA) has worked tirelessly over the years to develop an effective special interest group infrastructure. In response to the health care reform issue, the ANA formulated a position paper that states that the U.S. health care system needs restructuring, wellness promotion must become our emphasis, and universal access to health care services must be developed.

The ANA has been politically active in several other areas, including health care rationing. With limited resources, the question of health care rationing must be addressed. Those with adequate insurance worry about restrictions, and the uninsured or underinsured worry that they will be excluded. Rationing can mean limiting access to care or limiting contact to the more expensive providers.

RESEARCH BRIEF

Blegen, M., Goode, C., & Reed. L. (1998). Nurse staffing and patient outcomes. Nursing Research, 47(1), 43–50.

Hospitals today are faced with critical staff mix decisions. However, few studies have examined the effects of decreased numbers of staff registered nurses (RNs) on patient care outcomes. The purpose of this study was to examine the relationships among total hours of nursing care, registered nurse skill mix, and adverse patient care outcomes. Adverse outcomes were defined as unit rates of medication errors, client falls, skin breakdown, client and family complaints, infections, and deaths. Study sites included 42 inpatient units. The correlation among the variables were determined after controlling for client acuity.

Units with higher average client acuity had lower rates of medication errors and client falls but higher rates of the other adverse outcomes. With average client acuity on the unit controlled, the proportion of hours of care delivered by RNs was inversely related to the unit rates of medication errors, decubiti, and client complaints. Total hours of care by other nursing personnel were directly related to increased rates of decubiti, complaints, and mortality. An unexpected finding was that the relationship between the RN proportion of care was curvilinear; as the RN proportion increased, rates of adverse outcomes decreased up to 87.5%. Above that level, as RN proportion of care increased, the adverse outcome rates also increased. This finding was likely related to client acuity. The conclusion of the study was that the higher the RN skill mix, the lower the incidence of adverse occurrences on the client care unit.

Through the years, the ANA and state organizations have continued to support legislation that ensures basic health care services for everyone. To influence policy, nurses need to vote and be politically active in their states and know what bills are being considered. To be politically active, you can work on someone's campaign, run for political office, support candidates financially, or simply stay in contact with elected state and federal officials and provide them with information when needed.

New Nursing Opportunities

As health care changes, the practice of nursing must also change. Nurses must stay knowledgeable about health care trends to

BOX 2-4 NEW OPPORTUNITIES AND THE ACCOMPANYING SKILLS

Nurses can position themselves to accept the emerging roles in managed care systems. To assist in this process, the following seven areas of opportunity for nurses in a managed care environment and the skills needed to take on these new roles have been identified.

CONSUMER ADVOCACY

- Use of decision trees/tools
- Projection of statistical probabilities
- Negotiation skills
- Group interaction and facilitation
- Patient teaching using new media
- Understanding of principles of ethics

CHANGE AGENT

- Understand chaos theory/change theory
- Leadership skills vs. management skills
- Self-managed team abilities
- Grasp of organizational behavior and development theory

INDIVIDUAL GROWTH

- Self-empowerment
- Professional image
- New self-accountability for life-long learning and relevancy in a changing environment
- Computer literacy
- Networking ability
- Business-related skills: verbal and written presentation skills, communication technology familiarity, publication/media production, economics/finance forecasting skills
- Sensitivity to cost and quality, total quality management process, benchmarking, utilization management cost analysis, data integrity, tracking and manipulation, "best practices"

COMMUNITY-BASED CARE

- Cultural competence
- Assessment
- Population-focused care
- Innovative approaches to enhancing health of a community
- Epidemiology and environmental health
- Understanding concepts of risk

INFORMATION SYSTEMS

- Computer-related skills
- Informatics
- Decision support systems
- Ability to access and process data

ENTREPRENEURS/INTRAPRENEURS

- Understanding of contracts
- Abilities in innovative program development
- Marketing/selling
- Program budgeting
- Business plan development
- Problem identification and costing of solutions

PUBLIC HEALTH POLICY AND REGULATORY BODIES

- Legislative skills
- Knowledge of civics
- Understanding of administrative, legislative, and judicial roles of government
- Knowledge of key regulatory bodies related to nursing and health care
- Basic skill in legal interpretation and drafting

Source: ANA, 1996, p. 19.

---

make decisions about future careers. Those trends include growth in the health care workforce, economics as a driving force, changing demographics of the United States, transformation of individual providers into multilevel corporations with physicians becoming employees, the philosophical move from "everything for a few" to "an adequate amount for many," and the increased importance of ambulatory care and home health care (Huston & Fox, 1998). Some of the nursing roles related to these trends are discussed next. However, many future roles are yet to be created.

Advanced Practice Nurses

Advanced practice nursing is not a new category of nurses, but many of the traditional roles are changing. Nurse practitioners are moving into specialized areas such as geriatrics, acute care, and correction facilities health care. Clinical nurse specialists are becoming experts in case management, genetics, and comprehensive cancer care. Nurse anesthetists and nurse midwives are managing clients with specialized needs. Advanced practice nurses are prepared to work *with* physicians, not *for* them. As specialties develop, nurses are finding ways to become experts in those areas, and as more emphasis is placed on controlling health care costs, more providers will look to advanced practice nurses as providers of effective, quality, lower-cost care.

Entrepreneurs

In the future, more nurses than ever before will own nursing businesses. In areas like home health, health care management, insurance evaluation, nursing clinics, environmental evaluation, workplace health care, caregiver support, program evaluation, and respite care, the opportunities are endless. Nurses will be in a position to contract with larger systems for consulting services and the application of specialized knowledge and skills.

Data Management

Public and private agencies are looking for nurses who are skilled at creating and managing large databases containing client information. This field is known as *informatics*. Every health care organization is struggling with the need to maintain information in a safe but easily accessed manner. Data must be available for evaluation and decision making. Nurses with an understanding of client care data coupled with a working knowledge of computers, the workings of databases, and the use of evaluative statistics will be in the perfect position to fill these critical slots.

Research

We can no longer make decisions on the basis of what we have done before or what we think will work. Decisions must be based on data that can be seen, measured, and reproduced as needed, integrated with sound clinical practice experience. We are moving into an age of evidence-based client care. Consequently, client care research is more important today than at any time in the past. Nurse researchers try to develop an understanding of essential client care issues on which to base practice. They may be employees of an organization or working on a research project funded by the government or other organizations. Their work provides the structure for future practice that will "identify and apply the most efficacious interventions to maximize the quality and quantity of life for individual clients" (Sackett et al., 1997).

• •

Our ancestors tithed in the hope of life after death; we hope for more and better life before death.

Robert G. Evans

• •

• •

I don't know the key to success, but the key to failure is trying to please everybody.

Bill Cosby

• •

CONCLUSION

Some critics suggest that our health care system, which is supposed to guarantee access, innovation, and quality care, has instead become a system in crisis. A crisis exists in several areas: cost, availability, equity, efficiency, and responsiveness to public needs. This chapter contains a discussion of the history of our health care delivery system and descriptions of the changing components of that system. New roles for nursing are emerging as our health care system moves from one that was measured by the cost of its components to a system measured by the effectiveness of the care provided by its components.

CASE STUDY

A pregnant woman with severe epilepsy has presented to the health department from a local obstetrical practice. She had been working part-time at a local grocer until her seizures became unmanageable, and she is no longer employed. The client has been referred to the health department so that she can qualify for state funds for high-risk maternity care. The client's husband works for a local manufacturing company and has HMO coverage for both himself and his wife through a company-sponsored managed care plan. The deductible and co-payment are more than the couple can afford to pay, and they would like to find other resources to pay for the additional services needed to manage the epilepsy. The public health nurse checks with the state high-risk maternity care program and finds that the couple exceeds the income criteria and most likely will not qualify.

1. What are possible health and economic consequences if the client's health is not managed appropriately during pregnancy?

2. What system problems can you identify from the situation that result in ethical issues of treatment and care?

3. Who is responsible for seeing that this client receives appropriate care at an affordable cost?

CRITICAL THINKING ACTIVITIES

1. You are a 28-year-old single mother with three children. You are having pain in your stomach and trouble sleeping. You have no money and no insurance. How will you get someone to help you? What will you do if you need medication?

2. You are a 22-year-old single parent with two children ages 1 and 3. Your mother is unemployed and watches the children while you work. Your job does not provide you with insurance. Your pay is too high to allow you to be eligible for Medicaid and too low to allow you to afford insurance. What types of services do you need from the Health Department?

3. In a world of limited resources, developing equitable health policies involves many difficult decisions. How would you answer the following questions?

   - Should an 85-year-old man with debilitating emphysema be placed on a respirator?

   - Should a 78-year-old woman with breast cancer be put on chemotherapy?

   - Should major health insurance plans reimburse for experimental treatments?

   - Should an insurance plan be required to pay for a liver transplant for an alcoholic?

   - Should a baby with multiple incurable birth defects be placed in a neonatal intensive care unit?

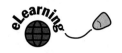 Explore Community Health Nursing on the web! To learn more about the topics in this chapter, access your exclusive web site: http://communitynursing.jbpub.com

REFERENCES

American Academy of Physician Assistants. (2002). *2001 AAPA Physician Assistant Census Report.* www.aapa.org

American Nurses Association (ANA). (1998). Managed care: Challenges and opportunities for nursing. *Nursing facts.* www.nursingworld.org/readroom/fsmgdcar.htm

Children's Defense Fund. (1998). *Children's Defense Fund: Healthy start FAQs.* www.childrensdefense.org/facts_america98.html

American Public Health Association (APHA). (1998). *Healthy people 2010 objectives.* Washington, DC: Author.

Fairbanks, J., & Wiese, W. H. (1998). *The public health primer.* Thousand Oaks, CA: Sage Publications.

Feldstein, P. (1999). *Health care economics.* Albany, NY: Delmar Publishing.

Fowkes, V. K., & Mentink, J. (1997). Nurses and physician assistants: Issues and challenges. In J. C. McCloskey & H. K. Grace (Eds.), *Current issues in nursing.* St. Louis: Mosby.

Herzlinger, R. (1997). *Market driven health care: Who wins, who loses in the transformation of America's largest service industry.* Redwood City, CA: Addison-Wesley.

Health Care Financing Agency (HCFA). (2002). *National health expenditure projections: 2001–2011.* www.hcfa.gov/stats/NHE-Proj/proj2001/default.htm

Health Care Financing Agency (HCFA). (1998). *National health expenditures projections: 1998–2008.* www.hcfa.gov/stats/nhe%2Dproj/proj1998/hilites.htm

Huston, C., & Fox, S. (1998). The changing health care market: Implications for nursing education in the coming decade. *Nursing Outlook, 46,* 109–114.

Johnson, C., & Broder, D. (1996). *The system: The American way of politics at the breaking point.* Boston: Little, Brown.

Keck, C. W., & Scutchfield, F. D. (1997). *Principles of public health practice.* Albany, NY: Delmar Publishers.

Lee, P. R., & Estes, C. L. (1997). *The nation's health* (5th ed.). Sudbury, MA: Jones and Bartlett.

Sackett, D. L., Rosenbergm W. C., Grant, J. A., Haynes, R. B., & Richardson, W. S. (1997). Evidence-based medicine: What is it and what it isn't. It's about integrating individual clinical expertise and the best external evidence. In P. R. Lee & C. L. Estes (Eds.), *The nation's health* (5th ed.). Sudbury, MA: Jones and Bartlett.

Salmon, M. (1997). Nursing practice in a political era. In J. C. McCloskey & H. K. Grace (Eds.), *Current issues in nursing.* St. Louis: Mosby.

Shi, L., & Singh, D. (1998). *Delivering health care in America: A systems approach.* Gaithersburg, MD: Aspen Publishers.

U.S. Bureau of the Census. (1995). Health insurance coverage by selected characteristics. *Annual demographic survey.* http://ferret.bls.census.gov/macro/031996/health/2_000.htm

U.S. Department of Commerce. (1997). *National health expenditures.* www.hcfa.gov/stats.nhe%2Doact/nhe.htm

U.S. Department of Labor. (1998). *1997 National employment and wage estimates.* http://stats.bls.gov/oes/national/oes_prof.htm

U.S. Health and Human Services. (1999). *National health expenditures projections: 1998–2008.* www.hcfa.gov/stats/nhe%2Doact/nhe.htm

U.S. National Center for Health Statistics. (1997). *National health statistics.* www.cdc.gov/nchswww/default.htm

U.S. National Center for Health Statistics. (1998). *National health statistics.* www.cdc.gov/nchswww/default.htm

Williams, S., & Torrens, P. (1999). *Introduction to health services.* Albany, NY: Delmar Publishers.

Chapter 3
Epidemiology of Health and Illness
Gail A. Harkness

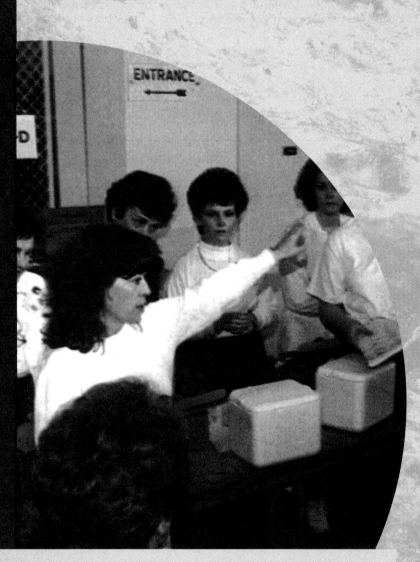

To understand the changes that can occur in the health of individuals or in various populations, it is necessary to identify the relationships between the biological and psychosocial phenomena that underlie health and illness. Epidemiology, the basic science of preventive medicine, has provided a process for understanding these relationships by studying different populations of people in various situations. Through study of health problems as they occur in groups or populations, many characteristics of specific illnesses or disabilities can be identified that may not be evident in the study of individuals alone.

QUESTIONS TO CONSIDER

After reading this chapter, answer the following questions:

1. What is the contribution of epidemiology to public health?
2. How do nurses use the principles of epidemiology?
3. How is the epidemiological process related to nursing and research?
4. What is the usefulness of rates in community health nursing?
5. What is the natural history of disease and levels of prevention?
6. What are *incidence* and *prevalence*?
7. What are the characteristics of a population by person, place, and time?
8. What are the characteristics of the four types of epidemiological research studies?
9. How can epidemiological research be used in community health nursing?

KEY TERMS

Adjusted rates
Case–control
Cross-sectional
Crude rates
Epidemic
Epidemic curve
Epidemiological triad
Incidence
Intervention
Morbidity
Mortality

Period prevalence
Point prevalence
Primary prevention
Prospective
Rate
Retrospective
Risk factors
Secondary prevention
Specific rates
Tertiary prevention

INDIVIDUAL WITHIN THE FRAMEWORK OF LIFE.

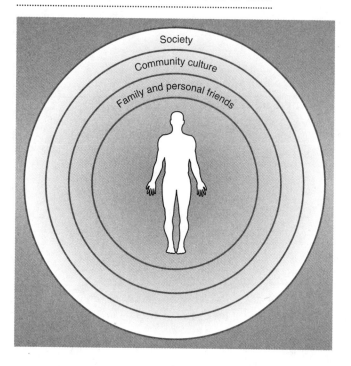

Health care for all individuals should be planned within the framework of family and personal friends, the immediate community culture where they live, and the larger world society. Any individual's health care needs cannot be completely or correctly defined unless these broader factors are analyzed and appropriately incorporated into a plan of care. Just as information must be collected about individuals in assessing health problems, data must be collected about groups, communities, and populations to assess the broader health needs of society.

For instance, the association between lung cancer and smoking might not have been ascertained by studying individual cases of lung cancer. Many smokers never develop lung cancer, and some nonsmokers do develop lung cancer. However, in 1950, Doll and Hill contrasted a group of lung cancer patients with a group of people who did not develop lung cancer. They clearly demonstrated that more people with lung cancer had smoked cigarettes than those people without the disease. This was substantiated by further research, and cigarette smoking is now considered a primary risk factor for lung cancer. This information has been the basis for national campaigns to decrease smoking among Americans. This example demonstrates the value of identifying certain characteristics or behaviors that increase risk of health problems even if the pathophysiology is not precisely known. Health care personnel can implement preventive health measures for both individuals and groups of people who are at high risk even if the causative factors are not known.

Epidemiology Defined

Epidemiology is the study of the distribution and the determinants of states of health and illness in human populations (Harkness, 1995). *Distribution* refers to the frequency of occurrence of states of health and illness; *determinants* refers to agents or factors that contribute to the cause of various states of health and illness. The word *epidemiology* is derived from the Greek word meaning epidemic: *epi*, upon; *demos*, people; and *logos*, treatise. The ultimate goal of epidemiology is to use the information obtained from the study of the distribution and determinants of states of health and illness to prevent or limit the consequences of illness and disability in humans and maximize their state of health. Although the influence of the environment on the occurrence of disease and the contagious nature of many diseases can be traced to Hippocrates, the techniques of modern epidemiological investigation were first developed in the mid-19th century.

William Farr, a physician from London, established the field of medical statistics. In 1839, he was appointed to the Office of the Registrar General for England and Wales. He set up a system for compilation of the numbers and causes of deaths and compared the deaths of workers in different occupations, the difference in mortality between men and women, and the effect of imprisonment on the frequency of death. He realized that studying the data from populations of people would provide much more information about human disease than studying individual cases (Humphreys, 1885).

During the mid-19th century, infectious diseases such as cholera and plague were still killing much of the population of Europe. The primary goal then was to limit the spread of these devastating diseases and prevent their recurrence. John Snow, another British physician, investigated the epidemic of cholera that took place from 1848 to 1854. His classic investigation of the outbreak clearly established the rate as a fundamental tool of epidemiology. Snow investigated cholera outbreaks associated with water supplied from two different water companies. He demonstrated statistically that cholera was associated with the water company that obtained their water from an area of the Thames River that was heavily polluted with sewage, and not with the company that obtained its water further upstream (Snow, 1855).

Florence Nightingale was a contemporary of Farr and Snow and was significantly influenced by their statistical methods. Nightingale is probably best known for her work at the British military hospital in Scutari. British and French troops had invaded the Crimea on the north coast of the Black Sea, supporting Turkey in its dispute with Russia. She and her 38 nurses found the conditions appalling. Buildings were infested with rats and fleas, streams of sewage flowed under the buildings, linens were filthy, and supplies were scarce. They initiated sanitary reforms, keeping records of illness and deaths. The figure on the following page shows a polar-area diagram designed by Nightingale to dramatize the needless deaths that occurred during the war and the effect of her reforms (Aiken, 1988; Cohen, 1984).

As a result of these early investigations, epidemiology traditionally has been associated with infectious diseases, with a focus

NIGHTINGALE'S POLAR-AREA DIAGRAM.

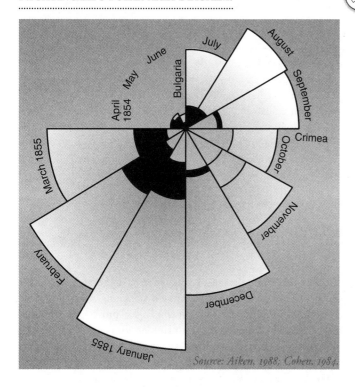

Source: Aiken, 1988; Cohen, 1984.

THE EPIDEMIOLOGICAL TRIAD.

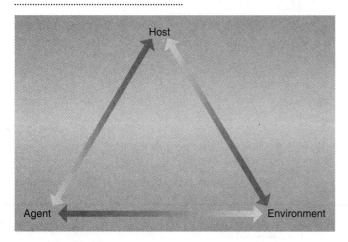

FYI

Florence Nightingale has been called one of the first epidemiologists as a result of her use of statistics to document health care needs.

epidemiological trial still remains a fundamental conceptual framework for the contemporary study of health problems.

Epidemiology can be considered both as a *methodology* used to study health-related conditions and as a *body of knowledge* that results from research into a specific health-related condition (Harkness, 1995). Using epidemiological research methodology to investigate health problems leads to the accumulation of a body of knowledge about that particular problem. (Epidemiological research methods are discussed later in the chapter.) Practitioners then can use this body of knowledge in their clinical decision making and in developing health services. For example, epidemiological research has associated hypertension, obesity, and smoking with increased incidence of heart disease. These are all potentially modifiable risk factors that often are associated with lifestyle and behavior choices. Nurses and other health professionals can use this information when assessing individual patients and helping them make choices about intervention techniques that may reduce their risk of heart disease. Also, community health nurses may initiate programs to identify hypertension at an early stage, to stop smoking, or to decrease weight in an attempt to decrease the risk of heart disease for the population as a whole.

Scope of Epidemiology

The scope of epidemiology has been expanded and therefore changed in recent years. Not only are the distribution and determinants of illness and disease investigated, but variables that contribute to the maintenance of health are also studied. The evolving changes in demographic characteristics, the patterns of disease, methods of control and prevention of health problems, and the need for maintaining wellness have contributed to this shift in the scope of epidemiology. *Healthy People 2010* uses determinants of health to derive the objectives for the nation. The depth of topics covered by the objectives reflect the diversity of critical influences that determine the health of persons who live in communities. Improved public health services, increased life expectancy, increased frequency of noninfectious disease and chronic degenerative conditions, and advances in technology are continually changing the health needs of society. (See Table 3-1 for a comparison of the leading causes of death in the United

on the **epidemiological triad**: agent, host, and environment. This model is based on the belief that health status is multifactorial, determined by the interaction of many agent, host, and environment characteristics, and not by any single factor. For example, factors influencing the development of a heart attack include heredity, high cholesterol levels, dietary excess, cigarette smoking, emotional stress, and many other factors. No one factor is considered a causative factor for the illness. Therefore, the

TABLE 3-1   COMPARISON OF THE LEADING CAUSES OF DEATH IN THE UNITED STATES BETWEEN 1900 AND 1996

1900	1996
1. Major cardiovascular-renal diseases	1. Diseases of the heart
2. Influenza and pneumonia	2. Malignant neoplasms
3. Tuberculosis	3. Cardiovascular accidents
4. Gastritis, duodenitis, enteritis, cholitis	4. Chronic obstructive pulmonary disease
5. Accidents	5. Accidents
6. Malignant neoplasms	6. Pneumonia and influenza
7. Diphtheria	7. Diabetes mellitus
8. Typhoid and paratyphoid fever	8. Other infections and parasitic diseases
9. Measles	9. Suicide
10. Cirrhosis of the liver	10. Chronic liver disease and cirrhosis

Bureau of the Census, 1998, p 100.

States over time.) Provision of present and future health care depends on (1) identifying health problems and needs, (2) collecting and analyzing data to identify factors that influence those health problems or needs, and (3) planning, implementing, and evaluating methods for prevention and control. These steps form the basis of the epidemiological process.

The Epidemiological, Research, and Nursing Processes

The epidemiological process, the research process, and the nursing process have all evolved from steps in the problem-solving process. All three processes have similar basic components: defining the problem, gathering data, analyzing the data, and evaluating the results. The research process focuses on obtaining new knowledge about a health condition. The epidemiological process and the nursing process are more focused on planning for control, for prevention, or for intervention activities that will help mediate a health condition (Table 3-2). The cyclical nature of the epidemiological process is illustrated in the figure on the following page.

Natural History of Disease

In 1958, Leavell and Clark, two public health physicians, championed the cause of preventive medicine by emphasizing that prevention is required at every phase of the disease

TABLE 3-2   SIMILARITIES BETWEEN THE EPIDEMIOLOGICAL PROCESS, THE RESEARCH PROCESS, AND THE NURSING PROCESS

EPIDEMIOLOGICAL PROCESS	RESEARCH PROCESS	NURSING PROCESS
Define problem	Define problem	**Assessment:**
Gather information from reliable sources	Review literature	Establish patient database
Describe problem by person, place, time	Conceptualize problem	
Formulate tentative hypothesis	Define variables	**Diagnosis:**
	Identify methodology	Interpret data
Analyze descriptive data to test hypothesis		Identify health care needs
		Select goals of care
Plan for control of the problem		**Planning:**
		Select process for achieving goals
Implement control plan	Collect data	**Implementation:**
		Initiate and complete actions to achieve goals
Evaluate control plan	Analyze data	**Evaluation:**
Prepare appropriate report	Publish report	Determine extent of goal achievement
Conduct further research	Conduct further research	

process. They called the course of any disease process as it develops in humans the "natural history of the disease" (see the figure on p. 52). During the prepathogenesis period, there are factors within individuals and their environments that may predispose or precipitate the disease. The initial interactions among agent, host, and environment occur during this period. For example, an individual may have an inherited predisposition to high cholesterol levels and may be obese, a smoker, and under excessive pressure at work in the prepathogenesis period. The period of pathogenesis begins when the host begins to respond with biological, psychological, or other changes. It is manifested by signs and symptoms that continue until the condition is resolved by recovery, disability, or death. If this individual is not able to modify the factors that predispose to disease, he or she is at high risk for a heart attack.

Leavell and Clark also identified levels of prevention for the prepathogenesis and pathogenesis periods: primary prevention, secondary prevention, and tertiary prevention.

Primary prevention includes activities that prevent a disease from becoming established and occurs during the prepathogenesis period. These activities include both health promotion activities and specific protection activities such as immunizations and protection from hazards and hygiene. Because no symptoms of illness exist, primary prevention programs are directed toward either the general healthy population or toward a group of healthy people who are known to be at high risk for a particular disease, illness, or injury. For example, public health organizations and voluntary agencies have emphasized the importance of regular exercise, a low-fat diet, and smoking cessation programs in an attempt to prevent coronary artery disease.

Secondary prevention includes activities designed to detect disease and provide early treatment. These activities involve early diagnosis, prompt treatment, and measures to limit disability. Screening programs for high cholesterol is an example of secondary prevention of coronary artery disease. If high levels are found, early treatment can be effective in lowering cholesterol levels.

Tertiary prevention includes the treatment, care, and rehabilitation of people with acute and chronic illness to achieve their maximum potential. If coronary artery disease is not prevented, a myocardial infarction may occur. A coronary artery bypass graft may be required, followed by a cardiac rehabilitation program.

Both secondary and tertiary prevention occur during the pathogenesis period. However, tertiary prevention is initiated after irreversible changes have resulted from the disease process. A detailed outline of the natural history can be created for any illness, and it becomes a helpful guideline for health professionals at all three levels of prevention.

Descriptive Epidemiology

Descriptive epidemiology focuses on the frequency and distribution of states of health within a population. By describing characteristics of groups of people who have or do not have certain illnesses, factors that are associated primarily with the people who have the illness can be identified. These are called **risk factors**. Generally, descriptive data can tell us what kind of people are at risk of developing certain health problems; what diseases, disabilities, or needs they have; how these problems are distributed in the community; who goes where for different kinds of

MODEL OF THE EPIDEMIOLOGICAL PROCESS.

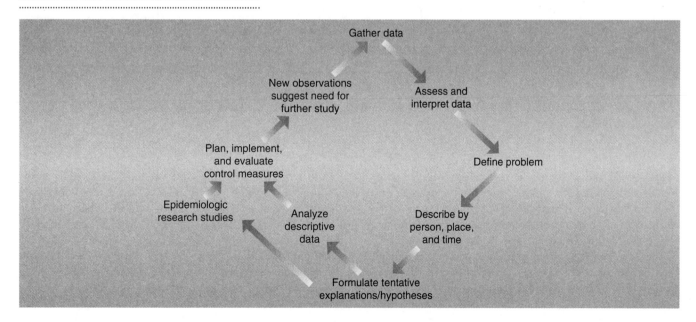

LEVELS OF APPLICATION OF PREVENTIVE MEASURES IN THE NATURAL HISTORY OF DISEASE.

The natural history of any disease of man		
Interrelations of agent, host, and environmental factors → Production of *stimulus* →	Reaction of the *host* to the *stimulus* — Early pathogenesis → Discernible early lesions → Advanced disease → Convalescence →	
Prepathogenesis period	Period of pathogenesis	

Health promotion	**Specific protection**	**Early diagnosis and prompt treatment**	**Disability limitation**	**Rehabilitation**
Health education	Use of specific immunizations	Case-finding measures, individual and mass	Adequate treatment to arrest the disease process and to prevent further complications and sequelae	Provision of hospital and community facilities for retraining and education for maximum use of remaining capacities
Good standard of nutrition adjusted to developmental phases of life	Attention to personal hygiene	Screening surveys		
Attention to personality development	Use of environmental sanitation	Selective examinations	Provision of facilities to limit disability and to prevent death	Education of the public and industry to utilize the rehabilitated
Provision of adequate housing, recreation, and agreeable working conditions	Protection against occupational hazards	*Objectives:* To cure and prevent disease processes		
	Protection from accidents	To prevent the spread of communicable diseases		As full employment as possible
Marriage counseling and sex education	Use of specific nutrients	To prevent complications and sequelae		Selective placement
Genetics	Protection from carcinogens	To shorten period of disability		Work therapy in hospitals
Periodic selective examinations	Avoidance of allergens			Use of sheltered colony
Primary prevention		Secondary prevention		Tertiary prevention
Levels of application of preventive measures				

Source: Leavell & Clark, 1965.

health service; and who provides the health services they need. Health professionals then use this information to set priorities for health programs, to find ways of using health resources more effectively, to plan strategies to meet emerging health care needs, and to evaluate the effectiveness of measures used to control or prevent specific disorders. However, it is important to emphasize here that descriptive epidemiology can be used to study states of wellness. For example, identifying factors such as diet and exer-

cise that are associated with healthy, community-dwelling elderly people older than 85 years of age can provide the information necessary to enhance wellness in other elderly populations.

Use of Rates
All epidemiological investigations depend on the ability to quantify the occurrence of a health problem. The most basic measure

RESEARCH BRIEF

Cook, R. L., Royce, R. A., Thomas, J. C., & Hanusa, B. H. (1999). What's driving an epidemic? The spread of syphilis along an interstate highway in rural North Carolina. American Journal of Public Health, 89(3), 369–373.

The purpose of this research study was to determine whether county syphilis rates were increased along I-95 in North Carolina during a recent epidemic. Data on syphilis cases, demographics, drug activity, and highways were used to conduct a longitudinal study of North Carolina counties from 1985 to 1994. Crude and adjusted incidence rates were calculated and adjusted for sociodemographic factors and drug use. A cross-sectional design was used. Ten-year syphilis rates in the I-95 counties greatly exceeded rates in non–I-95 counties: 38 versus 16 cases per 100,000 persons) and remained high even after adjustment for race, age, sex, poverty, urban area designation, and drug activity. Syphilis rates were stable until 1989, but increased sharply in I-95 counties after 1989. Increased drug activity in I-95 counties preceded the rise in syphilis rates. The authors offer possible explanations for these results: spread of syphilis through contact between truck drivers and local sex workers at truck stops and rest stops; cocaine distribution; and the use of crack cocaine, which increases risky behaviors such as higher numbers of sexual partners and less frequent condom use, owing in part to the exchange of sex for drugs. Although the authors do not state specifically which factors were responsible for the increase in syphilis rates along I-95, cocaine distribution along the highway seems the most likely explanation. Further study is recommended to determine the specific associations along I-95. A better understanding of the cause of the association has public health implications where more resources and interventions can be focused.

of frequency is to count the number of affected individuals. However, this may be misleading. The number of people in the population who could have been affected, but were not, should be taken into consideration. For example, five people in a community may have developed human immunodeficiency virus/acquired immunodeficiency syndrome (HIV/AIDS). The implications of this event would be interpreted very differently if those people came from a community of 500 people versus a community of 100,000 people. Also, the time frame in which the problem has occurred is important. The use of ratios, proportions, and rates provide a more valid description of health problems.

A *ratio* is a fraction that obtained by dividing one quantity by another quantity; it represents the relationship between the two numbers. The numerator is not included in the denominator. For example, the number of boys on a pediatric unit could be contrasted with the number of girls on the same unit using a ratio: 10 boys and 5 girls would result in a 2:1 ratio of boys to girls. A *proportion* is a type of ratio that includes the quantity in the numerator as a part of the denominator. Therefore, it is the relationship of a part to the whole. Dividing the number of boys on the pediatric unit by the total number of boys and girls on the unit results in a proportion: 10 boys out of 15 boys and girls would result in a proportion of boys equal to 67%.

A rate is a proportion that includes the factor of time. It is a measure of the quantity of a health problem in a specific population within a given period. Rates are the best indicators of the probability that a disease, condition, or event will occur; therefore, rates are the primary measurements used to describe occurrence. By using rates, it is possible to compare events that happen at different times and places and with different people. For example, rates make it possible to compare the occurrence of HIV/AIDS in two or more locations.

A rate consists of two parts: a *numerator* and a *denominator*. The numerator is composed of the number of cases of the health problem being investigated within a given period. The denominator is the population at risk during the same period. If the period is long, the population at risk is often estimated at a midperiod, such as midyear. There are four basic principles that apply to the calculation of rates:

1. *The numerator should include all events being measured; therefore, adequate information must be available.*

2. *Everyone in the denominator must be at risk for the event in the numerator.*

3. *A specific period must be indicated during which observations are made.*

4. *To make the rate a reasonable size to interpret and remove decimal points, the rate is multiplied by a base, usually a multiple of 10. Any base multiple of 10 may be chosen that results in a rate above the value of 1.*

The formula for rate calculation follows. Table 3-3 illustrates the calculation of rates that can be compared between cities.

$$Rate = \frac{\begin{array}{c} Number\ of\ conditions\ or\ events \\ occurring\ in\ a\ period\ of\ time \end{array}}{\begin{array}{c} Population\ at\ risk\ during\ the \\ same\ period\ of\ time \end{array}} \times Base\ multiple\ of\ 10$$

An example of the difference between rates and ratios is shown in the figure on p. 54. Fertility rates are defined as live births per 1,000 women age 15 to 44 years. Women experiencing live births are in the numerator, and all women of childbearing age are in the denominator. The abortion ratio is the

TABLE 3-3   **HYPOTHETICAL EXAMPLE OF THE CALCULATION OF RATES THAT CAN BE COMPARED BETWEEN TWO CITIES**

CITY A, 1998	CITY B, 1998
Number of hepatitis cases = 45	Number of hepatitis cases = 341
Population of City A = 153,000	Population of City B = 1,326,000
Hepatitis rate 45 × 100,000	Hepatitis rate 341 × 100,000
City A = 153,000	City B = 1,326,000
Hepatitis rate	Hepatitis rate
City A = 0.000294 × 100,000	City B = 0.00257 × 100,000
Hepatitis rate	Hepatitis rate
City A = 29.4 cases/100,000 people in 1998	City B = 25.7 cases/100,000 people in 1998

Counting only cases, City B has a higher frequency of hepatitis. However, when the population at risk is included in the rate calculation, City A has more cases per population than City B.

number of legal induced abortions per 1,000 live births. The numerator, the number of legal induced abortions, is not a part of the denominator, live births. Therefore, it is a ratio and not a rate. However, the number of legal induced abortions per 1,000 women of childbearing age is a rate, the abortion rate. The graph below shows the changes in the rates and ratio over a 22-year period (CDC, 1997a).

Incidence Rates

Incidence or occurrence rates are a form of rate that measures the occurrence of new illnesses in a previously disease-free group of people within a specific time frame, often a year. Therefore, it is a measure of the probability that people without a certain condition will develop the condition over a period of time. The nu-

FERTILITY RATE AND ABORTION RATIO AND RATE BY YEAR: UNITED STATES, 1972–1994.

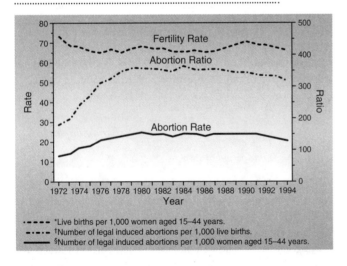

- - - - *Live births per 1,000 women aged 15–44 years.
- ·- · †Number of legal induced abortions per 1,000 live births.
———— §Number of legal induced abortions per 1,000 women aged 15–44 years.

merator of incidence rates include only the number of *new* conditions or events occurring within a period of time; therefore, the date of onset must be known. The general rules that apply to rates apply to incidence rates. Incidence rates and incidence ratios, especially **mortality** (death) rates, are often indices of the health of communities.

Incidence rates can be used to determine trends over time. For example, the figure on page 55 shows the rates of group B streptococcal (GBS) infection among infants in the United States (CDC, 1997c). This infection is the leading cause of bacterial disease and death among newborns in the United States and can cause illness and death in peripartum women and in adults with chronic medical conditions. Therefore, the incidence of this disease has been tracked in selected cities and their surrounding regions in different geographic locations. This incidence rate has been calculated as the number of infants infected per 1,000 live births. The figure shows that there is a decreasing incidence of GBS, and it is believed to be the result of improved measures of surveillance and widely publicized state-sponsored prevention activities (CDC, 1997c).

Prevalence Rates

Prevalence rates measure the number of people in a given population who have an existing health problem within a specified time frame. There are two types of prevalence rates. **Period prevalence** indicates the existence of a condition during an interval of time. **Point prevalence** refers to the existence of a condition at a specific point in time. Prevalence measures the amount of illness or **morbidity** that exists in a community as a result of the health problem under investigation. Many health care workers believe that prevalence rates are more important than incidence rates in determining the total burden of the illness on the community. Knowledge of the prevalence of a condition such as diabetes mellitus within a popu-

PREVALENCE OF SELF-REPORTED DIABETES BY AGE GROUP—UNITED STATES, 1980–1994.

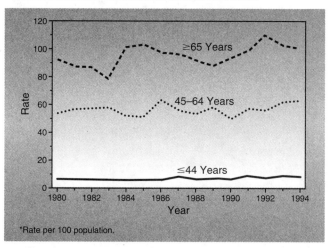

*Rate per 100 population.

(a)

AGE-ADJUSTED PREVALENCE OF SELF-REPORTED DIABETES BY RACE—UNITED STATES, 1980–1994.

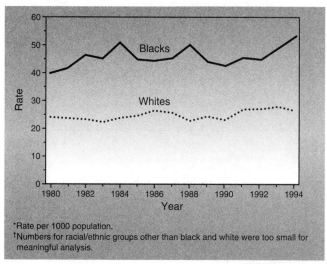

*Rate per 1000 population.
†Numbers for racial/ethnic groups other than black and white were too small for meaningful analysis.

(b)

FYI

The mortality rate of lung cancer has surpassed the mortality rate of breast cancer among women.

INCIDENCE RATE OF EARLY-ONSET GROUP B STREPTOCOCCAL (GBS) DISEASE BY YEAR AND SITE—SELECTED SITES, 1993–1995.

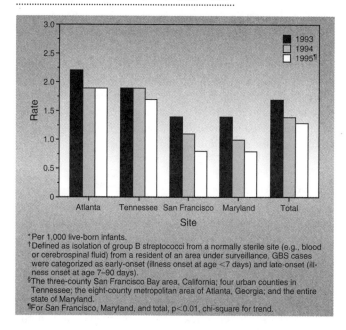

*Per 1,000 live-born infants.
†Defined as isolation of group B streptococci from a normally sterile site (e.g., blood or cerebrospinal fluid) from a resident of an area under surveillance. GBS cases were categorized as early-onset (illness onset at age <7 days) and late-onset (illness onset at age 7–90 days).
§The three-county San Francisco Bay area, California; four urban counties in Tennessee; the eight-county metropolitan area of Atlanta, Georgia; and the entire state of Maryland.
¶For San Francisco, Maryland, and total, p<0.01, chi-square for trend.

lation can lead to the prioritizing of facilities, services, and manpower to meet the special needs of diabetics in the community.

Prevalence is influenced by two factors: the number of people who have developed the condition in the past and the duration of their illness. The longer the duration of a condition, the higher the prevalence rate in the community. This is best illustrated with chronic diseases. For example, there are many more cases of diabetes in a community than would be indicated by calculation of the incidence rate, which reflects new cases only. Although the incidence rate for diabetes is low, people live for many years with the illness, and the duration is high. Therefore, in calculating prevalence rates, the numerator consists of the number of *existing* cases of the condition or event that occur within a specified period. For example, the existing cases of diabetes mellitus include new cases that were recently diagnosed plus those cases diagnosed in the past who are currently living with the illness.

Crude, Specific, and Adjusted Rates

Other common rates include crude, specific, and adjusted rates. **Crude rates** measure the experience of health problems in populations of designated geographic areas. These broad descriptive statistics may obscure significant differences in the risk of developing various conditions. Factors such as age, gender, ethnicity, and other demographic factors are not taken into consideration. Therefore, **specific rates** for subgroups of the population may be calculated. These more detailed rates are commonly calculated to describe the distribution of health problems by age, gender, ethnicity, and other demographic characteristics. **Adjusted rates** have been standardized, removing the differences in composition of populations, such as age. The figure on page 55 (part a) illustrates the prevalence of self-reported diabetes in three specific age groups. The rates are highest in those older than 65. Part b of the figure illustrates age-adjusted rates of self-reported diabetes by race (CDC, 1997f). In this example, age adjustment removes age as a factor in the calculation of the rates. Therefore, the differences shown reflect a rather dramatic increase in diabetes mellitus in African Americans. Knowledge of these factors can be helpful in assessing individual patients for their health care needs, as well as group needs for prevention and control programs.

Sources of Data

To describe a specific condition or event appropriately, it is necessary to collect data from reliable sources. Traditionally, epidemiologists have used the census of the population as a reliable source for the denominators in the calculation of rates. The census is required once every 10 years by the United States Constitution and is the basis for apportionment of seats in the House of Representatives. It has been performed every 10 years since 1790. The 21st census was completed in 1990. Through the years, the census has expanded, including characteristics of housing, nativity, migration, education, employment, income, and other information that is gathered from random samples of the population. Census information is analyzed and reported for the nation as a whole and in progressively small regions down to municipalities, census tracts, and blocks. Results are also reported in regions known as standard metropolitan statistical areas (SMSA). These regions are densely populated and are not necessarily bound by traditional state or county lines. The majority of the population of the United States lives within these areas.

Vital statistics are data collected from the continuous recording of events such as births, deaths, marriages, divorces, and adoptions, usually by state agencies. This information can be used to provide valid numerators and denominators for calculation of rates. The Centers for Disease Control and Prevention (CDC) in Atlanta collects all information regarding reportable diseases from state health departments. A sample of common reportable communicable diseases is found in Box 3-1. However, reportable diseases may vary somewhat from state to state. The CDC also collects information about other infectious and noninfectious health problems through a series of more than 100 national surveillance programs. The *Morbidity and Mortality Weekly Report (MMWR)* published by the CDC is the vehicle for distributing this information to health care professionals.

The National Health Survey, established in 1956, provides information about the health needs of the population of the United States. The National Center for Health Statistics is responsible for the ongoing surveys of households, physical examinations and laboratory reports, and health services providers. Most of this infor-

BOX 3-1 COMMON REPORTABLE COMMUNICABLE DISEASES

AIDS	Malaria
Amebiasis	Measles
Anthrax	Meningitis
Botulism	Meningococcal
Brucellosis	infection
Campylobacteriosis	Mumps
Chancroid	Pertussis
Chickenpox–zoster	Plague
Chlamydia	Poliomyelitis
Cholera	Psittacosis
Diptheria	Rabies
Encephalitis	Reye's syndrome
Food-associated	Rocky Mountain
illnesses	spotted fever
Giardiasis	Rubella
Gonorrhea	Salmonellosis
Granuloma inguinale	Shigellosis
Hemophilus	Syphilis
influenzae	Tetanus
Hepatitis A, B, non-A,	Toxic shock syndrome
non-B, unspecified	Trichinosis
Legionellosis	Tuberculosis
Leprosy	Tularemia
Leptospirosis	Typhoid fever
Lyme disease	Typhus
Lymphogranuloma	Yellow fever
venereum	

mation is prevalence data and is the only nationwide source of data on chronic illness, minor conditions, and functional problems.

The Behavioral Risk Factor Surveillance System (BRFSS) was established in 1984 to collect, analyze, and interpret behavioral risk factor data from all states. Information is gathered about health behaviors such as obesity, lack of physical activity, smoking, safety belt use, and screening programs for breast cancer and elevated blood cholesterol. These BRFSS data were used in the formulation of both national and state objectives for the year 2000 and are being used for the development of 2010 objectives. Data are published regularly in the *MMWR*.

Any health-related information that has been collected about a group of people can be a source of data used to determine the distribution of states of health. Often, health-related information is found in databases from health care institutions, disease registries, insurance companies, industries, accident and police records, private doctors offices, local surveys, and any other place where information is gathered. Community health nurses are likely to use these data when planning programs for groups of people with specific health needs and information about the population is needed. These records reflect only those conditions or events that are characteristic of the people that sought the services of that agency or participated in the survey. These data are helpful in establishing health services to meet their needs and in evaluating outcomes, but data must be interpreted carefully when applying the information to the community as a whole.

Person, Place, and Time

One of the first steps in investigating the distribution and determinants of a health care problem is to describe the problem (*what occurs*) in terms of person, place, and time. Descriptive epidemiology deals primarily with the study of the distribution of health problems. However, research studies that attempt to identify the determinants of a problem (*why it occurs*) depend on the accurate collection of descriptive data. Examining the information about person, place, and time can help identify the characteristics of people who develop a disease or illness and those who do not.

Person

Describing the person characterizes *who* develops the health problem. There are many variations among people according to genetic factors, biological characteristics, behavioral choices, and socioeconomic conditions. Because so many variations exist, incidence and prevalence rates should be calculated according to these factors. This can be done by examining individual case data

and examining specific and adjusted rates. Age is the most important characteristic affecting health status, followed by sex. Therefore, age-specific rates and sex-specific rates are usually calculated when describing a problem. Age-specific rates are calculated using the number of people in a given age group who have the problem being investigated in the numerator, and the population at risk in the given age group in the denominator.

An example of age-specific rates follows. The study was initiated following a 7-day period of intense environmental heat where maximum high daily temperatures in Dallas County, Texas, ranged from 101°F (38.3°C) to 106°F (41.1°C), and a series of deaths occurred. The figure on the following page is a bar graph that demonstrates that the average rate of heat-related deaths each year is greatest in the newborn to 4, 75 to 84, and 85+ age groups, as well as the very young and the elderly (CDC, 1997d).

Using this knowledge, community health nurses could initiate multiple actions, either for individuals in their care or for groups. When a heat wave is forecast, primary prevention messages about how to avoid heat-related illness should be disseminated to the public. The elderly should be encouraged to maintain their fluid intake and assisted to increase their time in air-conditioned environments, making use of shopping malls and public libraries, even for part of the day. Alcohol consumption should be discouraged because it may cause dehydration and increase the risk for heat-related illnesses. Parents of young children should be educated about the increased heat sensitivity of young children and their need for adequate fluids. Day-care centers could be primary sites for dissemination of information.

Often, specific rates are presented in table form, combining characteristics of persons and changes over time. Table 3-4 indi-

| TABLE 3-4 | **NUMBER OF REPORTED TUBERCULOSIS CASES, PERCENTAGE CHANGE IN NUMBER OF CASES, AND RATES*, BY SEX, AGE, AND YEAR—UNITED STATES, 1992 AND 1998** |

CHARACTERISTIC	NO. REPORTED CASES		% CHANGE FROM 1992 TO 1998	RATE	
	1992	1998		1992	1998
Sex[†]					
Male	17,433	11,413	−34.5%	14.0	8.6
Female	9,236	6,935	−24.9%	7.1	5.0
Age group (yr)[†]					
0–14	1,707	1,082	−36.6%	3.1	1.9
15–24	1,974	1,548	−21.6%	5.5	4.2
25–44	10,444	6,365	−39.1%	12.7	7.6
45–64	6,487	4,973	−23.3%	13.4	8.7
≥65	6,025	4,393	−27.1%	18.7	12.8
Total	26,673	18,361	−31.2%	10.5	6.8

*Per 100,000 population.
†Persons were excluded for whom sex (4 in 1992 and 13 in 1998) and age (36 in 1992) were not reported.

AVERAGE ANNUAL RATE OF HEAT-RELATED DEATHS BY AGE GROUP—UNITED STATES, 1979–1994.

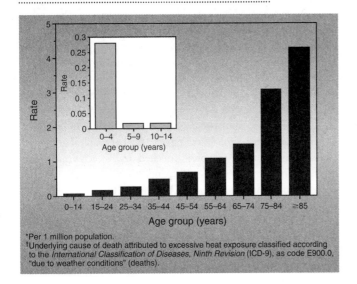

*Per 1 million population.
†Underlying cause of death attributed to excessive heat exposure classified according to the *International Classification of Diseases, Ninth Revision* (ICD-9), as code E900.0, "due to weather conditions" (deaths).

cates the number of reported tuberculosis cases, the age and sex characteristics of the cases, and the percentage change between 1992 and 1998 (CDC, 1999). This information shows that people older than 65 are the most vulnerable to tuberculosis. Nurses use this knowledge in establishing primary prevention programs and in assessing their elderly patients for signs and symptoms that may be indicative of the infection.

Place

Where the rates of the health problem are the highest or the lowest can be determined by examining the characteristics of place.

Understanding where illness occurs is a primary factor to be considered in planning prevention and control measures and making decisions about distribution of health care resources. Place can be a neighborhood, a health care facility, a town, a region, a nation, or any other natural or political boundary. The identification of health differences between urban and rural sectors or between similar localities are often helpful in investigating specific health needs of a community.

Place often is illustrated through the use of maps. For example, in an attempt to monitor progress to reduce the risk of severe adverse effects in children of mothers who consume alcohol, the CDC published the prevalence by state of reported frequent alcohol consumption among women of childbearing age. The figure below illustrates the prevalence of this risk factor (CDC, 1997b). State health departments have used these data to determine priorities for their health objectives for 2010. For example, Michigan, Iowa, and Pennsylvania have the highest prevalence rates and should have targeted primary prevention programs toward this risk factor. Community health nurses would participate in the various efforts to reduce alcohol consumption in this age group.

Time

When health problems occur can be described by identifying short-term fluctuations measured in hours, days, weeks, or months; by periodic changes that are seasonal or cyclical; or by long-term changes over decades that reflect gradual changes. Describing the time of short-term outbreaks of infectious diseases is often performed by developing an **epidemic curve**. These graphs provide indications as to the mode of transmission and spread of the organism. The figure on page 59 (top, left) is an example of an epidemic curve. It depicts an outbreak of viral gastroenteritis

PREVALENCE OF REPORTED FREQUENT ALCOHOL CONSUMPTION AMONG CHILDBEARING-AGE WOMEN (18–44 YEARS)—UNITED STATES, BEHAVIORAL RISK FACTOR SURVEILLANCE SYSTEM, 1995.

Reported consumption level	Pregnant women					All women				
	1991 (n = 1,053)	(95% CI†)	1995 (n = 1,313)	(95% CI)	p value	1991 (n = 26,105)	(95% CI)	1995 (n = 30,415)	(95% CI)	p value
Any drinking§	12.4	(9.5–15.2)	16.3	(13.1–19.4)	0.07	49.4	(48.4–50.3)	50.6	(49.7–51.6)	0.02
<7 Drinks per week	12.2	(9.4–15.0)	14.6	(11.5–17.6)	0.27	43.9	(43.0–44.9)	45.7	(44.8–46.5)	0.01
7–14 Drinks per week	—¶		0.9	(0.0–1.8)	—	3.4	(3.1–3.8)	3.0	(2.6–3.3)	0.04
>14 Drinks per week	0.1	(0.0–0.3)	0.3	(0.0–0.7)	0.28	1.4	(1.2–1.6)	1.1	(0.9–1.3)	0.04
≥5 Drinks on occasion**	0.7	(0.2–1.2)	2.9	(1.5–4.3)	0.003	10.5	(10.0–11.1)	10.5	(9.9–11.1)	0.96
Frequent drinking††	0.8	(0.3–1.4)	3.5	(1.9–5.1)	0.002	12.4	(11.8–13.1)	12.6	(12.0–13.3)	0.67

*Because weighted data are used in this analysis, results for 1991 may be slightly different from those reported previously. For consistency, national analyses were restricted to the 47 states that participated in the BRFSS in both 1991 and 1995.
†Confidence interval.
§Levels of any drinking may not add to the total prevalence of any drinking because some women did not respond to questions about consumption frequency and amount. One additional state was eliminated from the breakdown of any drinking because questions regarding consumption frequency and amount were not asked in that state in 1995.
¶Too few observations to calculate a reliable estimate.
**Five or more drinks on at least one occasion during the preceding month.
††Consumption of an average of seven or more drinks per week or five or more drinks on at least one occasion during the preceding month.

NUMBER OF CASES OF GASTROENTERITIS ASSOCIATED WITH EATING OYSTERS HARVESTED FROM LOUISIANA WATERWAYS, DECEMBER 1996–JANUARY 1997.

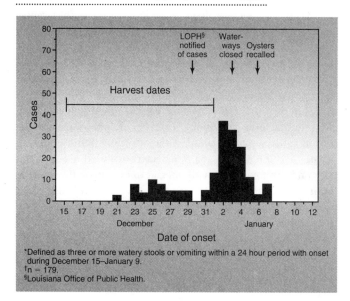

*Defined as three or more watery stools or vomiting within a 24 hour period with onset during December 15–January 9.
†n = 179.
§Louisiana Office of Public Health.

WEEKLY PNEUMONIA AND INFLUENZA (P&I) MORTALITY AS A PERCENTAGE OF ALL DEATHS IN 122 CITIES— UNITED STATES, JANUARY 1, 1993–FEBRUARY 15, 1997.

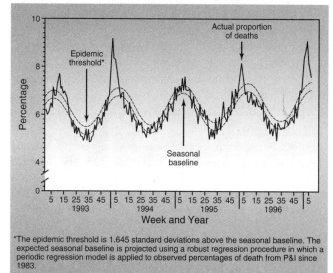

*The epidemic threshold is 1.645 standard deviations above the seasonal baseline. The expected seasonal baseline is projected using a robust regression procedure in which a periodic regression model is applied to observed percentages of death from P&I since 1983.

LIFE EXPECTANCY AT BIRTH BY YEAR OF BIRTH AND SEX— UNITED STATES, 1900–1996.

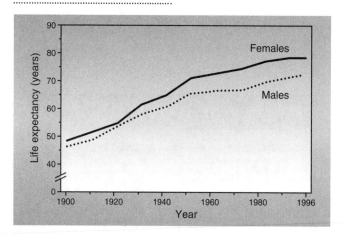

associated with eating oysters in Louisiana during December 1996 and January 1997 (CDC, 1997h). In this outbreak, 179 people became ill. The public health department was notified of the problem, contaminated oysters were identified, waterways closed, and the oysters recalled. The outbreak ended abruptly 2 days later. The only known source of the strain of gastrointestinal virus is feces from ill persons. Therefore, the probable source of the virus was oyster harvesters who admitted to routinely discharging sewage overboard. The oysters subsequently became contaminated with the virus and, after harvesting, were eaten by unsuspecting people in restaurants. Nurses working in public health agencies often are involved in identifying outbreaks such as this and may be involved in gathering and analyzing information and implementing control and preventive measures.

Periodic and *cyclical* changes also occur. For example, respiratory diseases are more common in the winter and spring (periodic), and hepatitis often increases in incidence every 7 to 9 years (cyclical). The figure above (right) reflects both periodic and cyclical changes in pneumonia and influenza mortality (CDC, 1997g). A seasonal baseline is developed, and variations from this baseline determine whether an epidemic is occurring.

These types of data are the evidence base for many of the control, prevention, and surveillance activities that are initiated by public health departments and community agencies initiated to keep the public healthy.

Long-term changes or trends over time are shown in the figure at right (CDC, 1997e). During the 20th century, significant changes in life expectancy at birth occurred. The figure includes

gender, a characteristic of persons to make the graph more meaningful. In a similar manner, the changes in trends of the mortality of various cancers can be seen when examined over decades (see figure above).

Analytic Epidemiology

Analytic epidemiology focuses on the determinants of health problems, or the *why*. When descriptive data are analyzed, the

FYI

The Framingham Heart Study is a prospective study that has continued to follow the health characteristics of a community for more than 30 years. Much of the information about risk factors for coronary heart disease that underlies preventive programs was obtained from the results of this study.

variations in person, place, and time often suggest tentative explanations or hypotheses. These hypotheses can then be tested through application of research methods in an attempt to find the reasons, or determinants, for these variations. This is a cyclical process because new knowledge may require further descriptive

or analytic analysis. Four types of studies are used in epidemiological analytic investigations: **cross-sectional**, **retrospective**, **prospective**, and **intervention** (experimental) studies. The basic characteristics of these studies are outlined in Table 3-5.

Ideally, the epidemiologist is seeking to establish a cause-and-effect relationship between the health problem or outcome that is being studied (dependent variable) and exposure factors (independent variables) that preceded it in time. Often, associations can be made between a condition and a specific factor, but a direct cause-and-effect relationship is weak or does not exist. More than one factor must be present for any illness to occur (multifactorial causation). Even in an infectious process, such as tuberculosis, presence of the organism alone is not sufficient to cause the disease. Characteristics of the agent, the host, and the environment all interact to determine the onset of the infection. The more factors that can be identified as contributors to a disease process, the weaker the cause-and-effect relationship will be.

RESEARCH BRIEF

Redelmeier, D. A., & Tibshirani, R. J. (1997). Association between cellular-telephone calls and motor vehicle collisions. The New England Journal of Medicine, 336(7), 453–458.

This epidemiological study of cellular phone use and motor vehicle collisions used a case-crossover design to study. The purpose of the research was to study whether using a cellular telephone while driving increases the risk of a motor vehicle collision. The sample included 669 drivers who had cellular phones and had been in accidents with significant property damage but no personal injury. Each person's cellular telephone calls on the day of the collision and during the previous week were analyzed using telephone bills.

A total of 26,798 cellular phone calls were made during the 14-month study period. The risk of a collision when using a cellular phone was four times higher than

the risk when a cellular telephone was not being used. The relative risk was 4.3 (95% confidence level, 3.0 to 6.5). The relative risk was similar for drivers who differed in personal characteristics such as age and driving experience. Of note, cellular phone calls made close to the time of the collision were particularly hazardous (relative risk, 4.8 for calls placed within 5 minutes of the collision, as compared with 1.3 for calls placed more than 15 minutes before the collision). Hand-free units offered no protection over handheld units (3.9 relative risk). Of the drivers, 39% used the cellular phones to call for emergency services, providing some advantage after the accident. The use of cellular phones in motor vehicles is associated with a quadrupling of the risk of a collision during the brief period of a phone call. There are implications from this study for education about risk reduction and the use of this new technology.

TABLE 3-5   CHARACTERISTICS OF EPIDEMIOLOGICAL ANALYTIC STUDIES

CROSS-SECTIONAL SURVEYS

Purpose	Describe health states and look for tentative hypotheses
Design	All data is collected at the same time
Data collection	Interviews, observation, questionnaires
Advantages	Flexible, broad, economical, uncomplicated; rapid results, large samples possible
Disadvantages	Superficial, cannot infer cause and effect

CASE-CONTROL OR RETROSPECTIVE STUDIES

Purpose	Determine whether a group with a health problem (case) differs in exposure from a group without the problem (controls)
Design	Select case and control samples according to specific criteria. The dependent variable (case or not) has already occurred
Data collection	Trace past experience to determine relevant exposure factors (independent variables)
Advantages	First step in hypothesis testing, inexpensive, relatively small samples can be used, results obtained quickly
	Good design for studying rare or chronic conditions
Disadvantages	Information about past exposure may not be available
	Selection of appropriate control groups may be difficult
	Incidence can only be estimated
	Temporal association between exposure and outcome may be difficult to determine
	Potential selection, recall, and observation bias

PROSPECTIVE, COHORT, OR LONGITUDINAL STUDIES

Purpose	Determine whether the incidence of the health problem varies between the exposed and nonexposed
Design	Samples chosen and observed forward in time
Data collection	Information on outcome variables obtained at specific intervals
Advantages	Incidence rates can be calculated directly
	Time sequence easier to obtain
	Effects of rare exposure can be investigated
	Multiple outcomes may be studied
Disadvantages	May extend over a long period
	Expensive
	Cases lost to follow-up

THERAPEUTIC OR PREVENTIVE TRIALS, INTERVENTION STUDIES

Purpose	Determine whether a group with particular characteristics will benefit from interventions when compared with a group or groups who do not receive the intervention
Design	Randomly choose and assign groups to either a study group or comparison group
	Introduce an intervention (independent variable) to the study group
Data collection	Collect data prospectively on a number of dependent variables
Advantages	Cause and effect can be examined
	Control over confounding variables
	Can conduct with small groups
Disadvantages	Possible reactivity (Hawthorne effect)
	Possible noncompliance with study protocols
	Observation bias, placebo effect

Source: Modified from Harkness, 1995.

CONCLUSION

Promoting and preserving the health of populations is a fundamental characteristic of community health nursing. Although nursing is a profession that focuses primarily on the individual, the person's health care needs cannot be completely or correctly defined unless family, personal friends, and the characteristics of the community and the society are considered. Epidemiology, the science of preventive medicine, provides a framework for studying and understanding these interactions. Epidemiology is the study of the distribution and the determinants of states of health and illness in human populations. The basic conceptual framework of epidemiology is the interaction among the agent, host, and environment—the epidemiological triad. Epidemiology is considered both as a methodology used to study health-related conditions and as an accumulated body of knowledge about a state of health. Nurses use the body of knowledge about a health problem in their clinical decision making and may become involved in epidemiological research methods to gather new health-related information.

Descriptive epidemiology examines the distribution of states of health in the population. The primary tool that is used in epidemiology is the rate, a proportion that includes the factor of time. Incidence rates measure the probability that people without a certain condition develop the condition during a specific time frame. The number of new conditions or events are measured. Prevalence rates measure the extent of an existing health problem within a specific period. These rates are often calculated according to characteristics of person (who), place (where), and time (when). Analytical epidemiology attempts to define the determinants of health problems (why) through rigorous research techniques. Types of analytical studies include cross-sectional, retrospective, prospective, and intervention studies.

CRITICAL THINKING ACTIVITIES

1. Using an example from your practice, identify two instances that illustrate how the epidemiological body of knowledge is used in clinical decision making.

2. Between January 1 and December 1, 1998, 25 new cases of tuberculosis were diagnosed in Boon Town, population 450,000. A prevalence survey taken the first week in January 1998 indicated that there were 250 cases on the list of active tuberculosis cases. There were 20 deaths due to tuberculosis recorded during this 1-year period. Using this information, calculate the following rates.

   - What was the incidence rate per 100,000 population for tuberculosis during 1998?

   - What was the prevalence rate per 100,000 population for tuberculosis during 1998?

   - What was the cause-specific death rate per 100,000 for tuberculosis in 1998?

3. Discuss how nurses could use the case-control research methodology to answer questions in their practice.

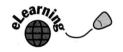 Explore Community Health Nursing on the web! To learn more about the topics in this chapter, access your exclusive web site:
http://communitynursing.jbpub.com

REFERENCES

Aiken, L. (1988). Assuring the delivery of quality patient care. State of the Science Invitational Conference: Nursing resources and the delivery of patient care (NIH Publication No. 89-3008, pp. 3–10). Washington, D.C.: U.S. Department of Health and Human Services, Public Health Service.

Bureau of the Census. (1998). Statistical abstracts of the United States, 1998, the national data book (118th ed., p 100). Washington, D.C.: U.S. Department of Commerce, Economics and Statistics Administration.

Centers for Disease Control and Prevention (CDC). (1997a). Abortion surveillance: Preliminary data—United States, 1994. *Morbidity and Mortality Weekly Report, 45*(51&52), 1123–1127.

Centers for Disease Control and Prevention (CDC). (1997b). Alcohol consumption among pregnant and childbearing-aged women—United States, 1991 and 1995. *Morbidity and Mortality Weekly Report, 46*(16), 346–350.

Centers for Disease Control and Prevention (CDC). (1997c). Decreasing incidence of perinatal group B streptococcal disease—United States, 1993–1995. *Morbidity and Mortality Weekly Report, 46*(21), 473–477.

Centers for Disease Control and Prevention (CDC). (1997d). Heat-related deaths—Dallas, Wichita, and Cooke Counties, Texas, and United States, 1996. *Morbidity and Mortality Weekly Report, 46*(23), 528–531.

Centers for Disease Control and Prevention (CDC). (1997e). Mortality patterns—preliminary data, United States, 1996. *Morbidity and Mortality Weekly Report, 46*(40), 941–944.

Centers for Disease Control and Prevention (CDC). (1997f). Trends in the prevalence and incidence of self-reported diabetes mellitus—United States, 1980–1994. *Morbidity and Mortality Weekly Report, 46*(43), 1014–1018.

Centers for Disease Control and Prevention (CDC). (1997g). Update: Influenza activity—United States, 1996. *Morbidity and Mortality Weekly Report, 46*(8), 173–176.

Centers for Disease Control and Prevention (CDC). (1997h). Viral gastroenteritis associated with eating oysters—Louisiana, December 1996–January 1997. *Morbidity and Mortality Weekly Report, 46*(47), 1109–1112.

Centers for Disease Control and Prevention (CDC). (1999). Progress toward the elimination of tuberculosis—United States, 1998. *Morbidity and Mortality Weekly Report, 48*(33), 732–736.

Cohen, B. (1984). Florence Nightingale. *Scientific American, 250*(3), 129.

Doll, R., & Hill, A. B. (1950). Smoking and carcinoma of the lung: Preliminary report. *British Medical Journal,* 2739.

Harkness, G. A. (1995). *Epidemiology in nursing practice.* St. Louis, Mosby.

Humphreys, N. A. (1885). *Vital statistics: A memorial volume of selections from the reports and writings of William Farr, 1807–1183.* London: Sanitary Institute of Great Britain.

Leavell, H. F., & Clark, H. G. (1965). *Preventive medicine for the doctor in his community: An epidemiologic approach.* New York: McGraw-Hill.

Leavell, H. R., & Clark, H. G. (1958). *Preventive medicine for the doctor in his community,* 3rd ed. New York: McGraw-Hill.

Snow, J. (1855). *On the mode of communication of cholera.* London: Churchill. (Reproduced in *Snow on cholera.* [1965]. New York: Hafner.)

Unit II

Factors Influencing Community Health

Chapter 4
Environmental Health

Carol J. Nyman, Patricia Butterfield, and Jean Shreffler

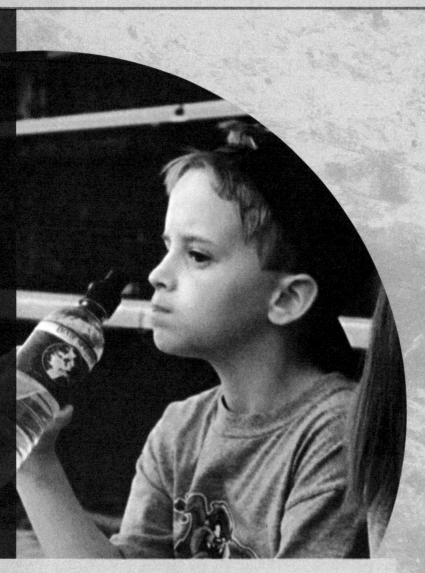

Only after the last tree has been cut down,
Only after the last river has been poisoned,
Only after the last fish has been caught,
Only then will you find that money cannot be eaten.

Cree Indian Philosophy

CHAPTER FOCUS

QUESTIONS TO CONSIDER

After reading this chapter, answer the following questions:

1. What specific global environmental threats impact public health?
2. What are current trends in disease and exposure in the environment?
3. What is the history of environmental health in the United States?
4. What is environmental health policy?
5. How does environmental health policy evolve?
6. What is the government's role in environmental health policy?
7. What are the specific roles of the community health nurse in promoting a healthy environment?
8. What is an exposure assessment, and how is it conducted?
9. What is the role of effective communication in the education of community residents?
10. What is upstream thinking, and how is it related to environmental health?
11. What are the key ethical principles related to the environment?
12. How does a community health nurse develop a clinical practice in environmental health?

KEY TERMS

Environmental health
Environmental justice

Risk assessment
Risk management

Social justice
Thinking upstream

Toxicology
Toxins

The impact of environmental agents on human health becomes fairly obvious when exposure levels are high and their effect on health is immediate. Nurses are most likely to observe such situations in emergency rooms and poison control centers. A frantic parent might call to report that their 3-year-old daughter was found playing with a bag of fertilizer in the garage. A young father, stripping woodwork in a spare basement room, is brought into the emergency room by his wife after being overcome by fumes from paint stripper. An elderly woman is found unconscious in her home after using her gas stove burners to heat her small apartment. In each situation, nurses and other health professionals organize a collective response to an immediate health crisis precipitated by an environmental agent. Detoxification procedures are initiated, and clinical efforts are focused on projecting target organ systems and maintaining system integrity.

In the previous scenarios, the link between environment and human health is readily apparent. It is easy to see that unfavorable consequences can result from a single exposure to a toxic agent. However, acute exposures comprise only the tip of the iceberg in the domain of environmental health. In most situations, associations between disease occurrence and exposure to one or more environmental factors are not easily traced; years or decades may have elapsed between exposure to the agent of concern and subsequent health effects. In addition, exposures may have occurred in small doses over time or may involve contact with a variety of compounds that interact with each other to cause incremental changes that ultimately culminate in disease. An additional complicating factor is that, for many environmental factors, incomplete and inconclusive science characterizes associations between exposure and the development of disease. Because of these and other considerations, environmental health is one of the most challenging and rapidly developing areas of community health nursing. Fortunately, for many nurses, it is also one of the most rewarding areas of practice.

Trends in Exposure and Disease

Health professionals and members of the general public are generally aware of the delicate balance that exists between the environment and global health. A goal of policy makers, both in the United States and elsewhere, has been to increase technology and encourage creative potential without compromising public health and safety. Unfortunately, despite our knowledge of the association between environmental contaminants and adverse health effects, our society continues to manufacture, use, and dispose of many potentially hazardous chemicals. In 1991, the U.S. industry reported the release of 3.39 billion pounds of potentially toxic chemicals into the air, water, and soil (EPA, 1993). The widespread use of chemicals with toxic effects highlights the importance of educating nurses who can formulate prevention programs to reduce opportunities of exposure in homes, workplaces, and public areas. Many cases of environmentally induced

illness can be prevented, but this requires actions that have not traditionally been recognized as within the scope of nursing (Kleffel, 1991, 1996).

••••••••••••••••••••••••••••

I have therefore come to believe that the world's ecological balance depends on more than just our ability to restore a balance between civilization's ravenous appetite for resources and the fragile equilibrium of the earth's environment; it depends on more, even, than our ability to restore a balance between ourselves as individuals and the civilization we aspire to create and sustain. In the end, we must restore a balance within ourselves between who we are and what we are doing. Each of us must take a greater personal responsibility for this deteriorating global environment; each of us must take a hard look at the habits of mind and action that reflect—and have led to—this grave crisis.

Al Gore, *Earth in the Balance: Ecology and the Human Spirit*, 1992

••••••••••••••••••••••••••••

The recently documented increases in the prevalence of asthma, in both children and adults, have been attributed to increasing air pollution in many urban areas. Approximately 50% of waterborne disease cases have been found to be due to chemical contamination (DHHS, 1991). New cases of renal and liver disease are diagnosed annually in this country with no known cause; organic solvents and heavy metals are both known to cause damage to these organs. These same agents have been implicated as neurotoxins causing central nervous system damage and have been hypothesized to contribute to the occurrence of several types of neurodegenerative and neurobehavioral disorders. About 200,000 infants are born annually with some form of birth defect; the cause of many of these defects is unknown. Although it is inappropriate and alarmist to suggest that environmental agents are the cause of increased disease throughout the world, it is equally inappropriate to fail to consider the single and multiple effects of environmental agents as potential agents in changing global disease patterns. Part of the role of professional nursing is to participate in research that helps further the scientific community's understanding of the cause and pathogenesis of cancer, neurological conditions, autoimmune disorders, and other diseases.

A World View

Citizens' concerns addressing environmental health issues have been voiced at a global level over the past decade. Depletion of the ozone layer, the greenhouse effect, acid rain, deforestation, and weather changes are now understood as problems for the world that no single nation can hope to address alone (Last, 1993). The relationships of industrialization and deforestation to the emergence of new diseases, and the reemergence of diseases previously thought to be under control (e.g., tuberculosis), is of special concern.

Emerging health concerns have been hypothesized to result from the consequences of natural environmental changes (e.g., warming Pacific coastal waters secondary to El Niño weather changes), intentional environmental manipulation (e.g., deforestation, amateur irrigation projects), and the introduction of new species to a geographic area (e.g., livestock into rainforest areas). Recent ecological changes associated with human health problems include the following:

- *Population movements and the intrusion of humans into new habitats, particularly tropical forests*
- *Deforestation, with new forest-farmland margins that expose farmers to new vectors of disease*
- *Irrigation, especially primitive systems that serve as breeding areas for arthropods*
- *Rapidly expanding urbanization, with vector populations finding urban breeding grounds in standing water and sewage*
- *Changes in technology and industrial practices, such as the overuse of antibiotics in modern medicine or the use of antimicrobial-supplemented animal feeds and their contribution to the development of drug-resistant microbes*

It is apparent that these problems will require a perspective that transcends country or provincial boundaries and mobilizes global concern and cooperation. Import policies in developed nations need to address the transfer of natural resources from developing countries, such as mineral wealth, oil, and exotic lumber. Environmentally sound practices in the mining, agriculture, and forestry industries need to be enhanced through cooperative efforts between industry and citizen groups. Several disease surveillance organizations have requested additional funding for the development of a system that coordinates global reporting of disease surveillance and control efforts. Better diagnostic techniques, prevention strategies, and risk factor analysis must be taught to health care professionals worldwide. More funding for basic and applied research related to the environment and infectious diseases can yield significant improvements in public health. Education for a global perspective is needed to address the issue of infectious disease within the context of shared environmental responsibility. As our planet moves from a national to an international perspective on health problems, it is easier to see that environmentally destructive practices in one country can eventually culminate in health problems in many other countries throughout the world.

A summary of an outbreak of Hantavirus, an emerging viral condition, is presented in Box 4-1. This outbreak has been partially attributed to the unseasonably wet spring that occurred in the western United States during 1993. In New Mexico and several other states, rainfall patterns lead to a significant increase in the deer mice population, which leads to an increased risk of ex-

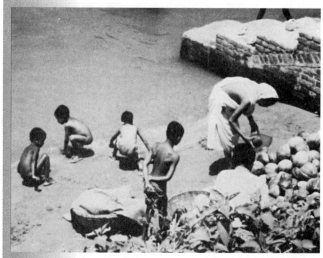

Children play in contaminated water of the Ganges in India.

posure to Hantavirus for persons residing in rural areas. Some scientists have hypothesized that global changes in weather patterns will lead to critical changes in disease occurrence over the next few decades.

The Environment and Health

Although many definitions of environment are used in the scientific literature, in this chapter the term *environment* refers to all external conditions or influences affecting living things (Valanis, 1996). Within this context, *environment* refers to more than biological and chemical hazards, including also dimensions of the social and cultural milieu. **Environmental health** refers to freedom from illness or injury related to toxic agents and other environmental conditions that are potentially detrimental to human health (Pope, Snyder, & Mood, 1995). Health care providers' roles in environmental health are expanding to include diagnosing and caring for people with exposures to chemical and physical hazards in their homes, workplaces, and communities through contaminated air, water, and soil.

Because environment is such a broad and pervasive concept, it can be difficult to define the boundaries of environmental health. The application of environmental health in clinical practice ranges from descriptions of hospital rooms to international and global perspectives on the health of the planet. Although a hospital room differs from a global ecology perspective in complexity as well as other dimensions, both views can provide insights into opportunities for health at the individual and collective level. Just as the scope of clinical practice varies from individual emergencies to situations in which a health care provider is charged with the health assessment of populations, so

BOX 4-1 AN OUTBREAK OF HANTAVIRUS

In May 1993, a healthy, athletic 21-year-old Navajo woman living on the reservation in New Mexico died from a respiratory ailment of acute onset. Five days later, on the way to her funeral, her 19-year-old fiancé, who had been feeling ill for several days, went into respiratory failure and could not be resuscitated. In late May, the woman's brother, who lived in a trailer near one the couple had shared, died of acute onset of a similar illness, as did his wife 5 days later. By early June, 24 cases with similar symptoms, including 12 deaths, had been reported in the area. Alert Indian Health Service personnel and Department of Health officials took immediate action, requesting assistance from the Centers for Disease Control and Prevention (CDC). Thanks in part to proactive epidemiology efforts and advances in molecular biology, within 4 weeks the CDC was able to identify the cause of death as pulmonary Hantavirus. This condition had not previously been seen in North America. The overall case fatality rate was 76%, with deaths in 13 of the first 17 confirmed cases (Duchin et al., 1994).

One of the strongest explanations for the appearance of this new and severe disease is environ-mental. The El Niño weather pattern had brought unusually wet weather to the area in the early 1990s. For 5 years, there had been a severe drought in the area, but in the winter of 1992-1993, there had been record snowfall followed by a rainy spring. The piñon nut harvest was unusually large, as was the mouse population. The University of New Mexico had done an ecological survey of the area that spring and was impressed to note a sudden population explosion among the deer mice—a tenfold increase since the previous year. The CDC discovered that deer mice were carriers of the Hantavirus, passing it in their urine and feces. With their numbers greatly increased, the deer mice were making more contact with humans by invading their homes, establishing a lethal connection with a new disease. The epidemiologist who did a survey of the initial victims' home after their deaths reported the presence of numerous mouse droppings (Garrett, 1994). Hantavirus may have been present in North America before 1993, but notable environmental and weather changes that occurred that year created a situation that brought humans, mice, and virus together in a profound way, allowing for the disease's presentation in humans.

too must the scope of environmental health assessment vary across situations.

Environmental Health Policy: Historical Perspectives

Consumer activism has resulted in the passage of laws and the establishment of regulatory agencies to safeguard public health. In the United States, examples of such agencies include the federal Committee on Consumer Interests, the Consumer Advisory Committee, and legislation addressing child safety and hazardous household products (Fine, 1988). Consumer advocate groups also initiated the formation of coalitions to inform and mobilize citizens around environmental health issues. Significant legislation and the establishment of federal and state agencies with the goals of protecting and improving the health of the environment also resulted from this movement. Examples of legislation passed during the 1960s and 1970s include clean air and water acts, occupational health and safety acts, toxic substances control acts, and the Poison Prevention Packaging Act. During these two decades, the Environmental Protection Agency (EPA), Occupational Health and Safety Administration, and Nuclear Regulation Commission were also established (Stevens & Hall, 1997).

Public and governmental actions addressing environmental health continue to this day, although some observers believe that responses have not been sufficient to reduce the health risks in the environment. Community right-to-know federal legislation, enacted in 1987, authorizes citizens' access to information addressing the presence, management, and release of hazardous chemicals in their community. Information addressing the storage and use of more than 300 chemicals was collected by the EPA, assembled into databases titled the Toxic Release Inventory, and made available to the public. The Pollution Prevention Act of 1990 authorized data collection activities addressing toxic chemicals that leave a community facility. These recent governmental efforts have greatly enhanced the ability of citizens to gain access to environmental data in their region. Such data can empower citizens to be vigilant on behalf of their community and respond quickly and effectively in the event of a hazardous materials incident or spill.

. . . .

They paved paradise and put up a parking lot.

Joni Mitchell, 1970

. . . .

However, despite recent advances in environmental information access, some environmental advocates point out that although some environmental risks have been minimized or eliminated, new risks have been identified but not sufficiently addressed. Citizen's advocacy groups have observed that regulatory and safety measures taken in the past have not been uniformly implemented or enforced; loopholes exist in others. In addition, some policy makers and legislators believe that environmental initiatives and laws are not in the best interests of the economy; thus, laws, standards, or initiatives have been cancelled, weakened, or not provided the support required to be effective.

Recent Environmental Health Issues

In the second half of the 20th century, awareness of the damage to the environment and its return impact on health grew dramatically. Population growth (see the following figures), urban spread, advanced technology, industrialization, and modern agricultural methods were the source of great progress but led to the creation of environmental hazards that may not have been observed previously. Each year, the EPA receives approximately 1,500 notices of intent to manufacture new substances. These new products are added to the EPA's inventory of toxic chemicals, which currently includes more than 65,000 chemicals (U.S. Congress, Office of Technology Assessment, 1990).

Although the health effects of many chemicals have been documented, many others have not been thoroughly studied.

Of additional concern is the cumulative effect of multiple chemicals on the human body over a lifetime. Studies of environmental carcinogenesis have primarily been conducted using animal bioassays to determine the incidence of cancer associated with exposure to a single agent (Garte, 1992). Although such tests have provided the bulk of scientific understanding of the dangers of selected agents, such as benzene, nitrosamines, and vinyl chloride, broader concerns exist about combinations of agents in the environment and possible synergism among health effects from multiple agents (Steingraber, 1997).

However, probably because of the rapid increase in chemical production and use since World War II, synthetically derived chemicals are often subject to irrational thinking about their dangers. Each environmental agent must be studied and understood; it is a profound mistake to conclude that all synthetic products are dangerous and those that are natural are safe. Some of the biggest threats to human health throughout the world originate from substances that predate the Industrial Revolution, including lead, mercury, and arsenic. Furthermore, chemical agents are often considered the sole source of environmental health threats; however, the scientific community has determined that physical agents (e.g., noise, vibration, ionizing radiation) and biological agents (e.g., bacterial contamination, fungal spores, viruses) also play significant roles in health problems of environmental etiology.

ESTIMATES OF WORLD POPULATION.

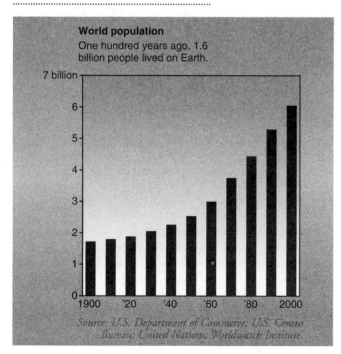

YEARS TAKEN TO REACH BILLION MARKERS.

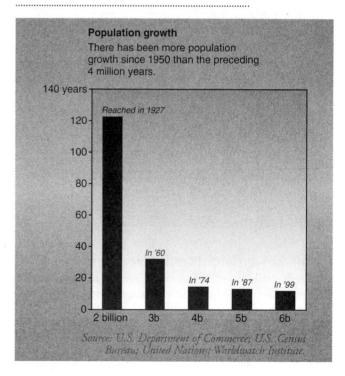

Historical Perspective on Environment and Health

The science of epidemiology has been closely linked to environmental health since the original work of John Snow in 1854. The same deductive processes in inquiry that Snow used to link cholera deaths to ingestion of contaminated Thames River water have since been duplicated countless times over the past century to link environmental agents with disease occurrence. Because the basic tenets of descriptive epidemiology (i.e., time, person, and place) have been so powerful a tool in establishing links between environmental agents and disease, this approach to scientific inquiry has stood the test of time for investigations of environmentally induced diseases at both local and global levels.

Some argue that epidemiological methods have been more effective in addressing infectious and acute diseases than chronic conditions. There may be some validity to this position, because links between exposure and disease are most easily made when the induction period is relatively brief. However, in recent years, chronic disease epidemiology has played an important role in furthering an understanding of relationships between environmental exposures and several types of cancer, neurological impairment, and autoimmune conditions. Examples in this area include associations between the following:

- *Asbestos and mesothelioma*
- *Prenatal exposure to diethylstilbestrol (DES, a form of estrogen given to pregnant women in the 1950s and 1960s to prevent miscarriage) and a rare form of cervical cancer*
- *Occupational exposure to vinyl chloride (used in the manufacture of polyvinyl chloride plastic pipe) and the development of liver cancer*

One of the biggest challenges in the area of chronic disease epidemiology is to establish evidence of exposure and exposure dosage for agents without biomarkers (i.e., a physiological fingerprint of exposure such as an elevated serum lead level indicating recent lead exposure). In these cases, exposure is most often estimated by using a questionnaire or interview guide. This method of ascertaining exposure can be problematic for exposures that may (or may not) have happened years or decades ago. Despite this and other challenges, epidemiological approaches to inquiry have been effectively used to explore associations between exposure and disease for many environmentally induced conditions both acute and chronic in nature.

Origins of Environmental Health Policy

Although concerns for environmental risks to health and safety have existed to some extent for centuries, the current widespread awareness and concern about these risks among public and private sectors is a relatively recent phenomenon. With the industrial revolution in the 1800s, the developed world, including the United States, focused on modernization and rapid production of goods and services. Concerns about depletion of natural resources or damage and hazards resulting from the products and wastes of industrialization were not yet realized or acted on. During this time, however, there was growing concern for working conditions and safety of workers, as reflected in the movement to organize and unionize the workforce to demand safe work environments, among other improvements. In the early decades of the 1900s, concerns about environmental health and safety were demonstrated by governments with the passage of laws to protect the public from hazardous goods in the marketplace. In the United States, for example, the Pure Food and Drug Law was passed in 1906 and the Food and Drug Administration was established in 1931 (Henson, Robinson, & Schmele, 1996). In the next several decades of the 1900s, war efforts and postwar industrial rebuilding consumed the energies of governments and the public. Again, the international production of war and postwar goods and services took precedence, and the lay public held a belief that their governments would protect them from environmental risks and hazards.

The birth of the consumer-driven environmental movement that continues today can be traced to the 1960s and 1970s. Multiple trends and events served to raise international consciousness that some aspects of the environment had become a growing risk to public health and safety. Disenchantment with postwar living conditions and the realization of the environmental effects of nuclear proliferation and war occurred after World War II. Public cynicism toward the government and other institutions occurred in this country during and after the Vietnam War era. Several widely read exposes of environmental hazards also were published during this time. One influential publication, *Silent Spring* (Carson, 1962), predicted the poisoning and destruction of the natural environment in the name of progress with the use of pesticides. Rachel Carson's book was history making in its effect on thought and policy making following its publication. Consumerism gained momentum during this time as a result of the efforts of national leaders and consumer advocate groups. All of these trends and events resulted in public concern and activism followed by governmental responses to citizens' growing environmental awareness.

Environmental Policy: Governmental and Public Roles

One of the primary purposes of government in a democratic society is to protect and safeguard the governed or the public. To fulfill this purpose, the government passes laws and enacts rules and regulations to prevent and reduce risks to the public. Government agencies and offices have been created to identify and monitor risks and hazards, monitor compliance with rules, and gather data to inform policy makers. Government initiatives have been implemented because of priorities of elected or appointed officials as well as in response to pressures from an environmentally conscious public.

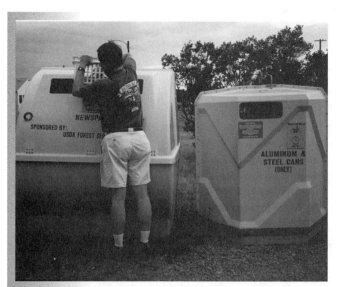

Recycling efforts have increased with significant environmental benefits.

Despite all of this governmental activity, our environment still poses hazards to the safety and health of the public, and in many cases, the dangers are more complicated now than ever before. Reasons for that increased risk include the following:

- *Environmental health has been addressed in a piecemeal fashion instead of in a potentially more effective comprehensive plan.*

- *Proposed policies and laws that improve the health of the environment are often perceived to be in conflict with what is in the best interest of business and the economy.*

- *Laws and policies cannot solve all environmental problems and risks without voluntary actions by individuals, groups, and organizations.*

- *Science has not been able to keep pace with potential environmental hazards and pollutants.*

- *In a world of finite resources, the costs of cleaning and protecting the environment are in competition with the costs of other desired and needed social programs.*

A discussion of nurses' actions to change local health policy on behalf of a disenfranchised group is summarized in the Case Study that follows.

At both the local and national levels, policy makers set national and state priorities among competing social programs, establish standards for environmental hazards and risks, take action against those who violate standards, and allocate billions of federal and state funds according to these established priorities. A broad set of population health goals to be achieved by the year 2000 was established by the U.S. Public Health Service (USPHS) 20 years ago and was reaffirmed with the publication of *Healthy People 2000* (DHHS, 1991) and *Healthy People 2010*

(DHHS, 2000). The *Healthy People 2010* objectives, which include environmental health as one of 28 priority areas, is the basis for federal and state policy formulation and action; selected objectives related to the environment are listed in the *Healthy People 2010* box on page 75.

The public plays an important role in setting the stage for policy decisions by expressing its values and in the actions it takes as an electorate. Policy makers are also influenced by organized interest groups and elected and appointed officials who represent these interests. In the environmental health arena, these groups have traditionally been organized into two factions: (1) businesses and industries that depend on the environment for raw materials and/or disposal of waste and (2) citizen groups and voluntary organizations that have an interest in preventing or limiting the extraction of raw materials or disposal of waste. Nurses can work to foster health communication between groups and direct the dialog to areas of common ground. In addition to participation of citizens, nurses can enlarge their role in environmental health policy making by increasing their political expertise and activity as professionals.

In the United States, policy makers and the public alike trust the nursing profession to be advocates for clients and to speak and act on behalf of the health of the population. Nurses are reliable and trustworthy sources of information about threats to health and also represent the largest group of health care professionals among the voting age population. By staying informed of current and accurate information on environmental risks, organizing and becoming actively involved with groups of nurses and others around environmental issues, and actively communicating with and lobbying policy makers as well as organized interest groups, nurses can effectively influence public policy. In the practice arena, nurses can also inform and mobilize citizen groups and other professionals to become actively involved in communicating and lobbying policy makers about environmental issues of concern to themselves and their communities.

Nursing and the Environment

Nursing's efforts to promote health by influencing environmental conditions predate the modern environmental movement by more than a century. Florence Nightingale, the founder of modern nursing, developed her theory of nursing with a strong emphasis on the individual's environment. Although the term *environment* did not appear in her published works, she addressed health using five environmental dimensions: (1) pure, fresh air; (2) pure water; (3) efficient drainage; (4) cleanliness; and (5) light, that is, direct sunlight (Nightingale, 1969/1860). To Nightingale, the environment was the surrounding context in which the individual lived; a person's health or illness was a direct result of environmental influences. Deficiencies in any of the five factors produced a health deficit. Nightingale also stressed the importance of a comfortably warm, noise-free environment

CASE STUDY

Health Policy Actions Result from Community Involvement

Pam and Steven are registered nurses practicing at a mobile clinic that provides health care for migrant farm workers and their families in a midwestern state. They discuss the numerous children with skin and respiratory complaints that they have recently seen at the clinic. A review of clinic records reveals that more than twice the expected number of children had been seen in the clinic presenting with skin irritations, headaches, or abdominal cramping. The nurses begin to gather more detailed interview data from mothers who bring their children to the clinic with these symptoms. They learn that mothers are bringing their infants to the fields because there is no affordable day care available in this area. Older children work with their parents picking vegetables. They discuss their observations with the clinic's medical director and a toxicology consultant from the Migrant Council. They learn that the symptoms they have observed are common in pesticide exposure or poisoning.

A team from the clinic and Migrant Council visit the local vegetable fields and find multiple exposure risks for children. Some mothers carry infants into the fields in cloth carriers as they pick crops. Other infants are left at the edges of the crop rows in child carriers and strollers. Children as young as 4 years old pick vegetables next to their parents. Rubber gloves and other protective coverings are not available in sizes small enough for child workers. Some children are observed picking pesticide-dusted vegetables and eating them unwashed for lunch. On review of applicable federal and state laws, they find that while regulations protecting children from pesticides in foods are strict and clear, they are much less clear regarding protection of adults or children who harvest that food. Laws regulating or providing for safety for agricultural child workers are also not clear.

The team meets to examine the data collected and formulate an approach. They decide that an immediate priority is to reduce the potential pesticide exposures in this local area. They plan to work with farm owners to provide low-cost or no-cost day care and child-sized protective equipment. They also plan educational programs for migrant parents, offered after hours in their housing areas, focused on reducing exposures. Because migrant workers travel after harvest to other agricultural areas, reducing the problem in this area alone will not protect the children as they move to other areas. The team identifies informal leaders in the group of migrant workers and provides them with training in community development so that they will be better able to advocate for safe working conditions on behalf of their group wherever they work. The team also contacts legislators and policy makers to advocate for improved regulations to protect migrant workers and their families from pesticide exposures.

Source: Adapted from Crenson, 1997.

and a good diet. Although originally written for a hospital environment, her concepts were broad enough to serve as a basis for public health nursing also and remain integral parts of nursing and health care.

• •

Within the last few years, a large part of London was in the daily habit of using water polluted by the drainage of its sewers and water closets. This has happily been remedied. But, in many parts of the country, well water of a very impure kind is used for domestic purposes. And when epidemic disease shows itself, persons using such water are almost sure to suffer.

Florence Nightingale, 1860

• •

Nursing has long noted the influence of the environment on health and has assumed the role of managing the interaction between clients and their environments. Often, nursing's approach has been to assist the client to adapt to the environment; thus, the focus for intervention was changing the individual or community client to facilitate a better match with the environment. An emerging role for nursing today is to intervene directly in environmental factors in an attempt to change unhealthy conditions and mobilize individuals or communities to do the same. Nurse scientists are conducting studies on environmental factors directly, such as water and air quality, policies, laws that influence health of the population, and conditions in workers' environments to improve understanding of healthful/unhealthful

HEALTHY PEOPLE 2010

Objectives Related to Environmental Health

Outdoor Air Quality

8.1 Reduce the proportion of persons exposed to air that does not meet the U.S. Environmental Protection Agency's (EPA's) health-based standards for harmful air pollutants.

8.4 Reduce air toxic emissions to decrease the risk of adverse health effects caused by airborne toxics.

Water Quality

8.5 Increase the proportion of persons served by community water systems who receive a supply of drinking water that meets the regulations of the Safe Drinking Water Act.

8.8 Increase the proportion of assessed rivers, lakes, and estuaries that are safe for fishing and recreational purposes.

Toxics and Waste

8.11 Eliminate elevated blood lead levels in children.

8.12 Minimize the risks to human health and the environment posed by hazardous sites.

Healthy Homes and Healthy Communities

8.16 Reduce indoor allergen levels.

8.20 Increase the proportion of the nation's primary and secondary schools that have official school policies ensuring the safety of students and staff from environmental hazards, such as chemicals in special classrooms, poor indoor air quality, asbestos, and exposure to pesticides.

Infrastructure and Surveillance

8.27 Increase or maintain the number of territories, tribes, and states, and the District of Columbia that monitor diseases or conditions that can be caused by exposure to environmental hazards.

Global Environmental Health

8.29 Reduce the global burden of disease due to poor water quality, sanitation, and personal and domestic hygiene.

Source: DHHS, 2000.

---

environmental conditions and the interventions that can improve them.

Just as it is a challenge to draw a circle around the concept of environmental health, so too is it difficult to delineate the unique role of nursing in addressing environmental health issues. Many professional disciplines, from wildlife biologists to microbiologists to engineers, consider environmental health problems within their domain of expertise. Environmental health is an area in which many different professionals are needed to prevent, minimize, and improve environmental problems. Both basic and applied research efforts are required to understand all of the implications of environmental health problems. Professional nurses are well suited to participate in collaborative efforts because they have historically functioned at the center of the health care team.

However, nursing efforts are focused exclusively on human health, in contrast to some professions, whose efforts are directed toward other species such as fish, large mammals, and plant life. Nursing interventions are directed toward preventing and minimizing the effects of environmental health problems on persons of all ages. That does not mean, however, that concerns about animal and plant life are dismissed or that health connections between species are not recognized.

Community health and occupational health are the nursing practice specialties often associated with health hazards in the physical environment. In view of the universal presence of environmental hazards, it is critical that nurses in all practice specialties have an understanding of environmental health (Pope, Snyder, & Mood, 1995). As client advocates, all nurses need to be concerned about the health of the environment because it is a major determinant of their clients' health.

It is important to consider the depth of inquiry when addressing the role of nursing in environmental health. What areas of inquiry contain the dimensions of environment that fall within the scope of nursing? Surely, given enough time and paper, one could generate a seemingly endless list of questions that relate human health to the environment. The challenge then lies in the ability to focus nursing assessment activities into areas that are most obvious to the clinical or research area of interest. One would expect to see overlapping areas of focus between environmental health, as it relates to professional nursing, and other professions such as toxicology, pharmacology, and the behavioral sciences. The goal then is not to stake out a new specialty area for nursing practice, but rather to integrate knowledge from nursing and other disciplines and apply this knowledge to the clients' needs for health promotion or restoration. A research study directed by nursing scientists is discussed in the Research Brief on this page.

Looking at the environment from a broad view, environmental factors are involved in almost all disease risks and include areas such as housing, nutrition, socioeconomic status, and lifestyle. Even the health of persons with genetic disorders can often be enhanced through nursing actions addressing personal and societal aspects of the environment. Environmental health includes a concern for not only the physical environment, but also the interrelated social, economic, psychological, and political environments. Such conditions as poverty, powerlessness, social injustice, and racism that arise from diverse environmental factors can reduce opportunities for health and contribute to illness just as certainly as do chemical or physical agents. A central goal of this chapter is to provide information that allows for a richer understanding of the connectedness among many features of the environment. Although information addressing physical agents predominates in this chapter, it is important to understand that aspects of the social and economic environment are also centrally linked to opportunities for health in civilizations throughout the world.

Roles of the Community Health Nurse

Nursing has a long history of identifying health risks and intervening directly on behalf of client health. The role of the nurse in providing pure water, a restful setting, and a hygienic hospital environment were among the early environmental concerns of the nursing profession. By the late 1800s and early 1900s, nursing became concerned with identifying and resolving communicable disease outbreaks, improper food handling, inadequate disposal of wastes, and unsafe water supplies (Tiedje & Wood, 1995). During the growing environmental awareness of the 1960s and 1970s, nursing expanded its environmental concerns to include identification and interventions related to exposures

RESEARCH BRIEF

Amaya, M. A., Ackall, G., Pingitore, N., Quiroga, M., & Terrazas-Ponce, B. (1997). Childhood lead poisoning on the US-Mexico border: A case study in environmental health nursing lead poisoning. Public Health Nursing, 14, 353-360.

Amaya and colleagues have documented high rates of exposure to lead, trace elements, and pesticides in Hispanic persons residing in United States–Mexico border communities. As one part of a larger study examining the serum lead levels in pregnant Hispanic women, a case investigation of a family with two children with elevated lead levels was conducted. Dust samples were collected both inside and outside the residence; additional samples were taken from water, paint, and cookware in the home. The evidence supported a hypothesis that primary exposure occurred from battery recycling and burning of electrical wire conducted on the premises by the father and grandfather of the children. Steps to ameliorate exposure pathways were undertaken by community health nurses working with the family. Monthly lead levels taken on both children declined over the next 4 months. Unfortunately, the family moved away without notice and was lost to follow-up 9 months after the initial event.

Such investigations capitalize on the risk communication skills of nurses working in border communities. Nurses' abilities to locate and intervene effectively with disenfranchised families are unsurpassed among health professions. Case-series and case-control studies by nurse scientists can yield important findings at the local and national levels, while furthering the role of nursing in the environmental health sciences. Elevated blood lead levels have been reported in approximately 8% of low-income children in El Paso County, Texas. Nursing research addressing the areas of risk communication, health care access, and intervention strategies with families at risk for lead exposure can lead to a significant reduction of persons affected by this serious health problem.

to toxins and chemicals from the home and community environments. More recently, nursing has acknowledged that the environment relevant to our clients' health is larger and more multifaceted than appreciated before. Accordingly, nursing's concerns have expanded to regional, national, and global physical environmental hazards as well as influences arising from the social, economic, psychological, and political environments.

BOX 4-2 STEPS IN AN ENVIRONMENTAL RISK ASSESSMENT

1. Hazard identification: Does the agent cause the adverse effect?
2. Exposure assessment: What exposures are currently experienced or anticipated?
3. Dose-response assessment: What is the relationship between the dose and incidence?
4. Risk characterization: What is the estimated incidence of the adverse effect in a given population?

Identification of Risks

Community health nurses often emphasize primary prevention activities that address environmental health because many environmentally induced illnesses are preventable through risk management activities. In concert with other professionals, community health nurses often conduct a systematic review of risks known as a quantitative **risk assessment**. Risk is the probability of injury, disease, or death for individuals or populations exposed to hazardous substances. It may be expressed numerically (e.g., "one in 1 million"), but this is often impossible and therefore risk may be expressed using terms such as *high*, *medium*, or *low*. The steps involved in a risk assessment are outlined in Box 4-2. **Risk management** involves developing and evaluating possible regulatory actions guided by the risk assessment plus other ethical, political, social, economic, and technological factors (U.S. Congress, Office of Technology Assessment, 1990).

Comprehensive Exposure Assessment

Community health nurses often participate in exposure assessments following the development of a case or suspected cluster of disease. Because of their methodical skills in home assessment, nurses are often called on to conduct comprehensive exposure assessments in homes or occupational settings. Strong interview, observation, and family assessment skills are needed by nurses to collect these data in a clear and systematic manner. Clues to potential solutions to environmental risks may occur during the course of community or home assessments, although the resolution of some risks may require the expertise of non-nursing professionals. Home visits often require follow-up conversations with toxicologists, industrial hygienists, or other scientists who have expertise with the exposures of interest.

Exposure assessments are much simpler when clients present with an acute illness, such as acute pesticide poisoning or in-

halation fever. Assessments become much more complex when the specific types of agents have not been considered a priori or when the induction period between exposure and disease occurrence is unknown. The greatest challenges occur in persons with chronic disease or disease of unknown cause or when exposure to small doses of multiple agents has occurred over years or decades. In these types of clinical situations, it is very unusual to make a link between disease and a specific type of exposure with a high degree of confidence. Unusual conditions and rarer forms of cancer, such as the association between asbestos and development of mesothelioma, are the exception and can often be narrowed down to a specific place and time in a one's life. Box 4-3 (pages 78–79) includes basic information addressing the components of a home assessment and environmental exposure history. As one would expect, data collection is customized to address the unique aspects of the exposures, setting, and persons involved in the situation.

Communicating Risk

Often, the most successful strategies for responding to environmental risks affecting a community involve empowering citizens to address the problem. If successful, these strategies result not only in the resolution of the immediate problem but also in the creation of a group able to address future threats. Nurses should be encouraged to become familiar with the principles of environmental risk communication. An increased availability of information to the public increases the possibility that the community health nurse will be sought for advice and further information. Nurses are trusted in a community, and the public values their opinions. It is professionally responsible to share science-based information with persons most affected. Nurses should understand the influence of the environment and environmental agents on human health based on knowledge of relevant epidemiological, toxicological, and exposure factors. Basic principles of risk communication can be used in many environmental health situations, ranging from a toxic spill incident to a neighborhood meeting to discuss groundwater contamination. Overall, risk communication focuses on telling citizens what is known about a risk situation in a clear and forthright manner. In addition, it is important to directly explain what information is not currently known and the process by which additional information will be communicated to all parties. Basic guidelines addressing the principles of risk communication are listed in Box 4-4 (page 80).

Infants and children have a unique vulnerability to being exposed to chemical agents. Communicating a balanced view of these risks to parents is a challenge for nurses in the community. An example of this challenge involves the practice of breast-feeding. For many years, nurses have played a significant role in policies and clinical actions that support breast-feeding practices in new mothers. This advocacy role has been based on scientific findings that breast milk is the ideal infant food because of the easy digestibility of milk proteins, the presence of maternal antibodies, and safety from contamination through the use of improperly sanitized bottles. However, over the past two decades, scientists have become increasingly aware that human breast milk also carries a host of potentially serious risks to infant health. The greatest area of concern has been physiological evidence that many chemicals to which the mother has been exposed are transferred into breast milk. Of special interest are the findings from studies that examine the metabolism and fate of chemicals that have extremely long half-lives (i.e., years and decades) within human populations. Such agents include poly-

chlorinated organic pollutants, including organochlorine pesticides, polychlorinated biphenyls (PCBs), and polychlorinated dibenzodioxins and dibenzofurans (PCDDs/PCDFs), as well as some forms of metals such as methylmercury. In most cases, persons ingest these agents in their diets, usually from contaminated fish and animal products such as meats, fats, cheese, and eggs. In large doses, many pesticide products and mercury compounds have affected neurobehavioral, neuromotor, and speech development (Kimbrough, 1995). Unfortunately, much less is known about the long-term effects of low-dose exposure in breast milk. For a variety of feasibility and methodological reasons, scientific studies of low-dose and early life exposures are extremely difficult

BOX 4-3 CONDUCTING A HOME ASSESSMENT AND ENVIRONMENTAL EXPOSURE HISTORY

AREAS OF VISUAL INSPECTION

Examine areas in the immediate vicinity of the home for the presence of the following:

- Water hazards
- Automobile, farm, or other large equipment
- Garbage/waste storage containers
- Garages, sheds, or other outbuildings for safety hazards
- Chemical storage areas
- Pets or livestock
- Areas where rats or mice could live around home or outbuildings
- General age and condition of home (e.g., presence of peeling paint, metal edges from siding)

   Consider whether any of the aforementioned items constitute a health threat to any family members or to the community in general.

QUESTIONS TO CONSIDER IN ASSESSING ENVIRONMENTAL AGENTS IN THE HOME

Ask family members about the following areas:

- Hobbies or crafts involving potential for lead exposure (e.g., stained glass, ceramic glazing)
- Potential for significant exposure to gasoline or diesel exhaust from car repair activities or from nearby traffic

- Safe storage of food (stored where vermin cannot contaminate food) and proper cooking and refrigeration facilities
- Storage and use of insecticides, lawn care products, fertilizers
- Home heating—type of furnace, use of wood stoves
- Use of cleaning products that are strong irritants
- Fumigants or other products used for tick or flea control in the home
- Storage of food in copper or brass containers (can contaminate food with lead or copper)
- Exposure to wood preservatives (e.g., pentachlorophenol) in log homes
- Potential for lead exposure through lead-based plumbing
- Source of water (municipal or private well)
- Any seasonal changes in water sources during the year (e.g., private well during the winter and water delivered to a cistern during the summer months)
- Recent home renovation activities such as sanding or stripping of old paint that could result in lead exposure to family members

QUESTIONS ADDRESSING SYMPTOMS RELATED TO ENVIRONMENTAL AGENTS IN THE HOME

Does any member of the family have symptoms that they attribute to an environmental exposure? If so, elicit

Continued

BOX 4-3 CONDUCTING A HOME ASSESSMENT AND ENVIRONMENTAL EXPOSURE HISTORY—CONT'D

the nature of symptoms, duration, fluctuations in symptoms over the day and from week to week, seasonal changes, related symptoms in other family members or others who spend extended time in the home.

ASCERTAINING AGENT-SPECIFIC DATA FROM INDIVIDUALS

Exposures

- Concurrent and past exposures to metals, dust, fibers, fumes, chemicals, biological hazards, radiation, noise, vibration
- Typical work day (job tasks, location, materials, agents used)
- Changes in routines or processes
- Other employees or household members similarly affected

Health and safety practices at work site

- Ventilation
- Medical and industrial hygiene surveillance
- Employment examinations
- Personal protective equipment (e.g., respirators, gloves, coveralls)
- Lockout devices, alarms, training, drills
- Personal habits (smoking, eating in the work area, handwashing with solvents)

Work history

- Description of all prior jobs, including short-term, seasonal, or part-time employment and military service
- Description of present job(s)

Environmental history

- Present and prior home locations
- Jobs of household members
- Home insulating, heating and cooling system
- Home cleaning agents
- Pesticide exposure (e.g., pet flea treatments, roach and ant sprays)
- Water supply
- Recent renovation/remodeling
- Air pollution, indoor and outdoor
- Hobbies: painting, sculpting, welding, woodworking, piloting, autos, firearms, stained glass, ceramics, gardening
- Hazardous wastes/spills exposure

Medical history

- Past and present medical problems
- Medications

Source: Adapted from Agency for Toxic Substance and Disease Registry, 1992.

---

to conduct. Such studies often help in the incremental advancement of scientific understanding but are not able to yield clear-cut answers to clinical questions (Gladen, Monaghan, Lukyanova, Hulchiy, Shkyryak-Nyzhnyk, Sericano, & Little, 1999; Hooper, 1999).

Infants and children are particularly susceptible to the toxic effects of chemical exposure for a number of reasons. Pound for pound of body weight, a child eats much more food than an adult. Youngsters between the ages of 1 and 5 years eat and drink three to four times more food and water than adults. In addition to increased food intake, there is evidence that compared with adult bodies, the metabolic pathways of children have a diminished ability to metabolize or detoxify chemical agents effectively. There is increasing evidence that children's daily activity patterns, such as playing on the ground and hand-to-mouth behavior, can also increase their exposure to environmental toxicants. Because of incomplete scientific evidence about the long-term consequences of exposure to chemical agents, primary prevention activities that reduce the opportunity of exposure provide the first and most important line of defense on behalf of children's health (Schmidt, 1999).

Assessment and Referral

A critical piece of comprehensive nursing practice is the identification of high-risk clients so that they can be referred for further evaluation and follow-up. To provide such care for these clients, nurses must have a good understanding of environmental health resources located within their geographic area. In many communities, professionals with environmental health expertise, such as industrial hygienists, physicians, and toxicologists, are located in

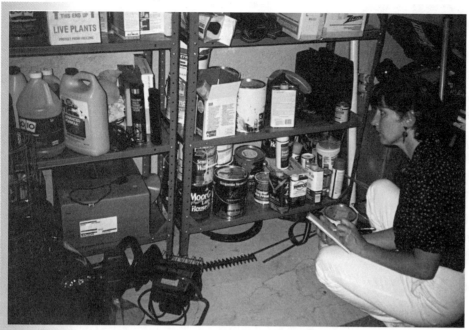

Chapter author, Dr. Patricia Butterfield, conducting a home environment exposure assessment.

BOX 4-4 BASIC GUIDELINES FOR RISK COMMUNICATION

Don't confuse people's understanding a risk with their acceptance of it—anger and resentment are often expressed when people are unwittingly exposed to an environmental hazard and feel that they have no control over the situation.

Avoid trivializing the risk or minimizing people's concerns. Frustration needs to be heard and acknowledged, not suppressed. It is important to listen attentively and respectfully to all concerns and respond in a clear manner with whatever information is currently available. Say what is known; also say what is not known. Gaining trust from the audience in a public meeting will not usually occur if people perceive that they are being patronized or placated. It is best to say what is currently known about the situation of concern and what is not known.

Often, health providers do not have all the information at hand or are waiting for additional information to come in (e.g., laboratory values or diagnostic tests from exposed persons). State clearly what information is not currently available and when that information will be available.

Respond to the different needs of different audiences. In an incident that involves a pesticide spill at a local school, the parents of schoolchildren will probably have different concerns than the janitor and physical facilities staff at the school. Think about your audience in advance—try to anticipate what questions you would have if you were in the audience and direct the discussion from that perspective.

Recognize that input from the public can help your agency make better decisions. Holding private meetings or trying to avoid public input is likely to fuel distrust in community members. By building in opportunities for affected persons to help remedy an environmental hazard situation, those persons gain a sense of control over the situation and feel like they are helping themselves and others. Think broadly about how to use citizens' help to get mailings out, set up phone trees, and form advocacy groups. If you do not allow citizens to work with you and your agency, they may begin to work against you.

Source: New Jersey Department of Environmental Protection, 1990.

the state health department. Other experts may be located in occupational health clinics in both hospital and community settings. For nurses working in agricultural communities, expertise in environmental health may often be found through contacts with county extension agents, pest management specialists, migrant and seasonal farm worker clinics, or agricultural medicine programs (Shreffler, 1996). It is essential that clients be referred to resources that are culturally and socioeconomically appropriate (Pope & Rall, 1995).

There is some evidence from applied research studies that both pediatric and adult clients are falling through the cracks of the health system when they are in need of specialized environmental health services. In a review of children residing in New York City, Markowitz, Rosen, and Clemente (1999) estimated that only 60% of high-risk children were being screened for lead poisoning; of those children who were found to have elevated lead levels, nearly 60% were not receiving timely follow-up by health care providers. In another recent study addressing the health consequences of lead exposure, elevated values were associated with an increased risk for hypertension later in life (Korrick, Hunter, Rotnitzky, Hu, & Speizer, 1999). A third environmental health study focused on persons at increased risk of developing lung cancer caused by both household radon exposure and cigarette smoking. Researchers developed statistical models of risk and determined that the most effective strategy to reduce the risk of radon-related cancer was smoking cessation. Stopping smoking was more effective in reducing cancer risk than directly reducing the levels of radon in the home (Mendez, Warner, & Courant, 1998). Although it is always optimal to reduce disease risk through all possible means (e.g., smoking cessation as well as radon reduction interventions), this study demonstrates the importance of addressing both environmental and behavioral means to minimize disease risk in exposed persons. Community health nurses are the health providers most familiar with their clients' home setting, lifestyle, work habits, and environmental exposures. Because of their unique presence in a variety of client settings, nurses may become aware of clients' environmental health risks and work toward directing them to an appropriate source of evaluation and treatment. A Case Study reflecting the need for ongoing assessment and education for families with asthma is presented in the box at right.

Upstream Thinking: Making Connections Between Environmental and Human Health

One of the most challenging areas in environmental health is linking a past exposure from 10 to 20 years ago with the development of a health problem. Even though we are intellectually aware that some agents have health consequences that may not be seen for years or decades, it can be difficult to take such a dis-

CASE STUDY

Asthma Management in a Young Girl

A community health nurse working in an urban area has been coordinating services with the school nurse practitioner at Northside Elementary, a primary school located in a low-income neighborhood. The nurse practitioner calls to request a home assessment for 7-year-old Lateesha. Lateesha is in the second grade, and the teacher notes that she has performed poorly in the classroom compared with her skill level during the previous year. In a phone interview, the mother states that she thinks the child's inattentiveness in the classroom results primarily from several recent colds that required Lateesha to miss school. The mother notes that Lateesha has missed 8 days of school so far this year and has had some difficulty with the make-up work following these absences.

When the nurse visits the home, she notes that Lateesha's mother, brother, sister, and grandmother live in a three-bedroom apartment near the school. When entering the home, the nurse notes that the room is very warm and sees an older model space heater in the kitchen area. The mother explains she wants to keep it warm for Lateesha's little sister, a 4-year-old who has complained that the apartment is too cool during winter. The nurse also notes several ashtrays in the living room and the presence of Tigger, the family cat. The mother informs the nurse that Lateesha has had four severe colds since October and that the last physician they saw at the clinic suggested that Lateesha has asthma. The mother received two types of inhalers for Lateesha following this clinic visit but notes that no one explained whether Lateesha is to use the inhalers every day or only after she develops a cold or breathing difficulties.

1. What should be the focus of the interventions of the community health nurse with this family?

tant and uncertain threat seriously. One conceptual approach that has been used in interdisciplinary public health efforts, referred to as *upstream thinking*, uses the analogy of a river to demonstrate connections between preceding exposures and later health consequences. This approach is based on an article by McKinlay (1979), who tells the story of a physician friend and his struggle to keep from feeling overwhelmed by the enormity of health problems that he encounters in clinical practice. The friend notes that he feels as if he is so caught up in rescuing individuals from the river that he has no time to look upstream to see who is pushing them in. In this analogy, the river represents illness and health providers' efforts to rescue people from illness. However, in this portrayal no one receives care until they are downstream in the river of illness, which precludes efforts to intervene before illness develops. McKinlay challenges providers to look upstream, where the real problems lie. The river analogy includes many concepts in community health nursing, including the natural history of disease and levels of prevention. The power of the upstream conceptualization of health lies in its simplicity and the ease with which one can connect the causes of disease with their consequences.

Upstream thinking lends itself well to health problems of environmental origin and can be helpful in guiding practice decisions that have long- and short-term consequences for our clients. Examples of environmental upstream nursing actions include the following:

- *Instructing a client to wear a respirator when stripping paint from an old home*
- *Encouraging farmers who work with pesticides to refrain from wearing their work boots into the house*
- *Developing a school policy to establish waiting periods for children to be off the playground following applications of fertilizers and herbicides*

In each situation, the nurse is acting from a primary prevention viewpoint to prevent or minimize the occurrence of an exposure. It is not even necessary to know the toxicology of all of the agents involved. Nurses can initiate an action and then seek guidance from experts in toxicology or other disciplines. The goal is to minimize the opportunity for harm by linking an understanding of nursing actions today with the prevention of harmful health effects in the future (Butterfield, 1990).

Ethical Principles Addressing Environmental Health Nursing

Nurses have a duty to safeguard clients from environmental hazards and risks regardless of clients' income, insurance status, or lack of access to care. The nurses' code of ethics addresses responsibilities to collaborate with other health professionals and citizens in promoting community and national efforts to meet the health needs of the public (ANA, 1985).

Justice is a highly valued ethical principle in most societies today and is one of the beliefs that guide the practice of nursing. The concept of fairness of opportunity is a value in the United States that is supported in laws that forbid discriminatory treatment that limits one's opportunities on the basis of unchangeable characteristics such as gender, race, or socioeconomic status. Social justice means fairness or equality in the distribution of the

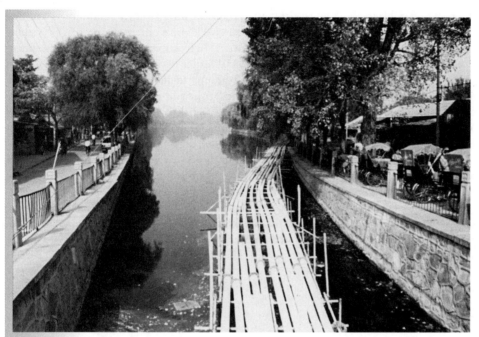

River in Hutong neighborhood in Beijing, China, demonstrating global clean-up efforts.

benefits and burdens of society. According to the principles of social justice, no one person or group should have a disproportionate share of the benefits available to a society nor of the burdens that are present.

When applied to environmental health, principles of social justice suggest that the ability to live in a healthy environment as part of the process for attaining or maintaining health should be available to all. Because health is of fundamental importance to having opportunities for life, liberty, and the pursuit of happiness, environmental risks that take place or are allowed to persist differentially that are based on gender, race, or socioeconomic status would not be consistent with justice or fairness of opportunity (Daniels, 1985). Justice is not served when some persons or groups have disproportionate shares of the benefits of healthy environments and others have disproportionate shares of the burdens of contaminated ones.

Most environmental hazards do not pose uniform or equal risks to the health of an entire population. Some widespread hazards, such as global warming, acid rain, and air or water pollution, involve an entire region or country, but most environmental health concerns involve different exposures within the same population. Some exposures occur because of behaviors or practices that could be considered changeable as a result of choices the individual makes. The decision to not wear protective gear when applying pesticides is an example of a choice that could easily be changed from health damaging to health protecting. Some exposures occur, however, because of unchangeable characteristics or circumstances of some individuals in the popula-

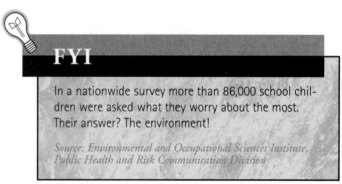

FYI

In a nationwide survey more than 86,000 school children were asked what they worry about the most. Their answer? The environment!

Source: Environmental and Occupational Sciences Institute, Public Health and Risk Communication Division

tion, such as socioeconomic status, race, powerlessness, age, or gender. Lead exposure, for example, is most common in children who live in low-income housing. The disposal of toxic waste into sites located near low-income neighborhoods whose residents lack the financial resources and power to prevent it is another example of disproportionate exposure to environmental hazards (Bullard, 1990, 1993).

The distinction between changeable and unchangeable courses of action may not always be clear-cut. For example, the training one receives about pesticide safety and the availability of safety equipment may affect the use of safety measures more than personal choice. Many environmental risks occur from exposures to toxic substances on the job. Some individuals may have the ability to change occupations to reduce risks, but many others cannot reasonably entertain such an option. It also may be possible to alter some risks such as living in low-income housing with lead-based paint. In this example, although residents' incomes and ability to relocate may be unchangeable, they can work to improve the safety in their current housing and influence landlords to correct or reduce environmental hazards such as removal of lead-based paint.

Nurses play a role in promoting environmental justice in several ways. Educating individuals on ways to reduce exposure to toxic substances is important. Giving information about contacts in health departments or work safety committees is helpful to individuals and groups. Helping groups organize and present a united voice to industries and politicians is important to people who may otherwise have been powerless to protest. Community health nurses know the strengths of their communities and are able to identify the people who could provide leadership to the group. Community health nurses are also already sensitive to their community's cultural or ethnic attributes, which may affect the process of seeking environmental justice. Activists concerned about environmental hazards and social justice have also begun to work with and for disadvantaged groups to increase their awareness of unequal environmental risks and possible strategies to improve them. Disadvantaged at-risk groups in a particular area may not be organized into a functioning community or have community or neighborhood organizations that can be readily mobilized for action. In this case, activists work with whatever organizations exist or form an informal group of concerned residents who may get others involved over time. An environmental hazard close to where people live is an issue that can be effective in organizing and mobilizing citizens to work together as a group.

CONCLUSION

The role of community health nurses in environmental health is evolving in several ways:

- *From illness treatment to illness recognition and prevention*
- *Toward a multidisciplinary foundation of basic and applied science*
- *Toward an emphasis on activities in which nursing excels, such as risk communication, community-based investigations, and client advocacy strategies*
- *Toward an integration of environmental health principles into all domains of nursing practice and research*

Knowledge of pollutants, whether physical, chemical, or biological, is characterized by incomplete science. The field is constantly changing, with the discovery of new hazards, but also innovative ways of minimizing hazard use and exposure. Nurses can participate in advancing environmental health science by participating in applied research activities on behalf of vulnerable groups or those disproportionately exposed to agents of concern.

Nurses have functioned at the fringe of power and politics, which has often been detrimental to the nursing profession, perhaps even to health care. In the field of environmental health, nurses are capable of making great contributions to the social, political, and economic forces that presently guide environmental health care policy. By broadening nurses' understanding of environment, new horizons in environmental health can be developed and expanded on behalf of the health of our clients, our nation, and our planet. The Case Study below uses a **thinking upstream** approach to explore nursing actions addressing social, economic, and political factors that culminate in the development of lead intoxication in children.

CASE STUDY

Broadening Nurses' Expertise in Environmental Health Clinical Practice—Thinking Upstream

Over the course of several years, a community health nurse was asked about water quality issues by clients attending the well-child clinic. These questions most commonly addressed parents' concerns about potable water contamination, and the nurse believed she was unqualified to answer these types of questions. After spending a few hours at home reviewing water quality information on the EPA's Internet home page, the nurse decided to seek some advice from the health department director about her lack of preparation to respond to clients' questions regarding environmental health. The director suggested that the nurse spend some time with a water quality specialist, who was located within another department, and authorized time for the nurse to work 1 week in that department. During her week with environmental health personnel, the nurse worked in the field when the environmental engineer inspected the installation of a private well west of town. She made a special

effort to talk with all of the people in the environmental health department so that she had a better understanding of the full range of expertise within the department. After working in the field, she visited the laboratory to observe testing procedures for water quality and to learn about the different water tests available to the public.

When she returned to the well-child clinic the following week, the nurse decided to allocate at least half an hour per day to developing a resource library on water quality issues in the clinic. She obtained educational brochures from the environmental health department; in addition, she established a system where nurses could give interested clients a plastic bottle for water sampling and have them send it directly to the laboratory for analysis. The nurse also asked the environmental engineer to make his phone number available to respond to any questions from clients about their water and septic systems.

Over the next year, the nurse provided continuing education for the nursing staff until they became more comfortable providing clients with specific information about water quality and differentiating between questions they could answer and those that were best re-

CASE STUDY—CONT'D

ferred to the engineers and scientists in the other department. Nurses came to understand that the prevention of problems held the key to long-term sustainability of water quality in their community and ecosystem. Many of the same principles of prevention that were so familiar to them in public health nursing could be applied equally well to actions to reduce opportunities for water pollution.

During the next few months, the nursing staff reached beyond its original contacts with the environmental health department and extended further into partnerships with other environmental information and advocacy groups in the area. They worked with the local university's pollution preven-

tion program to display and educate clients about the safe disposal of household products and solvents, to reduce solid waste, and to increase participation in recycling of paint and motor oil. Nurses found that they could often incorporate several minutes of "pollution prevention" instruction into many well-child visits and that parents were often appreciative of this information. The nurses worked to make other health departments aware of their efforts and presented a summary of their program at their annual public health association conference. As a culmination of their work, the nurses developed an Internet site to educate professional colleagues throughout the nation on their growing expertise in water quality and pollution prevention.

BOX 4-5 RESOURCES FOR ENVIRONMENTAL HEALTH INFORMATION

Agency for Toxic Substances and Disease Registry (ATSDR): Part of the U.S. Public Health Service. It conducts public health assessments, health consultations and investigations, health education, applied research, and emergency response. It maintains an exposure registry and toxicological profiles.

ATSDR
1600 Clifton Rd. NE (E-60)
Atlanta, GA 30333
(404) 639-0500
(404) 639-6204 (Division of Health Education)

Association of Occupational and Environmental Clinics: Conducts information sharing, education, and research through a network of clinics. It provides professional training, community education, exposure and risk assessment, clinical evaluations, and consultation services.

AOEC
1010 Vermont Ave NW
Suite #513
Washington, D.C. 20005
(202) 347-4976

Fax: (202) 347-4950
E-mail: aoec@dgs.dgsys.com
http://occ-env.med.mc.duke.edu/oem/aoec.htm

Nurses Environmental Healthwatch: Involved in educating nurses about environmental concerns and nursing's role in bringing about a safe, healthy environment.

Nurses Environmental Healthwatch
181 Marshall Street
Duxbury, MA 02332

Centers for Disease Control and Prevention (CDC): Protects the public health of the nation by providing leadership and direction in the prevention and control of diseases and other preventable conditions. It also responds to public health emergencies.

CDC
1600 Clifton Road, NE
Atlanta, GA 30333
(404) 639-3286

Consumer Product Safety Commission: Provides information on health and safety effects related

Continued

BOX 4-5 RESOURCES FOR ENVIRONMENTAL HEALTH INFORMATION—CONT'D

jurisdiction over chronic and chemical hazards in consumer products.

Consumer Product Safety Commission
East West Towers
4340 East West Highway
Bethesda, MD 20814
(301) 504-0580
(800) 638-2772

Environmental Protection Agency (EPA): Responsible for coordinated and effective governmental action on behalf of the environment.

EPA
401 M Street SW
Washington, D.C. 20460
(202) 260-2090

National Center for Environmental Health (NCEH): Preventing or controlling disease or injury related to the interactions between people and the environment outside the workplace.

NCEH
Mailstop F29
4770 Buford Highway NE
Atlanta, GA 30341-3724
(404) 488-7003

National Institute of Environmental Health Sciences (NIEHS): Principal federal agency for biomedical research on the effects of chemical, physical, and biological environmental agents on human health and well-being.

NIEHS
P.O. Box 12233
Research Triangle Park, NC 27709
(919) 541-7825

Pesticide Education Center: Seeks to educate the public about the hazards and health effects of pesticides. Works with the individuals or groups, conducts workshops.

PEC
P.O. Box 420870
San Francisco, CA 94142-0870
(415) 391-8511

Society for Occupational and Environmental Health (SOEH): Includes scientists, academicians, and industry and labor leaders seeking to improve the quality of working and living places.

SOEH
6728 Old McLean Village Drive
McLean, VA 22101
(703) 556-9222

CRITICAL THINKING ACTIVITIES

1. Take a walk or a drive around your own neighborhood and identify any potential environmental health risks. What kind of prevention interventions can be done to minimize exposure to these hazards? As a nursing student, what role can you play?

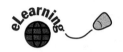 Explore Community Health Nursing on the web! To learn more about the topics in this chapter, access your exclusive web site: http://communitynursing.jbpub.com

REFERENCES

Agency for Toxic Substances and Disease Registry. (1992). *Case studies in environmental medicine (No. 26)—Taking an exposure history.* Atlanta: Author.

Amaya, M. A., Ackall, G., Pingitore, N., Quiroga, M., & Terrazas-Ponce, B. (1997). Childhood lead poisoning on the US-Mexico border: A case study in environmental health nursing lead poisoning. *Public Health Nursing, 14,* 353–360.

American Nurses Association (ANA). (1985). *Code for nurses with interpretive statements.* Kansas City, MO: Author.

Bullard, R. D. (1990). *Dumping in Dixie: Race, class, and environmental quality.* Boulder, CO: Westview Press.

Bullard, R. D. (1993). *Confronting environmental racism: Voices from the grassroots.* Boston: South End Press.

Butterfield, P. G. (1990). Thinking upstream: Nurturing a conceptual understanding of the societal context of health behavior. *Advanced Nursing Science, 12*(2), 1–8.

Carson R. (1962). *Silent spring.* Boston: Houghton Mifflin.

Clark N. M., Brosn, R. W., Parker, E., Robins, T. G., Remick, D. R. Jr., Philbert, M. A., Keeler, G. J., Israel, B. A. (1999). Childhood asthma. *Environmental Health Perspectives, 107* (Suppl. 3), 421–429.

Crenson, M. (1997, December 28). Kids at work in fields of unseen danger. *Missoulian,* p. A4.

Daniels, N. (1985). *Just health care.* Cambridge, MA: University Press.

Department of Health and Human Services, Public Health Service (DHHS). (1991). *Healthy people 2000* (Publication No. PHS-91-50212). Washington, DC: U.S. Government Printing Office.

Department of Health and Human Services, Public Health Service (DHHS). (2000). *Healthy People 2010. Conference edition.* Washington, DC: U.S. Government Printing Office.

Duchin, J. S, F. T. Koster, C. J. Peters, G. L. Simpson, B. Tempest, S. R. Zaki, T. G. Ksiazel, P. E. Rollin, S. Nichol, E. T. Umland, et al. (1994). Hantavirus pulmonary syndrome: A clinical description of 17 patients with a newly recognized disease. *New England Journal of Medicine, 330*(14), 949–955.

Eggleston, P. A., Buckley, T. J., Breysse, P. N., Wills-Karp, M, Kleeberger, S. R., Jaakkola, J. J. (1999). The environment and asthma in U.S. inner cities. *Environmental Health Perspectives, 107*(Suppl. 3), 439–450.

Environmental Protection Agency (EPA). (1993). *1991 toxics release inventory: Public data release* (EPA Pub. No. 745-R-93-003). Washington, DC: Office of Pollution Prevention and Toxics, EPA.

Fine, R. B. (1988). Consumerism and information: Power and confusion. *Nursing Administration Quarterly, 12*(3), 66–73.

Garrett, L. (1994). *The coming plague: Newly emerging diseases in a world out of balance.* New York: Penguin Books.

Garte, S. J. (1992). Environmental carcinogenesis. In Rom, W. N. (Ed.), *Environmental and occupational medicine* (2nd ed., pp. 105–123). Boston: Little, Brown.

Gladen, B. C., Monaghan, S. C, Lukyanova, E. M., Hulchiy, O. P., Shkyryak-Nyzhnyk, Z. A., Sericano, J. L., & Little, R. E. (1999). Organocholines in breast milk from two cities in Ukraine. *Environmental Health Perspectives, 107*(6), 459–462.

Gore, A. (1992). *Earth and the balance: Ecology and the human spirit.* Boston: Houghton Mifflin Co.

Henson, R. H., Robinson, W. L., & Schmele, J. A. (1996). Consumerism and quality management. In Schmele J. A. (Ed.), *Quality management in nursing and healthcare.* Albany, NY: Delmar.

Hooper, K. (1999). Breast milk monitoring programs (BMMPs): World-wide early warning systems for polyhalogenated POPs and for targeting studies in children's environmental health. *Environmental Health Perspectives, 107*(6), 429–430.

Kimbrough, R. D. (1995). Polychlorinated biphenyls (PCBs) and human health: An update. *Critical Review Toxicology, 25,* 133–163.

Kleffel, D. (1991). Rethinking the environment as a domain of nursing knowledge. *Advanced Nursing Science, 14*(1), 40–51.

Kleffel, D. (1996). Environmental paradigms: Moving toward an eccentric perspective. *Advanced Nursing Science, 18*(4), 1–10.

Korrick, S. A., Hunter, D. J., Rotnitzky, A., Hu, H., & Speizer, F. E. (1999). Lead and hypertension in a sample of middle-aged women. *American Journal of Public Health, 89*(3), 330–335.

Last, J. M. (1993). Global change: Ozone depletion, greenhouse warming, and public health. *Annual Review of Public Health, 14,* 115–136.

Markowitz, M., Rosen, J. F., & Clemente, I. (1999). Clinician follow-up of children screened for lead poisoning. *American Journal of Public Health, 89*(7), 1088–1089.

McKinlay, J. B. (1979). A case for refocusing upstream: The political economy of illness. In Jaco E. G. (Ed.), *Patients, physicians, and illness* (3rd ed., pp. 9–25). New York: The Free Press.

Mendez, D., Warner, K. E., & Courant, P. N. (1998). Effects of radon mitigation vs. smoking cessation in reducing radon-related risk of lung cancer. *American Journal of Public Health, 88*(5), 811–812.

New Jersey Department of Environmental Protection. (1990). *Improving dialogue with communities: A risk communication manual for government.* New Brunswick, NJ: Author.

Nightingale, F. (1969). *Notes on nursing.* New York: Dover. (Originally published by D. Appleton and Company, 1860).

Pope, A. M., & Rall, D. P. (Eds.). (1995). *Environmental medicine: Integrating a missing element into medical education.* Washington, DC: National Academy Press.

Pope, A. M., Snyder, M. A., & Mood, L. H. (Eds.) (1995). *Nursing, health and the environment: Strengthening the relationship to improve the public's health.* Washington, DC: National Academy Press.

Schmidt, C. W. (1999). Poisoning young minds. *Environmental Health Perspectives, 107*(6), A307–307.

Shreffler, M. J. (1996). An ecological view of the rural environment: Levels of influence on access to health care. *Advanced Nursing Science, 18*(4), 48–59.

Steingraber, S. (1997). *Living downstream: An ecologist looks at cancer and the environment.* Reading, MA: Addison Wesley.

Stevens, P. E., & Hall, J. M.(1997). Environmental health. In J. M Swanson & M. A. Nies (Eds.), *Community health nursing: Protecting the health of aggregates* (2nd ed., pp. 736–765). Philadelphia: W. B. Saunders.

Tiedje, L. B., & Wood, J. (1995). Sensitizing nurses for a changing environmental health role. *Public Health Nursing, 12*(6), 356–365.

U.S. Congress, Office of Technology Assessment. (1990, April). *Neurotoxicity: Identifying and controlling poisons of the nervous system* (Publication No. OTA-BA-436). Washington, DC: U.S. Government Printing Office.

Valanis, B. (1996). *Epidemiology in nursing and health care* (3rd ed.). Norwalk, CT: Appleton & Lange.

APPENDIX

ENVIRONMENTAL AGENTS AND THEIR ADVERSE HEALTH EFFECTS

Note: This table is not meant to be comprehensive, but to provide examples of several types of agents.

AGENT	EXPOSURE	ROUTE OF ENTRY	SYSTEM(S) AFFECTED	PRIMARY MANIFESTATIONS	AIDS IN DIAGNOSIS	REMARKS
METALS AND METALLIC COMPOUNDS						
ARSENIC	Alloyed with lead and copper for hardness; manufacturing of pigments, glass, pharmaceuticals; byproduct in copper smelting; insecticides; fungicides; rodenticides, tanning	Inhalation and ingestion of dust and fumes	Neuromuscular	Peripheral neuropathy, sensory-motor	Arsenic in urine	
			Gastrointestinal	Nausea and vomiting, diarrhea, constipation		
			Skin	Dermatitis, finger and toenail striations, skin cancer, nasal septum perforation		
			Pulmonary	Lung cancer		
ARSINE	Accidental byproduct of reaction of arsenic with acid; used in semi-conductor industry	Inhalation of gas	Hematopoietic	Intravascular hemolysis; hemoglobinuria, jaundice, oliguria or anuria	Arsenic in urine	
BERYLLIUM	Hardening agent in metal alloys; special use in nuclear energy production; metal refining or recovery	Inhalation of fumes or dust	Pulmonary (and other systems)	Granulomatosis and fibrosis	Beryllium in urine (acute); Beryllium in tissue (chronic); chest x-ray; immunological tests (such as lymphocyte transformation) may also be useful	Pulmonary changes virtually indistinguishable from sarcoid on chest x-ray
CADMIUM	Electroplating; solder for aluminum; metal alloys, process engraving; nickel-cadmium batteries	Inhalation or ingestion of fumes or dust	Pulmonary	Pulmonary edema (acute); Emphysema (chronic)		Also a respiratory tract carcinogen
			Renal	Nephrosis	Urinary protein	
CHROMIUM	In stainless and heat-resistant steel and alloy steel; metal plating; chemical and pigment manufacturing; photography	Percutaneous absorption, inhalation, ingestion	Pulmonary	Lung cancer	Urinary chromate (questionable value)	
			Skin	Dermatitis, skin ulcers, nasal septum perforation		
LEAD	Storage batteries; manufacturing of paint, enamel, ink, glass, rubber, ceramics, chemical industry	Ingestion of dust, inhalation of dust or fumes	Hematological	Anemia	Blood lead	Lead toxicity, unlike that of mercury, is believed to be reversible, with the exception of late renal and
			Renal	Nephrotoxicity	Urinary ALA	
			Gastrointestinal	Abdominal pain ("colic")	Zinc protoporphyrin; free erythrocyte protophyrin	
			Neuromuscular	Palsy ("wrist drop")		
				Encephalopathy, behavioral abnormalities		

Source: Tarcher, A. B. (Ed.). (1992). Principles and practice of environmental medicine. New York: Plenum Press.

Continued

AGENT	EXPOSURE	ROUTE OF ENTRY	SYSTEM(S) AFFECTED	PRIMARY MANIFESTATIONS	AIDS IN DIAGNOSIS	REMARKS
METALS AND METALLIC COMPOUNDS—cont'd						
LEAD cont'd			Central nervous system (CNS)			some CNS effects
MERCURY Elemental	Electronic equipment; paint; metal and textile production; catalyst in chemical manufacturing; pharmaceutical production	Inhalation of vapor; slight percutaneous absorption	Reproductive Pulmonary CNS	Spontaneous abortion (?) Acute pneumonitis Neuropsychiatric changes (erethism); tremor	Urinary mercury	Mercury illustrates several principles. The chemical form has a profound effect on its toxicology, as is the case for many metals. Effects of mercury are highly variable. Though inorganic mercury poisoning is primarily renal, elemental and organic poisoning are primarily neurological.
MERCURY Inorganic	Agricultural and industrial poisons	Some inhalation and gastrointestinal (GI) and percutaneous absorption	Pulmonary Renal CNS	Acute pneumonitis Proteinuria Variable	Urinary mercury	The responses are difficult to quantify, so dose-response data are generally unavailable.
Organic		Efficient GI absorption, percutaneous absorption, and inhalation	Skin CNS	Dermatitis Sensorimotor changes, visual field constriction, tremor	Blood and urine mercury (sensitivity?)	Classic tetrad of gingivitis, sialorrhea, irritability, and tremor is associated with both elemental and inorganic mercury poisoning; the four signs are not generally seen together. Many effects of mercury toxicity, especially those in CNS, are irreversible.
NICKEL	Corrosion-resistant alloys; electroplating; catalyst production; nickel-cadmium batteries	Inhalation of dust or fumes	Skin Pulmonary	Sensitization dermatitis ("nickel itch") Lung and paranasal sinus cancer		
ZINC OXIDE	Welding byproduct; rubber manufacturing	Inhalation of dust or fumes that are freshly generated		"Metal fume fever" (fever, chills, and other symptoms)	Urinary zinc (useful as an indicator of exposure, not for acute diagnosis)	A self-limiting syndrome of 24-48 hours with apparently no sequelae

Continued

AGENT	EXPOSURE	ROUTE OF ENTRY	SYSTEM(S) AFFECTED	PRIMARY MANIFESTATIONS	AIDS IN DIAGNOSIS	REMARKS
HYDROCARBONS						
BENZENE	Manufacturing of organic chemicals, detergents, pesticides, solvents, paint removers; used as a solvent	Inhalation of vapor; slight percutaneous absorption	CNS Hematopoietic Skin	Acute CNS depression Leukemia, aplastic anemia Dermatitis	Urinary phenol	Note that benzene, as with toluene and other solvents, can be monitored via its principal metabolite
TOLUENE	Organic chemical manufacturing; solvent; fuel component	Inhalation of vapor, percutaneous absorption of liquid	CNS Skin	Acute CNS depression Chronic CNS problems such as memory loss Irritation dermatitis	Urinary hippuric acid	
XYLENE	A wide variety of uses as a solvent; an ingredient of paints, lacquers, varnishes, inks, dyes, adhesives, cements; an intermediate in chemical manufacturing	Inhalation of vapor; slight percutaneous absorption of liquid	Pulmonary Eye, nose, throat CNS	Irritation, pneumonitis, acute pulmonary edema (at high doses) Irritation Acute CNS depression	Methylhippuric acid in urine, Xylene in expired air, xylene in blood	
KETONES Acetone(Methyl ethyl Ketone-MEK, Methyl n-proply Ketone-MPK, Methyl n-butyl Ketone-MBK, Methyl iso-butyl Ketone-MIBK)	A wide variety of uses as solvents and intermediates in chemical manufacturing	Inhalation of vapor, percutaneous absorption of liquid	CNS Peripheral nervous system (PNS) Skin	Acute CNS depression MBK has been linked with peripheral neuropathy Dermatitis	Acetone in blood, urine, expired air (used as an index for exposure, not for diagnosis)	The ketone family demonstrates how a pattern of toxic responses (i.e., CNS narcosis) may feature exceptions (i.e., MBK peripheral neuropathy)
FORMALDEHYDE	Widely used as a germicide and a disinfectant in embalming and histopathology, for example, and in the manufacture of textiles, resins, and other products	Inhalation	Skin Eye Pulmonary	Irritant and contact dermatitis Eye irritant Respiratory tract irritation, asthma	Patch testing may be useful for dermatitis	Recent animal tests have shown it to be a respiratory carcinogen. Confirmatory epidemiological studies are in progress
TRICHLORO-ETHYLENE (TCE)	Solvent in metal degreasing, dry cleaning, food extraction; ingredient of paints, adhesives, varnishes, inks	Inhalation, percutaneous absorption	Nervous Skin Cardiovascular	Acute CNS depression Peripheral and cranial neuropathy Irritation, dermatitis Dysrhythmias	Breath analysis for TCE	TCE is involved in an important pharmacological interaction. Within hours of ingesting alcoholic beverages, TCE workers experience flushing of the face, neck, shoulders, and

Agent	Exposure	Route of Entry	System(s) Affected	Primary Manifestations	Aids in Diagnosis	Remarks
HYDROCARBONS—cont'd						
TRICHLORO-ETHYLENE (TCE) cont'd						back. Alcohol may also potentiate the CNS effects of TCE. The probable mechanism is competition for metabolic enzymes
CARBON TETRACHLORIDE	Solvent for oils, fats, lacquers, resins, varnishes, other materials; used as a degreasing and cleaning agent	Inhalation of vapor	Hepatic Renal CNS Skin	Toxic hepatitis Oliguria or anuria Acute CNS depression Dermatitis	Expired air and blood levels	Carbon tetrachloride is the prototype for a wide variety of solvents that cause hepatic and renal damage. This solvent, like trichloroethylene, acts synergistically with ethanol
CARBON DISULFIDE	Solvent for lipids, sulfur, halogens, rubber, phosphorus, oils, waxes, and resins; manufacturing of organic chemicals, paints, fuels, explosives, viscose rayon	Inhalation of vapor, percutaneous absorption of liquid or vapor	Nervous Renal Cardiovascular Skin Reproductive	Parkinsonism, psychosis, suicide Peripheral neuropathies Chronic nephritic and nephrotic syndromes Acceleration or worsening of atherosclerosis; hypertension Irritation; dermatitis Menorrhagia and metrorrhagia	Iodine-azide reaction with urine (nonspecific since other bivalent sulfur compounds give a positive test); CS_2 in expired air, blood, and urine	A solvent with unusual multi-system effects, especially noted for its cardiovascular, renal, and nervous system actions
STODDARD SOLVENT	Degreasing, paint thinning	Inhalation of vapor, percutaneous absorption of liquid	Skin CNS	Dryness and scaling from defatting; dermatitis Dizziness, coma, collapse (at high levels)		A mixture of primarily alphatic hydrocarbons, with some benzene derivatives and naphthalenes
ETHYLENE GLYCOL ETHERS (Ethylene glycol monoethyl ether-Cellosolve, Ethylene glycol monoethyl acetate-Cellosolve acetate, Methyl- and butyl-substituted compounds such as ethylene glycol mono-methyl ether-methyl Cellosolve)	The ethers are used as solvents for resins, paints, lacquers, varnishes, gum, perfume, dyes, and inks; the acetate derivatives are widely used as solvents and ingredients of lacquers, enamels, and adhesives. Exposure occurs in dry cleaning, plastic, ink, and lacquer manufacturing, and textile dying, among other processes	Inhalation of vapor, percutaneous absorption of liquid	Reproductive CNS Renal Liver			Ethylene glycol ethers, as a class of chemicals, have been shown in animals to have adverse effects including reduced sperm count and spontaneous abortion, as well as CNS, renal, and liver effects

Agent	Exposure	Route of Entry	System(s) Affected	Primary Manifestations	Aids in Diagnosis	Remarks
HYDROCARBONS—cont'd						
ETHYLENE OXIDE	Used in the sterilization of medical equipment, in the fumigation of spices and other foodstuffs, as a chemical intermediate	Inhalation	Skin	Dermatitis and frostbite		Recent animal tests have shown it to be carcinogenic and to cause reproductive abnormalities. Epidemiologic studies indicate that it may cause leukemia in exposed workers
			Eye	Severe irritation; possibly cataracts with prolonged exposure		
			Respiratory tract	Irritation		
			Nervous system	Peripheral neuropathy		
DIOXANE	Used as a solvent for a variety of materials, including cellulose acetate, dyes, fats, greases, resins, polyvinyl polymers, varnishes, and waxes	Inhalation of vapor, percutaneous absorption of liquid	CNS	Drowsiness, dizziness, anorexia, headaches, nausea, vomiting, coma		Dioxane has caused a variety of neoplasms in animals
			Renal	Nephritis		
			Liver	Chemical hepatitis		
POLY-CHLORINATED BIPHENYLS (PCBS)	Formerly used as dielectric fluid in electrical equipment and as a fire retardant coating on tiles and other products. New uses were banned in 1976, but much of the electrical equipment currently used still contains PCBs	Inhalation, ingestion, skin absorption	Skin Eye Liver	Chloracne Irritation Toxic hepatitis	Serum PCB level for chronic exposure	Animal studies have demonstrated that PCBs are carcinogenic. Epidemiological studies of exposed workers are inconclusive
IRRITANT GASES						
AMMONIA	Refrigeration; petroleum refining; manufacturing of nitrogen-containing chemicals, synthetic fibers, dyes, and optics	Inhalation of gas	Upper respiratory tract	Upper respiratory irritation		
			Eye	Irritation		
			Moist skin	Irritation		
HYDROCHLORIC ACID	Chemical manufacturing; electroplating; tanning; metal pickling; petroleum extraction; rubber, photographic, and textile industries	Inhalation of gas or mist	Upper respiratory tract	Upper respiratory irritation		
			Eye	Strong irritant		
			Mucous membranes, skin	Strong irritant		

Continued

AGENT	EXPOSURE	ROUTE OF ENTRY	SYSTEM(S) AFFECTED	PRIMARY MANIFESTATIONS	AIDS IN DIAGNOSIS	REMARKS
IRRITANT GASES—cont'd						
HYDROFLUORIC ACID	Chemical and plastic manufacturing; catalyst in petroleum refining; aqueous solution for frosting, etching, and polishing glass	Inhalation of gas or mist	Upper respiratory tract	Upper respiratory irritation		In solution, causes severe and painful burns of skin and can be fatal
SULFUR DIOXIDE	Manufacturing of sulfur-containing chemicals; food and textile bleach; tanning; metal casting	Inhalation of gas, direct contact of gas or liquid phase on skin or mucosa	Middle respiratory tract	Bronchospasm (pulmonary edema or chemical pneumonitis in high dose)	Chest x-ray, pulmonary function tests	Strong irritant of eyes, mucous membranes, and skin
CHLORINE	Paper and textile bleaching; water disinfection; chemical manufacturing, metal fluxing; detinning and dezincing iron	Inhalation of gas	Middle respiratory tract	Tracheobronchitis, pulmonary edema, pneumonitis	Chest x-ray, pulmonary function tests	Chlorine combines with body moisture to form acids, which irritate tissues from nose to alveoli.
OZONE	Inert gas-shielded arc welding; food, water, and air purification; food and textile bleaching; emitted around high-voltage electrical equipment	Inhalation of gas	Lower respiratory tract	Delayed pulmonary edema (generally 6-8 hours following exposure)	Chest x-ray, pulmonary function tests	Ozone has a free radical structure and can produce experimental chromosome aberrations; it may thus have carcinogenic potential.

AGENT	EXPOSURE	ROUTE OF ENTRY	SYSTEM(S) AFFECTED	PRIMARY MANIFESTATIONS	AIDS IN DIAGNOSIS	REMARKS
IRRITANT GASES—cont'd						
NITROGEN OXIDES	Manufacturing of acids, nitrogen containing chemicals, explosives, and more; byproduct of many industrial processes	Inhalation of gas	Lower respiratory tract	Pulmonary irritation, bronchiolitis fibrosa obliterations ("silo filler's disease"), mixed obstructive-restrictive changes	Chest x-ray, pulmonary function tests	
PHOSGENE	Manufacturing and burning of isocyanates, and manufacturing of dyes and other organic chemicals; in metallurgy for one separation; burning or heat source near trichloroethylene	Inhalation of gas	Lower respiratory tract	Delayed pulmonary edema (delay seldom longer than 12 hours)	Chest x-ray, pulmonary function tests	
ISOCYANATES TDI (toluene diisocyanate) MDI (methylene diphenyldiiscyanate) Hexamethylene diisocyanate and others	Polyurethane manufacture; resin-binding systems in foundries; coating materials for wires; used in certain types of paint	Inhalation of vapor	Predominantly lower respiratory tract	Asthmatic reaction and accelerated loss of pulmonary function	Chest x-ray, pulmonary function tests	Isocyanates are both respiratory tract "sensitizers" and irritants in the conventional sense.
ASPHYXIANT GASES (simple asphyxiants: nitrogen, hydrogen, methane, and others)	Enclosed spaces in a variety of industrial settings	Inhalation of gas	CNS	Anoxia	O_2 in environment	No specific toxic effect; act by displacing O_2

Continued

Agent	Exposure	Route of Entry	System(s) Affected	Primary Manifestations	Aids in Diagnosis	Remarks
CHEMICAL ASPHYXIANTS						
CARBON MONOXIDE	Incomplete combustion in foundries, coke ovens, refineries, furnaces, and more	Inhalation of gas	Blood (hemoglobin)	Headache, dizziness, double vision	Carboxy-hemoglobin	
HYDROGEN SULFIDE	Used in manufacturing of sulfur-containing chemicals; produced in petroleum product use; decay of organic matter	Inhalation of gas	CNS Pulmonary	Respiratory center paralysis, hypoventilation Respiratory tract irritation	PaO$_2$	
CYANIDE	Metallurgy, electroplating	Inhalation of vapor, percutaneous absorption, ingestion	Cellular metabolic enzymes (especially cytochrome oxidase)	Enzyme inhibition with metabolic asphyxia and death	SCN in urine	
PESTICIDES						
ORGANOPHOS-PHATES (malathion, parathion, and others)		Inhalation, ingestion, percutaneous absorption	Neuromuscular	Cholinesterase inhibition, cholinergic symptoms: nausea and vomiting, salivation, diarrhea, headache, sweating, meiosis, muscle fasciculations, seizures, unconsciousness, death	Refractoriness to atropine; plasma or red cell cholinesterase	As with many acute toxins, rapid treatment of organophosphate toxicity is imperative. Thus diagnosis is often based on history and a high index of suspicion rather than biochemical tests. Treatment is atropine to block cholinergic effects and 2-pyradine-alsoxine methiodide (2-PAM) to reactivate cholinesterase

Agent	Exposure	Route of Entry	System(s) Affected	Primary Manifestations	Aids in Diagnosis	Remarks
PESTICIDES—cont'd						
CARBAMATES: (carbaryl [Sevin] and others)		Inhalation, ingestion, percutaneous absorption	Neuromuscular	Cholinesterase inhibition, cholinergic symptoms: nausea and vomiting, salivation, diarrhea, headache, sweating, meiosis, muscle fasciculations, seizures, unconsciousness, death	Plasma cholinesterase; urinary 1–naphthol (index of exposure)	Treatment of carbamate poisoning is the same as that of organophosphate poisoning except that 2-PAM is contraindicated
CHLORINATED HYDRO-CARBONS (chlordane DDT heptachlor chlordecone (Kepone) aldrin dieldrin uridine)		Inhalation, ingestion, percutaneous absorption	CNS	Stimulation or depression	Urinary organic chlorine, or p-chlorophenol acetic acid	The chlorinated hydrocarbons may accumulate in body lipid stores in large amounts.
BIPYRIDYLS (paraquat diquat)		Inhalation, ingestion, percutaneous absorption	Pulmonary	Rapid massive fibrosis, only following paraquat ingestion		An interesting toxin in that the major toxicity, pulmonary fibrosis, apparently occurs only after ingestion.

Chapter 5
Politics and the Law

Sharyn Janes, Karen Saucier Lundy,
and Heather Rakauskas Sherry

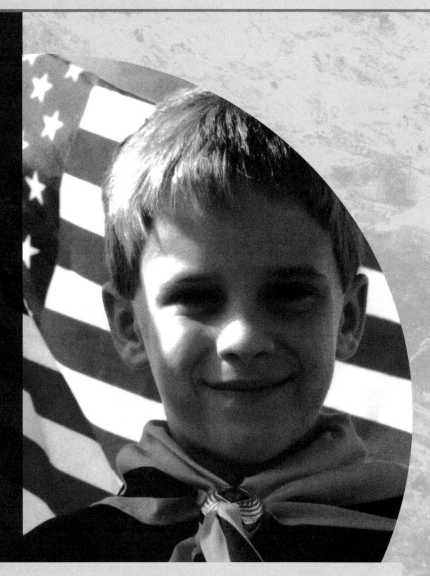

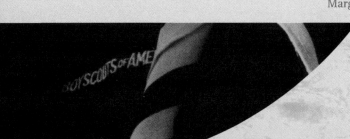

Never doubt that a small group of thoughtful, committed citizens can change the world; indeed, it's the only thing that ever does.
Margaret Mead

QUESTIONS TO CONSIDER

After reading this chapter, answer the following questions:

1. What is the role of the government in the health of its citizens?
2. How do the concepts of power and authority relate to public health regulation?
3. What is the history of governmental roles in health care?
4. What are the three branches of the federal government? What does each do in relation to health?
5. How is state government organized? How does it relate to health care?
6. What are the different kinds of laws?
7. What are the steps in the development of laws?
8. How can nurses be involved in the development of law and policy?
9. What are the primary issues related to regulation and licensure of nursing practice?
10. What settings are more likely to be influenced by legal issues in the practice of community health nursing and why?

KEY TERMS

Bill of Rights
Coercive power
Connection power
Constitutional law
Correctional nursing
Democracy
Equality
Executive branch
Expert power

Federal Register
Freedom
Information power
Judicial branch
Judicial or common law
Legislative branch
Legitimate power
Licensure

Lobbying
Malpractice
Negligence
Nurse Multistate Licensure
   Mutual Recognition Model
Nurse practice act
Police power
Political action committees
   (PACs)

Political power
Power
Preamble of the U.S.
   Constitution
Referent power
Regulatory process
Reward power
Statutory law
U.S. Constitution

While the political efforts of movers and shakers like Florence Nightingale, Lillian Wald, and Margaret Sanger are well documented, politics and policy have been historically seen as "outside" the scope of nursing. For most nurses, "political activism" meant voting in national and state elections. By the closing years of the 20th century, however, nurses began to realize that they could influence public policy by using nursing knowledge and skills. In 1992, acknowledging that decisions affecting nurses and their clients were being made in the national political arena, the American Nurses Association (ANA) moved its national headquarters to Washington, D.C. (Milstead, 1999).

Government Authority
Protection of the Public's Health

The early American colonists viewed health as controlled by divine intervention. They believed it was a result of self-care, and minimal governmental intervention was expected. Because health care was not a power granted to the federal government (such as defense or printing money), it developed into a power of the states or was left to the people themselves. Governmental health care and policies to provide funding and resources for health care were, for all practical purposes, nonexistent in the early days of the United States (Turnock, 1997).

As each new American colony was founded, the way in which it would be governed was a primary consideration. The specific problems and situations that each new colony faced varied so widely that each developed its own procedures and laws based on its own needs. From this evolved the idea of states' rights, which continues to play a critical role in the governance of health care policies, such as seat belt laws and immunization laws. Any attempts to limit the power of the states, either by the federal government or other states, is usually strongly opposed. Most states, for instance, will have similar laws about school attendance, drinking age, and immunizations, but the regulations themselves will vary considerably.

Federal law is based on the **U.S. Constitution**, which was ratified in 1789. The creators of the Constitution were careful to limit the federal government's involvement in the daily lives of citizens. The word *health* was never mentioned in the U.S. Constitution, making health care legislation problematic, because the Constitution therefore grants limited power in the creation of health laws. The Constitution has been amended 26 times. The first 10 amendments, known as the **Bill of Rights**, were adopted within 3 years of the Constitution's ratification. The Bill of Rights focuses on the protection of our most basic value: freedom. Freedom of speech, freedom of the press, and due process are all included. In recent years, the constitutional amendments have had relevance to health care issues. For example, the Fourteenth Amendment provides protection of personal liberty, such

as a woman's right to choose to have an abortion. It is important to note, however, that neither the U.S. Constitution nor state constitutions guarantee access to health care. States retain whatever power the U.S. Constitution does not specifically define in federal law. State power concerning health care is termed police power. The state can use its power to protect the health, welfare, and safety of its citizens by establishing boards of nursing and medicine and passing immunization laws (Kelly & Joel, 1996).

Power, Authority, and the Health of the Public

Politics is always about power—who gets it, how it is obtained, how it is applied, and to what purposes it is used (Bacharach & Lawler, 1980). The German sociologist Max Weber defined power as the ability to control the behaviors of others, even in the absence of their consent (Weber, 1947). Power then is the capacity to participate effectively in a decision-making process. If citizens cannot or do not affect the process, they are powerless (Lenski, 1984).

Power can be classified as either legitimate or illegitimate. Power is considered legitimate if people recognize that those who apply it have the right to do so. This includes elected government officials, aristocracy, and those believed to be inspired by God. Weber referred to legitimate power as authority (Bacharach & Lawler, 1980). A simple illustration of this authority is that if the police stop you for speeding and levy a fine against you, you will recognize the law and the person carrying out the law as legitimate and you will probably obey. A political system can exist only if the people see the authority as legitimate. Most persons must see it as desirable, workable, and better than alternatives. We may complain about our legal system and its excesses or our Congress members and their self-serving interests, but most of us believe that the system works to our benefit most of the time. Once the bulk of citizens in any society no longer consider the political system legitimate, it is doomed, for its power can then rest only on coercion, which will eventually fail. Most revolutions, such as the French Revolution, the Iranian Revolution, and the American Revolution, were preceded by an erosion of the legitimacy of the existing political system (Robertson, 1981).

• •

Among the Indians there have been no written laws. Customs handed down from generation to generation have been the only laws to guide them. Every one might act different from what was considered right if he choose to do so, but such acts would bring upon him the censure of the Nation. . . . This fear of the Nation's censure acted as a mighty band, binding all in one social, honorable compact.
George Copway (Kah-ge-ga-bowh), Ojibwa Chief, 1818–1863

• •

Concepts of Power

Political power is defined by Hewison (1994) as the "ability to influence or persuade an individual holding a governmental office to exert the power of that office to [effect] a desired change" (p. 1171). What allows some people to have more influence than others? Where does such power come from? Nurses can benefit from understanding these sources of power. French and Raven (1959) identify five power bases:

1. *Coercive power, which is the use of force to gain compliance, often born out of real or perceived fear or threat to self. Police often use coercive power.*

2. *Reward power, which involves giving something of value for compliance. Compliance then results from the perceived potential for reward or favor of someone in power. A politician may help constituents obtain money for a new hospital in exchange for their political support.*

3. *Expert power, which results from expert knowledge or skills. Bill Gates has considerable expert power because of his expertise in computers and systems.*

4. *Legitimate power, which results from a title or position, such as an elected judge or the surgeon general.*

5. *Referent power, which results from being closely associated with someone who is powerful; for example, the aide or spouse of a senator. This can also be referred to as reflected power.*

Hersey, Blanchard, and Natemeyer (1979) added two additional sources of power:

6. *Information power, which results from the desire for information held by one person from one who does not have access to the information. This is commonly seen in the diplomatic corps of the United States.*

7. *Connection power, which results from the belief that a certain person has a special connection to a person or organization believed to be powerful. Lobbyists often use this kind of power when working with legislators' staff assistants (Helvie, 1998).*

One primary way of gaining power as a nurse is through knowledge. Nurses can use their knowledge of politics, power, and the change process to introduce change favoring health in the legislative process. Nurses have historically had very little interest in achieving power. Others have too long been the "voice" of nursing, and nurses and their clients have suffered through lack of appropriate nurse advocacy (Huston, 1995).

Another way that nurses can achieve power is through affiliating with others who have similar interests in health. Through networking and using the power of numbers, nurses can effect change through those in power positions. Coalitions of people and organizations are most effective in bringing about change (Helvie, 1998).

....

When nurses fully understand the impact of policy in the health care arena, when nurses fully understand the importance of tying outcomes research to public policy and when nurses fully understand the politics of health care, and mobilize their numbers and influence behind the political process, only then will the health system thrive, and with nurses as key players.

Betty Dickson, Mississippi Nurses Association
Executive Director and Lobbyist

....

The idea of a nation-state is relatively new. The concept emerged in Europe only a few centuries ago, then spread to the Americas, and spread to most parts of Africa and Asia only during the 20th century. In the founding of the United States, a representative democracy was a new idea. **Democracy** comes from a Greek word meaning "rule of the people," and this is no doubt what Abraham Lincoln had in mind when he defined democracy as "government of the people, by the people, and for the people." Democracy in the United States requires that we recognize the powers of the government as being derived from the consent of the governed. We elect representatives who are responsible for making political decisions. According to Robertson (1981), "Representative democracy is historically recent, rare and fragile" (p. 488).

There are five basic conditions that must exist for a democracy to thrive:

1. *Advanced economic development: This almost always involves an urbanized, literate, and sophisticated population that expects and demands participation in the political process.*

2. *Restraints on government power: This involves institutional checks on the power of the state (Robertson, 1981).*

3. *Consensus on basic values and a widely held commitment to existing political institutions.*

4. *Tolerance of dissent.*

5. *Access to information: A democracy depends on its citizens to make informed choices. There must be a free press.*

....

Give me liberty or give me death!

Patrick Henry, 1775

....

Freedom versus Equality

Freedom is defined in the United States as freedom "of"—freedom of speech, freedom of the press, and so on. In more socialist societies, freedom is defined as freedom "from"—freedom from hunger, freedom from unemployment, freedom from exploitation by people who want to make a fortune. In the United States, we equate freedom with "liberty." Socialist societies equate freedom with "equality." In general, the more liberty that exists in a society, the less equality. Your liberty to be richer than anyone else violates other people's right to be your equal; other people's right to be your equal violates your liberty to make a fortune. In the United States, we have chosen to emphasize liberty, which evolves from our value system. This emphasis can lead only to social inequality. Socialist societies emphasize equality, thus limiting personal liberty (Robertson, 1981).

In health care we often fail to understand why laws cannot be easily passed to impose penalties on persons who engage in risky behavior, such as requiring helmets for motorcyclists or tubal ligations for women who have injured their children through neglect or abuse. The answer lies in our emphasis on freedom in the United States and the limited power of the state. Recognizing and understanding these basic concepts about our government can help us use our skills and resources in the political process much more efficiently.

••••••••••••••••••••••••••••

Eternal vigilance is the price of liberty.

Wendell Phillips, 1852

••••••••••••••••••••••••••••

Evolution of the Government's Role in Health Care

The **Preamble of the U.S. Constitution** states that one of the purposes of the federal government is to "promote the general welfare" of the people. This can be found in Article 1, Section 8. The federal government derives its power to become involved in health care activities from this simple declaration. Because of this very general statement, the degree of health care services provided by the federal government is often a source of conflict among the various constituents and political parties. As a capitalistic society, and lacking clear direction from the U.S. Constitution, the provision of health services for the general population has historically been the concern of private enterprise. Private physicians delivered services to clients, and clients in turn paid a fee for that service. This concept has been the foundation of medical care provision in the United States since the beginning (Miller, 1992).

The first involvement of the federal government in health care was highly specialized for government employees. As early as 1796, the Marine Hospital Service was established to provide care for sick and disabled seamen. In 1852, St. Elizabeth Hospital in Washington, D.C., was established to provide health care for federal employees. A landmark study, the Shattuck Report, written in 1850, recommended measures such as the creation of local and state boards of health; collection of vital statistics; and supervision of housing, factories, sanitation, and communicable disease control. Soon health departments in major cities became common. The Shattuck Report is considered the basis for the development of local and state health departments. Military personnel were soon cared for through the federal government,

---

BOX 5-1 1965: WHAT A YEAR FOR HEALTH LAW IN THE UNITED STATES!

- Drug Abuse Control Amendments of 1965 (Public Law No. 89-74)
- Federal Cigarette Labeling and Advertising Act (Public Law No. 89-92)
- Construction Act Amendments of 1965 (Public Law No. 89-105)
- Community Health Services Extension Amendments of 1965 (Public Law No. 89-109)
- Health Research Facilities Amendments of 1965 (Public Law No. 89-115)
- Water Quality Act of 1965 (Public Law No. 89-234)
- Heart Disease, Cancer, and Stroke Amendments of 1965 (Public Law No. 89-239)
- The Clean Air Act Amendments and Solid Waste Disposal Act of 1965 (Public Law No. 89-272)
- Health Professions Educational Assistance Amendments of 1965 (Public Law No. 89-290)
- Medical Library Assistance Act (Public Law No. 89-291)
- Appalachian Regional Development Act of 1965 (Public Law No. 89-4)
- Older Americans Act (Public Law No. 89-73)
- Social Security Amendments of 1965 (Public Law No. 89-97)
- Vocational Rehabilitation Act Amendments of 1965 (Public Law No. 89-333)
- Housing and Urban Development Act of 1965 (Public Law No. 89-117)

Source: Forgotson, 1967.

---

which eventually led to the Veterans Administration (VA). The VA is currently the largest health care system in the United States.

It was not until after World War II that the federal government ventured into health care and community health programs for the general population. In 1946, the Hill-Burton Act provided funds for building hospital facilities in many communities. Government funding for specific treatments for disease did not happen until the 1960s. Before the 1960s, the federal government primarily provided programs for the economically disadvantaged populations. The social welfare programs of the 1960s brought about the most dramatic changes in federal involvement in health care. The establishment of Medicare in 1965 was significant in that it became the first program to provide health services to citizens other than federal employees. The basic purpose of Medicare was to provide health care for the elderly. The Medicaid program was developed in 1965 and provided health care for low-income individuals. See Box 5-1 for a list of the most significant health legislation acts passed during the "turning point decade" of the 1960s.

The Civil Rights Act of 1964, although not directly related to health, provided fair access to health facilities for all races and genders. The Environmental Protection Agency (EPA) was created through the National Environmental Policy Act and is historically one of the most significant pieces of U.S. environmental health policy. In recent years, significant legislation has been passed, including the Americans with Disabilities Act in 1990. This act increased the opportunities for Americans with disabilities to be integrated into mainstream society by removing physical barriers and improving public accommodation and services.

Government

Federal Government

The federal government consists of three separate branches—Executive (Office of the President), Legislative (Congress), and Judicial (federal court system). All three branches have a powerful impact on the health care delivery system and nursing practice. Nurses should be aware of how the different branches of the government affect health care policy and the ways that nurses can have a voice.

Executive Branch

The **Executive branch** consists of the president, the vice president, the Office of Management and Budget, and the cabinet departments, whose leadership is appointed by the president and approved by Congress. The cabinet departments that have the greatest effect on health care policy and nursing education, research, and practice are the Department of Health and Human Services, the Department of Education, and the Department of Labor.

The Department of Health and Human Services

The Department of Health and Human Services (DHHS) is the federal agency most concerned with protecting the health of all Americans and providing essential human services, especially for those who are least able to help themselves. There are more than 300 programs under DHHS supervision, with a wide spectrum of activities and services. Some of these services include the following (DHHS,1999):

- *Medical and social science research*
- *Communicable disease prevention, including immunization services*
- *Financial assistance for low-income families*
- *Child abuse and domestic violence prevention*

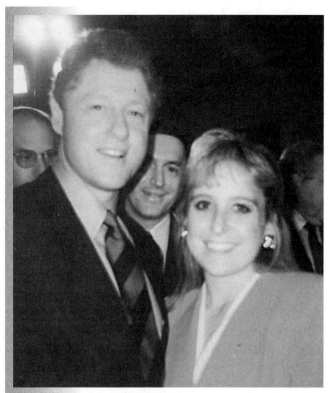

Chapter author, Heather Rakauskas Sherry, and President Bill Clinton.

- *Medicare and Medicaid*
- *Child support enforcement*
- *Food and drug safety*
- *Maternal and infant health improvement*
- *Services for older Americans*
- *Substance abuse treatment and prevention*

Box 5-2 lists a few of the health offices and services under the umbrella of DHHS.

BOX 5-2 U.S. DEPARTMENT OF HEALTH AND HUMAN SERVICES

Office of the Secretary of Health and Human Services
Office of the Assistant Secretary/Surgeon General
Administration on Aging
Administration for Children and Families
Health Care Financing Administration
Social Security Administration
Public Health Service

U.S. Public Health Service. The U.S. Public Health Service (PHS) is responsible for the administration of many of the most familiar federal health care agencies and services. The PHS is headed by the surgeon general of the United States, who is appointed by the president. The 200th anniversary of the PHS was celebrated in 1998. In 200 years, the PHS has grown from a handful of contract physicians to eight operating divisions within the DHHS, with more than 50,000 health care professionals and a 6,000-member, all-officer Commissioned Corp (Satcher, 1998). The operating divisions of the PHS are outlined in Box 5-3 and described below. Many nurses are employed by all divisions of the PHS, including a chief nurse, who holds the rank of rear admiral.

The mission of the Agency for Health Care Policy and Research (AHCPR) is to generate and distribute information that improves health care delivery. AHCPR funds cross-cutting research on health care systems, health care quality and cost issues, and effectiveness of medical treatments (DHHS, 1999). Along with the American Academy of Nursing, the AHCPR sponsors a nursing scholar in the agency to study the integration of clinical nursing care with issues of cost and access to health care (Bednash, Heylin, & Rhome, 1998).

The Agency for Toxic Substances and Disease Registry (ATSDR) monitors and funds research programs and interventions aimed at preventing health-related problems associated with exposure to toxic substances. Working with states and other federal agencies, the ATSDR conducts public health assessments, health studies, surveillance activities, and health education programs in communities near waste sites on the EPA's National Priorities List. Toxicological profiles have been developed for hazardous chemicals found at these sites (DHHS, 1999).

Services to prevent and treat mental health problems and substance abuse are provided through the Substance Abuse and Mental Health Services Administration (SAMHSA). Funding is provided through block grants to the states for substance abuse and mental health services, including treatment for more than 340,000 Americans with severe substance abuse problems

---

A CONVERSATION WITH...

At no other time in our nation's history has our country so needed the expertise of nurses in the development of health policy. As our nation struggles to reverse the tide of rising numbers of uninsured children and adults, to increase consumer involvement in health choices, and to care for our expanding aging population, we must turn to the expertise of our nation's nurses.

I have spent many years with nurses. In Congress, I worked closely with the American Nurses Association on issues of pay equity and equal rights. In 1984, ANA was the first group to endorse my candidacy for Vice President. In my 1992 race for the U.S. Senate, I reached out to a nurse, Judy Leavitt, to work on health policy and be a leader in my campaign. And again, in 1998, I turned to the nurses for their expertise in my U.S. Senate campaign.

—Geraldine Ferraro,
former member of the U.S. House of
Representatives (D–New York) and 1984 U.S.
Vice Presidential Candidate

Source: Mason, D. J., & Leavitt, J. K. (Eds.). (1998). Policy and politics in nursing and health care. Philadelphia: W. B. Saunders.

(DHHS, 1999). Funding for education and research is disbursed through SAMHSA's Center for Mental Health Services, Center for Substance Abuse Treatment, and Center for Substance Abuse Prevention (Bednash, Heylin, & Rhome, 1998).

The Centers for Disease Control and Prevention's (CDC) mission is to promote health and quality of life by preventing and controlling disease, injury, and disability. The CDC employs more than 7,000 people in 192 different occupations (CDC, 1998). The focus of the CDC is on the community as the client, allowing nurses to make significant contributions in a variety of areas. Nurses are involved in the establishment of infection control guidelines and the prevention of substance abuse, human immunodeficiency virus (HIV), and other sexually transmitted diseases, as well as in the areas of violence, adolescent and school health, women's health, infants' and children's health, and immunization (Bednash, Heylin, & Rhome, 1998). The CDC also guards against international disease transmission with CDC personnel stationed in more than 25 foreign countries (USDHHS, 1999).

The mission of the U.S. Food and Drug Administration (FDA) is to ensure safe food and cosmetics, safe and effective medicines and medical treatments, and safe products such as mi-

---

BOX 5-3 U.S. PUBLIC HEALTH SERVICE

Agency for Health Care Policy and Research

Food and Drug Administration

Agency for Toxic Substances and Disease Registry

Health Resources and Services Administration

Substance Abuse and Mental Health Services Administration

National Institutes of Health

Centers for Disease Control and Prevention

Indian Health Service

crowave ovens (Bednash, Heylin, & Rhome, 1998). FDA approval is needed before any experimental drugs can be tested or sold in the United States.

The Health Resources and Services Administration (HRSA) helps provide health resources for medically underserved populations. HRSA consists of the Office of Rural Health, the Bureau of Primary Care, the Bureau of Maternal and Child Health, the Office of Minority Health, and the Bureau of Health Professions. The Bureau of Health Professions contains the Division of Nursing, which oversees funding for undergraduate and graduate nursing education programs (Bednash, Heylin, & Rhome, 1998). A nationwide network of HRSA community and migrant health centers, as well as primary care programs for the homeless and residents of public housing, serve more than 8 million Americans each year. HRSA provides services to persons with HIV or acquired immunodeficiency syndrome (AIDS) through the Ryan White CARE Act programs, oversees the organ transplant system, and works to decrease infant mortality and improve child health (DHHS, 1999).

The Indian Health Service (IHS) provides comprehensive health services to Native Americans and Alaska Natives primarily living on reservations. In 1999, the IHS had 37 hospitals, 60 health centers, 3 school health centers, and 46 health stations. In addition, the IHS provided assistance to 34 urban Indian health centers. Services are provided to nearly 1.5 million Native Americans and Alaska Natives of 557 federally recognized tribes (DHHS, 1999).

The National Institutes of Health (NIH) funds and conducts health research through 19 different institutes and centers, including the National Institute of Nursing Research (NINR). The National Institute of Nursing Research began as an NIH center in 1986 and was elevated to institute status in 1993. The research funded through NINR focuses on health promotion and disease prevention, acute and chronic illness, and nursing systems (Bednash, Heylin, & Rhome, 1998).

Department of Education

The U.S. Department of Education provides billions of dollars each year for postsecondary education, including nursing education. Federal Family Education Loans (Stafford Loans), Pell Grants, Perkins Loans, and Federal Work Study programs are just a few of the sources of funding provided (Bednash, Heylin, & Rhome, 1998).

Department of Labor

The U.S. Department of Labor is responsible for enforcing the Fair Labor Standards Act (minimum wage and overtime), the Employee Retirement Income Security Act (employee benefit and retirement plans), and the Occupational Safety and Health Act (OSHA) (job safety and health). All these are important to nursing practice. The ANA has worked closely with the Department of Labor for nearly 20 years to ensure adequate funding for

the health and safety of nurses in the workplace through enforcement of OSHA standards (Bednash, Heylin, & Rhome, 1998).

Legislative Branch

The U.S. Congress is the legislative branch of the federal government. Congress has two houses with equal power: the Senate and the House of Representatives. The Senate has 100 members, two from each state. The House of Representatives membership varies according to the population. A representative is elected to represent a specific number of constituents, so states with larger populations have more representatives. The number of representatives a state has increases or decreases with corresponding changes in the state's population. The House of Representatives currently has more than 400 members. The sole legislative power of the federal government lies with the two houses of Congress. A partial list of the responsibilities of the U.S. Congress is outlined in Box 5-4.

Judicial Branch

The **judicial branch** of the federal government, known as the U.S. court system, consists of 94 federal district courts, 13 circuit courts of appeals, the U.S. Supreme Court, and several specialized courts to address customs, patents, military issues, and so on. A Supreme Court justice generally keeps his or her appointment until retirement or death. At that time, a replacement is appointed to the position by the president and approved by Congress.

Although the judicial branch of the government is not involved in making policy, the way in which the courts interpret the law may have a profound effect on health care, including

---

BOX 5-4 RESPONSIBILITIES OF THE U.S. CONGRESS

- Conduct hearings on issues that may generate federal legislation.
- Draft legislation.
- Estimate cost of proposed legislation.
- Enact legislation to create programs.
- Review legislated program operations.
- Determine the federal budget.
- Appropriate funds for federal operations.
- Decide entitlement policy (e.g., Medicare, Medicaid, Social Security).
- Confirms or rejects presidential nominations for high-level federal positions (e.g., cabinet members, federal judges).

Source: Bednash, Heylin, & Rhome, 1998.

" A CONVERSATION WITH... "

In 1991 I received a telephone call from Geraldine Ferraro asking me to come to New York City to be interviewed for a leadership position on her campaign for a United States Senate seat representing the state of New York. How did Gerry find me and why did she want a nurse to work on a major national campaign?

My connection to Gerry followed one of the most important principles of political involvement and influence—"use your connections." I had spent a sabbatical year at the ANA working in the governmental affairs department. While there, I collaborated with one of the women who had been involved in Gerry's nomination for vice president of the United States in 1984. She knew Gerry was considering a run for the U.S. Senate, so she called her to recommend my political skills to her. Gerry indicated a strong interest in working with me because of my involvement with ANA, the first group to endorse her candidacy for vice president. Gerry called me and hired me a week later.

For a year and half I worked as the upstate campaign coordinator. I was responsible for 54 of the 62 counties in the state, an area that covers over 40,000 square miles. I started with nothing except a great candidate. I had to organize an office, create a database of contacts, organize a grassroots network, raise thousands of dollars, and create fundraising and media events. Although I had been an active volunteer in numerous congressional and state legislative campaigns, I had never been a paid staff member. I did not have an appointed position in the political party, so I had to use all my communication skills, organizational skills, and nursing intuition to create a campaign presence in every one of the 54 counties under my leadership.

It helped to have a candidate with name recognition. When I called major democratic leaders and potential supporters I didn't have to introduce my candidate. I used my connections and those of Gerry to build a grassroots structure. I focused on women's organizations, women leaders, nurses and their organizations, other health professionals, and any other men and women throughout the state who wanted to volunteer for Gerry. Gerry's candidacy energized and excited the electorate, as it had when she ran for vice president. It wasn't hard getting volunteers; it was only

difficult organizing them to contribute in meaningful ways. Whether it was organizing events for fundraising, working with the media, conducting voter registration drives, or soliciting political endorsements, it took incredible planning and organizational skill and thousands of volunteer hours. I planned it all—over 200 events—supported by a grassroots structure of over 5000 volunteers from every profession, occupation, and interest group who held campaign events, gave money, and worked for Gerry in their home communities.

The nurses came out in droves. Nurses who had never been involved politically suddenly wanted to help Gerry and listen to her message. Because I had been active in both the ANA-PAC and New York State political activities, I was able to help Gerry receive an early endorsement by the ANA-PAC and encourage New York State Nurses Association to mobilize their members.

What was it like to work so closely for such a national and international "celebrity"? It was fun, grueling, exciting, challenging, and a once in a lifetime experience. What made it easy was Gerry. She was personable, caring, and in many ways very much like her constituents. She had experienced poverty as well as success; she was a

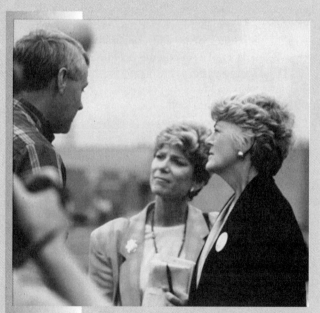

Judy Leavitt and 1984 vice presidential candidate, Geraldine Ferraro.

teacher and a lawyer; she was a mother, grandmother, and wife—so she knew about the issues and could relate to people throughout the country. She used me to draft her health platform and respected my expertise in teaching her about the issues. In addition, Gerry was able to bring the best political and media consultants to work with me and the campaign staff. Traveling with Gerry was the most fun of the entire year and a half. We would often spend two or three days alone traveling throughout the upstate counties, affording us an opportunity to become good friends. I was the oldest staff person, much closer in age to Gerry. That created a special bond that enabled me to have access

to her and engendered mutual respect. At each event, I would sometimes look around as she was speaking and think how lucky I was to be able to have the opportunity to help elect someone whom I admired and believed could have been a fine senator. Unfortunately that never happened. Gerry lost in the primary election by less than 10,000 votes out of 4 million cast. The country lost the chance to have a great senator. I gained a friend and stories for a lifetime.

—Judy Leavitt,
MEd, RN, Campaign Manager for Geraldine Ferraro,
Candidate for U.S. Senate in 1992

nursing practice. Nurses can affect the outcome of court cases by serving as expert witnesses or legal consultants (Bednash, Heylin, & Rhome, 1998).

State Government

Although the role of the federal government is in the forefront of American politics, the truth is that most of the policies and laws related to nursing practice are created at the state level. The creation and enforcement of nurse practice acts and the regulation of nursing practice through licensing occurs at the state level. In 1996, more than 100,000 bills were introduced in state legislatures across the country, with about 25% of them affecting nurses and nursing practice (Gaffney, 1998). State governments consist of the same three branches as the federal government: executive, legislative, and judicial.

Executive Branch

The executive branch of state government consists of the governor, the lieutenant governor, and the attorney general. Most governors are elected to 4-year terms and are eligible for reelection. The governor is responsible for presenting the state budget to the legislature and overseeing state spending. The governor's policy initiatives are often presented as part of the state budget proposal and may contain health-related programs. The lieutenant governor presides over state affairs in the absence of the governor and can influence health and social policies within the state. The attorney general represents the public's interests in legal cases coming before the court, not including the state supreme court. The attorney general's office is often called on to interpret the nurse practice act to clarify the intent of legislation or regulations (Gaffney, 1998).

State Agencies

State agencies may be divided into five different categories:

1. *Agencies led by elected officers such as secretaries of state, treasurers, and attorney generals*

2. *Agencies led by officers appointed by the governor or independent boards, such as secretaries of human services and commissioners of health*

3. *Professional licensing and regulatory boards, such as boards of nursing*

4. *Public authorities and corporations, such as higher education assistance authorities*

5. *Independent boards and commissions, such as councils of higher education and public utilities commissions*

The Department of Health is a state organization whose primary purpose is to oversee and maintain the health of the community. The director of the state department of public health is appointed by the governor. There are many different divisions within the department of public health, which may include data collection and surveillance, administration of Medicaid and other federally funded programs, public health programs, and hospital regulation (Gaffney, 1998).

Legislative Branch

State legislatures are the oldest part of the American government, existing long before the drafting of the U.S. Constitution. In fact, the Declaration of Independence was signed by representatives of the legislatures of the 13 colonies that became the original 13 states. State legislatures levy taxes, appropriate funding, and create and monitor agencies to carry out state business (Gaffney, 1998). Patterned after the federal legislature, all state legislatures (excluding Nebraska) are comprised of two houses: a Senate and a House of Representatives. In each state, the House of Representatives is larger than the Senate because senators represent larger districts within the state than members of the House. Therefore, each senator has a greater number of constituents.

Judicial Branch

State judicial systems are similar to that of the federal system. The state supreme courts serve to interpret the language of their state constitutions and apply it in the courtroom. In recent years, there has been an upheaval in state law related to health care. Many more malpractice suits are being brought against physicians, nurses, and hospitals by people who believe that they have been injured as a result of negligence or inappropriate action (Gaffney, 1998).

Local Government

Local governments are the link between citizens and the state and federal governments. Local governments distribute billions of federal and state dollars to local community agencies to provide services. The quality of life in a community is determined by how local government officials make decisions about the delivery of services. Some of the services provided and monitored by local governments are public health, public education, drinking water, sewage disposal, police protection, and solid waste management (Majewski & O'Brien, 1998).

The number, size, and type of local government varies throughout the country depending on state and regional culture, economics, and geography. The U.S. Census Bureau has divided local governments into four categories: counties, municipalities, towns and townships, and special districts (Majewski & O'Brien, 1998). Local governments are divided into the same branches of government (with variations) as the federal and state governments.

Different Types of Law

According to Webster's New World College Dictionary (Neufeldt, 1996), a law is a rule of conduct established and enforced by the authority, legislation, or custom of a given community, state, or other group. There are three types of laws in the United States: constitutional law, legislation and regulation, and judicial or common law.

Constitutional law is derived from federal and state constitutions and is the supreme law of the land. The U.S. Constitution is the highest legal authority that exists, and no other law, state or federal, may overrule it. A state constitution is the highest state law authority, but any provisions that conflict with the federal constitution will be invalidated by the courts. It is not considered a conflict, however, if state constitutions provide more expansive individual rights than those guaranteed by the federal constitution (Kaplan, 1985).

Legislation and regulation, known as **statutory law**, is established through formal legislative processes. Each time the U.S. Congress or state legislatures pass legislation, the body of statutory law grows (Betts & Waddle, 1993). Statutes are enacted by both federal and state governments. Local statutes, called *ordinances,* are enacted by local governing bodies, such as city and county councils (Kaplan, 1985).

Judicial or common law, known as case law, is derived from decisions made in the courtroom. Common law is based on the principles of justice, reason, and common sense rather than rules and regulations (Guido, 2001). Each time a judge or a jury makes a decision, the body of common law grows (Betts & Waddle, 1993). Decisions are made based on decisions from previous similar cases. Judges are bound by previous decisions (i.e., precedents) unless it can be shown that the previous rulings are no longer valid. Therefore, a decision made in a case with no predecessors is critical because it becomes a precedent-setting case.

Common law can be categorized as either civil or criminal. Civil law protects individuals and involves the enforcement of rights, duties, and other legal relations between private citizens (Betts & Waddle, 1993). For example, an individual can sue another individual or a company for not fulfilling the terms of a legal contract. Criminal law is a crime against the state and involves public concerns against unlawful behavior that threatens society (Betts & Waddle, 1993). Murder is an example of criminal law. Although the crime was committed against an individual, it threatens the security of society as a whole.

How an Idea Becomes a Law

In today's climate of health care reform, nurses must understand the legislative process to be able to influence the development of sound health care policy for their clients and for the profession of nursing (Abood & Mittelstadt, 1998). Because the legislative process is similar at both the state and federal levels, it is described at the state level in this chapter. Although the legislative pathway may differ slightly from state to state, the basic process is the same (Abood & Mittelstadt, 1998). The state of Florida is used as the example.

A bill can be introduced only by a member of the legislature. Legislators introduce bills for many reasons, which may include pleasing a constituent or a special interest group, declaring a position on an issue, getting publicity, or simply avoiding a political attack (Abood & Mittelstadt, 1998). Companion bills (or twin bills) are sometimes introduced by legislators in the Senate and House of Representatives to increase the likelihood that the bill will pass and become law.

During a legislative session, the House and Senate meet separately and attempt to pass legislation that has previously been considered by a number of legislative committees. Committees are often referred to as the "heart of the legislative process" because they allow legislators to break down into smaller groups to discuss pertinent issues (Florida Legislature, 1994a). This enables members to have more in-depth discussions than would be possible if all issues were discussed by the entire legislature. Committees are established by authority of rules, which are adopted separately by the House and the Senate. The Speaker of the House and the President of the Senate, both of whom are elected by each body and represent the majority party, designate a chair and a vice-chair for each committee and appoint legislators to serve as committee members. Legislators usually serve on more than one committee.

There are three basic kinds of committees: standing, select, and conference committees. Standing committees are established by both the Senate and the House of Representatives to manage their business. They can be distinguished from each other by the kind of issues that they consider. For example, the Florida House of Representatives has a standing committee on health care licensing and regulation, which is responsible for considering bills relating to that particular area. The staff of this committee is responsible for doing the fact-finding groundwork for legislation that is referred to the committee for consideration. For example, if the committee were considering a bill proposing a change in the requirements for registered nurse (RN) licensure, it would study the current licensure requirements, find out why the sponsor of the bill (one or more of the representatives) believes the change is necessary, examine what the effects of the proposed change might be, and hear testimony from nurses, as well as the broader health care community, to gain insight about how they feel about the proposed change. Once all these things are considered, the committee passes judgment on the proposed legislation.

If the bill passes the committee, it travels either to the next committee of reference (if there is more than one) or to the floor of the House or Senate to be voted on by the respective body as a whole. If the committee does not pass the proposed legislation (reports unfavorably on the bill), the legislation will die unless two thirds of the members vote to reconsider it. This is a very high percentage, and further consideration is unlikely to occur in this situation.

Committees wield significant power in the legislative process. The chair of each committee has a great deal of influence over legislation because he or she decides which bills will be heard by the committee. If a bill is not heard, it cannot be voted on and therefore cannot be passed. Committees also have the authority to amend proposed legislation, so the original bill may look very different by the time it reaches the floor of the House or Senate.

A second type of committee is the select committee. These types of committees are appointed to perform certain tasks and may last anywhere from a few minutes to several years. For example, on the opening day of each legislative session, the Senate president will appoint a select committee to inform the House of Representatives that they are ready to begin conducting business. The Speaker of the House will appoint a similar committee that completes the ritual. These select committees complete their ceremonial function in a few minutes. On the other hand, when an issue arises that merits special consideration, a select committee may be established to consider that particular issue in depth. For example, the 1999 Florida Legislature had to consider a comprehensive legislative package introduced by Governor Jeb Bush regarding education. Rather than refer the large number of bills to different standing committees, the Speaker of the House of Representatives appointed a Select Committee on Transforming Florida's Schools to consider the bills as a complete educational package. This committee consisted of members of the House of Representatives (from both political parties) and was chaired by the member who sponsored the legislation. It met for 2 weeks immediately before the legislative session, heard testimony from supporters and opponents, and was responsible for amending and voting on the bills in the package.

The third type of committee is a conference committee. Before the functions of this kind of committee can be described, it is necessary to further explain the process of how a bill becomes a law. For a bill to be signed into law and become an act that is sent to the governor for consideration, it must pass both houses of the legislature in identical form. This is often more difficult than it sounds. First, the bill must have a sponsor in both the House and the Senate. These "companion" bills may be identical, similar, or very dissimilar. When a bill makes it through the committee process and is considered on the floor of the House or Senate, it goes through an amendatory process. Once amended, the bill requires a majority vote to pass.

Let's use RN licensure requirements as a hypothetical example. The House bill, after completing the committee process, increases both the level of education needed to obtain an RN license and the competencies required to pass the licensure exam. On the floor, House members amend the bill to add two more competencies. The bill, as amended, passes with a majority vote and is sent to the Senate for consideration. The Senate takes up the House bill and agrees with the increased educational requirements but decides to amend the bill because it does not agree with the competencies that the House has chosen. In the amendatory process, the Senate removes three of the competencies required in the House bill and adds two new competencies from the original Senate bill. The House bill, as amended by the Senate, then passes the Senate with a majority vote and is sent back to the House. If the House does not agree with the changes made by the Senate, they may reach an impasse. This often results in the bill's demise. However, if the proposed legislation is important to the leadership in each house, the presiding officers may appoint a conference committee in an attempt to reach a compromise agreement.

If differences cannot be reconciled through the conference committee, the proposed legislation will fail. If the conference committee can reach an agreement, the House and Senate must vote on the compromise "as is," and no amendments can be offered. Usually, conference reports are submitted during the waning hours of a session, when time is short and legislators are unlikely to reject conference committee recommendations because it will most likely result in the failure of the bill (Florida Legislature, 1994a).

FYI

A conference committee is appointed every legislative session to consider the budget. This committee is always important because the budget is the only bill that the legislature is *required* to pass.

It is important to realize that many bills make it through the committee process but never get heard on the floor of the House or Senate. The presiding officers of each house, through the standing committees on rules and calendar, have control over which bills will be considered by the full House or Senate. Just as in committee, if a bill is not heard on the floor, it cannot be voted on and therefore cannot pass.

If a bill makes it through the committee process and passes both houses in identical form, it is called an *act*. Each act is sent to the governor for consideration, and he or she may either sign it into law, allow it to become law without his or her signature, or veto it. If an act is vetoed, the legislature may override it with a two-thirds vote in both houses. However, because the governor does not consider the acts until after the legislative session has adjourned, the legislature would be forced to either call a special session or wait until the next session to take action.

How Nurses Can Get Involved

Nurses can become involved in the political process at various levels. The first and most important thing is to be an informed voter. Nurses should watch the news, read the newspaper, surf the Internet, and be aware of what the candidates stand for on the national, state, and local levels. Nurses should also find out where candidates stand on the issues that are important to them as nurses. This can be accomplished with just a minimal amount of investigation. Nurses can contact the professional organizations to which they belong to find out which candidates they support. If a candidate is an incumbent, his or her voting record on issues of importance should be checked. Nurses must make phone calls, write letters, and ask questions!

Once legislators are in office, nurses should get to know them and make themselves and their views known to them. Box 5-5 contains some tips for effectively communicating ideas to legislators.

To have one of your ideas introduced as a bill, you must first find a sponsor in both the House and the Senate. The best scenario would be to approach a potential sponsor who is influential among legislators and who has a record of sponsoring successful legislation in your area of interest. This person will be likely to have more success in building coalitions among members than a less experienced legislator. It is also helpful if the legislator feels strongly about the issue because he or she will be more likely to fight for the proposed legislation.

Some legislative bodies place limits on the number of bills that can be filed by a particular member. It is necessary to investigate whether limitations exist and, if so, approach potential sponsors early. Timing can be crucial, especially if the issue of concern is a highly publicized one. Be aware of media coverage and strategically plan your moves.

Lobbying

The 1999 Florida Guide to Legislative Lobbyist Registration defines **lobbying** as "influencing or attempting to influence legisla-

---

BOX 5-5 TIPS FOR EFFECTIVE COMMUNICATIONS WITH LEGISLATORS

- Know who your legislators are and know how to contact them.
- Have a clear understanding of the legislative process.
- Contact your legislator about an issue that concerns you before the legislature takes action on it. (Although the legislative session may not begin until March, the committee process begins during the fall months. It is important to remember that all bills must first go through the committee process.)
- Use a variety of communication methods to contact your legislator, including telephone calls, letters, e-mail, fax, office visits, and so on. Be extremely careful to use correct spelling and grammar so that you do not lose your audience.
- Be polite, even if you disagree with the legislator's viewpoint on the issue. Your ability to effectively communicate your concerns diminishes if you go on the attack.
- Be prepared! Share with your legislator facts and figures that demonstrate the effect that a particular bill might have on your profession. Your opinions must be backed up with facts to be given any credence. You are the expert. Show it.
- Be concise and specific. It is important to remember that legislators must consider a large range of issues. Their time and attention are limited.
- Suggest a course of action and offer assistance. It is always beneficial to leave a one-page summary of your ideas with your legislator so that he or she may refer back to it or pass it on to legislative staff or other members.
- Establish a rapport with legislative aides and committee staff. These are the people who have direct and frequent contact with legislators and are responsible for providing them with a great deal of information.

Source: Florida Legislature, 1994b.

---

tive action or non-action through oral or written communication or attempting to obtain the goodwill of a member or employee of the Legislature" (p. 2). A lobbyist is a person who is employed and receives payment for the primary purpose of lobbying on behalf of another person, group, or governmental entity. Most states, if

CASE STUDY

Two Mississippi Nurses Lead the Way
Deborah Konkle-Parker, MSN, FNP

As a nurse practitioner working in an outpatient HIV clinic in Jackson, Mississippi, Debbie Konkle-Parker and other providers depended on the federal Ryan White AIDS Drug Assistance Program (ADAP), administered by the Mississippi Department of Health (MSDH), to help many of their clients get medicines. ADAP was used primarily to help clients who had no health insurance or whose medications exceeded the Mississippi Medicaid limit of five prescriptions per month.

In early April 1997, after several years of uneventful program usage, word was received from the health department that the Ryan White program was not accepting any more referrals for ADAP assistance. The recent addition of expensive protease inhibitors to the treatment regimen for HIV had depleted the entire year of federal ADAP funding by mid-March. This news came suddenly, without warning, and with no back-up plan for those with no other resources.

This sudden news sent providers and clients reeling, with no way to deal with this shortfall in services. A week later, there was a meeting of health care providers at the Mississippi Department of Health. At this meeting, the health care providers were informed that those individuals who were already receiving a protease inhibitor from ADAP would continue to receive medications, but all others would be cut off from the program. No more referrals were being accepted. This could literally mean the difference between life and death for many clients.

To deal with the problem, Debbie Konkle-Parker organized a problem-solving session to determine a way to cope with this change. She sent letters to concerned individuals, requesting their presence at a networking meeting. The meeting was attended by health care providers representing all disciplines, representatives from MSDH, representatives from the pharmaceutical industry, and persons with HIV/AIDS. The discussion at the meeting revealed that although most states provided funding from their state budgets to augment the federal ADAP dollars, Mississippi did not. It was decided that to change this policy, it was im-

portant to become an organized body to influence the legislators. The Mississippi HIV/AIDS Assembly was formed, with Debbie Konkle-Parker as its chair. The Mississippi HIV/AIDS Assembly consisted of two committees: (1) the AIDS Aware committee for mobilizing grassroots lobbying efforts around the state and (2) the Health Provider Network of interdisciplinary health care providers who could mobilize organizational lobbying efforts. Shortly after this meeting, the Mississippi State Department of Health found a way to temporarily redirect some of the money from other parts of the Ryan White program to re-enroll some clients who had been dropped from the program. But that effort was only putting a "Band-Aid" on the problem until further funding could be obtained.

The Health Provider Network set about the task of determining the direction of the work of the assembly, and the AIDS Aware committee gathered grassroots support for their efforts. The highest priority goal was supporting the Health Department's request of $500,000 from the state budget for ADAP. Although this amount was much less than what was actually needed, it was determined that politically this was an amount that reasonably could be requested by the Health Department. The Mississippi AIDS Assembly requested $2 million from the legislature, which was the estimate of how much money was actually needed to meet the extent of the problem in Mississippi.

Through these two committees, several different actions were taken, including providing speakers to bring attention to the issue for the public; maintaining a "silent" presence, including media coverage at a key budget hearing meeting; attending a meeting of the legislature's public health committee where bills were decided on before being brought to the floor; and applying consistent pressure on legislators to consider this issue. Multiple mailings went out to individuals throughout the state, encouraging personal communication with their legislators and a "spreading of the word."

The result of this year-long work was the first-ever state dedication of $750,000 to the Mississippi Ryan White AIDS Drug Assistance Program, with more to follow each year. This funding allowed a return of new referrals to the program and an immediate lessening of the waiting list of individuals needing medications.

Continued

CASE STUDY—cont'd

Connie Thompson, BSN, RN

As the infection control coordinator of a medical center in Jackson, Mississippi, Connie Thompson played a big role in the efforts of the Mississippi HIV/AIDS Assembly and eagerly joined in the excitement surrounding its legislative victory. But after the excitement faded away, Thompson realized that this was only the beginning. More funding and services were needed, not only for persons living with HIV/AIDS, but for persons living with any chronic disabling disease.

In August 1998, under the leadership of Thompson, a variety of Mississippi organizations and agencies joined forces in an effort to influence legislative health care issues for disabled persons. Eventually this group formed a coalition of more than 50 organizations and agencies known as the Coalition for Uninsured Mississippians, representing thousands of Mississippians with disabilities or chronic illnesses who are denied access to health insurance each year. These individuals—persons with cancer, heart disease, HIV,

diabetes, asthma, lupus, arthritis, and other diseases—earn a little more money, either from disability payments or job income, than the maximum allowed to qualify for Medicaid. However, they don't make enough money to be able to afford expensive private health insurance.

As a result, these men, women, and children are forced to make frequent visits to hospital emergency rooms for basic health care. Or worse, they do not seek care at all until a crisis occurs that requires inpatient hospitalization. Proper disease management with regular clinic visits for appropriate follow-up and networking for client care and services would maintain optimal health standards for these individuals. Quality of life for these persons would greatly improve and health care would be more cost-effective if they had access to health insurance.

The timing for the work of the coalition was a critical factor. The Federal Balanced Budget Act of 1997 offered states the option of allowing citizens with disabilities to purchase Medicaid on a sliding fee scale according to their income. In August 1998, the U.S. Department of Health and Human Services urged state governors, state legislators, and Medicaid directors to take advantage of this important new option. The Coalition for Uninsured Mississippians sought support from Mississippi's citizens for a legislative bill that would allow disabled persons with incomes below 250% of the federal poverty level to buy in to Medicaid coverage. The purchase of this coverage would

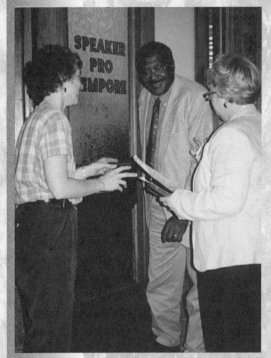

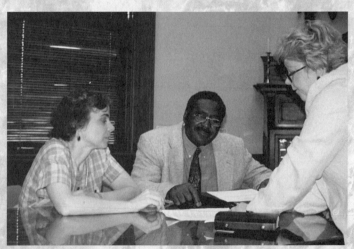

Connie Thompson, BSN, RN, and Deborah Konkle-Parker, MSN, RN, FNP, work with Robert G. Clark, Mississippi State Representative.

be based on a sliding scale fee. Both the Balanced Budget Act of 1997 and the encouragement from the U.S. Department of Health and Human Services were used to support the coalition's action.

Within 2 months of the coalition's initial meeting a petition supported by thousands of Mississippians had been sent to the co-chairs of the joint subcommittees of health and welfare of the state legislature. A statewide Forum for Effective Advocacy of Chronic Illnesses and Disabilities was held to discuss the issues, and a task force was formed to meet with the director of the division of Medicaid to look for solutions. Connie Thompson, as the fa- *cilitator of the Coalition for Uninsured Mississippians, was invited to serve on the attorney general's Partners for a Healthy Mississippi task force.*

As a result of the coalition's efforts, a bill to expand Medicaid coverage by authorizing a buy-in opportunity to workers who are disabled and earning less than 250% of the federal poverty was drafted and signed into law by the Mississippi legislature and the governor during the 1999 legislative session.

In both of the above scenarios, nurse-led public policy strategies, starting with simple problem-solving meetings, have achieved the goal of improving health care for some of Mississippi's poor and vulnerable citizens.

RESEARCH BRIEF

Monardi, F., & Glantz, S. A. (1998). Are tobacco industry campaign contributions influencing state legislative behavior? American Journal of Public Health, 88(6), 918–923.

This study examined the influence of tobacco industry campaign contributions on state legislators' tobacco voting records in six states. Data on campaign contributions to state legislators and legislators' tobacco control policy scores were analyzed using multivariate simultaneous equations regression models. The data analysis revealed that as tobacco industry contributions increase, the calculated policy scores tended to decrease (i.e., state legislators become more supportive of the tobacco industry's political agenda). These results were significant even after controlling for partisanship, majority party status, and leadership effects. The conclusion of the study was that tobacco industry campaign contributions significantly influence state legislators in terms of tobacco control policy making.

ployed by a home health agency would not be considered lobbyists unless their most significant work responsibility dealt with governmental affairs. However, this does not mean that the nurses cannot contact their legislators and actively support or oppose legislation that affects their home health agencies. It simply means that the nurses are not be required to register because they do not receive payment for the purposes of lobbying.

Lobbyists must adhere to many rules and regulations, which may vary widely from state to state. Therefore, it is important that nurses be aware of the rules, if any, that apply in their states. Regulations may also change from year to year, which makes it necessary to keep current. For example, in Florida, rules and regulations regarding the receipt of gifts from lobbyists are established in statute (Section 112.3148, Florida Statutes). Other states may not be so proscriptive and may outline rules only in policy manuals or employee handbooks. Some states may not even have rules for lobbyists, but most have some kind of regulation.

Best practices for lobbying as well as for concerned constituents include being aware of all applicable rules and restrictions, establishing a good rapport with legislators and legislative staff, and always backing up your position with hard data. If nurses adhere to these principles, their likelihood of successfully communicating their ideas will greatly increase.

Political Action Committees

Through the years, the ANA and various other specialty health organizations have taken leadership roles in mobilizing nurses in grassroots lobbying. This has required a significant effort to educate nurses about the political process and how to remain cognizant of the political issues that affect nursing and health. Because federal law requires that campaign contributions be kept as a separate fund and that no organizational membership be used for this purpose, many groups have created separate organizations for

not all, require lobbyists to be registered as such. This registration allows citizens to be informed about activities that are aimed at influencing government decision making. For example, when major legislation relating to health care is being considered, it may be beneficial to know which groups have hired lobbyists to promote their interests and monitor their activities and expenditures.

For example, home health agencies may hire lobbyists whose principal responsibilities are to represent the organization's interests to the legislature and other government agencies. Nurses em-

political activities. These organizations are referred to as **political action committees (PACs)**. Their work is completely separate from the rest of the organization's work. The primary purpose of a PAC is to endorse and support candidates for public office who support the legislative agenda of the organization or group making the endorsement (Curtis & Lumpkin, 1998). Nursing PACs exist at the federal and state level, most often through the ANA (ANA-PAC) and state nurses associations. ANA-PAC is the 30th largest federal PAC and in 1995 was identified as the second fastest growing federal health care PAC in the nation (Kelly & Joel, 1996).

Regulation and Licensing of Nursing Practice

The Regulatory Process

Although it is important for nurses to be involved in the legislative process, it is equally important for nurses to understand the **regulatory process**. According to Webster's New World College Dictionary (Neufeldt, 1996), *regulation* is "the act of controlling, directing, or governing according to a rule, principle, or system" (p. 1131). Once bills are passed into law by the legislative branch of government, they must be implemented by the administrative agencies of the executive branch (Abood & Mittelstadt, 1998; Loquist, 1999). Legislation is purposely expressed in broad terms to provide flexibility and adaptability of laws over time. Regulation is expressed in very specific terms describing how the administrative agency with jurisdictional authority will implement the law (Loquist, 1999). The legislative process is used to create policy and laws to address a particular issue when none exist. Regulation is used to clarify and interpret existing policy and laws and decide what methods will be used to enforce them (Loquist, 1999).

Regulations frame the way health policy is transposed into services and programs. Although regulations are a direct result of passed legislation, they are shaped into their final forms by the ongoing involvement of health care professionals and their professional organizations, third-party payers, consumers, and other special interest groups. Before a federal agency can implement a law, it must publish the proposed regulation or set of regulations in the *Federal Register*. The publication of the proposed regulations affords anyone with any interest in the regulations the ability to react to them before they become finalized. Commenting on proposed regulations before they are finalized is one of the most important, but often neglected, parts of the legislative process (Abood & Mittelstadt, 1998).

HEALTHY PEOPLE 2010

OBJECTIVES RELATED TO LAW

3.14   Increase the number of states that have a statewide population-based cancer registry that captures case information on at least 95% of the expected number of reportable cancers.

6.13   Increase the number of tribes, states, and the District of Columbia that have public health surveillance and health-promotion programs for people with disabilities and caregivers.

13.9   Increase the number of state prison systems that provide comprehensive HIV/AIDS, sexually transmitted diseases, and tuberculosis (TB) education.

13.10   Increase the proportion of inmates in state prison systems who receive voluntary HIV counseling and testing during incarceration.

15.24   Increase the number of states and the District of Columbia with laws requiring bicycle helmets for bicycle riders.

18.11   Increase the proportion of local governments with community-based jail diversion programs for adults with serious mental illnesses.

23.15   Increase the proportion of federal, tribal, state, and local jurisdictions that review and evaluate the extent to which their statutes, ordinances, and bylaws assure the delivery of essential public health services.

27.14   Reduce the illegal buy rate among minors through enforcement of laws prohibiting the sale of tobacco products to minors.

Source: DHHS, 2000.

The U.S. Constitution dictates that the government has a duty to protect its citizens. The Tenth Amendment to the U.S. Constitution provides the states with all the powers not specifically reserved for the federal government. Regulation of health care professions is one way that each state exercises its responsibility to protect the health, safety, and welfare of its residents.

Nursing practice in each state is governed by a nurse practice act, which includes the laws and regulations that control the requirements for entry into practice, the standards for acceptable practice, the standards for continuing competence, and the disciplinary actions taken for misconduct (Loquist, 1999). The state nurse practice act is the most important piece of legislature for nurses because it governs every facet of nursing practice (Guido, 2001).

Each state legislature designates a board of nursing to administer the nurse practice act. There are 61 boards of nursing in the United States and its territories. The most critical role of the board of nursing is to ensure the safety of the public by monitoring the competency of practicing nurses through licensure (Loquist, 1999).

Licensure

A license is "a formal permission authorized by law to do something" (Neufeldt, 1996, p. 779). Nurses must be licensed in a state in order to work as an RN, licensed practical nurse (LPN), or vocational nurse (LVN). **Licensure** provides the public with the greatest level of protection because it protects the title of RN or LPN and delineates the scope of nursing practice (Loquist, 1999). Requirements for licensure include proof of graduation from an approved academic program, a passing score on the licensing examination, and personal qualifications such as citizenship or visa permits, good physical and mental health, and good moral character (Barnum, 1997; Guido, 2001; Loquist, 1999).

All states administer licensing examinations using a standardized national test developed and administered by the National Council of State Boards of Nursing (NCSBN). Licensing examinations are called the National Council Licensing Examination for Registered Nurses (NCLEX-RN) and the National Council Licensing Examination for Practical Nurses (NCLEX-PN). Traditionally, nurses have been required to be licensed in the state in which they practice. If a nurse moves to a different state, he or she must obtain a license from the new state. A national examination makes seeking reciprocity (recognition of licensure from one state to another) an easy process if the nurse has a valid license in one state (Betts & Waddle, 1993; Guido, 2001).

In recent years, the use of telecommunication technology has transformed the health care delivery system and challenged the individual state licensing system. Mergers of health care systems have produced giant corporations that operate across state lines. Nurses serve as case managers for clients living in many different states and staff regional or national telephone advice and consultation hot lines (Hutcherson & Williamson, 1999; Loquist, 1999; Wakefield, 1999). As nurses began practicing in several states at the same time, separate licenses had to be obtained from each state. This policy is impractical and expensive.

In response to the licensing dilemma, the NCSBN adopted a new model for nursing regulation called the **Nurse Multistate Licensure Mutual Recognition Model**. According to the ANA, multistate licensure allows a nurse to practice in several states while holding a license in only one state. States enter into interstate compact agreements to coordinate activities associated with licensure. This mutual recognition model allows nurses to practice in states that have adopted an interstate compact with each other. The nurses are held accountable for compliance with the laws and regulations of each state's nurse practice act (ANA, 1998). In March 1998, Utah became the first state to pass legislation to adopt the Mutual Recognition Model (ANA, 1998). Other states are following, but not without controversy. Many nursing organizations, concerned with client safety and nursing standards, are questioning the appropriateness of the model (King, 1999).

State boards of nursing are responsible not only for ensuring the competency of nurses entering into practice, but also for monitoring the competence of those nurses already in practice. Most nurse practice acts have provisions that require employers to report any violations. Procedures for reporting misconduct, conducting investigations, and issuing sanctions are outlined in the regulations of each state's or territory's nurse practice act. Licensed nurses are responsible for knowing the laws and regulations that govern nursing practice in their states (Loquist, 1999).

Nursing Practice and the Law

The most common lawsuits filed against health care professionals involve the principles of **negligence** and **malpractice**, which fall under the classification of tort law. Torts are legal wrongs committed against another person or against the property of another person. The wrongdoing may be intentional or unintentional and must result in physical, emotional, or economic harm (Betts & Waddle, 1993; Guido, 2001).

Although the terms *negligence* and *malpractice* are often used interchangeably, there is a fine distinction between them. *Negligence* is a general term that describes the failure to act as any prudent or reasonable person would act in a specific circumstance. *Malpractice* is a more specific term that considers a professional standard of care as well as the professional status of the health care provider. To be liable for malpractice, the person committing the misconduct must be a professional acting in a professional role. Professional misconduct includes either doing something that should not be done (commission) or not doing something that should be done (omission) (Betts & Waddle, 1993; Guido, 2001).

For a nurse to be found guilty of malpractice in a court of law, the following must have existed:

- *A duty was owed to the client.*
- *There was a breach of the duty owed to the client.*
- *Harm was caused to the client.*
- *The harm was foreseeable.*
- *The action or inaction of the nurse caused the harm (Guido, 2001).*

CONCLUSION

Nurses in the community must remain current and informed about politics and law as related to public health nursing practice. The political system is ultimately about the distribution of power through formalized and complex systems of law, policy, and regulatory control mechanisms. Settings within the community have legal implications for the nurse, and there are emerging opportunities for nurses within the political/legal community. Furthermore, for nurses to maintain control of professional nursing practice, understanding and applying political knowledge helps secure our future in the health care delivery system.

CRITICAL THINKING ACTIVITIES

1. Do all three types of law apply to professional nursing practice? In what ways?
2. In what ways can nurses influence legislation that affects nursing practice?
3. What types of nursing situations may lend themselves to malpractice suits?
4. What steps can you take to avoid a lawsuit?

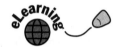

Explore Community Health Nursing on the web! To learn more about the topics in this chapter, access your exclusive web site:
http://communitynursing.jbpub.com

REFERENCES

Abood, S., & Mittelstadt, P. (1998). Legislative and regulatory processes. In D. J. Mason & J. K. Leavitt (Eds.), *Policy and politics in nursing and health care* (3rd ed., pp. 384–396). Philadelphia: W. B. Saunders.

American Nurses Association (ANA). (1998). *Multistate regulation of nurses.* www.nursingworld.org/gova/multibg.htm.

Bacharach, S. B., & Lawler, E. J. (1980). *Power and politics in organizations.* San Francisco: Jossey-Bass.

Barnum, B. S. (1997, August 13). Licensure, certification, and accreditation. *Online Journal of Issues in Nursing.* www.nursing world.org/ojin/tpc4/tpc4_2.htm.

Bednash, G. P., Heylin, G. B., & Rhome, A. M. (1998). Federal government. In D. J. Mason & J. K. Leavitt (Eds.), *Policy and politics in nursing and health care* (3rd ed., pp. 436–457). Philadelphia: W. B. Saunders.

Betts, V. T., & Waddle, F. I. (1993). Legal aspects of nursing. In K. K. Chitty (Ed.), *Professional nursing. Concepts and challenges.* Philadelphia: W. B. Saunders.

Centers for Disease Control and Prevention (CDC). (1998). *Fact book FY 1998* (DHHS Publication No. 1998-638-018). Washington, DC: U.S. Government Printing Office.

Curtis, B. T., & Lumpkin, B. (1998). Political action committees. In D. J. Mason & J. K. Leavitt (Eds.), *Policy and politics in nursing and health care* (3rd ed., pp. 546–554). Philadelphia: W. B. Saunders.

Department of Health and Human Services (DHHS). (1999). *Greetings from the Secretary. Donna Shalala.* www.hhs.gov/about/greeting.html.

Florida Legislature, Office of the Clerk. (1994a). *Citizen's guide to the legislature. How the committee process works.* www.leg.state.fl.us/citizen/documents/howcomm.html. Accessed May 1999.

Florida Legislature, Office of the Clerk. (1994b). *Citizen's guide to the legislature. Getting your voice heard: Tips for effectively communicating your ideas.* www.leg.state.fl.us/citizen/documents/howwrite.html. Accessed May 1999.

Florida Legislature, Office of the Clerk. (1994c). *Citizen's guide to the legislature. How an idea becomes a law:* www.leg.state.fl.us/citizen/documents. Accessed May 1999.

Forgotson, E. H. (1967). 1965: The turning point in health law—1966 reflections. *American Journal of Public Health, 57*(6), 934–935.

French, J. R., & Raven, B. (1959). The basis for social power. In D. Cartwright (Ed.), *Studies in social power.* Ann Arbor: University of Michigan Press.

Gaffney, T. (1998). State government. In D. J. Mason & J. K. Leavitt (Eds.), *Policy and politics in nursing and health care* (3rd ed., pp. 417–427). Philadelphia: W. B. Saunders.

Guide to Legislative Lobbyist Registration. (1999). Tallahassee, FL: Lobbyist Registration Office.

Guido, G. W. (2001). *Legal issues in nursing* (3rd ed.). Upper Saddle River, NJ: Prentice Hall.

Helvie, C. O. (1998). *Advanced practice nursing in the community.* Thousand Oaks, CA: Sage.

Hersey, P., Blanchard, K., & Natemeyer, W. (1979). Situational leadership: Perception and impact of power. *Group Organizational Studies, 4,* 418–428.

Hewison, A. (1994). The politics of nursing: A framework for analysis. *Journal of Advanced Nursing, 20,* 1170–1175.

Hutcherson, C., & Williamson, S. H. (1999, May 31). Nursing regulation for the new millennium: The mutual recognition model. *Online Journal of Issues in Nursing,* http://nursingworld.org/ojin/topic9/topic9_2.htm.

Huston, C. J. (1995, Fall). Nursing and political action in the twentieth century: From separation to fusion. *Revolution: The Journal of Nurse Empowerment,* 50–53.

Kaplan, W. A. (1985). *The law of higher education* (2nd ed.). San Francisco: Jossey-Bass.

Kelly, L. Y., & Joel, L. A. (1996). *The nursing experience* (3rd ed.). New York: McGraw-Hill.

King, S. E. (1999, May 31). Multistate licensure: Premature policy. *Online Journal of Issues in Nursing,* www.nursingworld.org/ojin/topic9/topic9_3.htm.

Lenski, G. E. (1984). *Power and privilege.* Chapel Hill, NC: University of North Carolina Press.

Lobbyist Registration Office. (1999). *Guide to legislative lobbyist registration 1999.* Tallahassee, FL: Florida Legislature.

Loquist, R. S. (1999). Regulation: Parallel and powerful. In J. A. Milstead (Ed.), *Health policy and politics. A nurse's guide* (pp. 105–146). Gaithersburg, MD: Aspen.

Majewski, J. V., & O'Brien, M. C. (1998). Local government. In D. J. Mason & J. K. Leavitt (Eds.), *Policy and politics in nursing and health care* (3rd ed., pp. 405–416). Philadelphia: W. B. Saunders.

Miller, D. F. (1992). *Dimensions of community health.* Dubuque, IA: Wm. C. Brown.

Milstead, J. A. (1999). Advanced practice nurses and public policy, naturally. In J. A. Milstead (Ed.), *Health policy and politics. A nurse's guide* (pp. 1–41). Gaithersburg, MD: Aspen.

Neufeldt, V. (Ed.). (1996). *Webster's new world college dictionary* (3rd ed.). New York: Macmillan.

Robertson, I. (1981). *Sociology* (2nd ed.). New York: Worth.

Satcher, D. (1998, May/June). Public Health Service: On the job for 200 years. *Public Health reports, 113,* 201–203.

Turnock, B. J. (1997). *Public health: What it is and how it works.* Gaithersburg, MD: Aspen.

Wakefield, M. K. (1999). Have license, will travel. *Nursing Economics, 17*(2), 114–116.

Weber, M. (1947). *The theory of social and economic organization* (ed. and trans. A. M. Henderson & T. Parsons). New York: Oxford University Press.

6

Transcultural Nursing and Global Health

Sharyn Janes

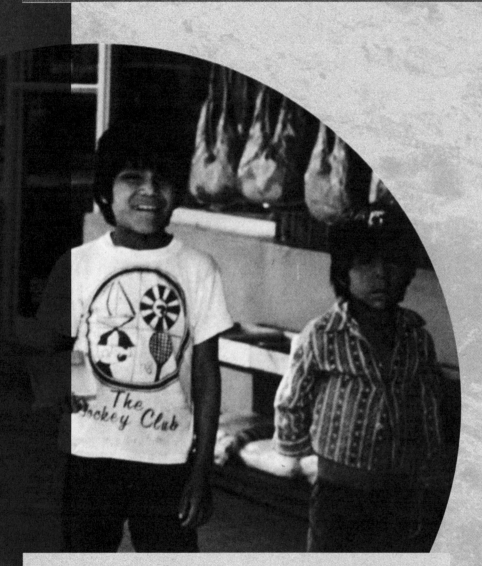

In a world connected by supersonic transports and cyberspace, nurses need to be alert to developments in the changing world. Nurses need to continually update and modify their nursing practices in accordance with changing global political, social, economic, and cultural realities.

CHAPTER FOCUS

Transcultural Concepts

International and Global Health

Role of International Agencies
The United Nations
The United Nations Children's Fund
The World Health Organization
The Carter Center

A Role for Nurses

Health Care and Nursing Around the World
Czech Republic
Cuba
Iran
Nepal
South Africa

Healthy People 2010: Objectives Related to Cultural Diversity and Care

QUESTIONS TO CONSIDER

After reading this chapter, answer the following questions:

1. What are the demographic trends affecting health care delivery and nursing in the United States?
2. What is culturally competent nursing care?
3. What are the principles of transcultural nursing?
4. What roles do international agencies play in world health efforts?
5. What roles do nurses play in global health?

KEY TERMS

The Carter Center
Cultural barriers
Cultural bias
Cultural ignorance
Cultural imposition
Cultural pain

Cultural shock
Cultural values
Cultural variations
Culturally competent care
Culture
Emic view

Ethnocentrism
Etic view
Generic care
"Health for All"
International health
Professional care

Stereotyping
The United Nations (UN)
The United Nations Children's Fund (UNICEF)
The World Health Organization (WHO)

Nursing is entering a new century and a new millennium with many new challenges and opportunities. The United States is the most culturally diverse country in the world. In 1994, *Time* magazine called the United States the "Universal Nation." Nurses are interacting with and caring for many immigrants, refugees, and travelers from many different cultures, as well as members of many different cultural groups living in the United States. Yet, the future holds still more diversity for the "Universal Nation" with the coming of enormous demographic, social, and cultural change. In the United States, the racial and ethnic profile of the population is changing. The white majority is shrinking as the population ages, but the underrepresented ethnic groups are younger and growing in number. In fact, in some states, like California, there is a "minority majority," with the white population accounting for less than half of the population (Spector, 2000). Spanish is the dominant language spoken in some regions of Texas, California, and Florida.

Nurses must use a wide variety of transcultural concepts, principles, and practices to help them function in many different cultural contexts. **Culture** is the learned, shared, and transmitted values, beliefs, norms, and lifeways of a particular group that guide their thinking, decisions, and actions in patterned ways (Leininger, 2001). Culture not only refers to race and ethnicity but may also refer to gender, religion and spirituality, sexual orientation, age, education, socioeconomic status, geographic region, or any characteristic that influences a person's worldview. Transcultural nursing focuses on holistic and comprehensive ways to know and serve people's health care needs. As nurses learn about the essential and desired care expectations of different cultures, they become aware of many different ways to provide culturally competent care (Leininger, 2001).

Until the 1960s, when Madeleine Leininger developed the theory of culture care diversity and universality, cultural factors were not included in health care and nursing, and often were not even recognized as important. With Leininger's development of the field of transcultural nursing, nursing and other health care professionals began to realize the role that culture plays in health behavior and practices, and thus in health care delivery. In the last three decades, many nursing leaders, such as Rachel Spector, Larry Purnell and Betty Paulanka, Joyceen Boyle and Margaret McAndrew, Joyce Giger and Ruth Davidhizar, have followed Leininger's lead and developed their own excellent models and approaches to culturally competent nursing care. However, due to limited space, this chapter will focus on the transcultural concepts and principles developed by Madeleine Leininger.

Trancultural Concepts

To provide culturally competent nursing care, it is important to understand several major concepts. A few definitions are presented

---

BOX 6-1 DEFINITIONS

Culture: The learned, shared, and transmitted values, beliefs, norms, and lifeways of a particular group that guide their thinking, decisions, and actions in patterned ways.

Cultural values: The powerful directive forces that give order and meaning to people's thinking, decisions, and actions.

Cultural variations: The subtle or obvious variables among and between cultures that make them unique with respect to traditional or nontraditional ways of living.

Cultural lifeways: The patterned ways of living of a particular individual or group.

Cultural imposition: The tendency to impose one's beliefs, values, and lifeways on another individual or culture, due largely to ignorance about a culture.

Ethnocentrism: The belief that one's own ways of living or doing are the best, most preferred, or superior to others.

Stereotyping: The undesirable tendency to prejudge and fix cultures into rigid and biased ways, due largely to ethnocentrism and racism.

Cultural blindness: The inability to recognize one's own values and lifeways or those of another culture, making culture invisible.

Cultural clashes: Major conflicts in valuing and understanding differences between cultures and variability among or within cultures.

Caring: Actions and activities directed toward assisting, supporting, or enabling another individual or group with evident or anticipated needs to improve a human condition or lifeway, or to face death.

Nursing: A learned humanistic and scientific profession and discipline focused on human caring.

Emic view: The insider's or local perspective about cultures, families, lifeways, and health care.

Etic view: The outsider's or external perspective about cultures, families, lifeways, and health care.

Culturally competent care: The deliberate and creative use of transcultural nursing knowledge and skills to assist or facilitate individuals or groups to maintain their well-being, recover from illness, or face disability or death.

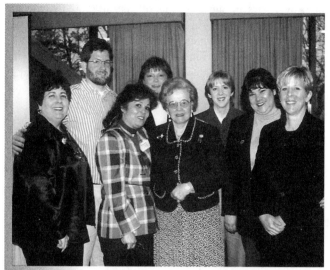

Dr. Madeleine Leininger (center), founder of Transcultural Nursing, with members of the Mississippi Chapter of the Transcultural Nursing Society.

in box 6-1; however, there are some that need to be discussed further with clinical examples provided to explain them.

The first concept is **culturally competent care**, which refers to using cultural knowledge in creative and meaningful ways to provide appropriate and beneficial care to members of diverse cultures. Nurses combine the traditional practices of their clients with their own professional nursing knowledge to provide mean-ingful, safe, and responsible care. Culturally competent care is nursing care tailored to include the cultural values and beliefs of the client into the care plan to the greatest extent possible (Leininger, 2001).

Cultural values are the powerful forces that direct the way that people think, act, and make decisions (Leininger, 2001). For example, older people in the South value their *country cookin'*, which consists of a wide variety of foods deep-fried in lard with lots of gravy and salt. This can pose a problem for an elder with hypertension and coronary artery disease. But, food choices are such an important cultural value that nurses must be creative in including as many of these foods as possible (or healthier variations of them) in the nutritional plan for Southern elders. Completely changing their diet will not be effective because elders believe that they've "lived this long eating these foods so it can't be that harmful."

Two concepts that are important for nurses to understand are emic and etic views. *Emic view* is what the local people or "insiders" see as important to know and believe (Leininger, 2001). For example, some cultures, such as many Asian American or Native American groups, believe very strongly that elders should be cared for by the family at home and NEVER live in a nursing home or extended care facility. Members of these cultural groups may even be offended if the nurse offers them institutionalized care as an option for their elder. On the other hand, many European Americans often believe that a nursing home or other care facility is the best place for their elders to receive the care and protection that cannot be offered in the home.

Etic view is an external or "outsider's perception of a culture" (Leininger, 2001). For example, if nurses don't understand the

HEALTHY PEOPLE 2010

OBJECTIVES RELATED TO CULTURAL DIVERSITY AND CARE

Access to Quality Health Services

1.8 In the health professions, allied and associated health professions, and the nursing field, increase the proportion of all degrees awarded to members of underrepresented racial and ethnic groups.

Educational and Community-Based Programs

7.11 Increase the proportion of local health departments that have established culturally appropriate and linguistically competent community health-promotion and disease-prevention programs for racial and ethnic minority populations.

Mental Health and Mental Disorders

18.13 Increase the number of states, territories, and the District of Columbia with an operational mental health plan that addresses cultural competence.

Source: DHHS, 2000.

religious or spiritual beliefs of clients that are different from their own religious or spiritual beliefs, these nurses are not able to offer supportive and appropriate care to the clients and families who are facing serious illness or death.

Concepts closely related to emic and etic views are generic and professional care. *Generic care* is the folk care or traditional health practices that cultures have used over time, while *professional care* is what is learned in nursing, medicine, or other health care educational programs. The differences in these care concepts need to be understood and integrated to provide culturally competent and beneficial care (Leininger, 2001). For example, some cultures are patriarchal and require the male head of the family to make all decisions related to health care for all family members. Nurses who understand this traditional health practice would include the family patriarchs in all health care decisions related to family members. This display of respect for the generic practices of the cultural group would help in developing cooperative working relationships between nurses, clients, and families.

Two other concepts that are closely related are ethnocentrism and cultural imposition. *Ethnocentrism* is the belief that one's own ways are superior to all others and should be the preferred ways of acting, believing, or valuing something (Sumner, 1906). An example of this is the Anglo-American nurse who thinks that all people living in the United States must speak English. Ethnocentrism implies that there is only one "right" way to think or act.

Cultural imposition occurs when one group of people force their cultural beliefs, values, and patterns of behavior on others. It is one of the most common problems encountered between cultures. An example of this is the Anglo-American nurse who imposes her belief that women should be equal partners with their husbands in making health care decisions for the family on a Mexican-American mother. This can cause conflict in the family and may lead to the family's total rejection of the nurse's care (Leininger, 2001).

Cultural bias means that a member of one cultural group strongly believes that all decisions must be based on his or her own values and beliefs. If nurses are unable to identify their own cultural biases, therapeutic interventions can not be provided for clients and families. Both nurses and clients may have cultural biases that need to be identified and discussed so that acceptable compromises can be developed (Leininger, 2001).

Cultural ignorance means that the nurse is lacking enough knowledge about a specific culture to provide safe and appropriate care. Cultural ignorance can lead to ineffective or even harmful care practices with non-therapeutic outcomes for clients (Leininger, 2001).

When a person is disoriented or unable to respond appropriately to a situation because of unfamiliarity or fear of what was experienced, that person is in a state of **cultural shock** (Leininger, 2001). For example, a nurse makes a home visit to a poor family of Mexican-American migrant farm workers. There are six children (ages 2 to 12) and four adults sleeping on the floor in a one-room shack. There is no indoor plumbing and the grandmother is cooking dinner in a pot on a coal stove on the front porch. Flies are on the open food containers and mosquitoes are coming in through the open door and windows. The nurse is overwhelmed by the family's living conditions so she promptly leaves the home and refuses to return. Because of her cultural shock, she is not able to assess the family's health and provide for their health care needs.

Cultural pain is the discomfort or suffering experienced by a member of a particular cultural group when insulting or offensive remarks are made by an outsider (Leininger, 2001). For example, a Muslim family experienced cultural pain when the nurse who was caring for their father said it was "ridiculous to say prayers at specific times each day when it shouldn't matter when you pray. God is always there, not only at certain times of the day." It was apparent to the family that the nurse did not understand or respect Muslim religious practices.

Cultural variation is the term used to describe slight or marked differences within cultural groups (Leininger, 2001). For example, Hispanic Americans share many cultural similarities in-

RESEARCH BRIEF

Jemmott, L. S., Maula, E. C., & Bush, E. (1999). *Hearing our voices: Assessing HIV prevention among Asian and Pacific islander women.* Journal of Transcultural Nursing, 10(2), 102–111.

This study was conducted to (1) assess the impact of human immunodeficiency virus/acquired immunodeficiency syndrome (HIV/AIDS) on the Asian/Pacific Islander community and to determine whether there were any changes in behavior as a result of HIV; and (2) identify their perception of risk, HIV risk behaviors, factors contributing to risk behaviors, barriers to HIV prevention, and kinds of prevention programs that would benefit their communities. The study also described culturally competent considerations when designing HIV prevention strategies for Asian/Pacific Islander women. The participants consisted of 22 low-income women, ages 18 to 44, living in a large metropolitan area. They were divided into two different groups and interviewed using focus interviewing techniques guided by the health belief model. The women had numerous concerns about their risk for HIV related to their cultural taboo about discussing sexual issues and condom use. Both groups stated that HIV prevention efforts must be tailored to the cultural needs of Asian/Pacific Islander women if they were to be successful.

CASE STUDY

As a community health nurse you are making home visits twice a week to Mrs. Mendoza, who lives in a rural community. Mrs. Mendoza is an 82-year-old Mexican American woman with a below-the-knee amputation of her left leg related to her diabetes mellitus. She lives with her 50-year-old son and two teenage grandsons. It is difficult to communicate with Mrs. Mendoza or to do any diabetic teaching because you do not speak Spanish and no one in the Mendoza household speaks English. During your first five visits, the neighbor who lives down the road was willing to come to Mrs. Mendoza's house during your visits to serve as your interpreter. However, on your sixth visit, you discover that the neighbor is not at home. Because you are unable to communicate with Mrs. Mendoza you go to each of her neighbors' houses looking for someone who can speak English but find none of them at home. Frustrated and behind schedule, you return to Mrs. Mendoza's house to learn that her son, who has been at home during all of your visits, is able to speak English fluently.

1. How do you feel when you learn that Mrs. Mendoza's son can speak English?

2. Why do you think he did not tell you he could speak English earlier?

3. What could you have done to make the situation different?

cluding language, values, and beliefs, but there are also major differences in the historical and cultural backgrounds of Cuban-Americans, Puerto Ricans, and Mexican-Americans.

Cultural barriers are obstacles in the paths of different cultural groups that inhibit their access to opportunities and subsequent achievement of their desired goals (Leininger, 2001). When clinics and other health care facilities do not provide information in all the languages spoken by the people they serve, access to health care and important health information is denied to cultural groups that do not speak the language of the dominant culture.

Putting labels on members of a culture that reflect perceived fixed characteristics (negative or positive) of that particular group without taking individual or group differences into account is known as **stereotyping**. Rigid stereotypes are not precise and often cause cultural pain (Leininger, 2001). Some examples of stereotyping include assumptions that all Native Americans are alcoholics, all Anglo-Americans are selfish and materialistic, all African Americans are militant, and all Asian Americans are either highly intelligent or passive and unwilling to learn new things.

· ·

In a real sense all life is interrelated. All men are caught in an inescapable network of mutuality, tied in a single garment of destiny.

Rev. Martin Luther King, Jr.

· ·

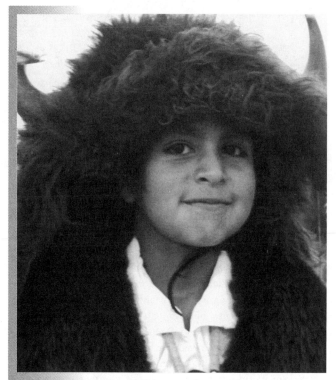

It is important for children to learn the ceremonies and rituals of their culture to develop a healthy sense of "self."

BOX 6-2 TRANSCULTURAL NURSING PRINCIPLES

1. All human cultures have diverse living, caring, and healing modes that nurses need to study and understand to work effectively with people of different cultures.

2. Care is a basic human need, and it is the essence and dominant focus of the nursing profession.

3. Understanding one's own culture is the first essential expectation to understand other cultures or subcultures.

4. People have the right to have their cultural values known, respected, understood, and used appropriately in nursing and health care services.

5. Transcultural nursing is concerned with the comparative values, beliefs, and practices of specific cultures in order to provide meaningful, safe, and specific health care practices.

6. Nurses use humanistic and scientific cultural care knowledge as they provide care to different cultures. Humanistic care aspects make people remain human, and scientific research findings about cultures and care guide nurses' decisions and actions.

7. Understanding culture care differences and similarities enables the nurse to respect clients and assist them to grow, function, maintain their well-being or health, and prevent illnesses and premature death.

8. Willingness to enter the client's world and become an active and interested participant is essential in maintaining effective nurse-client or nurse-family relationships.

9. Listening, respecting, and being attentive to what clients of different cultures say or do are essential to understanding them and providing meaningful and beneficial nursing services.

10. A nurse's ability to speak the client's cultural language opens the door to understanding what the client is seeking or experiencing.

11. If the client's cultural lifeways, values, and caring expressions do not immediately "make sense," the nurse must continue to make an effort to understand them.

12. In every culture, care, healing, and health practices are greatly influenced by clients' worldviews, environmental context, and social structure features (including the religious or spiritual beliefs, kinship ties, political-legal views, economic aspects, technologies, and specific cultural historical values).

13. Every culture usually has two major types of health care systems: generic (indigenous, traditional, folk) and professional (learned in schools). Nurses need to understand these to provide culturally congruent care.

14. Cultures have their own culturally defined ways to promote and maintain health, face death, and deal with unfavorable sociocultural conditions and crises.

15. Health care practices in Western and non-Western cultures have major differences that need to be understood when planning and providing care to clients.

Source: Leininger, 1995.

International and global health

At the dawn of the new millennium, we are living in a global society. The Internet puts us in instant contact with people from many parts of the world. Through e-mail and the World Wide Web we have immediate access to a wide variety of information in many different languages. Not only are we exposed to many cultures and ideologies, but, through rapid global transit, we are exposed to many diseases and illnesses that we had only heard or read about in the past. Travel time has been reduced to less than a day to get to the other side of the world.

Recent world events have given rise to a new global health concern—biological and chemical terrorism. Biological agents are infectious microbes or toxins used to produce illness or death. Terrorists may use biological agents to contaminate food or water supplies because they are very difficult to detect. Some chemical agents are also difficult to detect. They can be effective within a few seconds or it may take as long as hours or days (FEMA, 2002). It is feared that smallpox may be used as a form of biological terrorism. In that case, the effects would be devastating since most nations stopped manufacturing the smallpox vaccine after they believed smallpox to be eradicated in the late 1970s. The threat of biological or chemical terrorism affects all peoples and nations of the world and has become an international health priority.

Globalization is really not a new concept for nurses. It dates back to the days of Florence Nightingale. Her influence was felt in the British Empire and as far away as India, all of Europe, the Middle East, Australia, and North America. The health care challenges

A Conversation With...

Nursing students and others frequently ask me: How did transcultural nursing get started? In the 1950s I envisioned the field of transcultural nursing as an important and neglected area of study and practice. I was working as a child psychiatric clinical nurse specialist in a child guidance agency and discovered that children and families who came from different cultures could not be cared for or treated in the same way. I observed that children of African, Appalachian, German, Jewish, and other cultures clearly revealed differences in their eating, sleeping, playing, interaction, and sociocultural patterns. Because nurses were the major direct and continuous health care providers, they needed to understand these differences. I realized that my basic nursing program failed to prepare me to effectively deal with different cultures and types of care. I was culturally ignorant of the values, beliefs, and lifestyle practices of people. I had no idea how cultures could exert such a powerful force on people's health and well-being. I soon realized that nursing and other health care providers tended to treat all people alike, treating people as if they were mainly biophysical and psychological beings who were devoid of culture. Health care providers acted with limited knowledge and cultural influences on healing and well-being.

These realities led me to pursue graduate study in anthropology so that I could learn from scholars who had been studying cultures around the world for over 100 years. After learning from the experts in anthropology, I faced the challenge of how to develop the new field of transcultural nursing. One of the first tasks was to establish courses and programs in transcultural nursing, which entailed preparing faculty and practitioners to become transcultural nurse generalists and specialists in a field unknown to nurses. It also involved stimulating nursing leaders and organizations, as well as nursing students, to become interested in transcultural nursing knowledge and practices.

Almost five decades later, transcultural nursing knowledge is recognized as essential for teaching, research, practice, and consultation worldwide. Nursing students have been the strongest and most persistent promoters of transcultural nursing, along with patients who recognize that they have a right to have their cultures re-spected and given attention in health services. Schools of nursing, as well as many hospitals, clinics, and community agencies, are giving attention to diverse cultures in education and clinical services. This attention is necessary to meet accreditation requirements. Community health nurses continue to see the urgent need for transcultural nursing as they care for many families of different cultures. Since patients are increasingly dismissed from hospitals early, it is the role of community health nurses to maintain care services and relationships with cultural groups, including many new immigrants, refugees, and other newcomers to their communities.

In the early years there were nurses who were resistant to transcultural nursing. They were afraid to deal with cultural factors and wanted to protect themselves by not getting involved in areas they did not understand. Transcultural nursing education has helped many nurses face their fears and move forward to become more competent practitioners.

Transcultural nursing concepts, principles, theories, and research findings are guiding nurses to provide transcultural nursing services in the community, hospitals, clinics, hospices, and many other settings where nurses work. The Journal of Transcultural Nursing was established in 1988 and provides a rich source of transcultural nursing research findings and other information. In addition, many books, articles, and other publications focus on transcultural nursing to guide nurses in their practices.

The Transcultural Nursing Society, established in 1974, offers regional, national, and global conferences where nurses can meet with other transcultural nurses to share ideas and experiences and expand their worldview. In 1988 the Transcultural Nursing Society began to certify nurses to ensure that they could provide safe, competent, and effective care to people of diverse cultures. Today there are over 100 certified transcultural nurses (CTN), but many more are preparing themselves to meet the certification requirements. The Transcultural Nursing Society became the first organization to provide certification of nurses worldwide, which is a hallmark for future nursing directions.

—Madeleine Leininger

she faced were similar to many of the challenges faced by nurses today. Her systematic approach to nursing became the basis for modern nursing. In 1899, the nursing profession, realizing the importance of a global approach to nursing, established the International Council of Nurses (ICN), which was the first international organization for health care professionals. Today the ICN consists of over 100 national nursing organizations representing more than 1.5 million nurses. Through collaboration with international agencies focusing on global health, the nursing profession has advanced the agenda and policies that influence the health of the public and the welfare of nurses around the world (Kim, 2001).

Role of International Agencies

The United Nations

The United Nations (UN) was founded in 1945 when 51 nations came together after World War II to establish a commitment to world peace and security through international cooperation. Today, with a membership of 189 nations, the UN represents the interests of almost all of the countries of the world. When nations become members of the UN, they agree to accept the obligations of the UN Charter, which outlines the basic principles of international relations. However, the United Nations is not a form of world government. It does not make laws, but merely provides the means to help resolve global conflicts and formulate policies that affects all nations. All member nations, regardless of size, wealth, or political system, have an equal vote in the decision-making process. While the UN cannot force any member nation to act on any recommendations made, its decisions reflect world opinion and represent the moral authority of the community of nations (United Nations, 2002).

The United Nations has been working to combat intolerance in all its forms throughout the second half of the 20th century and into the 21st century. In 1948, the Universal Declaration of Human Rights was drafted by the General Assembly of the UN to outline the basic rights and freedoms to which all peoples of the world are entitled. Two International Covenants were developed, which most UN member nations consider to be legally binding. One addresses economic, social, and cultural rights and the other addresses civil and political rights. These two covenants, along with the Universal Declaration of Human Rights, constitute the International Bill of Human Rights (United Nations, 2002).

Through the years, the UN has established special organizations such as the United Nations Children's Fund to address various social and economic issues. There are also independent nongovernmental organizations (NGOs) that are related to the UN but are not under UN authority. These organizations have their own memberships, charters, budgets, and staffs. Two of these that will be discussed here are the World Health Organization and the Carter Center.

The United Nation's Children's Fund

The United Nations Children's Fund (UNICEF) was created in 1946 by the United Nations General Assembly to help European children in the aftermath of World War II. Today, UNICEF provides economic and humanitarian relief for the world's children without discrimination. The children in the world's poorest countries receive the highest priority. Special protection is ensured to children who are victims of war, disasters, extreme poverty, all forms of violence and exploitation, and those with disabilities (UNICEF, 2002).

Through programs aimed at ending hunger, controlling diseases, saving the environment, and securing human rights, UNICEF strives to improve the lives and health of all the world's children. An example is the worldwide focus on malnutrition, which is implicated in half of all child deaths. The effects of global malnutrition also affect millions of survivors who are left with physical and mental disabilities and a vulnerability to infectious and chronic diseases. UNICEF's nutrition programs have had much success in recent years. For example, 12 million children per year are having iodized salt added to their diets to prevent irreversible mental impairment. In addition, more than 60% of the world's children are receiving dietary vitamin A supplements to increase their resistance to disease (UNICEF, 1998; 1999).

••••••••••••••••••••••••••

During this final year of the 20th century, a child will be born, bringing the world's population to 6 billion. What lies ahead for this 6 billionth baby, no one can say. But for the majority of babies, the risks are high and the odds daunting. Half of the world's poor are children. Early death from preventable disease, illiteracy, or traumatic conflict often awaits them. For the 6 billionth child and for all children, the odds can and should be better.

Carol Bellamy, Executive Director of UNICEF, Progress of Nations, 1999

••••••••••••••••••••••••••

The World Health Organization

The World Health Organization (WHO) was organized in 1948 through a special agreement with the United Nations. Its goal is that all the peoples of the world should attain the highest possible level of health. Health is defined by WHO's Constitution as a state of complete physical, mental, and social well-being, not merely the absence of disease or infirmity. Dr. Gro Harlem Brundtland, Director-General of WHO, has developed the following strategic directions for WHO to advance global health in the 21st century:

1. *reducing excess mortality, morbidity, and disability, especially in poor and marginalized populations;*

2. *promoting healthy lifestyles and reducing risk factors to human health that arise from environmental, economic, social, and behavioral causes;*

3. *developing health systems that equitably improve health outcomes, respond to people's legitimate demands, and are financially fair; and*

4. *framing an enabling policy and creating an institutional environment for the health sector, and promoting an effective health dimension to social, economic, environmental, and development policy (WHO, 2002).*

In 1977, the World Health Organization set a goal that all people would attain a level of health by the end of the 20th century that would allow them to lead socially and economically productive lives. This led to the development of "Health for All by the Year 2000." Each country has developed their own national health goals based on the Health for All by the Year 2000 international objectives. The United States developed "Healthy People 2000," which was updated to "Healthy People 2010" in 2000. Specific "Healthy People 2010" objectives are listed in each chapter of this text.

The Carter Center

••••••••••••••••••••••••••

"We believe good health is a basic human right, especially among poor people afflicted with disease who are isolated, forgotten, ignored, and often without hope. Just to know that someone cares about them can not only ease their physical pain but also remove an element of alienation and anger that can lead to hatred and violence."

—President Jimmy Carter

••••••••••••••••••••••••••••

Former President Jimmy Carter and his wife Rosalynn founded the Carter Center in 1982. Located in Atlanta, Georgia, the Carter Center is a private, non-partisan, nonprofit organization connected to Emory University and governed by an independent board of trustees, chaired by Jimmy Carter. Its goal is to improve quality of life through programs developed to eradicate and control infectious diseases, health education projects to teach disease prevention and health promotion, and agricultural training to increase the food supply for poor families. The Carter Center has led a worldwide campaign to eradicate Guinea Worm Disease in Asia and Africa and control river blindness in Africa and Latin America. Their efforts have achieved a 98 percent reduction in Guinea Worm Disease and provided more than 35 million treatments for river blindness. Every year the Center's Mental Health Program assists in improving services and treatment for millions of people around the world suffering from mental illnesses (Carter Center, 2002).

A Role for Nurses

Nurses living and working in the 21st century need to expand their focus from one that concentrates on individuals and fami-

FYI

Of the 4.4 billion people in developing countries, nearly three-fifths lack access to safe sewers, a third have no access to clean water, a quarter do not have adequate housing, and a fifth have no access to modern health services of any kind.

More than 110 million active land mines are scattered in 68 countries, with an equal number stockpiled around the world. Every month more than 2,000 people are killed or maimed by mine explosions.

The three richest people in the world have assets that exceed the combined gross domestic product of the 48 least developed countries.

It is estimated that the additional cost of achieving and maintaining universal access to basic education for all, basic health care for all, reproductive health care for all women, adequate food for all, and clean water and safe sewers for all is roughly $40 billion a year—or less than 4% of the combined wealth of the 225 richest people in the world.

Source: UNDP, 1998a.

lies in local or regional settings to one that considers the effects of global health issues on their nursing practice. So many of the health conditions we see in our own communities, such as communicable diseases, poverty-related conditions, and violence, are directly related to global health problems and need to be understood in a global context in order to develop appropriate nursing interventions.

Health Care and Nursing Around the World

Czech Republic

Sharon L. Oswald and Elizabeth A. Simnons

The Czech Republic is a small Eastern European country bordered by Germany, Poland, Austria, and Slovakia. Until 1989, the Czech Republic was part of the Soviet state of Czechoslovakia. The current population of the Czech Republic is greater than 10 million, with an average life expectancy of 74 years of age and an infant mortality rate of 6.67 per 1,000 live births.

With the dismantling of the Soviet Union in 1989, the Czech Republic embarked on a rapid path of change from a socialist to a capitalist society. The Czech Republic went from the private sector representing less than 1% of the gross domestic product in 1989 to accounting for more than 56% in 1994 (Lastovicka, Marcincin, & Mejstrik, 1995). The privatization of industry contributed greatly to a sense of social cohesion throughout the country.

However, even with the general success of privatization, reform of the health care system has been met with criticism and resistance. Few have questioned the need for reforms; however, many have questioned the suitability of the methods used to change the system. Under the previous communist regime, the Czech health care system was characterized by universal coverage, national control, absence of competition, and inefficiencies. From World War II until 1992, health care was free to all citizens. The system, based on the national health service model, was hierarchical in nature and controlled by the government. The Czech Republic was split into regional health authorities, which in turn were further divided into district authorities. Although all health policies were established by the central government, committees headed by medical doctors controlled the regional and district authorities (Rubas, 1995; Zarkovic, Mielck, John, & Beckmann, 1994). The amount of money physicians and nurses received under this system depended on the type of health care institution, the hospital's capabilities, and the number of employees (Vyborna, 1994).

Just before privatization, the Czech health care system developed extensively and the number of nurses and physicians grew to approximately 4.7% of the Czech labor force. At the same time, hospital efficiency and equipment quality and reliability substantially deteriorated (Deppe & Oreskovic, 1996). The oversupply of health professionals, coupled with the lack of any concrete incentive to work, created a workforce overflowing with unmotivated, unproductive workers. In a country where medical personnel were paid barely livable wages, efficiency and customer service were not strong points. Furthermore, until 1993, hospitals were funded according to occupancy. Therefore, the incentive existed for administrators and doctors to keep the beds occupied (Earl-Slater, 1996), adding to the inefficiency of the system.

The transformation of the health system began in 1990, when the Czech parliament adopted a new health care system that was to guarantee access to health for all, privatization of health care providers, and community participation. In 1992, fundamental reform was initiated, beginning with a tax on wages to fund the new health care system and the introduction of compulsory health insurance. Health insurance was made mandatory for all citizens; however, the state theoretically assumed responsibility for those who were unable to pay. By design, the system was supposed to support the belief that health was not dependent on wealth and the wealthy were not responsible for the poor.

The Czech government established an insurance-based system that is administered by the newly formed General Health Care Insurance Office (GHIO), an independent insurance body. The GHIO was funded by a 13.5% tax on gross income, of which employers were required to pay two-thirds while their employees paid one-third. Working closely with the government, the GHIO was charged with redistributing the money collected from the mandatory tax. The GHIO holds approximately 84% of the insured market and is required by law to accept anyone who applies for insurance (Earl-Slater, 1996; Vyborna, 1994). Employer-backed private insurance companies were permitted for employee groups of 20,000 or more (Vyborna, 1994). Hospitals (state, municipal, and private) may contract with whichever insurance companies they choose.

An initial step toward health care reform was the decentralization of state-owned institutions (Vyborna, 1994). Community health centers (physician practices) were also privatized; however, restrictions were placed on the range of services that could be provided. In many cases, ownership of community health centers (physician practices) was transferred by the state to local town halls and leased back to individual physicians. In these cases, the state was responsible for the upkeep of the facilities. The other alternative was the sale of a health center to a private owner, a religious entity, or a nonprofit organization. In these situations, the owners were responsible for upkeep and equipment.

Since privatization, employment levels in companies throughout the Czech Republic have remained constant, including the health care industry. As a result, the overemployment of health care professionals in the 1980s continues to put a strain on hospital budgets. In addition, pricing for health services places some unpredicted pressures on hospital operating budgets. A point system has been developed to control escalation of health care costs. This system does not impose cost controls on the hospitals, but instead places budget controls on all health care facilities. If hospitals or other facilities are unable to stay within their budgets, government officials reduce funding as a form of punishment, rather than attempt to renegotiate the budget or examine problem areas. With hospital employment levels hovering well above American standards and reimbursement for services established at the whim of the government, hospitals have found it difficult to stay in business. This problem is compounded by the prorated system of reimbursement. Reimbursement decreases with each corresponding day a client remains in the hospital.

In addition, although nurses and physicians were the most vocal groups in support of health care reform, they were the first to stage a public protest against the direction that the reform efforts were taking. Nurses and physicians have played a positive role in changing the public's attitude toward health care. Three physician/nurse strikes resulted initially from requests for higher salaries. As a result, nurses' salaries have been increased by an average of 30%. The Ministry of Health created the post of director of nursing in 1991, primarily to facilitate changes in nursing education and to define the role of nurses in the changing health care system (Misconiova, 1992).

Although in theory the privatization effort seemed logical and consistent with the changing economic conditions, in practice it has proven problematic. Both economic and social problems have surfaced. As government officials and management concentrated on the operational problems, they limited their focus on economic issues, disregarding the social concerns. However, privatizing a social system is considerably more complex than privatizing business. Health care is a physiological need—any threat to that need will automatically lead to some form of resistance. In the Czech Republic, health care is considered an inalienable right. By 1996, there was a public cry for the end of privatization. What has resulted is a stagnated transformation. As of the summer of 1998, privatization remained at a standstill—but progress toward health care access and quality remains a primary goal of the new government.

Cuba

Juana Daisy Berdayes Martínez, Anayda Fernández Naranjo, and Alavara Leonard Castillo

Cuba, a Caribbean island nation with a population of 11 million, is located between the Caribbean Sea and the Atlantic Ocean approximately 90 miles off the coast of the United States. After the Cuban revolution in 1959, Cuba experienced many economic and social transformations, which led to the development of its current health care policy. The belief in the right to health care for all citizens and the duty of the state to guarantee it brought about the provision of free health services for all Cuban citizens. A process of reorganization and expansion of the national health system was initiated based on the primary care model. Several measures were taken to guarantee accessibility of health services for all. For example, new hospitals in rural zones and in mountains were constructed, greatly increasing the number of hospital beds nationwide. Health professionals no longer worked in private practices, but instead became part of the government's primary care system (Jardnes, Ouviña, & Aneiro Riba, 1991).

From its beginnings, the Cuban public health system has included the participation of the community in its historic evolution. In 1964, the first polyclinic was created to deliver comprehensive health care to communities. Community participation in health care was reinforced in 1975 with the creation of health advisory committees in each community. The health advisory committees are made up of people in the community who participate in analyzing the health of the community and facilitating collaboration between the health care system and community residents. In 1984, the new Cuban primary care model was introduced, with family physicians and nurses as essential components. Family practice physician offices, staffed by a physician and one or two nurses, began to spring up in every neighborhood. The principles of primary care proclaimed in Alma Ata in 1978 were applied in creative ways and adjusted to the economic and social conditions of Cuba. In this way, the truly humanistic dimensions of medicine and health care were applied to the care of people in their own communities, where they live, work, study, or play. As a result, Cuba met the WHO's "Health for All" 2000 objectives in 1985. Although Cuba is considered a developing country, its health indices are comparable to those of developed countries such as the United States. The life expectancy for Cubans is 75 years of age, and the leading causes of death are heart disease, malignant tumors, accidents, and cerebrovascular diseases.

Since 1989, with the economic collapse of the Soviet Union, with whom Cuba conducted 85% of its commercial trade, the living conditions of the population have deteriorated. In addition, the 40-year-old economic embargo of Cuba by the United States has contributed significantly to the economic depression. The health services that have been affected most are organ transplant and other technology programs, surgical activity, the availability of medications, and the acquisition and maintenance of medical equipment. Despite these resource limitations, the goals of the Ministry of Public Health are focused on maintaining free and accessible health care for all citizens and continuing the progress attained in the years since the revolution. Some of the future goals include expanding home care with medical and nursing surveillance for clients with acute conditions, increasing outpatient surgery services, and increasing emphasis on secondary and tertiary prevention.

The infant mortality rate, considered one of the best indicators of the health status of a population, has steadily decreased. Despite adverse economic conditions, the infant mortality rate was 7.8 per 1,000 in 1999, placing Cuba among the top 25 countries in the world with the lowest infant mortality rates. More than 99% of Cuba's children are born in hospitals or other health institutions. Vaccine-preventable diseases such as poliomyelitis, diphtheria, pertussis, measles, and tetanus have been controlled or virtually eliminated. In 1998, 98.5% of all children younger than 2 years of age were immunized.

At present, Cuba has 64,000 physicians (1 for every 170 inhabitants) and 82,527 nurses (17,568 of whom have baccalaureate degrees). More than 30,000 physicians and 32,000 nurses work in family practice settings in the community, with an emphasis on health promotion and illness prevention.

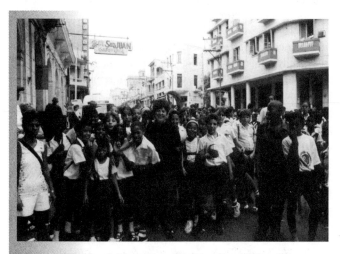

Chapter author, Dr. Sharyn Janes (center) with school children in Havana, Cuba.

Nurses working in communities are in privileged situations to identify and satisfy the needs or problems of families. By interacting with individuals and families in the community daily, the nurse is able to develop a holistic view of the health status of the community and its members. The work of the community health nurse corresponds to the needs of the population of the community where the family physician's office is located. The nurse works with the physician in a synchronized relationship. Together they provide health care for between 120 and 140 families, through office appointments and community visits to homes, day-care centers, schools, cafeterias, and so on (Eisen, 1996) During office visits, the nurse performs treatment procedures, immunizations, and physical examinations. Other activities include case management, health teaching, and research (Jardnes, Ouviña, & Aneiro Riba, 1991).

The physician-nurse team devotes half of each day to community visits, primarily home visits. The physical contact with the family environment allows the team to assess the environmental conditions in which the family lives, as well as the family's health practices, lifestyle, customs, and family relationships (Eisen, 1996).

Despite the difficulties encountered during recent years, Cuba offers a health system that is highly developed and effective. Because of the focus on primary care in the community, Cuba's main health indicators, such as an average life expectancy of 75 years of age, are comparable to those of industrialized countries, placing Cuba far ahead of the rest of Latin America and other developing countries around the world.

Iran

Marjaneh Fooladi

Iran, a country with a population of 60 million, is located in East Asia, bordered by the Gulf of Oman, the Persian Gulf, the Caspian Sea, Azerbaijan, Armenia, Turkmenistan, Pakistan, Afghanistan, Turkey, and Iraq. The average life expectancy in Iran is 70 years of age, and the infant mortality rate is 30 per 1,000 live births. Iran is a religious state known as the Islamic Republic of Iran. Shiite Islam is the official religion.

Since the Iranian Revolution of 1979, the health status of Iran has changed a great deal. Iran lost many of its devoted medical doctors, nurses, and medical technicians during the Eight Years War with Iraq because hospitals were one of the major war targets of Iraq.

The medical schools continue training doctors despite their losses in the war and those who fled to the United States. At the end of 1993, 73% of Iranians had access to health care, compared with 50% at the end of 1980 (the end of the revolution), and childhood immunizations for children younger than 12 years old reached 92% by the end of 1995.

The greatest success in the health care system during the postrevolution era has taken place in the rural and urban poor sections of the country. These sections were the most under-served areas during the prerevolution period. Today, these two sections have been so prosperous and well served in Iran that it serves as a model to other developing nations.

Another striking factor since the revolution is that women are encouraged to seek higher education, especially in medical schools. Today, 90% of women receive higher education, compared with 38% before the revolution (Friedman, 1996). Another noteworthy factor in the health care system is gender segregation. Gender segregation requires hospitals to segregate care given to men and women. In the present health care system, female nurses care for female clients and male nurses care for male clients. By the same token, female physicians care for female clients and male physicians care for male clients in most levels of health care, including primary, secondary, and tertiary (Iran gender segregation, 1998).

In many villages, however, life, death, health, and sickness are still attributed to God's will, and they are accepted in a spirit of fatalism. Accordingly, poor health is accepted, and medical aid is sought only when the illness interferes with one's daily work routine. A large number of Iranians believe in natural herbs, folk medicine, and the Holy Koran as curative means for illnesses. For instance, many Iranians use the *Book of Healing*, written by Avicenna (Abu Ali Cina, 980–1037 AD). This book contains descriptions of herbal medicine, dosages, and exercises, as well as general health rules. Because many medical problems are regarded as part of the supernatural, they are handled by religious leaders, whose services have been solicited in areas such as gaining someone's affection and love or ensuring the birth of a male child for couples who desire a son (Carter, 1978).

For serious illnesses, the family may consult a village herbalist or a medical doctor. Historically, in villages where there was not a medical doctor or health clinic, barbers were called to perform circumcisions and tooth extractions. Occult powers were given to midwives, who were viewed as specialists in the diseases of women and children (Carter, 1978).

In Iranian society, mothers carry a heavy load of responsibility on their shoulders as health care providers. The members of the family depend on mothers to handle their health problems and administer their everyday remedies. In return, mothers train their daughters in traditional medical lore, using magical formulas and herbs and preparing foods based on particular rules for certain illnesses.

Some of the most common terms for illness and their meaning as expressed by an Iranian client include the following:

- *Chashm e bad (evil eye)—believed to be a malicious spell cast on individuals through the eyes of another person or beast. People who believe their illness has resulted from evil eyes seek cure through praying and reading from the Holy Koran.*
- *Ghalbam gerefteh (distress of the heart)—indicates a feeling that the heart is being squeezed; it denotes severity from mild excitation of the heart or palpitation to fainting and*

heart attack. It also can be an expression that the individual is feeling blue or sad (Good, 1980).

- *Saram seda meekoneh (pounding in one's head)—expresses a general feeling that something is wrong; it may mean a feeling of anxiety (Good & Good, 1982).*

- *Balancing "hot" and "cold" foods—normally hot and cold categories are based on the Galenic-Islamic medical tradition (Good, 1980). These are not related to food temperature. Iranians put a great deal of emphasis on their diet. They include lots of fruits and vegetables in their diets, and they avoid excess fat. Culturally, they avoid processed foods, preferring to cook only with fresh ingredients. They refuse to eat incompatible foods at the same time. For example, fish and yogurt are incompatible. Honey and walnuts are considered hot, whereas cucumbers, watermelon, and yogurt are deemed to be cold.*

The following are a few home remedies commonly used by Iranians to prevent and treat symptoms of minor ailments:

- *Teas or herbs such as gole gohv zaboon are used for treatment of nervousness*

- *Nabbot (recrystallized sugar) is used to treat stomach upset and offset the cold foods*

- *Mint tea and cilantro seeds are used to induce relaxation and sleep*

- *Sucking quince seeds is used to relieve a sore throat*

- *Getting enough rest and exercise*

- *Keeping warm or dressing adequately (Hafizi, 1996; Lipson, 1992)*

Nepal

Debendra Manandhar

Nepal is a small country, with a population of 24 million, bordered by China and India. As a result of poverty and very limited access to health services, its health statistics are among the worst in Asia. The infant mortality rate is estimated to be 74 per 1,000 live births; the mortality rate of those younger than 5 is 189 per 1,000 live births; the maternal mortality rate is 8.5 per 1,000 women aged 15 to 49. The average life expectancy at birth is estimated to be 58 years.

The major causes of ill health lie primarily in widespread and extreme poverty and in an associated lack of basic infrastructures. This can be illustrated by the existing ratio of health personnel, hospitals, and hospital beds to population. There is just 1 doctor per 16,800 population, and even more important is the limited nursing staff, 1 nurse per 4,700 population. Similarly, there is 1 hospital per 161,948 population and 0.3 hospital beds per 1,000. These ratios are very low compared with the other South Asian countries (UNDP, 1998b).

Four health systems co-exist simultaneously in Nepal. These systems are divided into four broad categories: the home-

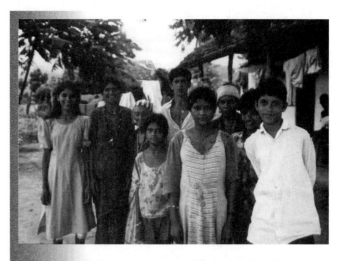

Hindu family in a mountain village in Nepal.

based system, the traditional faith healing system, the Ayurvedic (traditional Hindu) system, and the allopathic (modern Western) system.

Limited access to health services and the relatively low quality of public health institutions, along with the prohibitive costs of allopathic medicine and modern health services, force most households to rely on home remedies. The most common home remedies include folk remedies passed down from generation to generation and local herbs. Over-the-counter Western medicines, which are almost completely unregulated, are being used in increased numbers.

The failure of many home remedies invites intervention from community-level faith healers. Such healers base their treatment on an intimate knowledge of the sick person, divine invocation of ancestors, and herbal remedies. Healers often specialize in particular techniques, and specific healers are consulted according to the nature of the illness. The number of such healers is very large, indicating the legitimacy of the system. One study estimated the number of local faith healers at 400,000 to 800,000, which roughly translates to one faith healer for every six households. The significant role of local healers has been widely noted. The majority of sick persons in the rural areas who eventually visit the allopathic health clinic had first consulted a tradition faith healer. The majority of the women in rural areas use the services of faith healers for childbirth, partly because women prefer to deliver a baby at home.

The Ayurvedic (traditional Hindu) system of healing has been practiced in South Asia since ancient times. It is based on the physiological characteristics of the sick person, the symptoms of the illness, and a detailed pharmacological knowledge of herbs. The herbal treatments that households and local faith healers use are often borrowed from the Ayurvedic system. Most Ayurvedic healers work within the private domain, although there is some public support. Ayurvedic healing in the public sector is performed through one central Ayurvedic hospital with 50 beds, one 15-bed zonal hospital, 172 dispensaries in 55 districts, and a central drug-manufacturing unit (UNDP, 1998b).

Nepal began using a modern allopathic public health system at the end of 19th century. By 1955, there were 34 small-scale hospitals with a total of 623 beds and 24 dispensaries. An organized national public effort to spur the development of modern health services started in the mid-1950s. A large-scale malaria control program was launched in 1955; the leprosy and tuberculosis control projects were initiated in 1966; the smallpox eradication program was launched in 1968; and a family planning and maternal and child health board was established in 1968. In 1971, the Division of Basic Health Service was formed within the Department of Health to provide basic health to a maximum number of people. Small-scale public hospitals were established at various regional and district centers. In 1977, the successful smallpox eradication project was converted to the expanded program for immunization. Other health programs, such as nutrition support and diarrhea control, were integrated in 1980. Private and international nongovernmental organization initiatives also led to the establishment of rural health posts, clinics, hospitals, and drug retail outlets. One teaching hospital was also established within the public sector. Public health offices were established in all districts.

Significant steps were taken by the Nepalese government to expand the public health network in the mid-1980s and early 1990s. A national policy decision led to the formation of a unified group of volunteer community-based female health workers to provide basic health services, including health education and basic first aid treatment. At present, they number more than 42,000. Although their educational level is low, their achievements in terms of community sensitization to health-related issues and referrals to health care clinics are significant. Another national policy decision created an integrated institutional structure of public health at the local and regional levels. Implementation of this policy is leading to the establishment of community-level health posts in all parts of the country.

These governmental policies, together with expanding private initiatives, have led to a gradual rise in trained health personnel and health facilities at various levels. As of 1997, local clinics had been established in 3,187 of the 3,912 villages. A total of 75 public hospitals are functioning today in different regions. Approximately 40 hospitals and nursing homes have been established under private initiative. In addition, larger numbers of health clinics and laboratories have been set up in the private sector as well. In addition, there has been a significant increase in the number of health personnel and hospital beds per unit of population (UNDP, 1998b).

The formal health sector is organized through the Ministry of Health (MOH), with central offices of the various programs based in Kathmandu. The MOH is by far the largest single provider of formal health services. The MOH expenditure comprises nearly 50% of total expenditure on health care. Since its inception in the 1950s, the MOH has undergone almost continuous restructuring to become an integrated public health system with an emphasis on preventive care (UNDP, 1998b).

In every district, there is a District Health Office (DHO). Beside planning, management, and organization of health activities, the DHO is also made responsible for mobilizing all health and health-related institutions and supervising and monitoring the activities of these institutions regularly. At present, there are 1,196 physicians, 2,986 nurses, 240 Ayurved physicians, 130 Ayurved assistants, 1,186 health assistants, 4,015 village health workers, and 42,000 female community health volunteers in total for all districts combined in the country (UNDP, 1998b).

Private providers of health services in Nepal include private nonprofit providers, modern private for-profit providers, and traditional providers. The nonprofit providers are composed of nongovernmental organizations (NGOs) and international NGOs (INGOs). NGOs include small, local grassroots organizations as well as the national NGOs, such as Family Planning Association of Nepal, Nepal Red Cross Society, and so on. There are approximately 20 nonprofit hospitals with more than 1,000 beds. In most cases, the hospitals are run on a partial cost recovery basis. NGOs and INGOs provide support for governmental health services or parallel private health services.

The Nepal Social Welfare Council (SWC) estimates that NGOs operate about 235 primary health centers and that about 24% of all local rural health facilities are managed by NGOs. Forty percent of the budgets of NGOs that are registered with SWC are spent on health services, although health activities differ in scope and quality. The quality of health care services provided by NGOs is perceived to be better than those provided by the public sector. The strengths of NGOs include close contacts with local communities, nonbureaucratic structures, management flexibility, and higher staff motivation. Many of the NGOs have been experimenting with different methods of community financing schemes, which include sale and supply of drugs to retail outlets and community-based prepayment schemes.

Besides large local and international NGOs, many community-based organizations (CBOs) are involved in providing health care to communities. However, there is little documentation of the efforts of smaller grassroots level health CBOs.

Another kind of private sector provider is the for-profit organization. There has been significant growth in private nursing homes and clinics, especially in the urban areas. There are currently about 15 private for-profit hospitals and nursing homes with more than 200 beds.

Traditional healers are considered important private providers. Payment to the traditional healers is made both in cash and in kind. Many studies found the role of the traditional healers in the rural communities to be of great importance. In Nepal, there are still many remote places where it is almost impossible for the government to provide appropriate health care because of the mountainous terrain and local sociocultural beliefs. In such cases, traditional healers are the only source of health care.

Sadly, despite the growth in the health infrastructure in recent years, nearly 80% of the population are still not receiving health care services. Although the number of local clinics has increased, they are still ill equipped. The annual drug rations allocated to local clinics are adequate for only 3 to 6 months. Physicians and nurses often are absent from the rural-based clinics and regional and district hospitals. A major reason for this inadequate access to health care is related to poverty. The per capita health expenditure in Nepal is very low ($7) compared with other South Asian neighbors such as India ($21), Pakistan ($12), and Sri Lanka ($18).

South Africa
Ntombodidi Muzzen-Sherra (Zodidi) Tshotsho

South Africa, a country with a population of more than 40 million, is located in the most southern apex of the African continent. The average life expectancy in South Africa is 57 years of age, and the infant mortality rate is 52 per 1,000 live births. Before 1994, when the present government of South Africa was democratically elected, the majority of the population had limited or no access to health care services because of the legacy of apartheid. The laws and policies of the apartheid regime discriminated against the majority of South Africans on the basis of race and skin color. Between 35% and 55% of the South African population lived in poverty, with 53% of them living in rural areas. Poverty was rampant primarily because of the country's poor infrastructure and lack of resources in the rural areas, including poor transportation facilities.

Since the new government has been in place, many major changes have taken place in South Africa to ensure that health care services are accessible, affordable, and rendered in an equitable manner to the majority of the people. The National Department of Health published a *White Paper for the Transformation of the Health System in South Africa* on April 16, 1997, outlining a set of policy objectives and principles for the transformation of the health care system (Government Gazette No. 17910, 1997). The goals outlined in the white paper included the following:

- *Unifying the previously fragmented services at all levels into a comprehensive and integrated national health system (NHS)*
- *Improving equity, accessibility, and utilization of health services*
- *Extending the availability and ensuring the appropriateness of health services*
- *Developing health promotion activities*
- *Improving health sector planning and monitoring of health status and services*

The health services have been reorganized with an emphasis on planning and implementing health care services in ac-

cordance with primary health care principles. The responsibilities of health care services have been passed down from the national level to the provincial and district levels. The country is divided into nine provinces, with each one having its own department of health. A district health system for the delivery of services at the district level has been established in each province. Separate functions for all three levels of the health care system have been designated to avoid duplication of services and to ensure a well-coordinated comprehensive health care system.

Some of the roles of the National Department of Health include providing leadership for the formulation of legislation and health policy, building the capacity of the provincial health departments to provide effective health services, ensuring equity in the allocation of resources to the provinces and municipalities, developing a coordinated health information system, and forming partnerships with other national health departments and international agencies.

The mission of the provincial health departments is to promote and monitor the health of the people in the provinces and develop and support a caring and effective primary health care system. Some of the roles and functions of the provincial health departments include developing the capacity to deliver the full range of health services within the provinces, distributing resources (personnel, equipment, and facilities) to achieve accessible and cost-effective delivery of services, decentralizing all aspects of administration and management for services to allow local democratic participation in the control of health services, and achieving strategic, functional, and managerial integration of health services of both provincial and district health services.

Each province is divided into a number of functional districts. The main purpose of the district health system in South Africa is to decentralize responsibility for health care delivery and place it at the local level. This level of the health care system is responsible for the overall management and control of its own budget and the provision and purchase of a full range of comprehensive primary health care services within its area of jurisdiction. All services are rendered in collaboration with other governmental, nongovernmental, and private structures. In some provinces, district management teams are already in place and functioning well.

Equitable, accessible, and affordable comprehensive primary health care services in South Africa are slowly becoming a reality, as evidenced by a substantial increase in the number of clinics built since the inception of the new health care system; free health care services for children younger than 5 years of age and pregnant women; changes in the education and training of health care workers; meals provided at schools to reduce the prevalence of malnutrition among children; compulsory community service for newly qualified medical practitioners; control measures for alcohol, illicit drugs, and tobacco; HIV/AIDS prevention measures and services to reduce the personal and social impact of HIV/AIDS; and the Expanded Program on Immunization (EPI) to control the seven vaccine-preventable diseases common in children—childhood tuberculosis, diphtheria, pertussis, tetanus, polio, measles, and hepatitis B (Masakhane, 1998).

The transformation of health services in South Africa is not without problems, however, as some sectors of the community are critical of these changes and seem not to appreciate the principles on which the present health care system is based. High unemployment rates, poverty, and the upsurge of violence are only a few of the factors contributing to the limited successes of health care services. One of the biggest problems is the limited successes in controlling HIV/AIDS and tuberculosis. Despite the many problems, appreciable strides have been made in improving the health of the people in the rural areas. The rural areas are being provided with electricity, running water, telephones, and adequate housing (Sefularo, 1998).

••••••••••••••••••••••••••••••

It is important to recognize that the development of nursing and its status as a profession is very much related to its social contract. This contract varies around the world, but the overall theme is fairly consistent. Nursing is looked to for committed service to all peoples in need. Nursing is seen as responding to need, regardless of class, race, ethnicity, gender, or political affiliation. What this means is that nursing is fundamentally important to the pursuit of equity and social justice. It also means that nursing has a far-reaching impact that goes well beyond those individuals and families that nurses touch each day.

Marla Salmon, ScD, RN, FAAN,
Dean, Emory School of Nursing,
Atlanta, 1998

••••••••••••••••••••••••••••••

CONCLUSION

In today's world all nursing is transcultural and all health care is global. Our rapid transit travel systems allow us to circumvent the globe in a day. Our computer technology and television broadcast satellites enable us to witness world events as they are actually happening. The threat of biological and chemical warfare, in the wake of recent terrorist attacks, is a frightening reality. Never has it been more important for our health and survival as a nation and a planet to understand health care issues from a transcultural perspective. It is only through understanding, tolerance, and acceptance that we will be able to provide adequate and competent nursing care for the individuals and families we serve in communities all over the world.

CRITICAL THINKING ACTIVITIES

1. How many different cultural groups are there in your community? Who are they?
2. What are some of their traditions and values?
3. How are they different from you?
4. How are they like you?
5. Which groups or organizations in your community are working locally to improve people's lives?
6. Are nurses actively involved with any of these groups? If so, in what capacity?

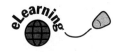 **Explore Community Health Nursing on the web!** To learn more about the topics in this chapter, access your exclusive web site: http://communitynursing.jbpub.com

REFERENCES

Carter Center. (2002). *Health Programs:* www.cartercenter.org/healthprograms

Carter, N. L. (1978). Social systems. In H. H. Smith (Ed.), *Iran: A country study.* Washington, DC: American University.

Deppe, H-U., Oreskovic, S. (1996). Back to Europe: Back to Bismarck? *International Journal of Health Services, 26*(4), 777–802.

Earl-Slater, A. (1996). Health care reforms in the Czech Republic. *Journal of Management in Medicine, 10*(2), 13–22.

Eisen, G. (1996). The primary attention in Cuba. The physician's team, the family nurse and the polyclinic. *Public Health Cuban Magazine, 22*(2), 117–124.

FEMA. (2002). *Backgrounder: Terrorism:* www.fema.gov/hazards/terrorism

Friedman, T. L. (1996). The talk of Tehran. *The New York Times, 145*(50542), p. 27.

Good, B. J., & Good, M. D. (1982). Toward a meaning: Centered analysis of popular illness categories: "Flight illness" and "heart distress" in Iran. In A. J. Marsella & G. M. White (Eds.), *Cultural conceptions of mental health and therapy.* Dordrecht: Reidel.

Good, M. D. (1980). Of blood and babies: The relationship of popular Islamic physiology to fertility. *Social Science and Medicine, 146,* 147–156.

Government Gazette No. 17910. (1997, April). *White paper for the transformation of the health system in South Africa.* Pretoria: South African Government Printing Office.

Hafizi, H. (1996). Iranians. In J. G. Lipson, S. L. Dibble, & P. A. Minarik (Eds.), *Culture and nursing care* (pp. 169–179). San Francisco: UCSF Nursing Press.

Jardnes J. B., Ouviña J., & Aneiro Riba, R. (1991). Education in the science of health in Cuba. *Public Health Cuban Magazine, 25*(4), 387–407.

Jemmott, L. S., Maula, E. C., & Bush, E. (1999). Hearing our voices: Assessing HIV prevention needs among Asian and Pacific Islander women. *Journal of Transcultural Nursing, 10*(2), 102–111.

Kim, M. J. (2001). Nursing in a global village. *CHART, 98*(4), 4–6.

Lastovicka, R., Marcincin, A., & Mejstrik, M. (1995). Corporate governance and share prices in voucher privatized companies. In J. Svejnar (Ed.), *Czech Republic and economic transition in Eastern Europe.* San Diego: Academic Press.

Leininger, M. (2001). Transcultural nursing care in the community. In K. S. Lundy & S. Janes (Eds.). *Community Health Nursing. Caring for the Public's Health.* Sudbury, MA: Jones & Bartlett Publishers.

Leininger, M. (1995). *Transcultural nursing: Concepts, theories, research, and practice.* Columbus, OH: McGraw-Hill.

Lipson, G. J. (1992). The health and adjustment of Iranian immigrants. *Western Journal of Nursing Research, 14*(1), 10–29.

Masakhane, J. (1998, October 29). List of healthy results. *Pretoria News,* p. 20.

Misconiova, B. (1992, September/October). Healing a sick society. *World Health,* 4–5.

Rubas, L. (1995, May 30). The intended reforms in health care Ministry of Health of the Czech Republic. Ministry of Health, Czech Republic Parliament, Prague.

Sefularo, M. (1998). Health and development of social welfare—North West Province. *Pretoria News,* p. 8.

Spector, R. E. (2000). *Cultural Diversity in Health & Illness (5th Ed.).* Upper Saddle River, NJ: Prentice Hall Health.

Sumner, W. G. (1906). *Foldways.* Boston: Ginn.

UNDP. (1998). *Nepal: Human development report.* Kathmandu: Author.

UNICEF. (1998). *The state of the world's children:* http://unicef.org/sowc98/silent.htm

UNICEF. (1999). *Progress of nations:* www.unicef.org/pon99/legcom2.htm

UNICEF. (2002). *UNICEF Mission Statement:* www.unicef.org/mission.htm

United Nations. (2002). *The UN in Brief:* www.un.org/Overview

Vyborna, O. (1994). *The reform of the Czech health care system.* Working paper. Co-sponsored by the Ford Foundation, in conjunction with Center for Economic Research and Graduate Education Charles University and Economics Institute of the Academy of Sciences of the Czech Republic.

World Health Organization. (2002). *Overview of WHO:* www.who.int/about/overview

7

Communicable Disease

Sharyn Janes and Gale A. Spencer

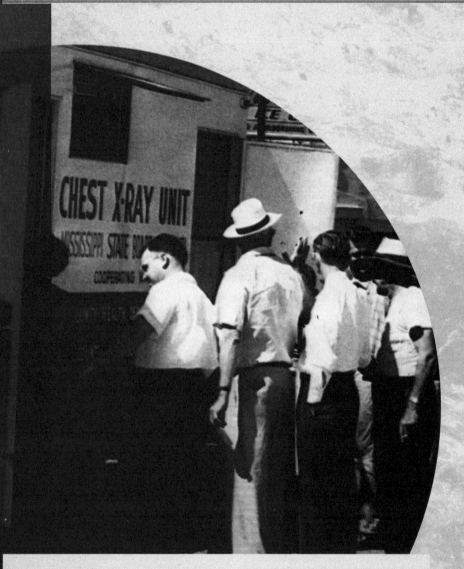

Some 1,500 people, mostly children and working age adults, will die in the next hour from infectious diseases, many that could be prevented for less than the cost of a few bottles of aspirin.

World Health Organization, June 17, 1999

QUESTIONS TO CONSIDER

After reading this chapter, answer the following questions:

1. What is the current infectious disease threat both in the United States and worldwide?
2. What are the reasons for the emergence of new diseases and the reemergence of diseases previously under control?
3. What are the factors that make up the chain of infection?
4. What are the different types of immunity?
5. How do vaccines aid in the prevention of communicable disease?
6. What is the role of the community health nurse in the prevention and treatment of infectious disease?

KEY TERMS

Acquired immunity	Immunity	Period of infectivity	Vector
Active humoral immunity	Incubation period	Personal surveillance	Virulence
Agent	Isolation	Quarantine	Zoonoses
Fomites	Passive immunity	Reservoir	
Herd immunity	Pathogenicity	Segregation	

The Problem of Communicable Disease

Communicable disease, or infectious disease, has always been a focus of community health nursing practice. In fact, at the end of the 19th century, when public health nursing emerged as a nursing specialty, communicable diseases were the leading cause of illness and death. During the early years of the 20th century, nurses continued to care for large numbers of adults and children who were sick or dying from a wide variety of infectious diseases. The typhoid epidemic in the early 1900s and the great influenza pandemic of 1918, which killed 20 million people worldwide (CDC, 1998a), are just two examples of infectious diseases that caused enormous suffering and death. Tuberculosis (TB) was a leading killer until well into the 1930s and 1940s, when TB sanitariums were overflowing. Nursing students in hospital schools in bigger cities were routinely tested for antibodies against TB, and most of them who came from rural areas tested positive. After a year in the urban hospital wards of the 1930s and 1940s, it was almost a certainty that nursing students would test positive for TB (Garrett, 1994).

The development of antibiotics, particularly penicillin, in the mid-1940s curbed the spread of bacterial infections and significantly decreased the number of deaths from infectious diseases like TB and typhoid fever. Vaccinations against diseases such as polio, whooping cough, and diphtheria, along with urban sanitation efforts and improved water quality, dramatically lowered the incidence of infectious diseases (CDC, 1998a). So although infectious disease still took an enormous toll in the rest of the world, a shift in leading causes of morbidity and mortality from infectious diseases to chronic diseases in industrialized nations like the United States caused attention to be focused on chronic conditions such as heart disease, cancer, and diabetes. Antibiotics became the "wonder drugs" of the latter half of the 20th century, and modern medicine triumphed. Or so we thought.

As early as the 1950s, penicillin began to lose its effectiveness against infections caused by *Staphylococcus aureus.* In 1957, and again in 1968, new strains of influenza originating in China rapidly spread throughout the world. During the 1970s, several new diseases were identified in the United States and elsewhere, including Legionnaires' disease, Lyme disease, toxic shock syndrome, and Ebola hemorrhagic fever. The 1980s brought human immunodeficiency virus/acquired immunodeficiency syndrome (HIV/AIDS) and a resurgence of TB, which rapidly spread throughout the world. By the 1990s, it was apparent that the threat of infectious disease was again a global reality (CDC, 1998a).

Now that we have entered the 21st century, we are again faced with infectious diseases that challenge medical and nursing practice. Some are old and familiar, like TB and influenza, and others are new and unfamiliar, like Ebola and hantavirus. Many of the new challenges are viral in origin, but the overuse and misuse of antibiotics over the last half century have also caused drug-resistant and often fatal strands of bacterial infections to emerge (Box 7-1). In fact, in much of the world, the most dangerous emerging diseases are not viral but bacterial or parasitic (Garrett, 1994).

The entire world is becoming much more vulnerable to the eruption and spread of both new and old infectious diseases. Infectious disease is a global problem brought about by recent dramatic increases in the worldwide movement of people, goods, and ideas. Not only are people traveling more, but they are traveling more rapidly and going to more places than ever before

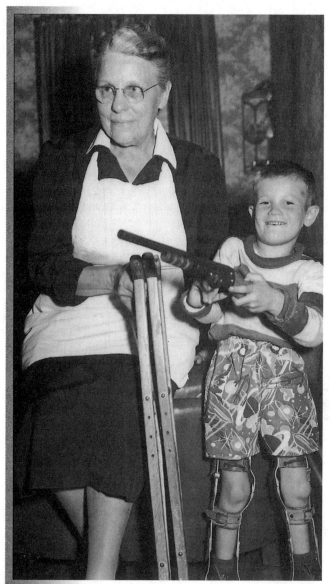

A home visit provided the public health nurse with an opportunity to assess a child with polio in familiar surroundings (circa 1951).

BOX 7-1 FACTS ABOUT ANTIBIOTICS AND ANTIBIOTIC RESISTANCE

- Alexander Fleming, a Scottish scientist, discovered the first antibiotic in 1928.
- Antibiotics became widely available in the 1940s.
- Two million pounds of antibiotics were produced in the United States in 1954. Today, more than 50 million pounds are produced.
- Antibiotics work by either killing bacteria or inhibiting their growth. They do not work on viral infections.
- People consume more than 235 million doses of antibiotics yearly. The Centers for Disease Control and Prevention estimates that 20% to 50% of that use is unnecessary.
- Antibiotic resistance occurs when bacteria causing a specific infection are not destroyed by the antibiotics taken to halt the infection. Unnecessary and improper use of antibiotics promotes the spread of antibiotic-resistant bacteria.

Source: Data from CDC, 1999a.

contributing factors are the emergence of new diseases, poverty, environmental changes, mass population shifts, and economic and social globalization. It is interesting to note that five of the six communicable diseases included on the list of the 10 deadliest diseases in the world were previously thought to have been contained, according to the World Health Organization's 1997 World Health Report (*Drug resistance*, 1998) (Table 7-1).

························

The single biggest threat to man's continued dominance on the planet is the virus.

Joshua Lederberg, Nobel Laureate

························

To address the increasing threat of infectious diseases, nurses must understand the problem from global and historical perspectives. There are many roles for nurses in the battle against infectious diseases. From a community health nursing perspective, primary and secondary prevention concepts must guide nursing practice. A holistic approach that includes health education, environmental health, political action, human rights, and cultural competency is the key. Communicable disease is, after all, not a new concept. Microbes have been an enemy of humans since ancient times. They did not disappear just because science developed drugs and vaccines or because Europeans and Americans cleaned up their cities and towns, and they certainly will not go away when humans choose to ignore or downplay their existence (Garrett, 1994). This chapter describes the present-day threat of infectious diseases and explores the role of community health nurses. Selected *Healthy People 2010* objectives related to communicable diseases are listed on the following page.

(Mann, 1994). Currently, one of every three people throughout the world dies from infectious diseases each year. Infectious diseases are the number one cause of death worldwide and are the sixth leading cause of death in the United States. Some of the

---

TABLE 7-1   **TEN MOST DEADLY DISEASES**

NAME OF DISEASE	COMMUNICABLE OR NONCOMMUNICABLE	DEATHS (IN MILLIONS)
1. Coronary heart disease	Noncommunicable	7.2
2. Cancer (all types)	Noncommunicable	6.3
3. Cerebrovascular accident	Noncommunicable	4.6
4. Acute lower respiratory infection	Communicable	3.9
5. Tuberculosis	Communicable	3.0
6. Chronic obstructive pulmonary disease	Noncommunicable	2.9
7. Diarrheal diseases	Communicable	2.5
8. Malaria	Communicable	2.1
9. HIV/AIDS	Communicable	1.5
10. Hepatitis B	Communicable	1.2

[1]Diseases in color represent reemerging infectious diseases.

Source: American Association for World Health, 1998c.

HEALTHY PEOPLE 2010

OBJECTIVES RELATED TO COMMUNICABLE DISEASES

Food Safety

10.1   Reduce infections caused by food-borne pathogens.

10.2   Prevent an increase in the proportion of isolates of *Salmonella* species from humans and from animals at slaughter that are resistant to antimicrobial drugs.

10.6   Improve food employee behaviors and food preparation practices that directly relate to food-borne illnesses in retail food establishments.

Immunization and Infectious Diseases

Diseases Preventable Through Universal Vaccination

14.1   Reduce or eliminate indigenous cases of vaccine-preventable disease.

14.2   Reduce hepatitis B.

14.5   Reduce invasive pneumococcal infections.

Diseases Preventable Through Targeted Vaccination

14.6   Reduce hepatitis A.

14.7   Reduce Lyme disease.

Infectious Diseases and Emerging Antimicrobial Resistance

14.9   Reduce hepatitis C.

14.11   Reduce tuberculosis.

14.15   Increase the proportion of international travelers who receive recommended preventive services when traveling in areas of risk for select infectious diseases: hepatitis A, malaria, typhoid.

Vaccination Coverage and Strategies

14.27   Increase routine vaccination coverage levels of adolescents.

14.29   Increase the proportion of adults who are vaccinated annually against influenza and ever vaccinated against pneumococcal disease.

14.30   Reduce vaccine-associated adverse events.

Source: DHHS, 2000.

Transmission of Infectious Agents

The role of nurses in the control of infectious disease prevention and treatment is based on an understanding of ways in which diseases are transmitted from one person to another. *Transmission* is "any mechanism by which an infectious agent is spread from a source or reservoir to a person" (Benenson, 1995, p. 544). There are three general modes of transmission: direct, indirect, and airborne.

Chain of Infection

The chain of infection is defined as the minimum requirements for an infectious or communicable disease to occur. Six factors make up the chain of infection: (1) an etiological agent or pathogen, (2) a source or reservoir of infection, (3) a means of escape from the source or reservoir (portal of exit), (4) a mode of transmission, (5) a portal of entry into the new host, and (6) a susceptible host.

The causative **agent** or pathogen is any substance or factor that can cause disease. Agents may be bacteria, virus particles, chemicals, or any other plant or animal substance that can cause illness, disease, disability, or death. Causative agents differ both in their ability to cause disease and in their ability to cause serious illness. **Pathogenicity** refers to the agent's capacity to cause disease in an infected host, whereas **virulence** defines the ability of the agent to produce serious illness. For example, both botulism and salmonella are highly pathogenic agents (they can easily cause disease), but botulism is much more virulent (it causes more severe disease).

The source of infection, or **reservoir**, is the habitat or medium in which the agent lives and/or multiplies. Reservoirs can be living things (e.g., humans, animals, insects) or inanimate objects (e.g., food, intravenous [IV] fluids, feces, surgical instruments, stuffed animals) that are conducive to the maintenance or growth of the agent. Reservoirs of infection are human beings, animals, and environmental sources. Humans become reservoirs of infection when the infectious agent has entered the body and established itself. There are three levels of infection in humans: (1) colonization, (2) inapparent infection, and (3) clinically overt disease.

Colonization occurs when the agent is present on the surface of the body or in the nasopharynx and multiplies at a rate sufficient to maintain its numbers without producing any identifiable evidence of a reaction in the person. Inapparent infection (subclinical infection) occurs when the agent is not only present but multiplies in the human reservoir. In an inapparent infection, the agent causes a measurable reaction; however, it does not cause the human to have symptoms of illness. Inapparent infections are usually identified only through laboratory testing (Benenson, 1995). Finally, clinical disease occurs when the agent is present in the human and causes physical symptoms. The time interval between initial contact with an infectious agent and the first appearance of disease symptoms is the **incubation period** (Benenson, 1995). The communicable period, or **period of infectivity**, is the time during which an infectious agent may be transferred directly or indirectly from an infected person to another person, from an infected animal to humans, or from an infected person to animals. All infected persons, including those with colonization, are reservoirs for the agent. Animal reservoirs are mainly domestic animals and rodents.

Zoonoses are animal diseases that are transmissible to humans under natural conditions. Animals transmit the disease directly to humans, but these diseases usually are not transmitted from human to human. Examples of zoonoses are bovine TB, rabies (although theoretically it can be transmitted by humans), and anthrax. Environmental reservoirs also transmit directly to humans. An example of an environmental reservoir is hookworm in soil. Inanimate objects such as food, surgical instruments, and human feces can also be reservoirs for diseases.

The agent leaves the reservoir through a portal of exit. Portals of exit and portals of entrance are similar. They include the following, listed in order, starting with the more common portals: respiratory, oral, gastrointestinal, reproductive, IV, urinary, skin, cardiovascular, conjunctival, and transplacental.

The last factor in the chain of infection is a susceptible host. The agent must enter a human host who is vulnerable to the specific disease agent. Susceptibility can be related to factors such as age, immunological status, lifestyle habits, or the presence of other infectious diseases or chronic illnesses.

Routes of Infection

The agent then must be transmitted to the next susceptible host through a mode of transmission. Transmission can be direct, indirect, or airborne.

Direct transmission consists of the direct and immediate transfer of an infectious agent from one infected host or reservoir to a portal of entry in the new host. This may be through direct contact that occurs through biting, kissing, or sexual intercourse or by direct projection of droplet spray into the conjunctiva of the eye or mucous membranes of the eye, nose, or mouth. The projection of droplet spray occurs with sneezing, coughing, talking, singing, or spitting, and is usually limited to a distance of approximately 1 meter (Benenson, 1995).

Indirect transmission usually occurs through a vector or by a vehicle. A **vector** is some form of living organism, usually an animal or an arthropod. Arthropods are insects such as flies and mosquitoes. Flies often carry organisms that are picked up on their feet or proboscis and transferred to food or water. When the organism is carried in this manner, it is called *mechanical vector-borne transmission* because the organism (or agent) does not multiply in the carrier. Mosquitoes, however, are often carriers of biological vector-borne transmission as multiplication and development of the organism occurs in the mosquito before the organism is transmitted to the new host through a bite (or inoculation). An example of this type of vector-borne disease is the transmission of malaria by the bite of a mosquito.

Vehicle-borne transmission is defined as contaminated inanimate objects, called **fomites**, which serve as an intermediate means by which an infectious agent is transported and introduced into a susceptible host through an appropriate portal of entry (Benenson, 1995). Examples of fomites are toys, bedding, soiled clothes, surgical instruments, and contaminated IV fluids. An example of a vehicle-borne disease is salmonella, which can be transmitted from a kitchen countertop contaminated while thawing raw chicken for dinner.

Airborne transmission occurs through droplet nuclei and dust, which are particles suspended in the air in which microorganisms may be present. Droplet nuclei result from the evaporation of fluid from droplets disseminated by coughing, talking, or sneezing between one infected person and another host. Droplet nuclei can remain suspended in the air for long periods in a dry state. During this time, some droplet nuclei retain their infectivity, while others lose their infectivity or virulence. The particles are very small and are easily breathed into the lungs, where they are retained. When these particles reach the terminal air passages, they begin to multiply and an infection begins in the new host (Benenson, 1995). Pulmonary TB and legionellosis (Legionnaires' disease) are two illnesses that are transmitted by droplet nuclei.

Dust particles in which microorganisms may be present can also become airborne and thus can be breathed into the lungs and cause infection. Contaminated bedding and clothes are examples of objects that can create dust that may carry infectious microorganisms from one infected person to another host. Dust particles contaminated with deer mouse feces may be one way to transmit hantavirus to human hosts.

The cycle of transmission can be broken by breaking the chain of infection—by eliminating the agent, eliminating the reservoir of infection, eliminating transmission at the portal of exit or the portal of entry, or eliminating susceptible hosts.

Susceptibility Versus Immunity

For a disease to be transmitted, the new host must be susceptible to that disease. The concept of immunity forms the basis of understanding host resistance to disease. **Immunity** is the increased resistance on the part of the host to a specific infectious agent (Valanis, 1999). There are two types of acquired immunity found in humans: active and passive.

Acquired immunity can occur after having had the disease or through vaccination. If a person is infected with the disease (with or without clinical signs and symptoms), the disease agent stimulates the body's natural immune system. However, if the person is inoculated with the agent (in a killed, modified, or variant form), the vaccination artificially stimulates the immune system (see Box 7-2 for a list of vaccine-preventable diseases). Both methods of acquired immunity result in active humoral immunity because the human body produces its own antibodies when the immune system is stimulated. **Active humoral immunity** is based on a B-lymphocyte response, which results in immunity that lasts for several years with diseases such as tetanus or a lifetime with diseases such as measles or mumps (Benenson, 1995). **Passive immunity** can be acquired either through the transplacental transfer of the mother's immunity to a disease to her unborn child or from the transfer of already-produced antibodies into a susceptible person (such as the use of immune serum globulin for persons exposed to hepatitis A). Passive immunity is based on a cellular, T-lymphocyte sensitization. Passive immunity is of short duration, lasting from days to months (Benenson, 1995).

Herd immunity is the resistance of a population or group to the invasion and spread of an infectious agent (Benenson, 1995).

BOX 7-2 VACCINE-PREVENTABLE

Adenovirus	Meningococcal
Anthrax	infections
Cholera	Mumps
Chickenpox (varicella)	Pertussis
Diphtheria	Plague
Hepatitis A	Pneumococcal
Hepatitis B	pneumonia
Haemophilus	Polio
influenzae	Rabies
Influenza	Tetanus
Japanese encephalitis	Typhoid
Measles	Yellow fever

Source: CDC, 1994.

Herd immunity is based on the level of resistance a population has to a communicable disease because of the high proportion of group members in the population who cannot get the disease because they have been previously vaccinated or have previously had the disease. Jonas Salk, one of the developers of the polio vaccine, suggested that if 85% of the population were immunized against polio (the herd immunity level), a polio epidemic would not occur (Timmreck, 1998). Herd immunity provides barriers to the direct transmission of infection through a group or population because the lack of susceptible individuals in the population stops the spread of infection.

Communicable Disease Prevention

One of the foundations of public health is the prevention and control of communicable disease. Timmreck (1998) states that the three key factors in the control of communicable disease are as follows:

1. *The removal, elimination, or containment of the cause or source of infection*

2. *The disruption and blockage of the chain of disease transmission*

3. *The protection of the susceptible population from infection and disease*

Approaches to the control of communicable disease should be based on the levels of prevention—primary, secondary, and tertiary.

Primary Prevention

Primary prevention activities are targeted at intervening before the agent enters the host and causes pathological changes. This level of prevention attempts to increase the host's resistance, inactivate the agent (source of infection), or interrupt the chain of infection.

A major focus of primary prevention is on increasing the resistance of the host. This can be accomplished through health education and/or immunization. Health education can target many subjects to increase the resistance of the host. It can identify a variety of activities that will improve the host's resistance, such as frequent handwashing, proper nutrition, adequate rest, and proper attire. Immunization is another method of primary prevention that increases the host's resistance. Immunization uses vaccines that are obtained either from the agent in a killed, modified, or variant form or from fractions or products of the agent (Valanis, 1999). Vaccines are available for many common infectious diseases.

Inactivating the agent involves stopping the agent by chemical or physical means. The protection of food has become particularly important in the last few years, with frequent food-borne illness outbreaks occurring as a result of improper storage, preparation, and handling. Proper temperatures must be maintained to inactivate the agent when storing, preparing, and cooking food. Proper food handling, which includes handwashing during preparation, is also important. Many bacterial agents (e.g., staphylococci, salmonellae, and *Escherichia coli*) can contaminate food and make the consumers of the food extremely sick. Irradiation of food (particularly beef and vegetables) has been suggested as a method of control, but this continues to be vigorously debated. Chemical methods are also used to inactivate agents. Chemical methods are used to chlorinate water supplies and to treat sewage, as well as to disinfect infectious or potentially infectious materials.

A common method of breaking the chain of infection is environmental control. Environmental control is aimed at providing clean and safe air, food, milk, and water; managing solid waste (garbage) and liquid waste (sewage); and controlling vectors (insects and rodents). Environmental control may target the reservoir, such as chlorination of a water supply. Environmental control may also be aimed at destroying the vector that transports the agent. One way a community may target the vector is to spray swamp areas (known to serve as reservoirs) with an insecticide to prevent mosquito-borne viral encephalitis. However, when this method is used, care must be taken to preserve the ecosystem as much as possible. Another method of breaking the chain of transmission is to encourage good personal hygiene and use of protective clothing. Methicillin-resistant *S. aureus* (MRSA) is an increasingly difficult nosocomial infection seen on medical and surgical floors in hospitals and in nursing homes. Health care providers must protect themselves and their clients by using proper hygiene and standard precautions when caring for all clients.

Primary prevention also includes restricting the spread of infection to human reservoirs and preventing the spread to other susceptible human hosts (Valanis, 1999). The four most commonly used methods are isolation, quarantine, segregation, and personal surveillance.

Isolation is the separation of infected persons during the period of communicability (Benenson, 1995; Valanis, 1999). These infected persons may be under one of several different types of isolation (strict isolation, contact isolation, respiratory isolation, tuberculosis isolation, enteric precautions, and drainage/secretion precautions). See Valanis's *Epidemiology in Health Care* (1999) or Harkness's *Epidemiology in Nursing Practice* (1995) for identification of types of isolation and diseases requiring precautions.

Quarantine is the restriction of healthy persons who have been exposed to a person with a communicable disease during the period of communicability. These persons are considered contacts of the infected human host. Quarantine prevents further transmission of the disease during the incubation period if the healthy contacts should become infected. Quarantine usually occurs for the longest usual incubation period of the disease. Quarantine is rarely if ever used today; however, before vaccination for diphtheria, it was often used in the United States.

Segregation is another method to control the spread of communicable disease. It is used to separate and observe a group of people who are infected with a specific disease. Segregation has been used in some countries to separate HIV-infected individuals from the general public in order to control the spread of AIDS. The United States still has public health laws that allow the segregation of persons with TB; however, those laws are rarely enforced, although in the early part of the 20th century, persons with TB were segregated from the general public in hospitals known as *sanitariums*. With the advent of new drug therapies and treatment, these sanitariums are no longer necessary.

Personal surveillance is close medical or other supervision of contacts and identified carriers of a specific disease without restricting their personal movement (Benenson, 1995). For example, public health officials continue to require personal surveillance of persons known to have had TB and to be carriers of typhoid.

As distinct from personal surveillance, disease surveillance is the continuing investigation of all incidence and spread of a disease that are relevant to effective control (Benenson, 1995). Public health surveillance is the systematic collection, analysis, interpretation, dissemination, and use of health information. Surveillance and data systems provide information on morbidity, mortality, and disability. Surveillance information is used to plan, implement, and evaluate public health programs to control communicable disease. To provide maximum benefits, surveillance data must be accurate, timely, and available in useful form (DHHS, 1991).

Although successful disease surveillance involves collaboration among federal, state, and local agencies, the U.S. Public Health Service (PHS) takes a leading role. PHS activities include collecting and analyzing health information at the national, regional, and when possible, state and local levels; providing data to federal, state, and local agencies for further analysis or use; assisting states and local agencies in conducting public health surveillance and evaluating data; and coordinating a network of federal, state, and local public health surveillance for diseases of public health importance (DHHS, 1991).

Secondary Prevention

Secondary prevention activities are targeted at detecting disease at the earliest possible time to begin treatment, stop progression, and initiate primary prevention activities to protect others in the community. Secondary prevention in infectious disease contributes to primary prevention because it restricts the infection to the human reservoir and prevents its spread to other susceptible individuals. Case finding and health screening are common activities used to accomplish this task. An example of case finding is following up on food handlers who may be infected during an outbreak of hepatitis. Screening for new cases of diseases can significantly decrease the spread of infection. Examples include screening for TB, through tuberculin testing, to detect and treat cases of TB among new immigrants; screening for herpes simplex virus type 2 in pregnant women to prevent infection to the infant

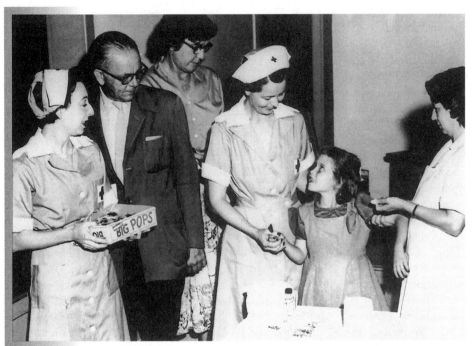

Nurses and physician administering Salk polio vaccine to a child (circa 1955).

during the birth process; screening for venereal diseases as a requirement for marriage licenses in some states; and administering gamma-globulin or immune serum after exposure to hepatitis.

Health education also plays a significant role in secondary prevention because it provides education about signs and symptoms, which enables individuals to identify illness and seek care early. Knowledge of health risk behaviors that contribute to the spread of disease may influence infected individuals to modify their behavior and thus assist in the prevention of the spread of disease.

Tertiary Prevention

Tertiary prevention limits the progression of disability (Timmreck, 1998). Hearing impairment from frequent ear infections, paralyzed limbs from polio, impaired vision from severe conjunctivitis, and shingles are just a few of the possible disabilities resulting from infectious disease. Treatment of symptoms and rehabilitation vary with each specific disease.

Control of Diseases

Vaccine-Preventable Diseases

Immunization is one of the most accepted and cost-effective preventive health practices in the United States. In the last 50 years, vaccines have prevented countless days of illness and hundreds of thousands of deaths. Most health care providers take for granted the rarity of vaccine-preventable diseases; many health care providers will never see a child with diphtheria, measles, or polio. Childhood immunization needs and practices are discussed

SABIN ORAL SUNDAY

POLIO PREVENTION PROGRAM

This Certifies That

Ruth Saucier

(NAME)

HAS RECEIVED SABIN ORAL POLIO VACCINE TYPE:

(1)   (3)   (2)

BRING THIS CARD FOR NEXT IMMUNIZATION. AFTER THIRD IMMUNIZATION, GIVE CARD TO YOUR FAMILY DOCTOR.

SABIN ORAL SUNDAY

POLIO PREVENTION PROGRAM

This Certifies That

Marshall Saucier

(NAME)

HAS RECEIVED SABIN ORAL POLIO VACCINE TYPE:

(1)   (3)   (2)

BRING THIS CARD FOR NEXT IMMUNIZATION. AFTER THIRD IMMUNIZATION, GIVE CARD TO YOUR FAMILY DOCTOR.

Vaccination cards from polio prevention program (circa 1956).

in chapter 21. Therefore, this chapter focuses on the vaccine-preventable diseases of adults and the need for adults to be immunized against them.

Adult immunization is extremely important. Approximately 70,000 adults in the United States die each year from vaccine-preventable diseases or their complications, compared with approximately 500 people (children and adults) who die of childhood vaccine-preventable diseases (Gardner & Schaffner, 1993; Thurm, 1998). Between 1980 and 1992, the number of deaths from infectious diseases rose 58% in the United States. Even when HIV-associated diagnoses are removed, deaths from infectious diseases still increased 22% during this period (DHHS, 2000). In fact, each year in the United States alone, at least 45,000 adults die from complications resulting from influenza, pneumonia, or hepatitis B, despite the availability of safe and effective vaccines to prevent these diseases. Approximately 90% of flu-related deaths occur in people age 65 and older (Thurm, 1998).

Hepatitis

Viral hepatitis encompasses several distinct infections. All are hepatatrophic and have similar clinical presentations. However, they differ in their cause and in some clinical, pathological, immunological, and epidemiological characteristics. Their prevention and control also vary (Benenson, 1995).

Hepatitis A

Hepatitis A is a highly contagious viral infection of the liver. In 1995, 31,582 cases were reported in the United States (CDC, 1995a). However, it is the most common vaccine-preventable disease in travelers (*Fact about hepatitis A for adults*, 1996). The hepatitis A virus (HAV) is found in the stool of infected people. The mode of transmission is person to person by the fecal-oral route. The infection is passed on by infected persons who do not wash their hands after having a bowel movement and contaminate everything they touch. Outbreaks have been related to contaminated water and to food prepared by food handlers who are infected with the hepatitis A virus. People are also infected with hepatitis A by eating contaminated raw shellfish, fruits, or vegetables.

People at risk for being infected with hepatitis A include the following (*Hepatitis learning guide*, 1998):

- *Those who share a household with someone who is infected with hepatitis A*
- *Individuals in a day-care center (adult employees or children) where a child or employee is infected with hepatitis A*
- *Those who travel to regions such as Africa, Asia (other than Japan), the Caribbean, Central and South America, Eastern Europe, the Mediterranean basin, and the Middle East*
- *Residents or staff of custodial institutions*
- *Homosexual men*

The symptoms of hepatitis A differ from person to person. Although many people infected with hepatitis A have no symptoms (particularly children), those with symptoms usually have an identifiable pattern. These symptoms include fever, nausea, vomiting, jaundice, diarrhea, fatigue, abdominal pain, dark urine, and loss of appetite. Respiratory symptoms, joint pain, and rash occasionally occur (*Facts about hepatitis A for adults*, 1996).

The incubation period is from 15 to 50 days, with the average time being approximately 28 days. The period of infectivity is during the last half of the incubation period, up to and including a few days after the onset of jaundice (Benenson, 1995).

Hepatitis A is prevented through the following means (Benenson, 1995):

- *Vaccination with the hepatitis A vaccine (with an initial injection providing protection for up to 1 year, with a booster dose [6 to 12 months after the first dose] providing prolonged protection)*
- *Education of the public about good sanitation and proper hygiene, with careful emphasis on handwashing*
- *Proper water and sewage treatment*
- *Education of employees in child day-care centers about the need for thorough handwashing after every diaper change and before feeding children or eating*
- *Immunization of child day-care employees*
- *Cooking shellfish to the proper temperature (85 to 90° C, or 185 to 190° F)*
- *Immunization with the hepatitis A vaccine of all travelers going to developing countries*

Hepatitis B

Hepatitis B is also a highly contagious virus that infects the liver. It is caused by the hepatitis B virus (HBV), which infects approximately 300,000 Americans annually. In the United States, more than 1 million people are chronically infected with HBV. Globally, there are an estimated 300 million HBV carriers (*Hepatitis learning guide*, 1998). The virus is found in the blood and body fluids of infected people. All persons who test positive for the hepatitis B antigen are potentially infectious. The mode of transmission can be person to person through sexual contact as well as through direct contact with blood or blood products resulting from sharing of needles or razors and from infected mother to infant during the birthing process. Hepatitis B is often described as a silent disease because it often infects people without making them feel ill. Infants are usually asymptomatic, and small children usually have a milder case of the disease. When symptoms do occur, the infected person will often complain of flulike symptoms, with loss of appetite, nausea and vomiting, stomach cramps, and extreme fatigue, which may progress to jaundice. Hepatitis B can progress to fulminating hepatic necrosis and death. Each year, 4,000 to 5,000 Americans die from hepatitis B (Benenson, 1995). Antiviral therapies are being used to treat active HBV with limited success.

The incubation period for hepatitis B is 45 to 180 days, with an average of 60 to 90 days. Hepatitis B occurs worldwide with little seasonal variation. Hepatitis B is prevented by the hepatitis B vaccine, which consists of a series of three intramuscular (IM) injections of the hepatitis B vaccine over 6 months. This vaccine is used to protect everyone, from newborn infants to older adults (*Facts about hepatitis B for adults*, 1997).

Hepatitis C

Hepatitis C is also a viral infection of the liver. It has been referred to as *parenterally transmitted hepatitis,* and before blood donor screening, it was the most common cause of posttransfusion hepatitis worldwide. Ninety percent of hepatitis C occurrence in Japan, the United States, and Western Europe is as a result of blood transfusions (*Hepatitis C*, 1997).

Hepatitis C virus (HCV) is found worldwide. The World Health Organization (WHO) estimates that up to 3% of the world's population is infected with HCV (*Hepatitis learning guide*, 1998). In the United States, hepatitis C currently accounts for 20% of acute viral hepatitis cases. Its occurrence is highest in IV drug users and hemophilia clients; moderate in hemodialysis clients; low in heterosexuals with multiple partners, homosexual men, health care workers, and family members of HCV clients; and lowest in volunteer blood donors (Benenson, 1995). The reservoir for the virus is in humans. The mode of transmission is indirect, spread through contaminated needles and syringes; however, this accounts for fewer than 50% of the infected cases in the United States. Transmission rates through household contact and sexual activity appear to be low, and perinatal transmis-

sion is uncommon. The route of transmission cannot be identified in more than 40% of infected clients (Benenson, 1995).

The incubation period of hepatitis C is from 2 weeks to 6 months, with most cases occurring within 6 to 9 weeks after infection. Most infected individuals with hepatitis C are asymptomatic (up to 90%); this includes even those with chronic disease (*Hepatitis C*, 1997). The most common symptoms are fatigue, nausea, vague abdominal discomfort, and jaundice. Severity ranges from inapparent cases (approximately 75%) to rare fulminating, fatal cases (Benenson, 1995). Although the disease appears to be less severe than hepatitis A or B in the acute stage, clients with chronic HCV infection develop chronic liver disease (occurring in more than 60% of adult clients). Of those developing chronic liver disease, 30% to 60% will develop chronic active hepatitis, and 5% to 20% will develop cirrhosis. There also appears to be an association between HCV infection and hepatocellular carcinoma (Benenson, 1995). Treatment with interferon is effective in approximately 20% of clients, and ribavirin has been shown to be somewhat effective as an antiviral agent against hepatitis C when used in combination with interferon (*Hepatitis C*, 1997).

Prevention measures for hepatitis C include the following (*Hepatitis C*, 1997; *Hepatitis learning guide*, 1998):

- *Universal screening of blood and blood products*
- *Effective use of standard precautions and barrier techniques*
- *Sterilization of reusable equipment and destruction of disposable equipment*
- *Public health education regarding the risks of using unsterilized equipment*

Because there is no vaccine against hepatitis C, prevention is the primary strategy against the virus.

Hepatitis D

Hepatitis D virus (HDV) is a defective, single-stranded RNA virus that requires the helper function of HBV to replicate. HDV is found worldwide, but its prevalence varies. Because it requires the HBV to replicate and to infect cells, it occurs either epidemically or endemically in populations with high rates of HBV infection (Benenson, 1995). Places where HDV is found to be endemic are Africa, southern Italy, Romania, parts of Russia, and South America. Populations that have high rates of hepatitis D are hemophiliacs, drug addicts, people with frequent blood exposures, residents in homes for the developmentally disabled, and male homosexuals. Humans serve as the reservoir for hepatitis D. The modes of transmission are similar to those of hepatitis B, with direct contact with blood or blood products the most efficient. Sexual transmission is less efficient than that of hepatitis B, and perinatal transmission is rare. The onset of hepatitis D is usually abrupt, with signs and symptoms similar to those of hepatitis B. Hepatitis D varies from being self-limiting to progressing to chronic hepatitis. Hepatitis D can be acquired either as a co-infection with hepatitis B or as a superinfection in persons with chronic HBV infection. When it is acquired as a co-infection, the person has a greater risk of severe acute disease, with a 2% to 20% chance of fulminant hepatitis. Chronic HBV carriers who acquire hepatitis D as a superinfection have a greater chance of developing chronic HDV infection. The superinfection with HDV has been found to increase the development of chronic liver disease with cirrhosis 70% to 80% compared with 15% to 30% of clients with HBV alone (*Hepatitis learning guide*, 1998).

The incubation period is approximately 2 to 8 weeks. Peak infectivity is thought to occur just before the onset of the illness. Symptoms are similar to those of hepatitis B and are identified as joint pain, abdominal pain, loss of appetite, nausea and vomiting, fatigue, and jaundice. No vaccine exists for HDV. The method of control is immunization with the hepatitis B vaccine; however, this is effective only in persons who are not already infected with HBV. For those infected with HBV, avoidance of any possible exposure to HDV is the only preventive measure (*Hepatitis learning guide*, 1998).

Hepatitis E

Hepatitis E is similar to hepatitis A in that there is no evidence of a chronic form. The fatality rate for hepatitis E is also similar to that of hepatitis A, except in pregnant women during the third trimester, when the fatality rate may reach 20%. Hepatitis E virus (HEV) is transmitted by the fecal-oral route. Contaminated water from feces of infected humans is the most commonly documented vehicle of transmission. Person-to-person transmission (seen in hepatitis A) does not appear to be a mode of transmission in hepatitis E, because secondary household cases are not common during outbreaks. The attack rate is highest in young adults; cases are uncommon in children and the elderly (Benenson, 1995).

The reservoir is unknown at this time, and an animal reservoir is possible. In the United States, as well as in most other industrialized countries, hepatitis E cases have been documented only among travelers returning from HEV-endemic areas (Benenson, 1995). HEV is endemic in Mexico, Central America, Asia, North Africa, the Middle East, and a few sub-Saharan African countries along the western coast (*Hepatitis learning guide*, 1998).

The incubation period is 15 to 64 days, with the mean incubation period ranging between 26 to 42 days (Benenson, 1995). Symptoms for hepatitis E are loss of appetite, nausea and vomiting, fever, fatigue, and abdominal pain. Many people who contract HEV have no symptoms. Prevention of hepatitis E relies primarily on the provision of clean water. Hygiene practice must be strict among travelers to prevent contracting hepatitis E when traveling in developing countries, such as avoiding drinking water and beverages with ice, uncooked shellfish, and uncooked fruits and vegetables (*Hepatitis learning guide*, 1998).

CASE STUDY

You are a nurse in a neighborhood-based clinic. In October, Mrs. Clark, a 75-year-old woman, comes into the clinic for her regular yearly physical examination. Mrs. Clark is in good health overall, with relatively few minor complaints. Last year, as part of her yearly visit, Mrs. Clark had been given an influenza vaccination. During this visit, however, Mrs. Clark tells you that she does not need to be vaccinated against influenza because she had gotten her "flu shot" last year. She also said, "I don't want the flu shot this year because I know somebody who got sick from it. I don't want to get sick."

1. Should you convince Mrs. Clark to get the influenza vaccination this year? Why or why not?
2. What other vaccines should you consider offering to Mrs. Clark?
3. What are the client education considerations for Mrs. Clark?

There is no vaccine and no identified treatment at this time; thus, prevention is very important.

Influenza

Influenza is another vaccine-preventable disease important in adults. Influenza is often called "the flu." It is an extremely contagious viral infection of the nose, throat, and lungs. In temperate zones, epidemics occur in the winter season, and in tropical zones, they occur during the rainy season. Influenza derives its importance from the rapidity with which epidemics occur, the high morbidity rate, and the severity of the complications that result from the infection. During major epidemics, the most severe illnesses and deaths occur in the elderly population and in those with debilitating diseases. In 1997, the flu vaccination rate for adults 65 and older was only 65.5% ("Immunizations lag," 1999).

There are three types of influenza viruses: A, B, and C. Type A is associated with widespread epidemics and pandemics, type B is associated with regional or widespread epidemics, and type C is associated with sporadic and minor localized outbreaks (Benenson, 1995). Occurrence is worldwide. The United States has an epidemic almost every year with type A, type B, or sometimes with both A and B.

Influenza symptoms are fever, myalgia, headache, sore throat, dry cough, and some gastrointestinal symptoms, such as nausea, vomiting, and diarrhea. Humans are the primary reservoir, with swine and avian reservoirs as likely breeding grounds for new strains. The mode of transmission is airborne, which is aerosolized or droplet material from the respiratory tract. The incubation period is very short, ranging from 1 to 3 days. People are infectious from 1 to 2 days before onset of symptoms to 4 to 5 days after onset (CDC, 1995b).

Most cases of influenza are preventable through a vaccine. Because the virus changes from year to year, it is necessary to be vaccinated yearly. The following people should receive a yearly vaccine: people 65 years and older, people with chronic disease (cardiac and/or respiratory), people who are immunocompromised, pregnant women who will be in their second or third trimester during the flu season, residents in long-term care facilities, health care workers, and adolescents receiving long-term aspirin therapy (who are at risk for Reye's syndrome) (*Facts about influenza for adults*, 1997; National Institute of Allergy and Infectious Diseases, 1997a).

Pneumococcal Disease

Pneumococcal disease is an acute bacterial infection. It is characterized by a rapid onset with shaking chills, fever, pleural pain, a productive cough, dyspnea, tachycardia, anorexia, malaise, and extreme weakness. Its onset is not as rapid in the elderly, and the first evidence is usually by x-ray examination. In infants and young children, the onset may be characterized by fever, vomiting, and convulsions. Pneumococcal disease is most severe in infants and elders, with higher death rates in both groups. The mortality rate is 5% to 10% with antibiotic therapy but can be as high as 60% for infants in developing countries where antibiotics are unavailable. The infectious agent is *Streptococcus pneumoniae* (pneumococcus). Its occurrence is worldwide, with peaks in the winter and early spring in temperate zones. However, it occurs in all climates and in all seasons (Benenson, 1995).

The reservoir for pneumococcal disease is in humans, and pneumoncocci are often found in the lungs of healthy people worldwide. The mode of transmission is airborne through droplets spread either by direct transfer or by indirect transfer when droplets have recently contaminated articles of clothes or bedding with discharge from the respiratory track. Person-to-person transmission is common. The incubation period is approximately 1 to 3 days.

Pneumococcal disease can be prevented through vaccination with polyvalent vaccine. Although this vaccine is not effective in children younger than 2 years of age (Benenson, 1995), it is safe in all others, and one immunization lasts most adults a lifetime against almost all the bacteria that cause pneumococcal disease. The following adults should be vaccinated: people 65 and older, people with chronic diseases, people who are immunosuppressed, residents of long-term care facilities, Alaska Natives, and American Indian populations (*Facts about pneumococcal disease for adults*, 1997). In 1997, the vaccination rate for adults 65 or older was only 45.5% ("Immunizations lag," 1999).

Routine Vaccines Indicated for Adults

All adults should be protected against many of the same diseases as adolescents and children. The tetanus and diphtheria (Td) vaccine should be given to all adults (Table 7-2). It is important for adults to be immunized against diphtheria and tetanus because 1 of every 10 people who get diphtheria will die from it, and 40 to 60 cases of tetanus occur each year, resulting in at least 10 deaths. Approximately 50% of Americans 50 years and older are inadequately immunized against tetanus and diphtheria (*Facts about adult immunization*, 1997).

Adults born before 1957 do not usually require the measles, mumps, and rubella vaccine because most of these adults have acquired immunity as a result of having the diseases during childhood. However, all adults born after 1957 should be immunized (see Table 7-2). Women of childbearing age should be given the rubella vaccine unless they have documentation of immunization after their first birthday. Currently, approximately 12 million women of childbearing age are susceptible to rubella. If rubella occurs during pregnancy, severe birth defects, miscarriages, and stillbirths can result (*Facts about adult immunization*, 1997). Although laboratory evidence of rubella immunity is acceptable, a stated previous history of rubella is unreliable and should not be accepted as proof of immunity. Before giving rubella immunization, the nurse should determine the likelihood of pregnancy during the next 3 months. The nurse should discuss with the woman her plans for reliable birth control during the following 3 months. Although there is no evidence that the rubella vaccine or other live viruses cause birth defects, the possibility exists. Thus, health care providers should not give any live vaccine to women known to be pregnant.

All adults without a reliable history of varicella disease (chickenpox) should receive the varicella vaccine. Adults who are either at highest risk for susceptibility or at high risk for exposing people to varicella should be targeted for varicella immunization (see Table 7-2). These adults include teachers, college students, military personnel, health care workers, and family members of immunocompromised persons. Although varicella is not considered a serious disease of childhood, adults are 25 times more likely to die from the disease. Adolescents and adults who develop varicella are 10 times more likely to require hospitalization and/or develop pneumonia, bacterial infections, and encephalitis (*Facts about adult immunizations*, 1997).

Emerging and Reemerging Infectious Diseases

Infectious diseases continue to be a problem for all people, regardless of age, gender, lifestyle, ethnicity, or socioeconomic status. New and mutated infectious diseases that have the potential to cause suffering and death and impose an enormous financial burden on individuals and society are always emerging. Two examples occurred in 1997, when a new strain of influenza that

TABLE 7-2   **ADULT IMMUNIZATION SCHEDULE**

VACCINE	TIMING OF IMMUNIZATIONS
Hepatitis A virus (HAV) for those at risk*	Two doses are needed to ensure long-term protection. Travelers to countries where the disease is common should get the first dose at least 4 weeks before departure.
Hepatitis B virus (HBV) for those at risk*	First dose; second dose 1 month later; third dose 5 months after second dose.
Influenza (flu)	Given yearly in the fall to people age 65 and older. Also recommended for people younger than 65 who have heart disease, lung disease, diabetes, and other chronic conditions, as well as for others who work or live with high-risk persons.*
Measles, mumps, rubella (MMR)	Two doses 1 month apart are recommended for adults born in 1957 or later if immunity cannot be proved.†
Pneumococcal	Usually given to those age 65 and older. Also recommended for people younger than 65 who have chronic illnesses such as those listed for influenza, and also for those with kidney disorders and sickle cell anemia.* A repeat dose 5 years later may be given for those at highest risk.*
Tetanus, diphtheria (Td) if initial series was not given in childhood	First dose; second dose 4 to 6 weeks later; third dose 6 to 12 months after the second dose; booster shot every 10 years.
Chickenpox (varicella)	Two doses are recommended for persons 13 and older who have not had chickenpox.‡

*Consult health care provider to determine level of risk.
†Should not be given to pregnant women or those considering pregnancy within 3 months of vaccination.
‡Should not be given to pregnant women or those considering pregnancy within 1 month of vaccination.

Based on the recommendations of the Advisory Committee on Immunization Practices, National Coalition for Adult Immunizations, CDC, 1997.

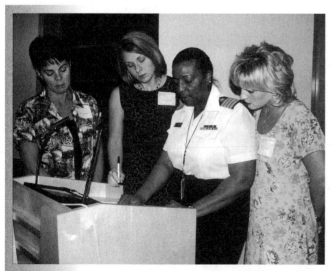

Mississippi nurses discuss immunization rates in their state with Captain Joyce Goff, RN (U.S. Public Health Service), Nurse Epidemiologist, at the Centers for Disease Control and Prevention, Atlanta.

had never been seen in humans began to kill previously healthy people in Hong Kong and strains of *S. aureus* with diminished susceptibility to vancomycin were reported in both Japan and the United States. If scientists cannot replace antibiotics that are losing their effectiveness, some diseases may become untreatable, as they were in the preantibiotic era (CDC, 1998a).

Everybody knows that pestilences have a way of recurring in the world; yet somehow we find it hard to believe in ones that crash down on our heads from a blue sky.
Albert Camus, 1948, *The Plague*

Emerging infectious diseases are diseases that have appeared for the first time or that have occurred before but are appearing in populations where they had not previously been reported. Reemerging infectious diseases are familiar diseases caused by well-understood organisms that were once under control or declining but are now resistant to common antimicrobial drugs or are gaining new footholds in the population and increasing in incidence (AAWH, 1997; Dzenowagis, 1997).

Concern about emerging and reemerging infectious diseases prompted a 1992 report issued by the Institute of Medicine (IOM) of the National Academy of Sciences. The report, "Emerging Infections: Microbial Threats to Health in the United States," concluded that emerging and reemerging infectious diseases are a major threat to the health of Americans and challenged the U.S. government to take action. The IOM report (1992) defines emerging or reemerging infectious diseases as those diseases whose incidence has increased within the last two decades of the 20th century or threatens to increase in the near future. Modern conditions that favor the spread of disease are listed in Box 7-3.

....

I think the weakest point in the United States is our false security that there will be no problems . . . we still have this feeling in the United States that we don't need to worry, that it's someone else's problem . . . but these diseases don't respect barriers. They don't respect borders.

Dr. David Heymann, Director of the Office of Emerging Infectious Diseases at the World Health Organization, 1997

....

> ### BOX 7-3 MODERN DEMOGRAPHIC AND ENVIRONMENTAL CONDITIONS THAT FAVOR THE SPREAD OF INFECTIOUS DISEASES
>
> - Global travel
> - Globalization of the food supply and centralized processing of food
> - Population growth and increased urbanization and overcrowding
> - Migration due to wars, famines, and other artificial or natural disasters
> - Irrigation, deforestation, and reforestation projects that alter the habitats of disease-carrying insects and animals
> - Human behaviors, such as intravenous drug use and risky sexual behavior
> - Increased use of antimicrobial agents and pesticides, hastening the development of resistance
> - Increased human contact with tropical rain forests and other wilderness habitats that are reservoirs for insects and animals that harbor unknown infectious agents
>
> *Source: CDC, 1998a.*

As a result of the IOM report, in 1994 the Centers for Disease Control and Prevention (CDC) and other health care groups launched a national effort to support public health efforts to control the negative impact of infectious diseases. As funds became available the CDC, in partnership with the IOM, state and local health departments, medical and public health professional associations, and international organizations implemented a plan titled "Addressing Emerging Infectious Disease Threats: A Prevention Strategy for the United States." The four major goals of the plan and the implications for nursing are described in Table 7-3.

Box 7-4 outlines some of the outcomes of the CDC's national effort to control the negative impact of infectious diseases 4 years later.

Food-Borne Disease

Infections caused by food-borne parasites or viruses are common. Each year in the United States, millions of people get sick from food-borne diseases and thousands die. In recent years, food-borne illness has become one of the fastest growing threats to community health in the United States (Foodborne illness, 1998; Mahon, Slutsker, Hutwagner, Drenzek, Maloney, Toomey, & Griffin, 1999). Much of the reason for this is that enormous quantities of food are being produced in central locations and then being widely distributed to all parts of the country (Mahon et al., 1999; Table 7-4). There have also been sharp increases in the number and types of food being imported from other countries. In response to these factors, the National Food Safety Initiative was created in 1997 to improve the safety of the nation's food supply (CDC, 1998a; Foodborne illness, 1998). The health care for people with food-borne illnesses can be very expensive.

> ### A CONVERSATION WITH . . .
>
> *With all our experience, we have not gone far on the road to eradicating disease. This knowledge keeps us humble. We have trouble outthinking a virus. Even smallpox humbled us until the very end. That virus seemed to have a better understanding of nature, human behavior, and ways to achieve immortality than the entire smallpox eradication team. The emergence and reemergence of infections must be approached with humility.*
>
> **—William Foege, MD**
> former director of the CDC
> and the Carter Center, Emory University, Atlanta
> Source: Foege, 1998.

TABLE 7-3   GOALS OF CDC PLAN OUTLINED IN *ADDRESSING EMERGING INFECTIOUS DISEASE THREATS: A PREVENTION STRATEGY OF THE UNITED STATES*

GOALS OF CDC PLAN (CDC, 1994) 1996)	ROLE OF NURSES IN CDC PLAN (COHEN & LARSON, 1996)
GOAL I SURVEILLANCE Detect, promptly investigate, and monitor emerging pathogens, the diseases they cause, and the factors influencing their emergence.	**GOAL I SURVEILLANCE** Support, explain, and circulate to the nursing community any recommendations made by CDC and their partner agencies focusing on the implications for nursing.
GOAL II APPLIED RESEARCH Integrate laboratory science and epidemiology to optimize public health practice.	**GOAL II APPLIED RESEARCH** Promote a population-based, epidemiological, systems approach for nursing practice and research.
GOAL III PREVENTION AND CONTROL Enhance communication of public health information about emerging diseases and ensure prompt implementation of prevention strategies.	**GOAL III PREVENTION AND CONTROL** 1. Collaborate with other professions and policy-making groups to support, endorse, and evaluate global strategies to prevent or reduce the threat of emerging infectious diseases. 2. Communicate with other nursing groups and recommend that they develop and disseminate policies and standards to prevent the spread of emerging infections. 3. Identify mechanisms to promote the appropriate prescription and use of antibiotics. 4. Address strategies to enhance host resistance and immunity. 5. Take a leadership role in initiatives to promote preventive strategies. 6. Take an active role in promoting science education for students in grades K through 12.
GOAL IV INFRASTRUCTURE Strengthen local, state, and federal public health infrastructures to support surveil-	**GOAL IV INFRASTRUCTURE** Serve as a clear voice to policy makers for support of public health, public education, public health infrastructure, and policies that protect the environment and promote ecological balance.

The yearly cost for food-borne illnesses in the United States is $5 to $6 billion in medical costs and lost productivity (National Institute of Allergy and Infectious Diseases, 1998a).

Foods can serve as a medium for growing bacterial pathogens or as a passive vehicle for transferring parasitic or viral pathogens. Most food-borne infections are directly related to foods of animal origin such as meat, fish, shellfish, poultry, eggs, and dairy products (Kaferstein & Meslin, 1998). Many food-borne bacterial diseases have emerged or increased during the last two decades. Some of the factors that bring about the multiplication and distribution of these bacteria in food are poor hygienic practices at the animal husbandry, slaughterhouse, and food processing levels as well as poor food preparation practices.

Prevention

There are three measures of protection against food-borne pathogens (Kaferstein & Meslin, 1998):

1. Prevention of contamination of food
2. Prevention of growth of pathogens
3. Prevention of the spread and survival of pathogens

BOX 7-4 SOME EXAMPLES OF THE IMPACT OF PREVENTION ACTIVITIES TO REDUCE MORBIDITY AND MORTALITY FROM EMERGING INFECTIOUS DISEASES FROM 1994 TO 1998

Decreased number of nosocomial outbreaks of multidrug-resistant tuberculosis from 9 between 1990 and 1993 to none in 1996 and 1997 as a result of the implementation of control measures in hospitals

Decreased incidence of hepatitis B by more than 60% from 1985 to 1996 primarily as a result of changes in high-risk behaviors and increased immunizations

Decreased incidence of hepatitis C by more than 80% from 1989 to 1996, primarily as a result of changes in high-risk behaviors and improved screening of the blood supply

Source: CDC, 1998a.

First, the quality of food at the production level must be improved. The environmental conditions under which food animals are raised and the use of fertilizers and pesticides for food plants must be monitored and controlled.

Second, food processing technology must be improved and used to prevent the survival and spread of food pathogens. Pasteurization, sterilization, and irradiation contribute significantly to food safety by reducing or eliminating disease-causing organisms.

Third, all food handlers must be educated in the principles of safe food preparation. This is probably the most critical line of defense, because most food-borne diseases are a result of one or more of the following (Kaferstein & Meslin, 1998):

- *Insufficient cooking of food*
- *Preparation of food too many hours before it is eaten, along with improper storage*
- *Use of contaminated raw food*
- *Cross-contamination where food is prepared*
- *Food preparation by infected persons*

Nurses' Roles in Prevention

Because many cases of food-borne diseases are a result of mishandling food in the home, community health nurses who visit families in their homes are in an excellent position to provide education for the persons in a family who are responsible for food handling and preparation (Kaferstein & Meslin, 1998). Female

---

TABLE 7-4 EXAMPLES OF MULTISTATE FOOD-BORNE OUTBREAKS IN THE UNITED STATES, 1994–1999

YEAR	ORGANISM	NUMBER OF STATES	FOOD SOURCE
1994	*Shigella flexneri*	2	Green onion, probably contaminated in Mexico
1994	*Listeria monocytogenes*	3	Milk, contaminated after pasteurization and shipped interstate
1995	*Salmonella enteritiditis*	41	Ice cream premix hauled in trucks that had previously carried raw eggs
1996	*Cyclospora cayetanensis*	20	Raspberries from Guatemala, mode of contamination unclear; cases also reported in the District of Columbia and two Canadian provinces
1996	*Escherichia coli O157:H7*	3	Unpasteurized apple juice, probably contaminated during harvest
1996	*Norwalk virus*	5	Oysters contaminated before harvest
1997	*Salmonella infantis*	2	Alfalfa sprouts, probably contaminated during sprouting
1997	*Cyclospora cayetanensis*	18	Raspberries imported from Guatemala, mesclun lettuce, and products containing basil; cases also reported in the District of Columbia and two Canadian provinces
1997	*Hepatitis A*	4	Strawberries from Mexico distributed through the USDA Commodity Program for use in school lunches
1998–1999	*Listeria monocytogenes*	22	Hot dogs and deli meats, probably contaminated while packaging

Source: CDC, 1998a, 1999d.

caregivers should be specifically targeted because they often prepare the food for infants and young children, elders, and others who are unable to cook for themselves.

School nurses can be successful in reducing the incidence of food-borne infections by educating children in the schools about the concepts of food safety. Educating children is not only an effective way to communicate safe food handling procedures to parents but is also a way to implant the principles of safe food preparation in the minds of future adults (Kaferstein & Meslin, 1998). School nurses should monitor school food programs and educate school food services personnel about proper handling and storage of foods. Educational programs should also be provided for teachers because of the amount of "food treats" that are served in the classrooms, especially in elementary schools.

Common Food-Borne Diseases in the United States

Campylobacteriosis

Campylobacteriosis, caused by bacteria of the genus *Campylobacter*, is one of the most common diarrheal diseases in the United States. The symptoms (diarrhea, abdominal pain, fever, nausea, and vomiting) usually develop within 2 to 5 days after exposure and typically last 1 week. Most people infected with *Campylobacter* will recover with no treatment except for drinking plenty of fluids for the diarrhea. However, in more severe cases, an antibiotic such as erythromycin can be used. Most cases of campylobacteriosis are a result of handling or eating raw or undercooked poultry. Most cases occur as isolated, sporadic events, although small outbreaks have been reported. More than 10,000 cases are reported to the CDC each year. However, because many cases are undiagnosed or unreported, campylobacteriosis is estimated to affect more than 2 million people every year, approximately 1% of the population (CDC, 1998b).

Listeriosis

Listeriosis, caused by the bacterium *Listeria monocytogenes*, has been recognized as a serious public health problem in the United States. The symptoms are fever, muscle aches, and sometimes nausea or diarrhea. If the infection spreads to the nervous system, headache, stiff neck, confusion, loss of balance, or seizures can occur. *L. monocytogenes* is found in a variety of raw food, such as uncooked meats and vegetables, as well as in processed foods that become contaminated after processing. The disease primarily affects pregnant women, newborns, and adults with weakened immune systems. An estimated 1,100 people become ill from listeriosis each year, and 250 of them die. Most deaths occur among immunocompromised and elderly clients. Infected persons are treated with antibiotics (CDC, 1999b).

Salmonellosis

Salmonellosis, caused by many different kinds of *Salmonella* bacteria, is a diarrheal disease that has been known for more than 100 years. The symptoms (diarrhea, fever, and abdominal cramps) usually develop within 12 to 72 hours after exposure and usually last 4 to 7 days. Salmonellosis usually does not require any treatment, but if the client becomes severely dehydrated or the infection spreads from the intestines to other body parts, rehydration with IV fluids and antibiotic therapy may be necessary. *Salmonella* can be transmitted to humans by eating foods contaminated with animal feces. Many raw foods of animal origin are frequently contaminated, but fortunately, thorough cooking kills *Salmonella*. Foods may also be contaminated by the unwashed hands of an infected food handler. Approximately 40,000 cases of salmonellosis are reported in the United States each year, but the actual number of cases may be 20 or more times greater (CDC, 1998c).

Escherichia coli O157:H7

Escherichia coli O157:H7 is an emerging cause of food-borne illness. *E. coli* O157:H7 is one of the hundreds of strains of the bacterium *E. coli*. Most strains of *E. coli* are harmless and live in the intestines of healthy humans and animals, but *E. coli* O157:H7 produces a powerful toxin that can cause severe illness. The combination of letters and numbers in the name refers to specific markers on the surface of the bacterium that distinguishes it from other types of *E. coli*. The symptoms of *E. coli* O157:H7 are bloody diarrhea and abdominal cramps, although sometimes there are no symptoms. Most people recover in 5 to 10 days without antibiotics or other specific treatment. In about 2% to 7% of infections, particularly among young children and elders, hemolytic uremic syndrome develops. This complication causes destruction of the red blood cells and kidney failure. Hemolytic uremic syndrome is a life-threatening condition usually treated with blood transfusions and kidney dialysis. With intensive care treatment, the death rate for hemolytic uremic syndrome is 3% to 5%. About one-third of persons with hemolytic uremic syndrome have permanent abnormal kidney function and may require long-term dialysis. Most cases of *E. coli* O157:H7 are associated with eating undercooked, contaminated ground beef; drinking raw milk; or swimming in or drinking sewage-contaminated water (CDC, 1999c).

Vector-Borne Diseases

A *vector* is an "animal, particularly an insect, that transmits a disease-producing organism from a host to a non-infected animal" (Neufeldt, 1996, p. 1478). Vector-borne diseases were responsible for more human disease and death from the 17th century through the early 20th century than all other causes combined (Gubler, 1998). In the late 1800s, mosquitoes were discovered to transmit such diseases as malaria, yellow fever, and dengue from human to human. By 1910, other major vector-borne diseases, such as African sleeping sickness, plague, Rocky Mountain spotted fever, Chagas' disease, sandfly fever, and louse-borne typhus, all had been shown to be transmitted by blood-sucking arthropods (Gubler, 1998).

TABLE 7-5	SUCCESSFUL GLOBAL VECTOR-BORNE DISEASE CONTROL/ELIMINATION PROGRAMS		
DISEASE		**LOCATION**	**YEAR(S)**
Yellow fever *(Aedes aegypti)*		Cuba	1900–1901
Yellow fever		Panama	1904
Yellow fever		Brazil	1932
Anopheles gambiae infestation		Brazil	1938
A. gambiae infestation		Egypt	1942
Louse-borne typhus		Italy	1942
Malaria		Sardinia	1946
Yellow fever		Americas	1947–1970
Malaria		Americas	1954–1975
Malaria		Global	1955–1975
Yellow fever		West Africa	1950–1970
Onchocerciasis		West Africa	1974–Present
Bancroft's filariasis		South Pacific	1970s
Chagas' disease		South America	1991–Present

Source: Gubler, 1998.

Most prevention programs have centered on vector control. Through a global effort during the 20th century, most of the vector-borne diseases in the world had been effectively controlled, primarily by the elimination of arthropod breeding sites and limited use of chemical insecticides (Table 7-5). However, the benefits of vector-borne disease control programs were short-lived. Vector-borne diseases such as Lyme disease and malaria began to emerge and reemerge in different parts of the world during the 1970s, and the numbers have greatly increased over the last three decades. Although the reasons for the resurgence are complex and poorly understood, two factors have been identified: (1) the diversion of financial support and subsequent loss of public health infrastructure and (2) reliance on quick fix solutions such as insecticides and drugs (Gubler, 1998).

Lyme Disease

In the 1990s, Lyme disease was listed as the most important emerging infection in the United States, accounting for 90% of vector-borne illness (Herrington, Campbell, Bailey, Cartter, Adams, Frazier, Damrow, & Gensheimer, 1997). First identified in 1975, when unusually high numbers of children living in Lyme, Connecticut, were diagnosed with juvenile arthritis, the annual number of reported cases of Lyme disease increased 25-fold between 1982 and 1998, with a total of 103,000 reported cases. The disease has steadily been moving into many different geographic regions in the United States (Pinger, 1998). In 1996, 45 states reported cases of Lyme disease to the CDC (Herrington et al., 1997). More than 16,000 cases were reported in the United States in 1996, and in 1997, there were more than 12,500 cases reported (CDC, 1999e).

The disease is caused by infection with the spirochete *Borrelia burgdorferi*, transmitted by infected *Ixodes scapularis* ticks in the northeastern, mid-western, and southern states and *I. pacificus* on the west coast (Herrington et al., 1997; National Institute of Allergy and Infectious Diseases, 1998b). These ticks generally feed on white-tailed deer and the white-footed mouse. The recent increase of the white-tailed deer population in the northeast and the influx of humans living in rural areas have probably contributed to the increased incidence of Lyme disease (National Institute of Allergy and Infectious Diseases, 1998b).

The symptoms of Lyme disease are multistage and multisystem. Early disease symptoms include a red rash resembling a bull's-eye forming over the tick bite and systemic flulike symptoms such as headache, muscular aches and pains, and fatigue. If untreated, symptoms can progress to include heart problems such as an irregular heart rate, shortness of breath, or dizziness; neurological problems such as meningitis, Bell's palsy, numbness, pain, or weakness in the limbs, or poor muscle coordination; and arthritis that shifts from joint to joint, with the knee being most commonly affected. About 10% to 20% of untreated clients develop chronic arthritis (National Institute of Allergy and Infectious Diseases, 1998b; Pinger, 1998).

Most cases of Lyme disease can be treated with antibiotic therapy. The earlier the treatment is begun, the more successful the treatment will be. However, early diagnosis is difficult because many of the disease symptoms mimic those of other disorders, and the distinctive bull's-eye rash is absent in more than 25% of those infected (National Institute of Allergy and Infectious Diseases, 1998b). It is important for the nurse to interview clients presenting with flu symptoms thoroughly to determine

RESEARCH BRIEF

Shankar, A. H., Genton, B., Semba, R. D., Baisor, M., Paino, J., Tamja, S., Adiguma, T., Wu, L., Rare, L., Tielsch, J. M., Alpers, M. P., & West, K. P., Jr. (1999, July 17). Effect of vitamin A supplementation on morbidity due to Plasmodium falciparum in young children in Papua, New Guinea: A randomised trial. Lancet, 354, 203–208.

A team of researchers in New Guinea followed 480 children between the ages of 6 and 60 months for 1 year. In the part of New Guinea where the study was done, 55% of preschool children carry *Plasmodium falciparum*, the parasite that causes malaria. The children were randomly assigned to groups that received high-dose vitamin A or a placebo every 3 months. By the end of the study, children who had received vitamin A had a 30% reduction in clinical episodes of malaria sickness and a 36% reduction of *P. falciparum* levels in the blood. In the age group normally experiencing the highest malaria sickness rate (12 to 36 months old), there were 35% fewer malaria attacks, 68% lower levels of *P. falciparum* in the blood, and 26% fewer enlarged spleens (a common result of malaria) in the children receiving the vitamin A. Although vitamin A reduced the number of acute clinical episodes of malaria, no statistical differences were found between the percentage of children in both groups who became infected with the malaria parasite. The researchers concluded that vitamin A supplements could be a cost-effective nonpharmacological treatment for malaria but would not be an effective method of primary prevention.

BOX 7-5 FACTORS CONTRIBUTING TO THE RESURGENCE OF MALARIA

- Increased resistance of malaria organisms to drugs currently used for treatment
- Civil wars in many countries, forcing large populations to relocate to different geographic regions
- Changing rainfall patterns and water development projects (e.g., dams, irrigation systems), which create new mosquito breeding places
- Poor economic conditions resulting in reduced health budgets and inadequate funding for drugs
- Changes in mosquito biting patterns, from indoor to outdoor biters

Source: Nchinda, 1998.

whether possible exposure to deer ticks could have occurred, particularly in warm weather months.

Malaria

Malaria is one of the oldest known diseases, with the first recorded case appearing in 1700 BC in China. In ancient Chinese, it was called "the mother of fevers" (The mother of fevers, 1998). Malaria is the most important of all vector-borne diseases because of its global distribution, the numbers of people affected, and the large numbers of deaths (Gubler, 1998). Worldwide, 10% to 30% of all hospital admissions and 15% to 25% of all deaths of children younger than 5 years of age are attributed to malaria. Each year, approximately 300 million people are infected by it, and as many as 2.7 million die, most of them residing in developing countries. The death toll includes more than 1 million children younger than 5 years of age (Liese, 1998; The mother of fevers, 1998).

Today, cases of malaria are reported in more than 100 counties throughout the world. Although more than 90% of cases occur in sub-Saharan Africa, the disease is also found in parts of Asia, the western Pacific, and Central and South America (Box 7-5). About 40% of the world's population, totaling more than 2 billion people, are currently at risk (The mother of fevers, 1998). Air travel has brought the disease to the doorsteps of industrialized countries, resulting in increased illness and death among travelers to areas with endemic disease (Nchinda, 1998). Although malaria is not endemic to the United States, it is the most common imported disease in the United States, with approximately 1,000 suspected cases being imported each year (Gubler, 1998). In recent years, clusters of malaria have occurred in California, New Jersey, New York, Texas, and Michigan, and 1,200 cases were reported to the CDC in 1995 (Pinkowish, 1998). Although malaria is not a widespread problem in the United States, nurses should be alert for imported malaria infection in their clients who travel abroad.

Malaria in humans is caused by a protozoon of the genus *Plasmodium* and the four subspecies, *falciparum, vivax, malariae,* and *ovale* (Nchinda, 1998). *P. falciparum* causes the most severe form of the disease in humans (Molyneux, 1998). The disease is transmitted through the bite of *Anopheles* mosquitoes (Marsh & Waruiru, 1998; Nchinda, 1998). Once inside the human host, the malaria organism enters the bloodstream and travels directly to the liver, where it hides and multiplies. After about 2 weeks, the newly produced organisms burst out of the liver into the bloodstream, where they attack red blood cells. These new malaria organisms rapidly reproduce in the bloodstream over the next few days until there are tens of millions of them. It is at this point that the human host begins to feel symptoms of illness (Marsh & Waruiru, 1998).

The first signs of illness are usually fever and malaise, often accompanied by a severe headache. At this stage of the illness, many people think they are experiencing the flu. Other malaria symptoms, such as vomiting, diarrhea, or coughing, might lead nurses or other health care providers to suspect gastric upset or respiratory infection. Malaria is a great imitator, making it important for nurses to suspect any fever as a potential case of malaria for clients who have recently traveled to a country where the disease is known to exist. Early diagnosis and rapid treatment are the keys to the secondary prevention efforts necessary to keep the disease from progressing to a complicated or severe state (Marsh & Waruiru, 1998).

West Nile Virus

West Nile Virus is a flavivirus commonly found in Africa, West Asia, and the Middle East. The first case of West Nile Virus was discovered in the West Nile District of Uganda, Africa, in 1937. It appeared in Egypt and Israel in the 1950s where it was recognized as a cause of severe human meningoencephalitis. In recent years it has emerged in the temperate regions of Europe and North America with the first case in the United States occurring in 1999. The virus is spread by infected mosquitoes and can infect humans, horses, many types of birds, and a few other kinds of animals (CDC, 2002a).

Humans generally experience a mild form of the disease, characterized by flu-like symptoms that generally last only a few days and do not appear to cause any long-term negative effects. However, in rare cases, humans can develop severe neurological diseases—West Nile encephalitis, West Nile meningitis, or West Nile meningoencephalitis. These illnesses are often very severe and can be fatal. Avoiding mosquito bites is the best form of protection from the virus. Treatment is mainly supportive, often involving hospitalization, intravenous fluids, respiratory support, and prevention of secondary infections for people with severe symptoms (CDC, 2002a; Petersen & Marfin, 2002).

Zoonoses

Many of the infectious diseases that have emerged or reemerged in the past few years have been zoonotic. Zoonoses are diseases that are caused by infectious agents that can jump from species to species—jumping from vertebrate animals to humans (Murphy, 1998; Neufeldt, 1996). Throughout time, humans have interacted with the other animals that share this earth. Whether domesticated work animals, animals raised or hunted for food, family pets, or unwanted household pests, animals and their products are an integral part of our daily lives (Meslin & Stohr, 1998). A variety of both domestic and wild animals carry viruses, bacteria, or parasites that can be transferred to humans either through direct contact with the animals and their waste products or through food products of animal origin (Heymann, 1998). Zoonotic diseases seem to be increasing at rapid pace for several reasons: Global human populations are increasingly bringing people into closer contact with animal populations; modern air travel has made it possible to travel to the other side of the world in a matter of hours; enormous environmental changes have been brought about by human activity; and bioterroristic activities are increasing, with the infectious agents of choice being zoonotic (Murphy, 1998).

Hantavirus

Hantavirus pulmonary syndrome was first recognized in the southwestern United States in 1993 when several deaths occurred from acute respiratory distress syndrome (Hantavirus infection, 1993; Toro, Vega, Khan, Mills, Padula, Terry, Yadon, Valderrama, Ellis, Pavletic, Cerda, Zaki, Wun-Ju, Meyer, Tapia, Mansilla, Baro, Vergara, Concha, Calderon, Enria, Peters, & Ksiazek, 1998). Initial symptoms include fever, muscle aches and pains, gastrointestinal upset, and headache. Cardiac dysfunction follows, with a 40% to 60% mortality rate (Toro et al., 1998).

Deer mice are the primary reservoir hosts for the southwestern U.S. hantavirus. Infection can occur when saliva or feces particles are inhaled in aerosol form during direct contact with the mice or when dried materials contaminated by mouse excreta are loosened, directly introduced into open wounds or eyes, or ingested in contaminated food or water. Humans can also become infected through deer mouse bites (Hantavirus infection, 1993). Avoidance of contact with the deer mouse population is the best way to prevent infection and control disease. Risks can be controlled through environmental hygiene practices that deter deer mice from inhabiting home and work environments (Hantavirus infection, 1993).

Pet Diseases

Pets, especially cats and dogs, are considered members of the family by many people worldwide. People give their pets names, share their food, and sometimes even share their beds with them, all in exchange for unconditional love (De Menezes Brandao & Anselmo Viana da Silva Berzins, 1998). Unfortunately, pets can be a source for zoonotic diseases. However, if pets are well nourished, properly vaccinated, and regularly examined by a veterinarian, there is little to fear (Chomel, 1998).

Cat-scratch fever, caused by *Bartonella henselae*, is generally a benign local inflammation of the lymph nodes transmitted through a break in the skin caused by a cat scratch. However, in people with weakened immune systems, it causes bacillary angiomatosis, a life-threatening vascular disease in which tumors are formed from blood cells. The organism is transmitted from cat to cat primarily by fleas (Chomel, 1998).

In countries where plague is endemic, cats can become infected or carry fleas from infected rodents they may have killed. Several cases of bubonic and pneumonic plague in humans in the United States have been associated with pet cats (Chomel, 1998).

Pets can carry infectious agents such as *Campylobacter* or *Salmonella*, which can cause diarrheal and gastrointestinal illness. Puppies and kittens with diarrhea pose the greatest risk. Reptiles are also carriers of a wide variety of *Salmonella* species. Pet turtles and iguanas have been linked to several severe, and even fatal,

FYI

Rabies and the Vampire Legend

The vampire legend began in Hungary around 1721 to 1728, at approximately the same time that a major rabies epidemic was occurring in dogs and other animals. Neurologist Juan Gomez-Alonso of Xeral Hospital in Vigo, Spain, said that clients with rabies often have a tendency to bite others and cannot tolerate mirrors or strong smells. When exposed to mirrors or garlic, they will often have spasms of the facial and vocal muscles causing hoarse sounds, bared teeth, and frothing at the mouth of bloody fluid.

Rabies occurs in men seven times more frequently than in women, and most vampire legends involve male vampires. Men with rabies suffer from insomnia and tend to wander at night, and because the disease affects the limbic system, which regulates emotions and behavior, they also become hypersexual.

In the 1700s, corpses were often exhumed to see if the person was a vampire. The signs of being a vampire included a lifelike appearance and blood flowing from the mouth. However, rabies can leave bloody liquid draining from the mouth long after death, and burial in the cold, humid climate of Eastern Europe preserved corpses for months or years.

Source: Adapted from IntelliHealth News, 1998.

cases of *Salmonella* among young children worldwide. It is easy to see why handwashing is extremely important after handling pets and before eating (Chomel, 1998).

Rabies

Rabies is probably the best known and most feared of the zoonoses because the disease is almost always fatal in humans once symptoms occur. The WHO estimates that more than 50,000 deaths from rabies occur a year, but the figure may actually be higher because of the large number of deaths worldwide that go unreported. In the United States, the number of rabies-related deaths has declined from more than 100 annually in 1900 to only one or two per year in the 1990s. Modern prevention efforts have proven almost 100% effective, with U.S. deaths occurring only in people who do not recognize their risk and fail to seek medical treatment (CDC, 1999f).

The virus is usually transmitted through bites from infected animals, but in rare cases, it can also be transmitted through infected licks on mucous membranes, inhaled infected bat secretions, and corneal transplants from undiagnosed human donors. Reservoirs for infection are domestic dogs and cats as well as many wild animals such as skunks, raccoons, foxes, wolves, and bats (Wilde & Mitmoonpitak, 1998). Before 1960, most rabies cases were in domestic animals, but now, more than 90% of cases occur in wild animals (CDC, 1999f). Efforts by U.S. wildlife agencies have helped control rabies in wild animal populations in recent years.

After entering the host, the rabies virus multiplies slowly at the portal of entry. It then invades the surrounding nerve tissue and slowly migrates to the spinal cord and brain. Once there, it multiplies, causing a rapid death. The incubation period can range from a few days to many years (Wilde & Mitmoonpitak, 1998). Rabies in humans is preventable by immediately cleansing all animal bites with soap and water and using rabies immune globulin and vaccine as indicated (Benenson, 1995; Wilde & Mitmoonpitak, 1998). Current rabies vaccinations are the best protection for pets and other domestic animals, thus significantly reducing the risk of exposure for humans.

Parasitic Diseases

Parasitic diseases, although more common in developing countries, have been on the rise in recent years in the United States. According to *Webster's Dictionary* (Neufeldt, 1996, p. 981), a *parasite* is an animal that lives on or in an organism of another species, from which it derives sustenance or protection without

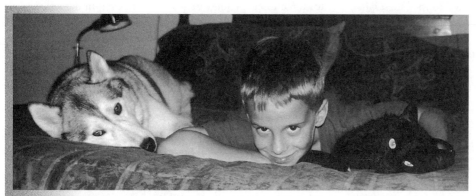

In American households, pets are members of the family. Children are especially vulnerable for exposure to infectious agents carried by pets.

benefit to, and usually with harmful effects on, the host. The most common parasites are helminths (worms and flukes) and one-celled protozoans.

Helminths

Pinworm infection (enterobiasis) occurs worldwide and is the most common helminth intestinal infection in the United States, with the highest prevalence in school-aged children, followed by preschoolers. The prevalence is low in adults except for mothers of infected children. Pinworm infection often results in no symptoms, but in some persons, there may be perianal itching and disturbed sleep. Diagnosis can be made by applying cellophane tape to the perianal region early in the morning before bathing or defecating. Transmission occurs by direct transfer of infective eggs from the anus to the mouth or indirect transfer through contaminated clothing, bedding, food, or other fomites. Treatment with oral vermicides and disinfection of clothing and bedding is usually effective (Benenson, 1995).

Roundworm infection (ascariasis) occurs worldwide, with the highest prevalence in children between 3 and 8 years of age living in moist, tropical countries. Typically, no symptoms occur. Live worms, passed in stools or occasionally through the mouth or nose, are often the first sign of roundworm infection. Transmission occurs by ingestion of infective eggs from soil contaminated with human feces or from uncooked produce contaminated with soil containing infective eggs; it is not transmitted directly from person to person. Treatment with oral vermicides is usually effective (Benenson, 1995).

Hookworm infection (ancylostomiasis) is widely endemic in tropical and subtropical climates but can also occur in temperate climates. Approximately 1 billion people (about one-fifth of the world's population) are estimated to be infected with hookworms. In persons with heavy infections, there is severe iron deficiency, which leads to severe anemia. Children with heavy, long-term infection may have hypoproteinemia and may be delayed in physical and mental development. Light hookworm infections generally produce no clinical symptoms. Diagnosis is made by finding hookworm eggs in feces. Transmission occurs by larvae in the soil penetrating the skin, usually of the foot. The larvae then enter the bloodstream and travel to the lungs, where they enter the alveoli and migrate up the trachea to the pharynx. They are swallowed and reach the small intestine, where they develop into mature half-inch worms in 6 to 7 weeks. They attach to the intestinal wall and suck blood. Treatment with vermicides is usually effective (Benenson, 1995; CDC, 1998d).

Protozoans
Giardiasis

Giardiasis is a disease caused by *Giardia lamblia,* a microscopic, one-celled parasite that lives in the intestines of humans and animals. This parasite is found in every part of the United States and every region of the world. In recent years, giardiasis has become one of the most common water-borne diseases in the United States. Transmission is through the fecal-oral route or through ingestion of contaminated food or water from swimming pools, lakes, rivers, springs, ponds, or streams. The most common symptoms of giardiasis are diarrhea, abdominal cramps, nausea, fatigue, and weight loss. Symptoms usually appear within 1 to 2 weeks after exposure and generally last 4 to 6 weeks, but they can last longer (CDC, 1998e).

Persons at risk for giardiasis are child care workers, children in diapers who attend day-care centers, international travelers, hikers, campers, or anyone who drinks untreated water from a contaminated source. Because chlorine does not kill *G. lamblia,* several community outbreaks have been linked to contaminated community water supplies (CDC, 1998e).

Giardiasis is difficult to diagnose and may require examination of several stool specimens over several days. The pharmacological treatment for giardiasis is metronidazole (Flagyl). Nurses can help prevent giardiasis outbreaks in their communities by teaching clients in community settings to wash their hands after using the bathroom and before handling food, to wash and peel all raw vegetables and fruits, and to avoid drinking water from any source unless it has been filtered or chemically treated (Benenson, 1995; CDC, 1998e).

Cryptosporidiosis

Cryptosporidiosis, often called *crypto,* is a disease caused by *Cryptosporidium parvum,* a microscopic, one-celled parasite. Although not a new disease in the developing world, cryptosporidiosis made its first major appearance in the United States in 1993, when 400,000 people became ill with diarrhea after drinking contaminated water. Today, crypto has become a major threat to the U.S. water supply. Transmission is through the fecal-oral route or through ingestion of food or water contaminated with stool, including water in recreational parks or swimming pools (CDC, 1998f, 1998g).

Immunocompromised persons are most at risk for crypto infection, particularly HIV-positive persons or persons receiving chemotherapy for cancer treatment. Other persons at risk for infection are child care workers, children in diapers who attend day-care centers, persons exposed to human feces by sexual contact, and caregivers of persons infected with crypto. The most common symptoms are watery diarrhea and cramps, which in some cases can be severe. Weight loss, nausea, vomiting, and fever may also occur (CDC, 1998g, 1998h; Guerrant, 1997).

Currently, no cure exists for crypto, but some drugs (e.g., paromomycin) may reduce the severity of the symptoms. Oral rehydration powders and sports drinks can help prevent dehydration. Nurses can help at-risk populations reduce their risk by teaching them to wash their hands often with soap and water; to avoid sex that involves contact with stool; to avoid touching farm

HEALTHY PEOPLE 2010

OBJECTIVES RELATED TO SEXUALLY TRANSMITTED DISEASES

Bacterial STD Illness and Disability

25.1 Reduce the proportion of adolescents and young adults with *Chlamydia trachomatis* infections.

25.2 Reduce gonorrhea.

25.3 Eliminate sustained domestic transmission of primary and secondary syphilis.

Viral STD Illness and Disability

25.4 Reduce the proportion of adults with genital herpes infection.

25.5 Reduce the proportion of persons with human papillomavirus.

STD Complications Affecting Females

25.6 Reduce the proportion of females who have ever required treatment for pelvic inflammatory disease.

25.7 Reduce the proportion of childless females with fertility problems who have had a sexually transmitted disease or who have required treatment for pelvic inflammatory disease.

25.8 Reduce HIV infections in adolescent and young females aged 13 to 24 years that are associated with heterosexual contact.

STD Complications Affecting the Fetus and Newborn

25.9 Reduce congenital syphilis.

25.10 Reduce neonatal consequences from maternal sexually transmitted diseases, including chlamydial pneumonia, gonococcal and chlamydial ophthalmia neonatorum, laryngeal papillomatosis (from human papillomavirus infection), neonatal herpes, and preterm birth and low birth weight associated with bacterial vaginosis.

Personal Behaviors

25.11 Increase the proportion of adolescents who abstain from sexual intercourse or use condoms if currently sexually active.

25.12 Increase the number of positive messages related to responsible sexual behavior during weekday and nightly prime-time television programming.

Community Protection Infrastructure

25.13 Increase the proportion of tribal, state, and local sexually transmitted disease programs that routinely offer hepatitis B vaccines to all STD clients.

25.14 Increase the proportion of youth detention facilities and adult city or county jails that screen for common bacterial sexually transmitted diseases within 24 hours of admission and treat STDs (when necessary) before persons are released.

25.15 Increase the proportion of all local health departments that have contracts with managed care providers for the treatment of nonplan partners of clients with bacterial sexually transmitted diseases (gonorrhea, syphilis, and chlamydia).

Personal Health Services

25.16 Increase the proportion of sexually active females aged 25 years and younger who are screened annually for genital chlamydia infections.

25.17 Increase the proportion of pregnant females screened for sexually transmitted diseases (including HIV infection and

Continued

HEALTHY PEOPLE 2010—cont'd

bacterial vaginosis) during prenatal health care visits, according to recognized standards.

25.18   Increase the proportion of primary care providers who treat clients with sexually transmitted diseases and who manage cases according to recognized standards.

25.19   Increase the proportion of all sexually transmitted disease clinic clients who are being treated for bacterial STDs (chlamydia, gonorrhea, and syphilis) and who are offered provider referral services for their sex partners.

Source: DHHS, 2000.

animals; to avoid touching the stool of pets; to wash and/or cook food; to be careful when swimming in lakes, rivers, pools, or hot tubs; to drink safe water; and to take extra precautions when traveling, particularly to developing countries (CDC, 1998f, 1998g, 1998h).

Sexually Transmitted Diseases

Approximately 15 million Americans become infected with sexually transmitted diseases (STDs) each year with over 25% of these infections occurring in adolescents. The overall disease rates for STDs in the United States are overwhelming. Rates for some STDs such as gonorrhea are higher in the United States than in some developing countries and are significantly higher than in most other developed countries in the world (CDC, 2001). The number of identified STDs continues to grow in the United States with eight new STDs appearing in the last two decades (Janes, St. Lawrence, St. Lawrence, Aranda-Naranjo 2001).

Sexually transmitted diseases are almost always transmitted through sexual activity. STDs are present in people representing all socioeconomic levels, ages, genders, ethnicities, and religions, although some subpopulations are at higher risk than others. Sexually active adolescents and young adults, men who have sex with men (MSM), and illicit drug users have higher rates of STDs than the general population (Janes, et al, 2001).

There are more than 25 organisms that can be transmitted through sexual activity causing dozens of different clinical presentations (Janes, et al, 2001). Five of the most common STDs are described in this chapter.

Chlamydia

Chlamydia is the most common STD in the United States with 3 million infections annually, a decline from 4 million annual infections during the 1980s. Seventy-five percent of women and 50 percent of men have no symptoms. While chlamydia is easily cured with antibiotics, it may be one of the most dangerous STDs for women because many cases go unrecognized and thus untreated. As many as 40 percent of women with untreated

BOX 7-6 CLINICAL PRESENTATIONS OF SEXUALLY TRANSMITTED DISEASES

In the case of sexually transmitted diseases (STDs), one organism does not cause one identifiable syndrome. Instead, similar presentations can be caused by different STDs. For example, pelvic inflammatory disease (PID) can be caused by gonorrhea, chlamydia, or other bacteria. Genital ulcers can be caused by herpes, chancroid, or syphilis, as well as by other infections. Some STDs, such as syphilis or HIV/AIDS, have many different clinical presentations and mimic many other health problems. Some diseases that were at one time not perceived as being particularly serious now are known to lead to very serious outcomes. For example, human papillomavirus infection (HPV) was widely associated with genital warts but not regarded as a serious condition until after it was discovered that HPV also causes several types of cancers.

chlamydia develop pelvic inflammatory disease (PID), and one in 5 women with PID become infertile (CDC, 2001).

Chlamydia is widespread among people who are sexually active, regardless of ethnicity, age, or gender. However, 40 percent of chlamydia cases are reported among adolescents between the ages of 15 and 19 years old. The prevalence of chlamydia among adolescent females exceeds 10 percent. While the data for adolescent males are more limited, the prevalence rate for young men is estimated to be more than five percent. The prevalence of chlamydia appears to be higher among underrepresented racial and ethnic groups, probably because of limited access to screening and treatment programs. For the same reason, chlamydia prevalence is highest in the southern states. In 1999, seven out of 10 states with the highest rates were in the southern United States (CDC, 2001).

Gonorrhea

Gonorrhea rates declined steadily in the United States from the mid-1980s to the mid-1990s, but steadily increased in the late 1990s and continue to increase, especially among adolescents and young adults. An estimated 650,000 cases of gonorrhea are reported each year in the United States, but it is estimated that these statistics represent only half the number of actual infections. The reported gonorrhea rate in the United States is the highest of any industrialized country. The United States has eight times more gonorrhea than Canada and 50 times more than Sweden (CDC, 2001).

While gonorrhea rates were once substantially higher among men than among women, the gap has considerably narrowed. Gonorrhea is one of the major causes of PID in women, often leading to infertility and ectopic pregnancies. In recent years, there are indications that cases of rectal gonorrhea may be on the rise among gay and bisexual men after a significant decline in the mid-1980s because of increased condom use. In addition, studies have shown that gonorrhea can facilitate HIV transmission, indicating that a resurgence of gonorrhea will most likely lead to a resurgence of HIV (CDC, 2001).

Gonorrhea rates have been increasing in all regions of the country since 1997, but remain highest in the southern states. This may be due to the higher level of poverty in the southern states as compared to other regions, as well as limited access to health care and preventive services in many rural areas. The high prevalence rates of gonorrhea may be contributing significantly to growing HIV epidemic in the south (CDC, 2001).

Syphilis

Syphilis rates are the lowest in the United States since reporting began in 1941 (CDC, 2001). The discovery of penicillin and the initiation of a national STD control program in the 1940s nearly eliminated syphilis in the United States in 1957; but since then, there have been national epidemics every seven to 10 years (St. Louis & Wasserheit, 1998). In 1999, the concentration of syphilis in only 20 percent of counties in the United States (see Figure 7-1) along with low rates of syphilis overall (see Figure 7-2) prompted the CDC to initiate the National Plan to Eliminate Syphilis in the United States.

Syphilis is a bacterial disease that progresses in stages, with different clinical presentations at each stage:

1. *Primary—ulcer or chancre at site of infection;*

2. *Secondary—rash, lesions on skin or mucus membranes;*

3. *Tertiary—cardiac, neurological, ophthalmic, or auditory lesions (Janes, et al, 2001).*

The disease is curable in the early stages and progression is preventable. The genital ulcers caused by syphilis can increase the susceptibility to HIV transmission two to five times. Untreated syphilis can be transmitted from mother to fetus causing birth defects affecting all systems, including severe neurological abnormalities (CDC, 2001).

African Americans and other underrepresented ethnic groups are disproportionately affected by syphilis. Syphilis rates are used as a glaring illustration of existing gaps in minority health status. The southern states have the highest concentration of syphilis cases reported. In 1999, the rate of syphilis in the South at 4.5 cases per 100,000 people was higher than any other region of the country (CDC, 2001).

Human Papillomavirus (HPV)

There are an estimated 20 million transmissible cases of Human Papilloma virus (HPV) at any given time in the United States. Each year, approximately 5.5 million Americans acquire a genital HPV infection. In recent years, studies have indicated that HPV may be the most common STD among young people who are sexually active (CDC, 2001).

There are 30 different types of HPV that can cause infection. Some of these may cause genital warts, but others can cause subclinical infections that are invisible or are difficult to see (CDC, 2001). An estimated 50 percent of people infected with HPV are unaware of their infection and thus are unknowingly spreading the virus to others (Janes, et al, 2001). Genital warts can be treated, but there is no treatment for the more common subclinical infections. This has become a major public health concern because of the connection between some types of HPV and cervical, penile, and anal cancer. In fact, recent research has suggested that as high as 80 percent of cervical cancers are associated with specific types of HPV infections (CDC, 2001).

Genital Herpes

There are two types of herpes simplex virus (HSV), both of which can cause genital herpes. While herpes simplex virus type 1 (HSV-1) can cause genital herpes, it most often causes fever blisters and cold sores around the mouth area. Herpes simplex virus type 2 (HSV-2) is the most common cause of genital herpes, but it can also cause sores around the mouth area (Janes, et al, 2001). As many as one million people in the United States become infected with genital herpes every year (CDC, 2001). Genital herpes infection produces recurrent painful ulcers, which can be treated but not cured. Nearly 80 percent of people with genital herpes never develop symptoms or do not recognize them (Janes, et al, 2001).

While Genital herpes (HSV-2) is prevalent among all age groups, in recent years the disease has increased most dramatically among adolescents and young adults. From the late 1970s to the early 1990s, herpes prevalence increased by 30 percent. The prevalence has remained fairly stable during the 1990s and

Primary and Secondary Syphilis   Counties with Rates Above and Counties with Rates Below the Healthy People Year 2000 Objective, United States, 1999

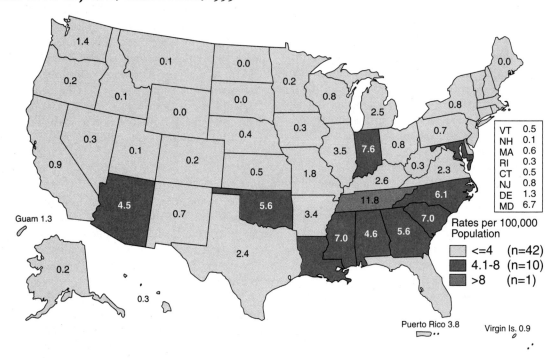

Note: The total rate of primary and secondary syphilis for the United States and outlying areas (including Guam, Puerto Rico and Virgin Islands) was 2.5 per 100,000 population, the Healthy People year 2000 objective is 4.0 per 100,000 population.

Primary and Secondary Syphilis   Rates by State: United States and Outlying Areas, 1999. Source: CDC, 2001

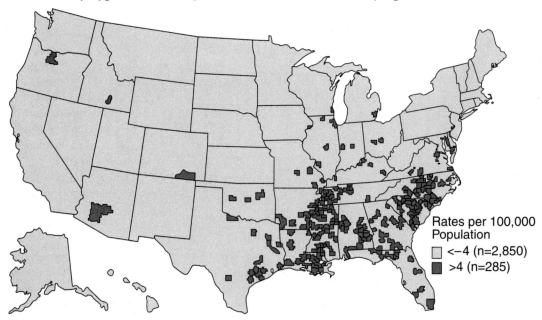

currently remains at about 19 percent of the U.S. population between the ages of 14 and 49 years old (McQuillan, 2000). Genital herpes infects one out of four women, as compared to one out of five men. Perhaps this is because male-to-female transmission, as with most other sexually transmitted diseases, is more efficient than female-to-male transmission. Genital herpes infection is equally common in both urban and rural areas in the United States and there are no significant differences by geographic location (CDC, 2001).

If I were going to imagine a real terror it would be a deadly virus that kills 100% of its victims, but incubates so slowly, say a decade, that millions of people are infected before they know it. It would be a virus that is transmitted sexually, attacking young adults while it takes advantage of our social inhibitions and bigotry about sex.

Dr. Joe McCormick, Chairman,
Community Health Sciences Department,
Aga Khan University, Pakistan

HIV/AIDS

The most significant emerging disease in the world during the last 20 years is HIV/AIDS. AIDS is the life-threatening, late clinical stage of infection with HIV. The disease was first recognized as a distinct syndrome in 1981, and the virus was first isolated in 1983 (Benenson, 1995).

As of June 30, 2001, the cumulative number of reported AIDS cases in the United States was 793,026. The total number of deaths from AIDS in the United States was 457,667 (CDC, 2002b). By the end of 2001, the total estimated number of global HIV/AIDS cases had exceeded 40 million and an

BOX 7-7 WHY WE SHOULD CARE
20 YEARS OF AIDS—1981 TO 2001

The figures in color following each year's entry represent the cumulative number of AIDS-related deaths that had occurred in the US from the beginning of the pandemic to the end of that year.

1981: The Centers for Disease Control and Prevention (CDC) diagnoses the first cases of AIDS-related diseases among young gay men. 159

1982: The CDC formally establishes the term "Acquired Immune Deficiency Syndrome (AIDS)" and identifies four risk factors associated with AIDS: male homosexuality, intravenous drug abuse, Haitian origin and hemophilia A. 625

1983: The CDC adds female sexual partners of men with AIDS as the fifth risk group.
Human Immunodeficiency Virus (HIV) is identified as the cause of AIDS. 2,137

1985: Actor Rock Hudson openly states that he has AIDS and dies later in the year.
After being prohibited from attending school because he has AIDS, Indiana teenager Ryan White advocates against discrimination or stigma associated with AIDS.
The Food and Drug Administration approves the first HIV antibody test. HIV screening of blood donations begins in US. 12,652

1987: The FDA approves the first antiretroviral medication, zidovudine (AZT), as an AIDS treatment.
The AIDS Memorial Quilt is displayed on the National Mall in Washington, DC.
The World Health Organization (WHO) establishes the Special Programme on AIDS, which later becomes the Global Programme on AIDS and then UNAIDS. 41,262

1988: WHO declares the first World AIDS Day on December 1.
National Institutes of Health (NIH) establishes the Office of AIDS Research (OAR), restructures its AIDS research program, and establishes the AIDS Clinical Trials Group (ACTG). 62,451

1989: Ryan White dies. Congress creates the National Commission on AIDS. 90,218

Continued

BOX 7-7 WHY WE SHOULD CARE
20 YEARS OF AIDS—1981 TO 2001

1990: Domestic and international non-governmental groups boycott the 6th International AIDS Conference in San Francisco in protest of the US immigration policy regarding HIV/AIDS status.
Ryan White CARE Act is authorized. *121,952*

1991: Star basketball player, Earvin "Magic" Johnson, announces that he is HIV-positive. *158,911*

1992: Tennis star Arthur Ashe announces that he has AIDS. *200,391*

1993: The FDA approves the female condom for sale in the US. *245,662*

1994: AIDS becomes the number one cause of death for all Americans between the ages of 25 to 44.
The Public Health Service recommends that HIV-positive pregnant women use AZT to reduce mother-to-child transmission.
Pedro Zamora, a young gay man living with AIDS, appears in the cast of MTV's popular show, The Real World; he dies later this year at age 22. *295,339*

1995: The Joint United Nationals Programme on HIV/AIDS (UNAIDS), an organization that oversees the efforts of seven UN programs focusing on AIDS, is established. *345,331*

1996: The FDA approves the viral load test, which measures the amount of HIV in blood.
The number of new AIDS diagnoses declines for the first time in the history of the pandemic.
Evidence of the efficacy of Highly Active Antiretroviral Therapy (HAART) is presented. *382,261*

1997: AIDS-related deaths in the US decline by more than 40% compared to 1996 rates, largely as a result of anti-retroviral therapies. *403,206*

1998: The Congressional Black Caucus calls on the US Department of Health and Human Services Secretary Donna Shalala to declare HIV/AIDS a public health emergency.
Congress approves $156 million for the Minority HIV/AIDS Initiative to address the disproportionate rate of HIV infection in certain racial and ethnic groups. *419,638*

1999: US announces $100 million in funding to sub-Saharan Africa and India through the Leadership and Investment in Fighting an Epidemic (LIFE) Initiative. *430,246*

2000: US and UN Security Councils declare HIV/AIDS a security threat.
President Clinton implements the Millennium Vaccine Initiative to develop vaccines for HIV, TB and malaria.
UNAIDS, WHO and other health groups join with pharmaceutical manufacturers to discuss price decreases for AIDS drugs in developing countries. *438,795*

2001: The UN General Assembly, under the leadership of UN Secretary-General Kofi Annan, convenes a special session to discuss HIV/AIDS. Goals that were set include—

2002-2010: Establishing a global AIDS fund with a target of $10 billion per year.

2003: Increasing the availability of medicines for HIV.

2004: Promoting youth's access to HIV/AIDS eduction and involving adolescents in the planning of HIV/AIDS prevention programs.

American Association for World Health
1825 K St, NW, Ste 1208
Washington, DC 20006
www.aawhworldhealth.org

HEALTHY PEOPLE 2010

OBJECTIVES RELATED TO HIV

13.1   Reduce AIDS among adolescents and adults.

13.2   Reduce the number of new AIDS cases among adolescent and adult men who have sex with men.

13.3   Reduce the number of new AIDS cases among females and males who inject drugs.

13.4   Reduce the number of new AIDS cases among adolescent and adult men who have sex with men and inject drugs.

13.5   Reduce the number of cases of HIV infection among adolescents and adults.

13.6   Increase the proportion of sexually active persons who use condoms.

13.7   Increase the number of HIV-positive persons who know their serostatus.

13.8   Increase the proportion of substance abuse treatment facilities that offer HIV/AIDS education, counseling, and support.

13.9   Increase the number of state prison systems that provide comprehensive HIV/AIDS, sexually transmitted disease, and tuberculosis (TB) education.

13.10 Increase the proportion of inmates in state prison systems who receive voluntary HIV counseling and testing during incarceration.

13.11 Increase the proportion of adults with tuberculosis (TB) who have been tested for HIV.

13.12 Increase the proportion of adults in publicly funded HIV counseling and testing sites who are screened for common bacterial sexually transmitted diseases (STDs) (chlamydia, gonorrhea, and syphilis) and are immunized against hepatitis B virus.

13.13 Increase the proportion of HIV-infected adolescents and adults who receive testing, treatment, and prophylaxis consistent with current Public Health Service guidelines.

13.14 Reduce deaths from HIV infection.

13.15 Extend the interval of time between an initial diagnosis of HIV infection and AIDS diagnosis in order to increase years of life of an individual infected with HIV.

13.16 Increase years of life of an HIV-infected person by extending the interval of time between an AIDS diagnosis and death.

13.17 Reduce new cases of perinatally acquired HIV infection.

Source: DHHS, 2000.

---

estimated 3 million people had died from AIDS in that year alone (CDC, 2002b).

HIV can be transmitted from person to person through unprotected sexual contact, through direct contact with blood or blood products through sharing needles or razors, and from mother to baby during gestation or the birthing process (Benenson, 1995).

Tuberculosis

TB is the leading cause of death worldwide from an infectious agent. Approximately 2 billion people, one-third of the world's population, are infected with TB, with about 3 million deaths occurring annually (AAWH, 1998b; National Institute of Allergy and Infectious Disease, 1997b; Torres, 1998).

Historically, TB has been one of the great scourges of humankind. It was a leading killer in the United States until the advent of antibiotics in the 1950s. For the next 30 years, TB was on a steady decline, at least in the developed countries (AAWH, 1998b; Grimes & Grimes, 1995). The 1980s, however, saw a sharp increase in TB cases, which has been primarily the result of the development of multidrug-resistant strains of the disease (AAWH, 1998b; Grimes & Grimes, 1995). Other reasons for the upsurge include the spread of TB in institutional living facilities such as shelters and correctional facilities, a declining public health infrastructure, increased

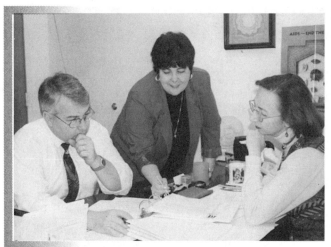

Chapter author Dr. Sharyn Janes (center) plans a statewide HIV education program for health care providers with Craig Thompson (left), Director of the STD/HIV Division of the Mississippi State Department of Health, and Cheryl Hamill, RN, Director of the Resource Center of the Delta Region AIDS Education and Training Center at the University of Mississippi Medical Center.

TUBERCULOSIS CASE RATES, UNITED STATES, 1997.

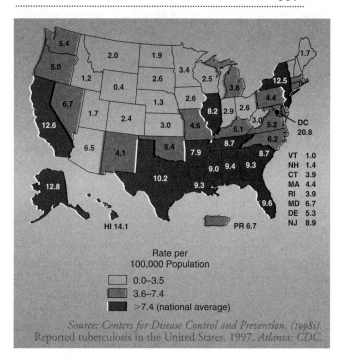

Rate per 100,000 Population

□ 0.0–3.5
▨ 3.6–7.4
■ >7.4 (national average)

*Source: Centers for Disease Control and Prevention. (1998i).
Reported tuberculosis in the United States, 1997. Atlanta: CDC.*

immigration from regions where TB is endemic, and the HIV/AIDS pandemic (Clark, Cegielski, & Hassell, 1997).

TB continues to be a major health problem in the United States, where an estimated 10 to 15 million people are infected, with about 10% of these people expected to develop active disease (Torres, 1998). Although the number of reported TB cases in the United States has shown a steady decline again in the past few years, cases are still high among high-risk groups such as the incarcerated, the homeless, elders, and HIV-infected persons, as well as underrepresented racial and ethnic groups and immigrants from countries with high TB rates and inadequate control measures (AAWH, 1998b; National Institute of Allergy and Infectious Diseases, 1997b; Torres, 1998).

TB is caused by *Mycobacterium tuberculosis* and is transmitted by droplets in the air. It usually affects the lungs (pulmonary), which accounts for 75% of all cases, although other body organs may be involved (extrapulmonary) about 25% of the time (National Institute of Allergy and Infectious Diseases, 1997; Torres, 1998). TB can live in an infected person's body and not cause illness. This is called *inactive* TB or TB infection. Approximately 5% of people with inactive TB develop active TB or TB disease later in life. Only about 10% of all persons infected with TB actually develop active TB. Symptoms of active TB include fatigue, weight loss, fever, chills, and night sweats. Symptoms of pulmonary TB also include a persistent cough, chest pain, and bloody sputum (Torres, 1998).

TB is both preventable and curable. Prevention is focused on treating persons with inactive TB infection prophylactically with anti-TB medications such as isoniazid (INH) for 6 to 12 months. It is extremely important for infected persons to complete the preventive therapy treatment both to prevent progression to active disease and to prevent the development of drug-resistant organisms (Torres, 1998).

Treatment for persons with active TB disease commonly includes such drugs as INH, rifampin, pyrazinamide, ethambutol, and streptomycin. These drugs are usually prescribed in various combinations. It is important that persons with active TB take the medication therapy prescribed for at least 6 months (Torres, 1998).

Multidrug-resistant TB disease (MDR-TB) may occur when medications are not taken consistently for the 6 to 12 months necessary to completely destroy the *M. tuberculosis* organism. In some U.S. cities, more than 50% of TB clients fail to complete their prescribed course of therapy. Many of these clients are homeless persons, drug addicts, or other persons living in poverty, who may not be reliable about taking their medications. Many individuals with TB may feel better after only a few weeks of therapy and stop taking their medications because of unpleasant side effects. MDR-TB is difficult to treat. Even with treatment, the death rate for MDR-TB clients is 40% to 60%, the same as for clients who receive no treatment (National Institute of Allergy and Infectious Diseases, 1997b; Torres, 1998).

The best method of treatment for persons in high-risk circumstances is direct observed therapy (DOT). DOT is a community-based prevention program in which a nurse or other health care provider is paired with a person infected with TB to ensure that the client follows the prescribed treatment plan. DOT programs have been successful in curing 95% of clients with pulmonary TB (Tor-

REPORTED TUBERCULOSIS CASES BY RACE/ETHNICITY, UNITED STATES, 1997.

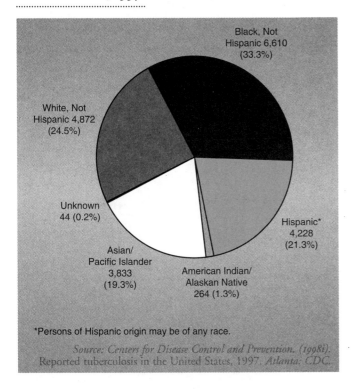

*Persons of Hispanic origin may be of any race.

Source: Centers for Disease Control and Prevention. (1998i). Reported tuberculosis in the United States, 1997. Atlanta: CDC.

res, 1998) and have the potential to save millions of lives worldwide over the next few years (DOTS: A breakthrough, 1998).

The HIV/TB Connection

The WHO estimates that 4.4 million people worldwide are co-infected with HIV and TB, with an estimated 80,000 to 100,000 of them living in the United States. Worldwide, TB is the leading killer among people infected with HIV. TB is listed as an AIDS-defining opportunistic infection for people who are infected with HIV. TB often occurs early in the course of HIV infection and may be the first indication that a person has HIV (HIV-related conditions, 1999; National Institute of Allergy and Infectious Diseases, 1997b). In the United States, approximately 8% of people co-infected with HIV and TB develop active disease each year. In comparison, otherwise healthy people infected with *M. tuberculosis* have approximately a 10% lifetime risk of developing active TB (National Institute of Allergy and Infectious Diseases, 1997b).

Early diagnosis and treatment of TB are critical for HIV-infected clients because the risk for drug-resistant TB is higher among people with HIV infection compared with other groups (MMWR, 1998; Moore, McCray, & Onorato, 1999). For people with HIV infection, the death rate for MDR-TB is as high as 80%. Because TB symptoms are the same as the symptoms for many other HIV-related opportunistic infections, TB is easy to overlook initially. HIV-infected clients may not react to tuberculin skin testing because their immune systems are suppressed

(HIV-related conditions, 1999; National Institute of Allergy and Infectious Diseases, 1997b). A comprehensive health history is an essential tool for assisting nurses and other health care providers to identify TB exposure risks in HIV-infected clients.

Global Disease Eradication Efforts

Despite the emergence and reemergence of infectious diseases in recent years, significant advancements in the elimination or eradication of some diseases that have existed for centuries have occurred through a united global effort. The eradication of smallpox by 1979 is thought to be the greatest triumph of modern public health (Garrett, 1994). The WHO, in collaboration with other international public and private health organizations, has targeted seven other communicable diseases for eradication in the beginning of the 21st century. These diseases are polio, measles, leprosy, river blindness, Chagas' disease, guinea worm disease, and lymphatic filariasis. According to the WHO, these crippling and sometimes deadly diseases can be eliminated in parts of the world and even completely eradicated worldwide within a generation. The methods being used to accomplish this goal are immunization and vaccination, drug therapy, community training, health education, and national disease surveillance efforts (Wittenberg, 1998).

All of the great efforts in the eradication of infectious diseases in the 20th century, however, may not be the great triumph we once thought. Now, in the early years of the 21th century, we are facing what may be one of our greatest political and public health challenges—bioterrorism. There have been isolated incidents of biological terrorism in recent years, including several deaths in 2002 caused by anthrax sent through the federal mail system in the United States. The Centers for Disease Control and Prevention (CDC) has formed a Bioterrorism Preparedness and Response Office to help target areas for initial preparedness efforts, including planning, improved surveillance and epidemiologic capabilities, rapid laboratory diagnostics, enhanced communications, and medication and treatment stockpiles (Rotz, Khan, Lillibridge, et al., 2002).

While there are many biological agents that may pose a threat to public health, one of the biggest threats is the reemergence of smallpox, because of its person-to-person transmission capability and its high mortality rate. For decades the only remaining smallpox organisms left in the world were stored in secured laboratories in the United States and the Soviet Union. In the aftermath of the political and economic collapse of the Soviet Union, much of the Soviet stores cannot be accounted for, making the threat of smallpox as a biological weapon a global issue. Many nations have designed models for large-scale vaccination clinics. The goal of the model developed by the United States is to vaccinate one million people over ten days (Rotz, et al., 2001). Nurses will be important to the success of the vaccination effort. In response to a potential need, many nurses are becoming certified disaster nurses through the American Red Cross and other available training programs.

CONCLUSION

Community health nurses have played a significant role in the prevention, control, and treatment of communicable diseases throughout recent history. Nurses' skills and knowledge will continue to be a vital part of global eradication efforts well into the 21st century.

CRITICAL THINKING ACTIVITIES

1. As a nurse working with the WHO, what actions would you take to eliminate the reservoir for a vector-borne diseases such as malaria? What kind of actions would you take to eliminate the reservoir for an airborne disease such as legionellosis?

2. Discuss the differences between active immunity and passive immunity. Give two examples of each kind of immunity. How long does immunity last for each example?

3. Identify one infectious disease and discuss primary, secondary, and tertiary prevention methods appropriate for that disease on the community level.

4. Compare and contrast the five viral types of hepatitis. Identify similarities and differences regarding the following:

   • Occurrence in the world

   • Infectious agent

   • Reservoir

   • Incubation period

   • Methods of control

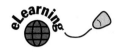 **Explore Community Health Nursing on the web!** To learn more about the topics in this chapter, access your exclusive web site: http://communitynursing.jbpub.com

REFERENCES

Adult Immunization Schedule. (1997). *National coalition for adult immunization:* www.medscape.com/NCAI/.

American Association for World Health (AAWH). (1997). *Emerging infectious diseases: Reduce the risk.* Washington, DC: Author.

American Association for World Health (AAWH). (1998b). *TB alert.* Washington, DC: Author.

American Association for World Health (AAWH). (1998c). Drug resistance opens new door for old threats. *AAWH Quarterly, 12*(1), 4–5.

American Association for World Health (AAWH). (2001). *I care. . . Do you?* Washington, D.C.: Author.

Benenson, A. S. (Ed.). (1995). *Control of communicable diseases in manual* (15th ed.). Washington, DC: American Public Health Association.

Centers for Disease Control and Prevention (CDC). (1994). *Addressing emerging disease threats: A prevention strategy for the United States.* Atlanta: U.S. Department of Health and Human Services.

Centers for Disease Control and Prevention (CDC). (1995a). Summary of notifiable diseases, United States 1995. *Morbidity and Mortality Weekly Report, 44*(53), 3.

Centers for Disease Control and Prevention (CDC). (1995b). *Epidemiology and prevention of vaccine-preventable diseases.* Atlanta: U.S. Department of Health and Human Services.

Centers for Disease Control and Prevention (CDC). (1998a). *Preventing infectious diseases: A strategy for the twenty-first century.* Atlanta: U.S. Department of Health and Human Services.

Centers for Disease Control and Prevention (CDC). (1998b). *Campylobacter.* Atlanta: U.S. Department of Health and Human Services: www.cdc.gov/ncidod/diseases/bacter/campyfaq.html.

Centers for Disease Control and Prevention (CDC). (1998c). *Salmonellosis.* Atlanta: U.S. Department of Health and Human Services: www.cdc.gov/ncidod/diseases/foodborn/salmon.html.

Centers for Disease Control and Prevention (CDC). (1998d). *Hookworm infection.* Atlanta: U.S. Department of Health and Human Services: www.cdc.gov/ncidod/dpd/hookworm.html.

Centers for Disease Control and Prevention (CDC). (1998e). *Giardiasis.* Atlanta: U.S. Department of Health and Human Services: www.cdc.gov/ncidod/dpd/giardias.html.

Centers for Disease Control and Prevention (CDC). (1998f). *Cryptosporidiosis: A guide for persons with HIV/AIDS.* Atlanta: U.S. Department of Health and Human Services: www.cdc.gov/ncidod/diseases/crypto/hivaids.html.

Centers for Disease Control and Prevention (CDC). (1998g). *Cryptosporidiosis.* Atlanta: U.S. Department of Health and Human Services: www.cdc.gov/ncidod/dpd/crypto.html.

Centers for Disease Control and Prevention. (1998h). *Cryptosporidiosis: Control and prevention.* Atlanta: U.S. Department of Health and Human Services: www.cdc.gov/ncidod/dpd/control.html.

Centers for Disease Control and Prevention (CDC). (1998i). *Reported tuberculosis in the United States, 1997.* Atlanta: U.S. Department of Health and Human Services.

Centers for Disease Control and Prevention (CDC). (1999a). *Antibiotic resistance. A new threat to your and your family's health.* Atlanta: U.S. Department of Health and Human Services: www.cdc.gov/ncidod/dbmd/antibioticresistance/default.html.

Centers for Disease Control and Prevention (CDC). (1999b). *Listeriosis.* Atlanta: U.S. Department of Health and Human Services: www.cdc.gov/ncidod/diseases/foodborn/lister.html.

Centers for Disease Control and Prevention (CDC). (1999c). *Escherichia coli O157:H7.* Atlanta: U.S. Department of Health and Human Services: www.cdc.gov/ncidod/diseases /foodborn /e_coli.html.

Centers for Disease Control and Prevention (CDC). (1999d). *Update: Multistate outbreak of Listeriosis.* Atlanta: U.S. Department of Health and Human Services: www.cdc.gov/od/oc/media/pressrel/r990114.html.

Centers for Disease Control and Prevention (CDC). (1999e). *Lyme disease: Introduction.* Atlanta: U.S. Department of Health and Human Services: www.cdc.gov/ncidod/dvbid/lymeinfo.html.

Centers for Disease Control and Prevention (CDC). (1999f). *Rabies: Introduction.* Atlanta: U.S. Department of Health and Human Services: www.cdc.gov/ncidod/dvrd/rabies/introduction/intro.html.

Centers for Disease Control and Prevention (CDC). (2001). *Tracking the hidden epidemics: Trends in STDs in the United States 2000.* Atlanta: U.S. Department of Health and Human Services.

Centers for Disease Control and Prevention (CDC). (2002a). *West Nile Virus.* Atlanta: U.S. Department of Health and Human Services: www.cdc.gov/ncidod/dvbid/westnile.htm

Centers for Disease Control and Prevention (CDC). (2002b). *Divisions of HIV/AIDS Prevention.* Atlanta: U.S. Department of Health and Human Services: www.cdc.gov/hiv/stats.htm

Chomel, B. B. (1998). Diseases transmitted by pets. *World Health, 51*(4), 24–25.

Clark. P. A., Cegielski. J. P., & Hassell, W. (1997). TB or not TB? Increasing door-to-door response to screening. *Public Health Nursing, 14*(5), 268–271.

Clinton, H. R. (1993). Nurses in the front lines. *Nursing & Health Care, 14*(6), 286–288.

Cohen, F. L., & Larson, E. (1996). Emerging infectious diseases: Nursing responses. *Nursing Outlook, 44*(4), 164–168.

De Menezes Brandao, M., & Anselmo Viana da Silva Berzins, M. (1998). When does a pet become a health hazard? *World Health, 51*(4), 20–21.

Department of Health and Human Services (DHHS). (1991). *Healthy People 2000: National health program and disease prevention objectives.* Washington, DC: U.S. Government Printing Office.

Department of Health and Human Services (DHHS). (2000). *Healthy People 2010: Conference edition.* Washington, DC: U.S. Government Printing Office.

DOTS: A breakthrough in TB control. (1998). *World Health, 51*(2), 14–15.

Drug resistance opens new door for old threats. (1998). *American Association for World Health Quarterly, 12*(1), 4.

Dzenowagis, J. (1997). Using electronic links for monitoring diseases. *World Health, 50*(6), 8–9.

Facts about adult immunization. (1997). Bethesda, MD: National Coalition for Adult Immunization: www.nfid.org/factsheets/adultfact.html.

Facts about hepatitis A for adults. (1996). Bethesda, MD: National Coalition for Adult Immunization: www.nfid.org/factsheets/hepaadult.html.

Facts about hepatitis B for adults. (1997). Bethesda, MD: National Coalition for Adult Immunization: www.nfid.org/factsheets/hepbadult.html.

Facts about influenza for adults. (1997). Bethesda, MD: National Coalition for Adult Immunization: www.nfid.org/factsheets/influadult.html.

Facts about pneumococcal disease for adults. (1997). Bethesda, MD: National Coalition for Adult Immunization: www.nfid.org/factsheets/pneuadult.html.

Foege, W. H. (1998). Controlling emerging infections: Lessons from the smallpox eradication campaign. *Emerging Infectious Diseases, 4*(3), 412–413.

Foodborne illness. (1998, July/December). *AAWH Quarterly, 12*(3–4), 8.

Gardner, P., & Schaffner, W. (1993). Immunization of adults. *New England Journal of Medicine, 328,* 1252–1258.

Garrett, L. (1994). *The coming plague. Newly emerging diseases in a world out of balance.* New York: Farrar, Straus, and Giroux.

Grimes, D. E., & Grimes, R. M. (1995). Tuberculosis: What nurses need to know to help control the epidemic. *Nursing Outlook, 43*(4), 164–173.

Gubler, D. J. (1998). Resurgent vector-borne diseases as a global health problem. *Emerging Infectious Diseases, 4*(3), 442–449.

Guerrant, R. L. (1997). Cryptosporidiosis: An emerging, highly infectious threat. *Emerging Infectious Diseases, 3*(1).

Hantavirus infection—Southwestern United States: Interim recommendations for risk reduction. (1993, July 30). *Morbidity and Mortality Weekly Report, 42,* 1–13.

Harkness, G. A. (1995). *Epidemiology in nursing practice.* St. Louis: Mosby.

Hepatitis C. (1997). Geneva: World Health Organization.

Hepatitis learning guide. (1998). Abbott Park, IL: Abbott Diagnostics.

Herrington, J. E., Campbell, G. L., Bailey, R. E., Cartter, M. L., Adams, M., Frazier, E. L., Damrow, T. A., & Gensheimer, K. F. (1997). Predisposing factors for individuals' Lyme disease prevention practices: Connecticut, Maine, and Montana. *American Journal of Public Health, 87*(12), 2035–2038.

Heymann, D. L. (1998). Zoonoses—disease passed from animals to humans. *World Health, 51* (4), 4.

HIV-related conditions. Focus on: Tuberculosis (1999, June/July). *HIV Frontline. A Newsletter for Professionals Who Counsel People Living with HIV, 37,* 6.

Immunizations lag among older adults. (1999, April). *The Nation's Health. The Official Newspaper of the American Public Health Association, 29*(3), 24.

Institute of Medicine. (1992). *Emerging infections: Microbial threats to health in the United States.* Washington, DC: National Academy Press.

IntelliHealth news. (1998, September 21). Rabies may explain the vampire legend. *The PointCast Network.*

Janes, S., St. Lawrence, J., St. Lawrence, J. B., & Aranda-Naranjo, B. (2001). Sexually Transmitted Diseases and HIV/AIDS. In K. S. Lundy & S. Janes (Eds.). *Community Health Nursing. Caring for the Public's Health.* Sudbury, MA: Jones & Bartlett Publishers.

Kaferstein, F. K., & Meslin, F. X. (1998, July/August). Keeping foods of animal origin safe. *World Health, 51*(4), 28–29.

Liese, B. H. (1998, May/June). A brake on economic development. *World Health, 51*(3), 16–17.

Mahon, B. E., Slutsker, L., Hutwagner, L., Drenzek, C., Maloney, K., Toomey, K., & Griffin, P. M. (1999). Consequences in Georgia of a nationwide outbreak of salmonella infections: What you don't know might hurt you. *American Journal of Public Health, 89*(1), 31–35.

Mann, J. M. (1994). Preface. In *The coming plague. Newly emerging diseases in a world out of balance.* New York: Farrar, Straus, and Giroux.

Marsh, K., & Waruiru, C. (1998). What is malaria? *World Health, 51*(3), 6–7.

McQuillian, G. M. (2000). *Implications of a National Survey for STDs: Results from the NHANES Survey.* Paper presentation at Infectious Disease Society of America Conference. September 7–10, 2000, New Orleans. LA.

Meslin, F. X., & Stohr, K. (1998). Animals that infect humans. *World Health, 51*(4), 5.

MMWR. (1998, October 30). Prevention and treatment of tuberculosis among patients infected with human immunodeficiency virus: Principles of therapy and revised recommendations. *Morbidity and Mortality Weekly Report, 47*(RR-20), 5.

Molyneux, M. (1998). Severe malaria. *World Health, 51*(3), 8–9.

Moore, M., McCray, E., & Onorato, I. M. (1999). Cross-matching TB and AIDS registries: TB patients with HIV co-infection, United States, 1993–1994. *Public Health Reports, 114,* 269–277.

Murphy, F. A. (1998). Emerging zoonoses. *Emerging Infectious Diseases, 4*(3), 429–435.

National Institute of Allergy and Infectious Diseases. (1997a, December). *Flu.* Washington, DC: Department of Health and Human Services.

National Institute of Allergy and Infectious Diseases. (1997b, March). *Tuberculosis.* Washington, DC: Department of Health and Human Services.

National Institute of Allergy and Infectious Diseases. (1998a, January). *Foodborne diseases.* Washington, DC: Department of Health and Human Services.

National Institute of Allergy and Infectious Diseases. (1998b). *Lyme disease. The facts, the challenge.* Washington, DC: Department of Health and Human Services.

Nchinda, T. C. (1998). Malaria: A reemerging disease in Africa. *Emerging Infectious Diseases, 4*(3), 398–403.

Neufeldt, V. (Ed.). (1996). *Webster's new world college dictionary* (3rd ed.). New York: Macmillan.

Petersen, L. R., & Marfin, A. A. (2002). West Nile Virus: A Primer for the Clinician. *Annals of Internal Medicine, 137*(3), 173–179.

Pinger, R. L. (1998). Lyme disease: An emerging health threat. *The Community. The Official Jones and Bartlett Community Health Newsletter, 1,* 1–2.

Pinkowish, M. D. (1998, August 15). Infectious diseases: Still emerging in 1998. *Patient Care,* 32–35, 39–40, 42, 47, 51–52.

Rotz, L. D., Kha, A. S., Lillibridge, S. R. Ostroff, S. M. & Hughes, J. M. (2001). Public health assessment of potential biological terrorism agents. *Emerging Infectious Diseases, 8*(2). Available at: www.cdc.gov/ncidool/eid/vol8no2/01-0164.htm.

Shankar, A. H., Genton, B., Semba, R. D., Baisor, M., Paino, J., Tamja, S., Adiguma, T., Wu, L., Rare, L., Tielsch, J. M., Alpers, M. P., & West, K. P., Jr. (1999, July 17). Effect of vitamin A supplementation on morbidity due to Plasmodium falciparum in young children in Papua New Guinea: A randomised trial. *Lancet, 354,* 203–208.

Shute, N. (1998). Hepatitis C: A silent killer. *U.S. News & World Report, 124*(24), 60–66.

St. Louis, M. E., & Wasserheit, J. N. (1998). Elimination of Syphilis in the United States. *Science, 281,* 353–354.

The mother of fevers. (1998, March/April). *World Health, 51*(2), 12–13.

Thurm, K. (1998, November). Adult immunizations save lives. *Closing the Gap. A Newsletter of the Office of Minority Health.* Washington, DC: Department of Health and Human Services.

Timmreck, T. C. (1998). *An introduction to epidemiology.* (2nd ed.). Boston: Jones and Bartlett.

Toro, J., Vega, J. D., Khan, A. S., Mills, J. N., Padula, P. Terry, W., Yadon, Z., Valderrama, R., Ellis, B. A., Pavletic, C., Cerda, R., Zaki, S., Wun-Ju, S., Meyer, R., Tapia, M., Mansilla, C., Baro, M., Vergara, J. A., Concha, M., Calderon, G., Enria, D., Peters, C. J., & Ksiazek, T. G. (1998). An outbreak of hantavirus pulmonary syndrome, Chile, 1997. *Emerging Infectious Diseases, 4*(4), 687–694.

Torres, M. (1998, July). Tuberculosis update. *National Council of La Raza Center for Health Promotion Fact Sheet.*

Valanis, B. (1999). *Epidemiology in health care.* (3rd ed.). Stamford, CT: Appleton & Lange.

Wilde, H., & Mitmoonpitak, C. (1998). Canine rabies in Thailand. *World Health, 51*(4), 10–11.

Wittenberg, R. L. (1998). From the president. Efforts toward eliminating seven diseases from the globe. *American Association for World Health Quarterly, 12,*(2), 2.

Unit III

Approaches to Community Health Nursing Practice

8

Nursing Informatics in Community Health Nursing Practice

Russell C. McGuire

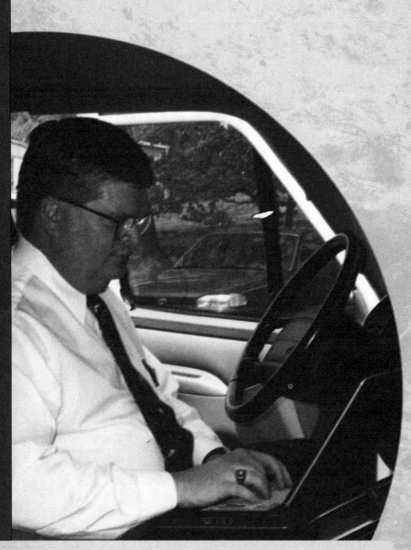

The worlds of health care, communication, and information technologies are ever evolving, separately and together. As nurses in the community expand their practice definition to embrace new information technologies, opportunities for improved health care to populations seem endless. This evolution is seen as a merger of health care technology with information and communications technology, fostering the design and implementation of health care management information systems in a variety of clinical practice settings.

QUESTIONS TO CONSIDER

After reading this chapter, answer the following questions:
1. What is nursing informatics?
2. How is the science of informatics used in nursing practice in the community?
3. What are the benefits of informatics?
4. How is client information managed using informatics?

5. What are some computer applications used in community health nursing?
6. How are management and network systems used in community health nursing practice?
7. What are the community health nursing benefits to using telehealth?

KEY TERMS

Database
Distributed data processing (DDP)
Electronic mail (e-mail)

Electronic spreadsheets
Health management information systems (HMIS)
Network client care

Nursing classification systems
Nursing data
Nursing informatics
Nursing information

Nursing information systems
Nursing knowledge
Telemedicine/telehealth

The clinical practice settings involved in this new technology include both the acute care and community-based practice environments. Organizations such as hospitals, and community-based agencies such as public health departments and home health agencies use information and communications technologies to collect, store, retrieve, analyze, and present client care data in the care delivery settings.

Health care continues to be a human endeavor that is necessarily complex in nature. Decisions related to client care continue to increase in complexity, with the need for rapid, accurate information for clinical decision making as a priority for effective care. Clinical decisions are just as complex and critical in the community-based nursing settings. As a response to these informational needs, systems have been designed to meet the clinical information requirements of community-based practice. Public health, home health, hospice, and other providers of community-based nursing care have the opportunity to use information and communications technologies in the provision of nursing care. This chapter explores how information and communications technologies, coupled with nursing science, can provide answers to complex clinical scenarios in community health nursing.

The Science of Nursing Informatics

The science of nursing informatics is a combination of information, communications, and nursing sciences. According to Saba and McCormick (1996), **nursing informatics** is a "branch of informatics particularly concerned with nurses' use of computer technology and the management of information that facilitates nursing practice and enhances nursing knowledge" (p. 222). The emergence of the specialty known as *nursing informatics* is not a recent phenomenon. Nurses have been using computers since the 1950s, and nursing informatics emerged as an advanced specialty in the 1980s. In 1989, Graves and Corcoran devised a conceptual framework based on a definition of nursing informatics. This conceptual framework describes the relationship among computer science, information systems science, and nursing science. Graves and Corcoran believe information management processing of nursing data is achieved through the collection of data, the transformation of nursing data into nursing information, and finally into nursing knowledge. Nursing informatics came of age in the 1980s, and characteristics of what constitutes nursing data have emerged.

. . . .

The best way to predict the future is to invent it.

Alan Kay

. . . .

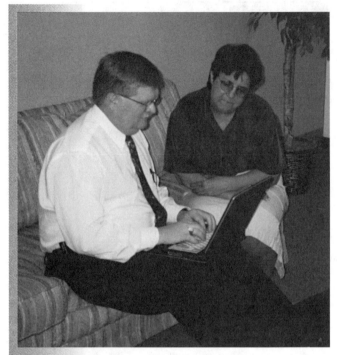

Chapter author, Russell McGuire, using a laptop computer during home health visit.

Nursing informatics uses nursing science and computer and communications technologies to produce effective and efficient client outcomes for individuals and communities. Through the collection of individual data elements, nursing as a professional discipline builds on its unique knowledge base. The transition from raw data to knowledge is a three-phased process. **Nursing data** is the raw form of elements that make up nursing information. For example, client name, gender, and diagnosis are each considered raw nursing data elements. When a nurse forms relationships between the raw data elements, **nursing information** emerges as a more fully developed picture of the client's clinical status is formulated. The nurse then acts on this information by formulating a set of interventions to deal with the particulars of a specific client care situation. *Nursing information* is related data elements that now are in a form that can be subjected to analysis and interpretation. Nursing information readily lends itself to archiving or storage in computer databases that allow for relational groupings of the data. Relational grouping of nursing information then allows for aggregation of information and the systematic study of nursing-related phenomena. Sets of nursing information that conform to theoretical and conceptual frameworks are known as **nursing knowledge**. When enough nursing information is collected, analyzed, and interpreted, aggregation of this information can be synthesized into nursing knowledge. It is nursing knowledge, when fitted to a logical, systematic set of standards, that provides the knowledge base of the discipline.

RESEARCH BRIEF

Wilson, R., & Fulmer, T. (1998). Home health nurses' initial experiences with wireless. pen-based computing. Public Health Nursing, 15(3), 225–232.

The community health care delivery environment continues to evolve along with the introduction of newer, more efficient information and communications technology. This research explores the change process as it is related to the implementation and use of information system technologies and their use in community-based nursing practice. Major changes in how home health agencies deliver services have been brought about by the Balanced Budget Act of 1997 and the implementation of a prospective payment system (PPS). Information technologies assist the home health nurse in providing care through electronic data collection, analysis, and presentation of clinical results. These technologies include the computer and telephone systems.

The experiences of nurses using wireless, pen-based units for their home health practice is documented by Wilson and Fulmer (1998). The Visiting Nurse Service of New York conducted focus group interviews to determine what the initial reactions of home health nurses were to their use of wireless, pen-based computers. Open-ended questions were used in the interviews, and subsequent concept analysis was performed to determine what major themes existed among the nurses' collective experiences with the computer use in the home. Wilson and Fulmer found several main themes in their analysis that shed some light on how home health nurses accept new technology use in their daily practice. These themes include (1) readiness—the transition from their use of manual documentation systems to automated documentation, (2) the perception of additional weight and an extra item to carry into and out of the home, (3) the perception of problems and concerns with data transmission, (4) viewing the computer as an assistive technology in their daily practice, (5) nurses as system trouble shooters, and (6) computers needed by their professional colleagues to communicate patient-related issues. The researchers found that understanding transition issues in implementing computer technology in home health are aided by eliciting opinions from practicing staff nurses as they implement change within their practice setting.

Computerized information systems used in the community health nursing practice setting can assist in the development of nursing knowledge through the automated process of collecting, storing, retrieving, analyzing, interpreting, and eventually presenting client-related data. These data than can be used in an intervention effort to meet individual, family, and community health needs.

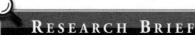

Learning is what most adults will do for a living in the 21st century.

Perelman

The accumulation of nursing data, information, and subsequently, nursing knowledge in this fast-paced era of electronics has fostered the use of information systems throughout health care. **Health management information systems (HMIS)** are used to collect, store, and process health-related data in a health care facility. In a health care system such as the community health care setting, elements of care delivery such as nursing, medicine, laboratory, radiology, and administration use information systems to coordinate and manage care for achieving more

RESEARCH BRIEF

Levy, S., & Williams, B. (1999). Attitudes to information technology. Nursing Standard 13(52), 1–13.

This research study was conducted in six hospitals of a Scottish National Health Service Trust, which provides both acute mental health and community services. The study explored the attitudes of health practitioners toward using computers within clinical settings. The study was carried out before the implementation of an information system; participants included nurses and nurse midwives. The study found that a large majority of nurses and midwives have positive attitudes toward computer use in their practice areas. Many indicated that the manual practice of documentation is inefficient. Many also remained unconvinced that computerized systems would record workload accurately and thus become effective clinical and management tools. The study also found that senior staff members possessed a greater degree of conviction regarding the potential benefits of computer use in the delivery of care.

efficient and better client-related outcomes (Sebastian & Stanhope, 1999). **Nursing information systems**, which are a part of the health management information system, continue to evolve at a fast pace. This pace is accelerated because of the development of faster processing computer equipment, advances in data transmission, and increases in information systems' efficiency and data manipulation effectiveness.

Zielstorff, Hudgings, and Grobe (1993) describe characteristics related to nursing information systems. These characteristics apply to nursing information systems in any nursing clinical practice settings. Several assumptions that pertain to the information systems used in all nursing practice settings are discussed by Zielstorff and her colleagues. These assumptions are necessary for understanding how the profession of nursing can support development of effective nursing information systems. These assumptions are outlined in Box 8-1.

Community Health Nursing and Nursing Informatics

In community-based nursing practice, the implementation of nursing information systems must be integrated with data systems that collect client data for other disciplines. The profession of nursing leads the way in data collection, the use of standardized language classifications, and design support for automated systems that can assist in supporting the integration of other health care disciplines. This integration of nursing information is useful in community health nursing when multiple disciplines are responsible for the care of the client and his or her caregivers, and when coordination of care is paramount in achieving expedient and successful outcomes.

Nursing informatics deals with the collection, manipulation, analysis, and interpretation of several levels of data, information, and knowledge. Community-based nursing deals with the same levels of data for which computer technology, nursing informat-

ics, and communications technology are used to transform data into knowledge. The first level of data is related to clients and their caregivers. Data such as client sociodemographic status, medical history, physical examination results, integrated health care assessments, and treatment plans are examples of client-level data or information. The second level of data is specific to the organization or agency. Examples of this level of data are an organization's productivity indicators, policies, and procedures, as well as the availability of community resources associated with a specific client's or caregiver's health care needs. The third level of data is domain specific. Domain-specific data are associated with care provided across the continuum of health care services delivery and are related to the client and caregiver responses (outcomes) to community health nursing interventions. Domain-specific data include the medical diagnosis and subsequent nursing diagnosis, the efficiency and applicability of specific nursing interventions and the subsequent client outcomes, and the data related to the specifics of providing care such as drug interactions with prescribed medications.

Benefits of Nursing Informatics for Community Health Nursing

The combination of nursing and information systems management produces several benefits for nurses practicing in the community. These benefits include (1) the management of client-level data; (2) the use of standardized nursing language to communicate what nurses do and how clients and their families respond to care; (3) provision of care in an efficient and productive manner; and (4) the use of information systems for research, health promotion, and illness prevention in the community.

Nursing Classification Systems

The different levels of data and subsequent levels of information and knowledge relevant to the practice of community-based nursing have been discussed thus far. To facilitate an understanding of how nursing languages are used to describe nursing practice and how standardized nursing languages are important in the context of automated nursing information systems, the discussion briefly turns to the evolution of **nursing classification systems**. It is important to remember that community health nurses use language as a medium for describing the client's clinical status, the appropriateness of the clinical care environment, the support systems available to the client, and the client's level of response to nursing intervention. To facilitate the use of language for communicating what nurses do, several professional nursing organizations have created initiatives to implement standardized nursing languages into clinical practice.

The American Nurses Association established the Steering Committee on Databases to Support Nursing Practice in 1990. The purpose of this committee was to develop policy to support the development of nursing classification systems, the uniformity

---

BOX 8-1 MAJOR ASSUMPTIONS AND NURSING INFORMATION SYSTEMS

- Nursing information systems are to be considered a part of an integrated client record system.
- Health care and thus nursing are information-intensive endeavors.
- The major resource in health care delivery is client-level data.
- The integration of systems is necessary for the successful implementation of nursing information systems.

Source: Zielstorff, Hudgings, & Grobe, 1993.

TABLE 8-1   SUMMARY OF NURSING CLASSIFICATION SYSTEM FEATURES

NAME	MAJOR FEATURES
NANDA: North American Nursing Diagnosis Association (Warren & Hoskins, 1995)	Research-based nursing diagnosis system having nine different diagnosis patterns (exchanging, communicating, relating, valuing, choosing, moving, perceiving, knowing, and feeling).
Visiting Nurses Association of Omaha Community Health Problem and Intervention System (Martin & Scheet, 1995)	Three major components: (1) problems classification, (2) intervention scheme, (3) problem rating scale for outcomes. Developed for and researched in community-based nursing practice settings (home health, public health, school nursing, and clinic settings).
HHCC: Home Health Care Classification (Saba & McCormick, 1996)	Developed to provide a standardized language system for coding/categorizing the services provided by nurses in the home health practice setting. Coding scheme for nursing diagnosis, interventions, and outcomes that are easily coded for computer data collection and retrieval.
NIC: Iowa Intervention Project: Nursing Intervention Classification (McCloskey & Bulechek, 1996)	Large data set of research-based nursing interventions dealing with six domains (physiological basic and complex behavioral, safety, family, and health systems). Interventions have a specific label, are defined, and have a set of actions or activities performed by the nurse while providing client care.
NOC: Iowa Outcomes Project: Nursing Outcomes Classification (Johnson & Maas, 1997)	The classification contains 218 outcomes, which are listed in alphabetical order. Each NOC outcome has a specific definition, a list of indicators that are used in the evaluation of client status, scale of measurement, and a list of references used in development of the outcome. Five-point Likert type scales were developed for use with the outcomes to measure client status in relation to the outcome.

of nursing data sets, and the implementation of a national data set. In 1992, the committee gave its support for the Unified Nursing Language System (UNLS). The UNLS is recognized by the National Library of Medicine for inclusion in the Unified Medical Language System. The Steering Committee on Databases to Support Nursing Practice currently recognizes five nursing taxonomies: (1) the North American Nursing Diagnosis Association (NANDA), (2) the Visiting Nurses Association of Omaha Community Health Problem and Intervention System, (3) the Home Health Care Classification (HHCC), (4) the Iowa Intervention Project: Nursing Intervention Classification (NIC), and (5) Iowa Outcomes Project: Nursing Outcomes Classification (NOC). A brief summary of each classification system is provided in Table 8-1.

The use of standardized nursing classification systems as described in Table 8-1 provides community health nurses with a uniform description of problems, interventions, and related outcomes while providing care to clients and their caregivers. In the community health nursing practice setting, the use of standardized nursing languages can (1) facilitate the appropriate selection of nursing interventions for cost-effective and clinically effective health care delivery; (2) assist in predicting client and caregiver outcomes; (3) foster transdisciplinary communications; (4) assist community health nursing managers in appropriate allocation of financial and personnel resources; (5) promote reimbursement for nursing services; and (6) articulate community health nursing's worth to health care policy planners at the state, federal, and international levels (Grier & McGuire, 1999).

Client Information Management

Health care is data intensive. Much of the collection of client-related clinical data takes a considerable amount of time and effort. The management of client-level data provides the community health nurse with an accurate assessment of clients' and their caregivers' situation for the purpose of planning, implementing, and evaluating care. Information systems allow for the organization of myriad data collected during an individual's admission to a community health care facility. This information can be stored for future retrieval, and the aggregation of this information can be analyzed for the benefit of the community.

Efficiency and Time Benefits

The use of nursing information systems can provide community health nurse managers and staff with efficiencies in productivity. The collection of client- and caregiver-centered information is often a time-consuming endeavor and uses financial and personnel resources. Savings in time are often demonstrated by the use of computer systems for communicating information over distance, over time, and to multiple users of the data. Clinical information can be shared with several users at the same time. An example is sharing laboratory results with a nurse practitioner at a remote community clinic at the same time the practitioner is consulting with a physician in a large tertiary center.

Information systems are used to manage health care information for population groups. Bargstadt (1998) described several benefits of information systems use in the community setting. These benefits include (1) collecting data to demonstrate clinical effectiveness of community health nursing care delivery to a specific population, (2) analyzing the collected clinical data for statistical comparison, (3) determining the cost-effectiveness of community health nursing programs on the care of clients and caregivers, and (4) using cost-effective data collection for outcome measurement.

Computer Applications in Community Health Nursing

Computer and communications technologies continue to grow rapidly in utilization with the community health care practice setting. This use will continue to grow in all segments of health care and will become more efficient and effective in meeting the goals of a community health care facility for information leading to sound clinical and financial decision making. Computer applications that support good communications and organization of clinically related data are available.

Electronic Mail

Computers have long been able to communicate with one another. In the past, communication between computer users had been an interactive endeavor; that is, both the sender and the receiver of the communication had to be at their respective terminals for the communication to take place. With today's **electronic mail** (**e-mail**) applications, the sender and receiver need not be at their respective computer terminals because the message can be sent in a "store and forward" manner. Depending on the type of operating system and e-mail software package, the typical e-mail system (e.g., Microsoft's Messaging) sets up a computerized mailbox that receives the incoming message and stores it for viewing by the receiving computer user when it is convenient. The received message can be read on the computer's monitor, saved for future reference, or printed. Messages can be configured with an "attached" or inserted file such as a word processing document, presentations, animation, sound bites, or electronic spreadsheets. In the community-based practice setting, messages of a critical nature (e.g., client status, critical laboratory reports, or case management information) can be sent to physicians or nurse practitioners from sources such as the laboratory, radiology department, health information systems departments, and remote sites such the public health department of home health agency.

Databases

Community-based health care delivery is data intensive. Client charts contain massive amounts of data that individually are just

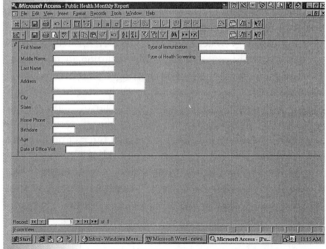

Example of a database entry screen.

single pieces of unrelated information. When data are used in this unrelated manner, analysis is difficult to perform. But when data are combined in a structure that demonstrates relationships between data elements, powerful data analysis can begin. A **database** software package such as Microsoft's Access gives the computer user the ability to generate records that have data elements grouped together for relational value. These individual records can be grouped, and further delineation of the data elements can be achieved. For example, a public health nurse might want to construct a monthly report of all pediatric clinic clients of a certain age or age group, data related to their visits, the immunization status of each client, and the type of health screenings that have been performed. If these data are first entered into a database program, age, dates of office visits, types of immunization, and types of health screening could be "queried" or selected by the nurse for the monthly report (see the figure on p. 182).

This type of database is known as *relational* because each data element in the database can be selected (or not selected) for report generation. Simple data analysis can then be performed on the individual and aggregate client care level.

Electronic Spreadsheets

Electronic spreadsheets assist the computer user with "crunching" or manipulating of large amounts of numerical data. The software displays a series of rows and columns in a gridlike depiction of a spreadsheet. This grid is displayed on the computer's monitor. Each box created by the intersection of a row and column is known as a *cell*. Individual numbers or formulas can be entered into the cell to calculate results for a given problem. For example, a home health nursing manager may want to know how many skilled nursing visits are a percentage of the total number of visits performed by all the professional staff in the agency. A column of cells is named "skilled nursing visits," and each of the registered nurses' monthly visits is entered in the cell next to their individual names. At the end of the column, the nurse manager designates one cell to enter a formula to (1) add all the cells that contain the registered nurses' monthly visits and (2) place the total number of professional visits for the agency into (3) a formula that would calculate a percentage (see the figure at top right). Sophisticated statistical analysis, supported by user-defined formulas that are a part of the spreadsheet software, can generate reports with graphs of a meaningful nature. Spreadsheet data can be "exported," that is, moved from one type of computer application to another.

For example, a nurse manager may want to perform some sophisticated statistical analysis that involves comparisons between two groups of clients. After collecting the desired data and entering these data into an electronic spreadsheet, the nurse manager can export the spreadsheet data file to a statistical package such as SPSS (Statistical Package for Social Sciences) for complex statistical comparisons.

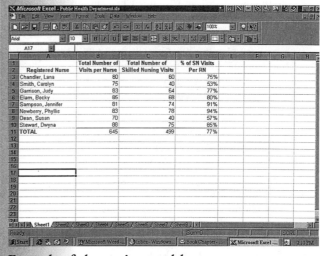

Example of electronic spreadsheet.

Internet Applications in Community-Based Nursing Practice

As computer networks have become more established throughout the nation, and for that matter the world, additional opportunities for sharing data, information, and knowledge have presented themselves to health care providers. The establishment of the Internet has enabled many health care practitioners to communicate and thus share community health–related data. The Internet is the product of a communications network known as the *ARPAnet*, a network of American defense computers. This network was developed in the late 1960s to counter the detrimental effects of nuclear warfare on computer and communications technology. It was first used to link various major university academic computer centers where United States defense research was being conducted. As the academic centers proliferated and began to link to one another, the Internet became a conglomeration of academic, commercial, governmental, and personal web sites used for the exchange of information, services, and research. The Internet affords the computer user the luxury of communicating with health care professional from around the world. The Web has become a wonderful resource for communications, research, and education for community-based nurses and the clients and caregivers they serve. There are thousands of web sites easily accessed by computer users throughout the world.

Health Care Delivery System Management Software

Health care information systems software designers have developed many different financial and business solutions for various health care delivery settings. From the 1970s through the present, software developers focused most of their development on hospital software that dealt with financial issues such as cost, revenues, payer mix, and diagnosis-related group (DRG) identification and coding. Decision support systems were mostly aimed at answering business questions. Recently, an emphasis on clinical data collection and presentation has emerged in the development of software applications for health care. With the advent of managed care, prospective payment, managed care reimbursement, and increased competition in the health care industry, special health care application software has been and continues to be designed for the community-based practice setting.

Software applications and computer systems (as well as networks) are being developed from a clinical perspective. Outpatient clinics, public health departments, free-standing and hospital-based home health agencies, and schools are all excellent practice settings that have elements of information systems development. One example is the development of a home health information system by the Atlanta-based health information system vendor McKesson HBOC. The product, Pathways Homecare, which is based on a relational database, gives the home health nurse the opportunity to collect client care data at the point of care—the home setting. Sociodemographic data, client assessments, visit notes, clinical pathways used for specific disease states, generation of Medicare forms for billing purposes, and agency financial management have been incorporated into the application. The Windows-based Pathways Homecare has a user-friendly graphical interface that lends itself well to "point and click" data entry and manipulation within the software application.

Networked Client Care

Computers used in a stand-alone configuration are powerful, productive business, academic, and clinical tools. The power of computers is enhanced or increased when linked together. When linked together, computer users can share application software and files, communicate, and therefore increase productivity. Community-based health care delivery systems use networks (the linking of computer and communications technologies) to transfer data, images, and video (medical video and health care teleconferencing).

For this transmission of data, networks have been designed and implemented in many health care setting. Stallings and Van Slyke (1998) describe three types of networks that are used extensively in community-based health care practice: (1) wide area networks (WAN), (2) local area networks (LAN), and (3) wireless networks.

Wide area networks are used by health care facilities for data transmission and data communications over a long distance. For example, WANs are used for data transmission between several health care facilities and their central office. Local area networks connect computer users who are generally within the confines of an office complex or the same build-

ing. Wireless networks use radio frequency or infrared technology for data transmission. This type of network allows for greater mobility in hardware use within a facility. An outgrowth of network development is client-server computer architecture. As computer technology migrated from massive mainframe systems to smaller personal computers, the linkage of these personal computers to one another lead to client-server technology. The server, a computer (either a powerful minicomputer, a large-capacity personal computer, or a mainframe) is connected to several personal computer workstations. These "clients" can use application software that resides on the server. An example of this relationship can be demonstrated by the use of a database that resides on the server. A computer user at a remote workstation queries the relational database, asking the server for specific records. Instead of the server sending all the records to the computer user, the server sends only the records that are specified by the client workstation user.

Certain advantages are gained by using client-server technology in the community-based nursing practice setting. First, the system configuration is composed of several powerful machines that give the community health nurse a considerable amount of computer power at lower cost than traditional mainframe, centralized, "closed" computing systems. Second, the client-server computer architecture is considered to be open systems technology. Community health care program planners can choose from among several hardware and software vendors to configure their computer system based on specific organizational and clinical needs. Finally, the computer system can grow and be enhanced when the community health care organization's needs change. An example of this can be demonstrated in the community-based nursing practice setting.

Most community-based practice settings are influenced by external factors such as federal and state government health care reimbursement programs. As these programs change their reimbursement strategies and their regulations, different reporting and documentation requirements are generated for the service provider. When the community health care organization has an open systems architecture as a base for the computer system, new hardware (if needed) and software (for the new reporting requirements) can be installed easily with the existing system's configuration.

The advent of client-server technology has led to more use of a network concept known as **distributed data processing** (**DDP**). In the DDP configuration, a community-based health care organization uses smaller computers as workstations at sites that can be situated within a single building or from off site, remote computing sites. These smaller competing sites are connected via telecommunications lines (POTS, T1 or T3, fiberoptic, or even satellite). The figure on p. 185 depicts a DDP configuration.

The advantages of developing and maintaining distributed data processing configuration are numerous. The remote sites

DISTRIBUTED DATA PROCESSING.

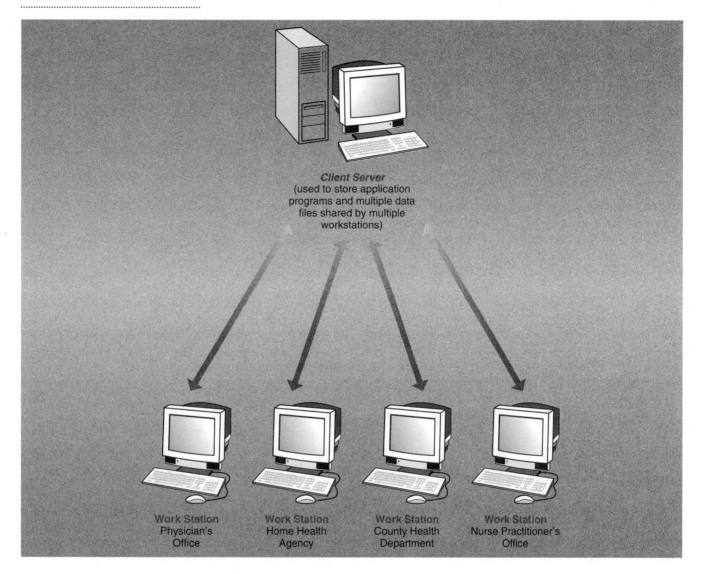

(e.g., off-site health department offices) can respond more quickly to service demands if data processing capabilities are available at the remote sites. Backup systems are more often available to the entire community health care organization, minimizing downtime caused by equipment or software failure. As health care service demands change within a community (as a result of external factors such as changes in Medicare, Medicaid, or managed care penetration) a community-based organization can change the DDP configuration incrementally, often without great expense to the organization. Finally, the computing needs of nurse executives, managers, and staff can be tailored easily within the DDP configuration. Analysis of client care data and

more productivity at staff levels can be realized when a DDP system is developed, implemented, and maintained.

Communication Technology and Community Health Nursing

Much of the United States is considered rural in geography, and thus there are inherent challenges to providing access to health care services. Lack of access to health care facilities and to limited numbers of health care providers tends to decrease opportunities for service provision. Distance to health care facilities and access to skilled health care providers are but two challenges to individuals seeking health care services in both rural and inner-city environments. **Telemedicine/telehealth** is the delivery of medical services over telecommunications lines and is paving the way for providing specialized, skilled services in areas that would otherwise be without.

The following discussion demonstrates how current telehealth applications are being used in the community-based practice setting. As with all information and communications technology, these applications are evolving into faster, less expensive methods for delivering community-based health care services.

Telehealth Care Benefits

An example of the benefit that telehealth can provide can be demonstrated in home health care. Home health care is one of the fastest-growing industries in the United States. Along with this growth has come a certain amount of scrutiny with regard to reimbursement practices. In an effort to control cost, the federal government is in the process of converting from a cost-based reimbursement system to a prospective payment system based on the Balanced Budget Act of 1997. Managed care also is increasing in market penetration. As a response to the increased pressures to remain financially viable, home health care agencies are looking at many innovative technologies to supplement, enhance, and complement care. Crist, Kaufman, and Crampton (1996) discussed the advances of telemedicine and its application within home health agencies.

There are three basic types of data transmitted from the home setting to a central home health office via telecommunications. Data, which are generally client specific, can be sent from a remote site to the home health agency's central station. This can include data elements such as blood pressure, blood oxygen, pulse, temperature, blood glucose, weight, electrocardiograph results, and other measurements. The second type of data that can be collected and transmitted is audio (e.g., heart and lung sounds). Voice data can include anything from voice conversation to stethoscope sounds and messages. The third and final type of data transmitted through telecommunication is image. It can take the form of still image (i.e., still-frame photograph) or full-motion video.

Community Health Nursing Benefits of Telehealth Care

Crist and her colleagues describe a telemedicine system that has been evaluated in the Cincinnati area. This system was primarily developed for home use but could also be used in the hospital, physician's office, or nursing home. The device is a user-friendly computer-based device used to communicate daily with clients and their caregivers to support their health care needs. The system was designed using touch screen and audio to coach clients through treatment protocols. Other features available from the unit are vital signs devices, which include thermometer, pulse oximetry, blood pressure cuff, and electrocardiograph; digital stethoscope to record heart, lung, and gastrointestinal sounds; a medication reminder system to increase client compliance with medication administration; real-time telephone communication for scheduling activities; video transmission of client to nurse, nurse to client; and touch screens that allow for coaching to assist the client in routine medical procedures, which can include procedures such as dressing changes, medication administration, and the taking of vital signs.

The system provides for the hookup of future devices such as a blood glucose monitor, a scale for obtaining weight, an intravenous (IV) pump, and a ventilator. The system can be customized to meet the particular needs of the client during installation and also has an alarm function for changes in client status. This system allows for 24-hour response to client needs and care management with necessary skilled visits. The central nursing station accumulates health care data such as vital signs, request for medication, communication events, and requests for assistance on each client for which a home-assisted nursing care (HANC) unit is installed. A unique feature of the system is the ability of the home health agency to change client protocols as client conditions change. The key factor to the successful application of the HANC network is the ability to customize the telecommunications systems for a particular client's needs.

Gains in staff productivity by using the HANC system were demonstrated in a cost-effectiveness study. Crist and her colleagues describe their research findings in a summary of retrospective chart review showing weekly savings for treatment therapy such as IV therapy ($2,207), wounds ($1,890), and diabetes ($1,807). They projected possible cost savings through the use of the telemedicine technology of approximately $255,000 per year for a total of 43 clients.

The Future of Informatics and Telehealth

The advent of telemedicine/telehealth brings a considerable amount of opportunity to community-based nursing practices. Client monitoring, client and caregiver education, transdisciplinary case conferences, and professional health care education are being achieved. Several researchers in telehealth see a future role for telecommunications in home care as an alternative to traditional in-home visits. Warner (1996) believes telehealth is a technological answer to proposed prospective payment systems being considered by Medicare. She bases this on the fact that agencies can be expected to be reimbursed at a fixed schedule rather than by the number of visits. Warner views the role of telecommunications as reducing unnecessary emergency room visits, reducing unnecessary/unscheduled physician office visits, providing early nursing intervention and prevention of repeat hospitalizations, and educating the client about early symptoms and managing these symptoms through a link to medical information (p. 792). The use of telehealth technology will enable the nurse to capture vital signs data (temperature, pulse, and blood pressure) at various times throughout the day without physically having to interact with the client. This collected data can then be used to revise the client's individualized care plan.

Warner envisions a nursing visit conducted through a telehealth system as encompassing the following: The nursing personnel places a call to the client's station using the client's home telephone number with two-way video communications and interactive audio; the nurse then interacts with the client, which consists of assessment, education, monitoring, and implementation of functions that would normally be made in person. Warner states that some telehealth systems allow the nurse to remotely control camera functions to get a closer view of wound sites and infusion sites as well as scanning the client's environment. Most systems will allow for an electronic capture of data elements necessary for a clinical record as well as still-frame photo and full-motion video. According to Warner, quality-of-care issues will also be met through enhanced productivity by replacing the travel time that nurses have in making their daily caseload assignments. Telehealth systems would also allow nurses to make visits in adverse weather conditions and in high-risk neighborhoods where safety is often threatened.

The use of telehealth systems can provide a telecommunications information system that is interactive between the nurse and the client, using text, video, audio, and/or graphics. Warner also advocates a telehealth utilization by diagnosis, with less severe acuities being matched with technologies that are also less technical. She places the complexity of client statuses on a continuum from less to more complex, more acute illnesses such as congestive heart failure, recovery after acute myocardial infarction, chronic obstructive pulmonary disease, and diabetes being on the higher end of the continuum and resulting in the need for more technical intervention. Warner discusses several factors that are related to determining when telehealth is appropriate for a particular client. A primary consideration should be the stability of the individual's disease processes. It is also necessary that the client possess sufficient cognitive ability, hearing, and vision to use the system or to have a caregiver to provide assistance In addition, consideration must be made for the client's and caregivers' feelings and beliefs with regard to allowing the system in their home (e.g., apprehension about technology, cost, or loss of privacy) (p. 794).

The future of nursing informatics will be based on supporting the individual practicing nurse's requirements for assessing, implementing, evaluating, and redefining care across all practice settings and teaching practicing clinicians how to use information and communication technologies. Gassert (1998), in her presen-

RESEARCH BRIEF

Kinsella, A., & Warner, I. (1998). Telehealth and managing congestive heart failure. Caring, 17(6), 14–18.

In anticipation of delivering alternative visit services in a prospective payment environment, Kinsella and Warner (1998) describe how telehealth applications aid community-based nurses in extending their services to patients with congestive heart failure (CHF). Basic telehealth technology can assist the home health nurse with providing quality care services at the same time they reduce cost associated with an in-person visit. These basic tools induce the use of (1) blood pressure cuffs with telecommunication capability, (2) scales with scanning capabilities, (3) computer software packages that assist CHF patients and their caregivers with meal planning, and (4) telephonic reminder programs for medication compliance and supportive messaging. Other medical technologies with telecommunications capabilities include the use of vital signs monitoring equipment, electronic scales, patient education via multimedia, and automated critical pathways. Each of these technologies, when used appropriately by skilled nursing clinicians, are cost-effective, cost-efficient tools that provide care to patients and their caregivers.

tation to the American Medical Informatics Association, envisioned meeting these needs and those of clients and communities through a national nursing informatics agenda. Her two-part agenda includes (1) a strategic direction for preparing nurses in the use of information and communication technologies through the education of nursing students, practicing nurses, and nursing faculty and (2) strategies that impact client care, including preparing nurses for information and communication use at the undergraduate, graduate, and continuing education levels; developing funding and programs for teaching specialized nursing informatic skills and, with other health care providers, developing collaborative programs in telecommunications that "will enhance the quality of clinical practice for populations at risk and contribute to the education of health providers" (p. 266); increasing nursing faculty exposure to information and communication technology use in nursing individual clients, communities, and caregivers; and developing the use of public and private resources such as the Internet to increase accessibility of health care knowledge resources for health care providers and the public (p. 267).

CONCLUSION

The use of information and communications technology in support of community nursing functions will continue to increase and offer community health nursing leaders and staff care for the clients and family caregivers they serve. The specialty of nursing informatics offers strategies for using technologies such as those discussed in this chapter to (1) collect individual- and community-related data, (2) store and retrieve this data for clinical decision making (through the process of converting raw data into nursing information and ultimately into nursing knowledge), and (3) provide in-depth analysis of data for increasing productive service delivery while providing quality care.

Nursing informatics uses computer and communication technologies to collect information in a readily understandable format. To assist nurses in using computers to describe the care they render in a community-based practice setting, standardized nursing languages such as NANDA, NIC, NOC, HHCC, and Omaha were developed and continue to be added to through research efforts. Standardized languages in computer systems are used to assess clients and their communities, describe the care community health nurses perform, and are a basis for communications between community health nurses and other health care providers.

The use of computer applications such as e-mail, databases, and spreadsheets can provide community health nurses with tools to increase their productivity and knowledge. E-mail can be used to coordinate communications among health care providers in the community. Databases have been used to collect and organize massive amounts of client- and community-related data to be used in research and business analysis. Spreadsheets can be used to perform complicated mathematical or statistical calculations that support clinical decision making. Information and communication systems continue to offer exciting, new ways for community health nurses to maintain a cost-effective presence in the community even when distance is a challenge. The use of telemedicine/telehealth provides the community health nurse with several strategies for maintaining visual and/or audio contact with clients and family caregivers.

The future of nursing informatics and telehealth is bright and promising. Innovations in nursing science combined with advances in information and communication technologies will provide community health nurses and planners with tools that will increase their contact with the communities they serve.

CRITICAL THINKING ACTIVITIES

1. You have been chosen to introduce your home health nursing staff to e-mail and the Internet. Detail what you would do to develop a program for the staff, outlining the benefits and uses of this technology in community health in an ambulatory-surgical center.

2. Develop an e-mail message for new nurses who will be converting to an electronic client care system in 6 months. How will you evaluate the effectiveness of your communication?

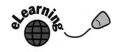 **Explore Community Health Nursing on the web! To learn more about the topics in this chapter, access your exclusive web site:** http://communitynursing.jbpub.com

REFERENCES

Bargstadt, G. (1998). Use of nursing information systems in the community setting. In S. Moorhead & C. Delaney (Eds.), *Information systems innovations for nursing* (pp. 213–226). Thousand Oaks, CA: Sage Publications.

Crist, T., Kaufman, S., & Crampton, K. (1996). Home telemedicine: A home health care agency's strategy for maximizing resources. *Home Health Care Management Practice, 8*(4), 1–9.

Gassert, C. (1998). The challenge of meeting patient's needs with a national nursing informatics agenda. *Journal of the American Medical Informatics Association, 5*(3), 263–286.

Graves, J., & Corcoran, S. (1989). The study of nursing informatics. *Image: The Journal of Nursing Scholarship, 21,* 227–231.

Grier, M., & McGuire, R. (1999). Nursing informatics: A means for change. In J. Lancaster (Ed.), *Nursing issues in leading and managing change* (pp. 533–553). St. Louis: Mosby.

Johnson, M., & Maas, M. (1997). *Iowa outcomes project: Nursing Outcomes Classification (NOC)* . St. Louis: Mosby.

Martin, K. S., & Scheet, N. J. (1995). The Omaha System: Nursing diagnosis, intervention, and client outcomes. *An emerging framework: Data systems advances for clinical nursing practice* (pp. 105–113). Washington, D.C.: American Nursing Association Publication, June. #NP-94.

McCloskey, J., & Bulechek, G. (1996). *Iowa intervention project: Nursing Intervention Classification (NIC)* (2nd ed.). St. Louis: Mosby.

Saba, V., & McCormick, K. (1996). *Essentials of computers for nurses* (2nd ed.). New York: McGraw-Hill.

Sebastian, J., & Stanhope, M. (1999). Managing resources. In J. Lancaster (Ed.), *Nursing issues in leading and managing change* (pp. 505–531). St. Louis: Mosby.

Stallings, W., & Van Slyke, R. (1998). *Business Data Communications* (3rd ed.). Upper Saddle River, NJ: Prentice Hall.

Warner, I. (1996). Telehealth home care. *Home Health Care Nurse, 14*(10), 791–796.

Warren, J. J., & Hoskins, L. M. (1995). NANDA's nursing diagnosis taxonomy: A nursing database. *An emerging framework: Data systems advances for clinical nursing practice* (pp. 49–59). Washington, D.C.: American Nurses Association Publication, June. #NP-94.

Zielstorff, R., Hudgings, C., & Grobe, S. (1993). *Next-generation nursing information systems: Essential characteristics for professional practice.* Washington DC: American Nurses Association.

9

Health Education in the Community

Lucy Bradley-Springer

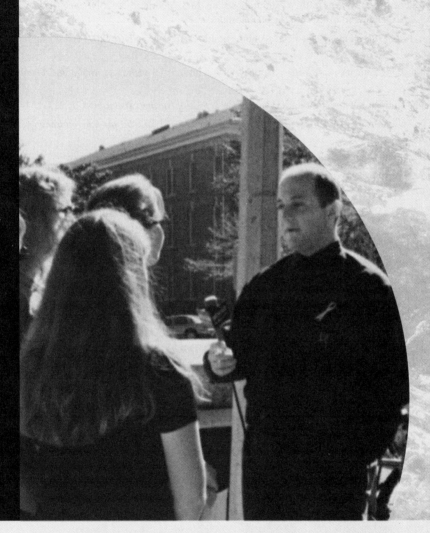

You may ask, "Why should I teach? Why would I want to change people's behaviors? I went to nursing school to give client care, not to teach. If I'd wanted to teach, I wouldn't have spent all this time learning to put catheters in and how to fill out care plans." The short answer is that teaching is an essential part of nursing. Nurses teach because it is a part of client care. The longer answer is that teaching clients improves health care. Education positively influences health outcomes when clients experience fewer complications and faster recoveries; learn to care for themselves, increasing autonomy and self-confidence; and are better prepared to resume their usual lives.

QUESTIONS TO CONSIDER

After reading this chapter, answer the following questions:

1. What is health education, and how does it differ in community settings?
2. What are behavior concepts and theories in education?
3. How are behavioral concepts and theories used to provide direction for health education programs?
4. What are principles of education, and how can they be integrated into health education practice?
5. What are the various situations in community health nursing in which education for behavior change can be incorporated into nursing care at the individual, group, and community levels?
6. What are the ethical issues in health education that have emerged from the current health care environment?

KEY TERMS

Absolutism	Behavior change	Domains of learning	Paternalism
Adherence	Benefits	Empowerment	Readiness
Advocacy	Cognitive dissonance	Health education	Self-efficacy
Autonomy	Community-based teaching	Learning goals and objectives	Teaching
Barriers	Compliance	Learning theories	
Behavior change theories	Discharge teaching	Motivation	

·····················

Wisdom is not a product of schooling, but the lifelong attempt to acquire it.

Albert Einstein

·····················

The purpose of health education is to change behaviors that put people at risk for injury, disease, disability, or death (Glanz, Lewis, & Rimer, 1990). This may sound blunt, but whether you call it modifying behavior or influencing behavior (Rankin & Stallings, 1996), it all boils down to the same thing: Nurses teach clients, families, groups, and communities with the primary goal of getting people to change behaviors in ways that focus on disease prevention, illness intervention, and health promotion. The mission of health education is to "reduce current and future suffering" by addressing "individual and social factors that contribute to health problems" (Guttman, Kegler, & McLeroy, 1996, p. i). This chapter explores the topic of health education: its theoretical bases, its application, the problems associated with it, and the community heath nurse's role in health education.

Health education can also increase the knowledge, skills, and confidence needed to make decisions. It improves continuity of care, decreases the risk of problem recurrence, and uses resources more efficiently. Educated clients and their families are better able to cope and more likely to recognize problems before they become severe. All of these benefits help nurses do their jobs because knowledgeable clients have fewer complications and present with fewer of the acute emergencies that require more complex care (Hunt, 1997).

Initially, health education concentrated on crisis management ("What do you need to know now that you've got a colostomy?"). However, the health care system in the United States is evolving. The emphasis is now on cost containment, health maintenance, and managed care (Damrosch, 1991). Over the past decade, health education has had to adjust to support

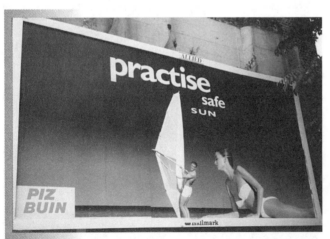

Public education campaign in Great Britain for prevention of skin cancer.

"

client care in the midst of all these changes. Today health education includes disease prevention ("How do you keep from getting tuberculosis?" or "How can you decrease your risk of a stroke from hypertension?") and health promotion ("How can you change to a healthier diet?") as well as continuing to deal with acute care issues. In addition, whether the focus is on reducing the rates of childhood infections or the deaths from cancer, health education and community-based programs are essential components of attaining every goal in the *Healthy People 2010* agenda (DHHS, 2000). Selected *Healthy People 2010* objectives related to health education are included in a box at the end of this chapter (p. 211).

Although nurses are not the only health care professionals capable of teaching, their knowledge, skills, and access to clients, especially in the community, make them particularly well suited to this complex task (Spellbring, 1991).

Theoretical Bases

When dealing with complex issues, it is wise to work from a theoretical base. Theories describe, explain, and predict behaviors within a functional framework (Glanz, Lewis, & Rimer, 1990). Theories about health education and behavior change can help nurses understand behavior and thereby help them develop useful strategies that influence people's health.

Concepts

Theories are based on concepts that are used to form the propositions that give structure to a theory. Some important concepts that support client autonomy in health education are defined in Table 9-1. In addition, it would be helpful to discuss absolutism and paternalism, two concepts that have lost favor in health education not only because they tend to stifle autonomy, but also because they have not been found to be effective.

Absolutism is a tactic we have all used. When absolutism is used in health education, the teacher basically says, "This is what you must do." Absolutism requires absolute **adherence** to specific, prescribed strategies (Cates & Hinman, 1992), and we have all done it because, as nurses, we know that smoking is not healthy and eating broccoli is. Absolute health care messages are

TABLE 9-1	IMPORTANT CONCEPTS FOR HEALTH EDUCATION THEORY

CONCEPT	DEFINITION
Advocacy	Process in which clients are informed and supported so that they can make the best decisions possible (Spellbring, 1991); advocacy is a primary nursing function.
Barriers	Those individually determined things that associate cost with a particular behavior (Palank, 1991); costs can be thought of in terms of money, time inconvenience, difficulty, risk, or interpersonal effort. Not having child care, for example, is a barrier for a mother who needs to attend a Narcotics Anonymous meeting.
Benefits	Those individually determined things that reinforce or reward a particular behavior (Palank, 1991); in other words, one person may see weight loss as a main benefit of exercise, but another may see meeting friends at the gym as the primary benefit.
Cognitive dissonance	Tension or discomfort that accompanies actions that oppose personal beliefs (Rankin & Stallings, 1996); for example, a person who lectures co-workers about good nutrition eats chocolate cake and feels guilty about it.
Empowerment	Process of helping people develop the abilities to understand and control their personal situations; can be applied at individual, group, and community levels (Israel, Checkoway, Schulz, & Zimmerman, 1994).
Motivation	Complex concept that refers to those "forces acting on or within an organism that initiate, direct, and maintain behavior" (Redman, 1997, p. 7).
Readiness	Motivation to perform a particular action at a particular time (Redman, 1997).
Self-efficacy	Personal conviction of ability to carry out specific behaviors in order to achieve a desired end (Damrosch, 1991; Palank, 1991); the "I know I can do this" feeling.

usually well intentioned. They are based on evidence that, if used consistently and correctly, the prescribed methods will make people healthier. The problem is that complete compliance with any behavior is difficult. Think, for instance, about the last time you tried to lose weight or start exercising regularly. Were you always able to meet your goals? Did you always skip dessert? Did you show up at the gym every morning? Demanding absolute compliance with absolute behaviors is risky because most people cannot meet such high standards. When they fail to meet these standards, they can lose confidence in their abilities to change and give up (Strang, 1992). Maybe you have given up on some of your goals. Hopefully, you knew that missing a workout session or eating a piece of chocolate cake did not spell disaster. Hopefully, you chalked it up to experience and moved forward in your behavior change program. If you didn't, maybe it was because you believed an absolutist message: Do it right or don't do it at all. You can see how this would make health education and behavior change difficult.

Absolutism is perpetuated in an atmosphere of paternalism. **Paternalism** occurs when health care providers (or other "experts") decide what the client should do (Rankin & Stallings, 1996). Although this also is usually done with altruistic motives, it is counter to the concept of promoting client autonomy. Paternalism and absolutism demand compliance. Compliance carries the expectation that clients will do exactly what providers tell them to do. If they don't, they are labeled "noncompliant," a term that implies client responsibility for failure (Rankin &

Stallings, 1996). The nursing philosophy of holistic client care supports individuals in their efforts to make health decisions and behavior changes. Absolutism, paternalism, and demands for compliance are all counter to this philosophy.

Learning Theory

Much health education is based on **learning theories** that have been developed over the past several decades. These theories are usually familiar to nurses, but some of the more important learning theory contributions to health education are briefly discussed here. The behavioral theorists, including Pavlov, Thorndike, and Skinner, showed how teachers could connect a stimulus to a desired response. This leads to a conditioned change in behavior that occurs every time the stimulus is presented. A client could, for instance, learn that brushing her teeth in the morning is associated with taking her birth control pill. Developmental theories, on the other hand, state that individuals need to acquire competence at one level of a developmental process before moving to the next level. Piaget showed that children go through specific developmental stages in their intellectual abilities, Erikson defined the psychosocial stages of growth and development, and Maslow explained a hierarchy of human needs where basic needs (e.g., food and shelter) must to be met before working on higher level needs (e.g., social connections and self-actualization). In addition, Rogers contributed the concept of learner-centered care in which the client learns to make decisions and solve problems (Hunt, 1997; Spradley & Allender, 1996).

Adult learning theory provides important information for health education. This theory holds that motivation to learn is based on four assumptions (Knowles, 1973):

1. *Adults perceive themselves to be self-directed: They want to have a say in what they learn.*

2. *Adults have a variety of life experiences and are insulted if these experiences are ignored: The wise teacher will build on these experiences.*

3. *Adults learn better when they see an immediate need: They are goal directed.*

4. *Timing education to coincide with an immediate need is more effective because the learner will see the immediate goal and be ready to learn.*

Behavior Change Theory

Theories that specifically address behavior change and health education incorporate ideas from these learning theories. **Behavior change theories** provide direction for nurses who teach in a variety of situations. A brief overview of some of these theories is provided in Table 9-2.

TABLE 9-2	OVERVIEW OF SELECTED THEORIES ABOUT HEALTH BEHAVIOR

THEORY AND KEY COMPONENTS	CASE STUDY

Health belief model: Individuals are more likely to take action to improve health if:
  They perceive themselves to be at risk for a problem (susceptibility)
  The problem is seen as serious enough to warrant action (severity, perceived threat)
  The expected benefits of the action outweigh the anticipated costs (e.g., in terms of overcoming barriers related to time, effort, money)
  There is a personal sense of ability to perform the required actions (self-efficacy) (Mirotznik, Feldman, & Stein, 1995; Rosenstock, 1990)
	Nina's mother and sister both died of breast cancer. Nina took care of her mother during the terminal phases of the disease, and she has told friends, "That was the most horrible thing I ever had to do." Nina was concerned about her own risk, so she talked to her nurse practitioner (NP). The NP gave Nina information about breast cancer, did a breast examination, scheduled Nina for a mammogram, and taught Nina how to do breast self-examination (BSE).
	Follow-up: Nina sees breast cancer as a terrible disease, and she feels that she may be at risk. She is motivated to protect her health but has trouble remembering to do BSE. Doing it actually frightens her: What if she should find a lump? At her next clinic visit, her NP provides Nina with a chart, watches her do BSE in the office, and discusses her concerns about finding a lump. The NP is able to assure Nina that she is doing everything right. Nina establishes a habit of BSE that works for her.

Harm reduction model: Health risks can be decreased by having clients ask, What is healthier, safer, or less risky than what I am doing now? and What steps am I willing and able to take in order to be healthier, safer, or less risky? Basic principles include the following:
  Most people are competent to make informed decisions about health behaviors; they are the only ones who know what will work for them in their specific situations.
  Needs are diverse and can be met in diverse ways; offering people a spectrum of potential behaviors is better than demanding that they adopt an absolute requirement.
  Incremental steps that provide chances for success work better than trying to make large, difficult changes where the risk of failure is high.
	Bob, who smokes two packs of cigarettes a day, arrives at Occupational Health for his annual physical. He tells the nurse that he exercises regularly and feels "as healthy as a horse." He denies any smoking-related problems, saying, "Smoking is my only vice and I really like it. It relaxes me. I tried to stop smoking once and it was a disaster, so why bother? But I am worried about smoking around my kids—they've been sick a lot lately." The nurse asks, "What do you think would be healthier for your kids?" Bob lists ideas ranging from quitting smoking all together to not smoking in the house. The nurse then asks, "Which of these things do you think would work best for you?" Bob decides to try smoking only in his office at home where "the kids can't come anyway."
	Follow-up: The nurse helped Bob explore his options without taking over and telling him what to do. He was then able to choose a behavior that he thought would work in his situation. Bob sees the nurse several months later and says, "Hey, you know how we talked about smoking only in my office to protect my kids? Well it's working real well. The kids haven't been sick as often and I'm not smoking as much either. I'm down to a pack and a half a day." By helping Bob see his options and by not demanding that he quit smoking, the nurse gave

TABLE 9-2	OVERVIEW OF SELECTED THEORIES ABOUT HEALTH BEHAVIOR—CONT'D

THEORY AND KEY COMPONENTS	CASE STUDY

People may need social support, education, referrals, and assistance to make changes (Bradley-Springer, 1996; Caplan, 1995).
 	
Goal-setting theory: Setting goals can help people change health-related behaviors by focusing effort, persistence, and concentration on the goal. The following steps are used:
  Determine the client's commitment to change.
  Analyze the tasks required to make changes: Complex tasks need to be broken down into subgoals (strategic analysis); simple tasks can be motivated by a simple goal.
  Assess the client's self-efficacy for performing required behaviors and help with skill development as needed.
  Goals should be difficult enough to require significant effort; they should be optimistic as well as realistic.
  Provide feedback on progress (Strecher et al., 1995).
	him the support he needed to make positive changes. Bob will now feel good about talking to the nurse if he wants to make further changes.
	At her last dental checkup, Ana's dentist pointed out that she had beginning gum disease and suggested that Ana start flossing. Ana said, "I know I should floss. I know how to do it. I floss for 2 or 3 days, but then I miss a day and I give up. I don't want to lose all my teeth like my mother did. I just can't keep it up." The dentist suggests that Ana set a goal of flossing every other day.
	
	Follow-up: Ana was committed to making a change and already possessed the required skills. By suggesting a specific, attainable goal, the dentist provided additional motivation. At her next checkup Ana says, "It worked! I'm flossing almost every day now. When I miss a day it's not that big a deal because I know I will be able to floss the next day." During her oral examination, the dentist is able to tell Ana that her gums look much better.

Theory of reasoned action: Behavioral intention to act is based on a combination of the following:
  Personal beliefs and evaluations about what will happen if the behavior is used (perceived chance of success)
  Personal attitudes and values about the behavior
  Feelings about what key people (family, friends, health care providers) in the person's life think about the behavior
  Motivation to change behavior (Carter, 1990)
  All things being equal, people are expected to act in accordance with their intentions (Miller, Wikoff, & Hiatt, 1992).
	Sue, a nursing student, has been dating Jack for 2 years. They plan to get married after she graduates. They have discussed having a family and agree that they do not want children for several years. Sue and Jack want to become sexually active. They visit the Student Health Center, where a nurse explains birth control options. Jack encourages Sue to use birth control pills (BCPs). Sue is worried because some of her friends have told her that BCPs caused them to gain weight.
	Follow-up: Although Sue is worried about weight gain, she believes that BCPs are effective and easy to use. She is clear that she does not currently want a pregnancy. She has Jack's support. Sue rarely misses taking her vitamin pills, so she is sure that she can remember to take the pills every day. This model predicts that Sue is likely to use BCPs consistently and correctly.

Social learning theory: Individual behavior, personal factors, and the environment create a triad of components that interact to influence health behaviors:
  A change in one component of the triad has an effect on all components (reciprocal determinism).
  Personal factors include behavioral capability, self-control, self-efficacy, internal
	Jose is a depressed 13-year-old who has just entered a new school. He hasn't made any friends at the new school, a problem he blames on being 20 pounds overweight. The people Jose admires most at school all seem to be thin. He also notices that they are active in after-school activities. Jose's mother reminds him that he is a good swimmer and encourages him to join the swim team.
	Follow-up: Jose's desire to lose weight is influenced by the rewards that he sees being given to slim people. His perception of his weight and his emotional response to it create a desire to change that is sup-

Continued

TABLE 9-2   **OVERVIEW OF SELECTED THEORIES ABOUT HEALTH BEHAVIOR—CONT'D**

THEORY AND KEY COMPONENTS	CASE STUDY
reinforcements, emotional coping response, and a belief that performing a behavior will lead to expected outcomes. The environment (everything external to the individual) and the situation (the individual's perception of the environment) provide opportunities to observe behaviors performed by others in the environment (vicarious learning) (Perry, Baranowski, & Parcel, 1990).	ported by his mother and his swimming ability. Jose knows that swimming can help. He tries out for the team and discovers that he can do the butterfly stroke better than anyone else. He joins the team, and in addition to exercising regularly and losing weight, Jose makes new friends and develops a more optimistic outlook.
Diffusion theory: New ideas, practices, or services (innovations) to improve health move from a resource (innovation developer) to the population (innovation users or adopters). Diffusion is more likely to occur if the innovation is cost-efficient, low risk, simple, flexible, and compatible with the social, economic, and value systems into which it is introduced. Innovations that are reversible (I can go back to where I was if I don't like it) and appear to be better than currently used methods have a better chance of being adopted. Diffusion can fail if the innovation does not work, if information about the innovation is not communicated well, if the potential user does not have the necessary resources for implementation, or if the innovation is in opposition to the user's value system. In addition, there may be a problem if components of the implementation process are abbreviated. An example of this would be when education about the innovation is omitted to save money. Maintenance of an innovation takes additional effort; without this, the adopted program can lose momentum and fade away (Orlandi, Landers, Weston, & Haley, 1990).	Injection drug users (IDUs) who do not share equipment to inject drugs are not at risk of infection with blood-borne diseases such as hepatitis B, hepatitis C, and human immunodeficiency virus (HIV). Activists in Metrotown, a community of 300,000, wanted to implement a needle and syringe exchange program (N/SEP) so that IDUs would have access to sterile injecting equipment. They gathered support from the city council, the health department, and law enforcement before setting up N/SEP sites around town. During the first week, only two IDUs brought in equipment to exchange. **Follow-up:** Activists (resource) did a good job in Metrotown of involving the established power systems. No doubt they convinced all of these entities that N/SEPs would be cost-effective, simple, reversible, and better than allowing used injecting equipment to accumulate on the streets of the city. The activists were less effective in communicating the benefits of N/SEPs to the intended users of the program. IDUs need to know that obtaining sterile equipment will decrease the risk of disease, will be easily accessible, and will not put them at risk for being targeted by the police. Although Metrotown has made a difficult public health decision, it will not be successful unless the innovation diffuses to the intended users.
Social marketing theory: Public acceptance of programs to improve health can be enhanced through marketing techniques. Marketing functions on a number of well-developed principles: Participants are offered benefits that are valued as being worth the cost (e.g., measured in effort, money, time). The consumer (client) is the central concern.	Everyone at Russell High School (RHS) is shocked when three students, all with blood alcohol levels over the legal limit, are killed in a car accident. The principal forms a committee of students, teachers, and administrators to develop a program to decrease drunk driving. After assessing the situation at RHS, the committee proposes a plan to encourage the use of designated drivers. The program is kicked off at an assembly where student leaders (athletes, class officers, cheerleaders) describe the program. They all wear t-shirts that say, "I care about my friends. I'm a designated driver." Students are regularly

TABLE 9-2	OVERVIEW OF SELECTED THEORIES ABOUT HEALTH BEHAVIOR—CONT'D

THEORY AND KEY COMPONENTS	CASE STUDY
Communication (in the form of advertising, public relations, direct marketing, promotion, and face-to-face encounters) is the key to getting information to the consumer. The marketing process has six stages that occur in a cycle: (1) analysis; (2) planning; (3) development, testing, and refinement of the plan; (4) implementation; (5) assessment of effectiveness; and (6) feedback to analysis (completing the cycle). Marketing strategies must be modified to function in situations in which social issues and health are the central concerns (Novelli, 1990).	reminded about the program in newspaper articles, intercom announcements, and student-lead discussions in homeroom classes. **Follow-up:** RHS used marketing strategies focused on consumers (students) to develop a program that would meet the objective to decrease drunk driving. Although the adults on the planning committee had some reservations about a program that seemed to condone drinking, they paid attention to the analysis provided by student representatives and approved the program. A survey done 3 months later showed that 40% of RHS students had been designated drivers, resulting in a significant decrease in drunk driving rates. An additional, unforeseen benefit was a decrease in the overall rate of drinking, a direct result of designated driving being seen as "cool."

The transtheoretical model, so called because it borrows from many other theories, provides new and helpful insights for health education. The central premise of the transtheoretical model is that people progress through a series of stages when they attempt to change behaviors. There are five stages of change: precontemplative, contemplative, preparation, action, and maintenance (Prochaska, Redding, Harlow, Rossi, & Velicer, 1994). Progression through the stages is rarely linear. People will change their minds, will hesitate, and may relapse several times before behavior change is permanent. Ten different processes are used to enhance progression through the stages of change:

1. *Consciousness raising (increasing the level of awareness)*
2. *Dramatic relief (experiencing and expressing feelings)*
3. *Environmental reevaluation (assessing how the environment affects the situation)*
4. *Self-reevaluation (assessing how a person thinks and feels about the situation)*
5. *Self-liberation (believing in the ability to change)*
6. *Helping relationships (caring and trusting relationships)*
7. *Social liberation (seeing social changes that support personal changes)*
8. *Counterconditioning (substituting more healthful behaviors for less healthful behaviors)*
9. *Stimulus control (restructuring the environment)*
10. *Reinforcement management (getting rewards)*

Table 9-3 gives an overview of the transtheoretical model, including examples of the 10 processes and interventions appropriate in each stage.

The Health Education Process

Health education is a process of planned teaching and support activities that help people learn (Spellbring, 1991). The education process follows the format of the nursing process, including assessment, planning, implementation, and evaluation (Rankin

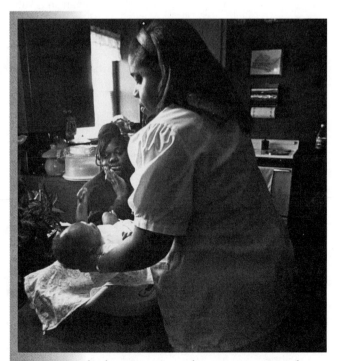

A nurse in the home setting educates a new mother about newborn care.

TABLE 9-3   OVERVIEW OF THE TRANSTHEORETICAL MODEL (ALSO KNOWN AS THE STAGES OF CHANGE THEORY)

STAGE: CLIENT'S PERSPECTIVE	CASE STUDY AND INTERVENTIONS
Precontemplative: Unaware of or unwilling to consider the problem; defensive about the change issue, resistant to information about the behavior, and reluctant to initiate a behavior change program; not considering change within the next 6 months; has little confidence in ability to change; sees many reasons not to change	During a routine physical, Sam, a 26-year-old lawyer, says, "You know, I was listening to the radio on the way over here and a woman was talking about having AIDS (consciousness raising). This whole thing scares me (dramatic relief). It's not just gay guys anymore. I know that I've had some risks, but the things I do are a part of my life and the people I hang with (environmental reevaluation)." **Stage-specific interventions:** Raise awareness of the issue through community-appropriate public education and media programs. Provide information and feedback to increase individual awareness of physical, social, economic, and psychological problems related to the commission or omission of specific behaviors. Discuss the positive aspects of change. Do not spend time discussing details of specific change tactics or programs: You're wasting your time if it is clear that the client is not ready to think about changing.
Contemplative: Ambivalent; responds with "Yes, but . . . "; may see reasons to change as well as reasons to remain the same; indecisive, aware that a problem exists and more open to information, but still unsure of ability to change; intends to change behavior within next 6 months	Sam's nurse encourages him to continue talking about his concerns and those behaviors that make him think he has been at risk. He says, "Well, I have some crazy friends. I go out with them every Saturday. We compare notes on how much sex we get. We dare each other to do things like using a prostitute or having anal sex or coming on to a gay guy. I'm not proud of some of the things I've done. Maybe I'm getting too old for this (self-reevaluation)." **Stage-specific interventions:** Tip the balance in favor of change. It is important to see this stage as the time when the client will develop a commitment to change. It is still too early to look at strategies. The aim is to analyze risks and rewards of the behavior and to provide information. Clarify goals and discuss incentives to change. It is now time to emphasize negative aspects of not changing. A discussion of the risk for harm is appropriate.
Preparation: Expresses desire to do something to initiate change; some experimentation with new behaviors may already be occurring; thinks change may be possible; seriously planning change within next 30 days but has not set specific goals	When asked how this makes him feel, Sam responds by saying, with a sigh, "I guess I should think about being more careful. I don't want to get anything bad, especially AIDS. I need to change my act (self-liberation)." **Stage-specific interventions:** Now is the time to get down to details. Help the client find change strategies that are acceptable, accessible, appropriate, and effective. Encourage the client to experiment with a strategy: "Try it next time, see how you like it," or "Find out how your family/partner/friends react when you do it." Be available to the client to discuss issues related to moving into the action stage. Help the client establish specific objectives. In Sam's case, this could be limiting nights out with his friends to once a month.
Action: Engages in action to create desired change; feels developing confidence in personal self-efficacy; thinks reasons to change outweigh reasons not to; behavior modified to meet goal(s) for 6 months	Over the course of the next 6 months, Sam and the nurse meet several times to discuss his progress. During this time, Sam says, "I've talked about this with my friend Mia. She just listens and never acts like I'm a bad person even when I tell her bad things I've done (helping relationship). Since I've started talking about it, I've had people tell me that I'm right to be concerned and that I should be more careful—even some of my buddies agree (social liberation)." Sam begins to take specific actions to decrease his risks. He begins to use condoms and decides to have sex only when he wants to and not "on a dare" (counterconditioning). **Stage-specific interventions:** Be aware that this is not an easy process. Support change efforts. Clients will need continuing encouragement, help with problem solving, and a place to simply vent frustrations.

TABLE 9-3	OVERVIEW OF THE TRANSTHEORETICAL MODEL (ALSO KNOWN AS THE STAGES OF CHANGE THEORY)—CONT'D

STAGE: CLIENT'S PERSPECTIVE	CASE STUDY AND INTERVENTIONS
Maintenance: Challenged to continue change; feels expanding self-efficacy; continues behavior change for more than 6 months	As Sam becomes comfortable with his new behaviors, he reports that other things are changing. He says, "I realized that my problems were related to my friends. They didn't understand why I wanted to change. They called me a wimp. So I decided to quit hanging out with them (stimulus control). The good thing is that I feel better about myself. Mia even told me that she's noticed that I seem happier (reinforcement management)." **Stage-specific interventions:** Help the client maintain change. Problem solving and unconditional support for the client are extremely important during this stage. Relapse prevention efforts can include interactive discussions, role-playing, and "what if" sessions in which the client identifies risks for relapse and develops workable strategies.
Relapse (not a stage): An important event that can occur at any time in the change process; if relapse occurs, the client may express anger and question ability to maintain change; may be embarrassed or ashamed; may blame self or others (including health care providers) for relapse	Sam returns to clinic a year later. When asked about how he's doing, he blurts out, "I blew it. I ran into Jake a few weeks ago and we went for a drink. Before I knew it, we'd picked up a couple of women. I ended up in a strange apartment and no one ever thought about using condoms. I'm really embarrassed about this—especially after I made such a big deal out of being careful with my friends. Maybe I wasn't meant to be safe. Maybe I'm supposed to get the clap or HIV or something else that's just as bad. I can't even face Mia." **Stage-specific interventions:** Clients may get "stuck" in relapse if they resort to self-incrimination or self-blame. Help the client renew the change process at an earlier stage without getting demoralized. Explain that relapse is common and may occur many times before behavior change is permanent. Point out specific instances of success that show the client's abilities to change. Provide referral to needed services. Sam, for instance, may need a work up for sexually transmitted disease.

Source: Adapted from Bradley-Springer, 1996.

& Stallings, 1996). While these steps are being taken, meticulous documentation should occur. The next section presents detailed information about each step in the education process, but before that, some important general points about education need to be made.

Education is client centered. An important question for the nurse to continually ask is, "How does *this* problem (e.g., diagnosis, stressor, need to change) affect *this* client?" To truly make the process client centered, nurses must remember that people live in complex social and culturally defined environments. Therefore, the involvement of family and significant others can help promote learning. In some cases, family involvement is essential, especially when health education is directed to children, clients with sensory deficits, or clients who are physically unable to perform the necessary skills. In general, involving others can provide social and emotional supports that help people make behavior changes (Rankin & Stallings, 1996). Unfortunately, clients do not always have healthy support structures, or they simply may not want others involved. In these cases, the nurse

should not force the issue. Instead, referrals to community resources and support groups should be considered.

It does not do to leave a live dragon out of your calculations if you live near him.

J. R. R. Tolkien

Assessment

The task of assessment is to gather information. This can result in a huge amount of information that the nurse uses to determine needs and priorities. Obviously, educational needs cannot be determined without looking at the entire client. Learning needs evolve from a knowledge of the client's overall health problems (actual and potential). In most cases, some of the needs discovered through assessment will have a cognitive, skill, or attitudinal component that must be addressed through education (Rankin & Stallings, 1996).

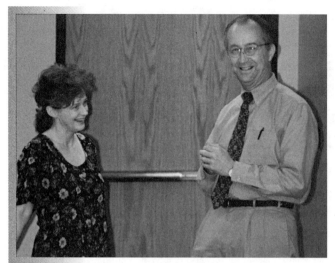

Chapter author Lucy Bradley-Springer and Kevin Morrisroe, RN, do a role play on Risk Assessment at a class in New Mexico.

Assessment requires active nurse-client interaction. This can be time-consuming, but the nurse can use assessment time to develop rapport with the client and significant others (Redman, 1997). Building a good working relationship during this phase will increase the amount of information the client reveals and will make the rest of the education process more enjoyable for both the client and the nurse. This is especially important in community health settings where nurses need to establish long-term relationships with individuals in the community. Table 9-4 lists some areas that need to be discussed during a health education assessment.

Data can be collected from a variety of sources, including direct observation, client records, other members of the health care team, and professional literature. The best way to get the client's point of view, however, is through an interactive interview. Client disclosure of information is enhanced by the following tactics (Rankin & Stallings, 1996):

- Establish an environment of trust. *This may require some time at the beginning of the conversation. Start by introducing yourself and telling who you are. ("Hi. I'm Faith Diaz, and I'm an RN from the home health agency.") Establish that you have experience in the area you will be addressing with the client. ("I've been working with people who've had your kind of surgery for 2 years.") Describe the intention of the interview and make it clear that questions are asked to help the client. As we all know, some of the questions that nurses need to ask can be embarrassing. Assure the client that there are health care reasons for asking each question and that all answers are confidential.*

- Choose the right time. *Be sure that you have time to adequately assess the client's needs. Ask if this is a good time for the client. Be sure the client is not in pain or anxious about*

an anticipated event. *If you know that your time is short, introduce the assessment session by saying, "I know you are anxious about your wound care. I only have 15 minutes to spend with you right now, and I need to ask you a few questions. Your answers will help me plan how I will teach you about your wound. I'll come back this afternoon, and we'll go over everything in detail. First, I'd like to know if you've ever had a wound like this before . . . "*

- Choose the right place. *The location of an interview should be comfortable and private. If it is not, the client (and the nurse) may concentrate more on the room temperature or the hard chairs or the constant interruptions than on the interview. If possible, do the interview on the client's "home turf." This can be in the client's home or a private room at the clinic. Asking questions in a known environment helps the client feel safe (Hunt, 1997).*

- Use open-ended questions. *Going through a list of "yes/no" questions does not provide the depth of information needed to develop effective, individualized teaching plans. Asking the client to describe her problems doing exercises after a mastectomy, for example, will get a lot of those "yes/no" questions answered without your even asking them. The client will also benefit from the experience of telling her story to an interested listener. Remember, clients (as adult learners) have unique perspectives that they need to share with you and that you should build into your teaching plan.*

- Use active listening skills. *Ask for clarification, summarize, and use open body language (nod, smile; do not act like you have to leave). These listening skills enhance interactions and ensure that you understand the client's meanings.*

When the interview is complete, summarize the main points and thank the client for spending time with you. Tell the client what you intend to do with the information and describe the next steps in the planning process. If you cannot continue the process at this time, tell the client when you will return.

Planning

During planning, the nurse and client discuss learning needs and potential goals. This is a negotiation process: The nurse provides input that the client uses to make decisions about specific interventions. The result of this process is a list of learning objectives. Hopefully, the list will not be too long, but some clients have many problems. In that case, it is best to prioritize the list by having the client choose those problems (1) that are most pressing (cause the most discomfort for the client) and (2) the client is most willing to work on (an estimate of readiness). Limiting the teaching session to one or two objectives is less intimidating than trying to make a large number of changes at the same time (Kreuter & Strecher, 1996).

Learning goals and objectives are established in the initial part of the planning phase. Goals and objectives provide an agreed-upon direction for implementation and a guide for eval-

TABLE 9-4 ASSESSMENT VARIABLES

WHAT TO ASSESS	ASSESSMENT QUESTIONS
Client understanding of the problem in question	What do you think is the cause of this problem? Why do you think it is happening now?
Client perception of need to change	How does the problem affect you? Has this problem limited your activities in any way?
Motivation to change: severity of problem and risks caused by the problem	How severe is the problem? Is it a short-term or a long-term problem? What harm could this problem cause you? What are the 2 to 3 main difficulties that you have because of this problem? What do you fear most about the problem? Why do you want to solve this problem?
Readiness to change	What would you like do to about the problem in the next few days (weeks)? What are the most important things that you would like to have happen?
Self-efficacy	How do you usually approach problems? How would you like to approach this problem? What do you think you can do about the problem? Have you tried to deal with this problem before? If so, what did you do and how did it turn out?
Perceived benefits to change	How would you feel if you solved this problem? If you didn't have the problem, what would be better in your life?
Perceived barriers to change	What has kept you from dealing with this problem in the past? Do you see things that may prevent your dealing with this problem? If so, what are they?
Psychosocial issues	Who gives you the most support? Would you like her or him to be in on our teaching sessions? Also assess housing, economic status, educational background, community resources, cultural and religious contributions to health care, native language, and so on.
Learning skills	How do you learn best? Would you like reading materials or videotapes or group sessions or private counseling or . . . ?

Source: Adapted from Kreuter & Strecher, 1996; Palank, 1991; Rankin & Stallings, 1996; and Redman, 1997.

uation. Goals are broad statements of the desired outcome: Jason will manage insulin administration to control his blood sugar, for example. Objectives are specific, detailed statements. They describe behaviors that will help meet a goal. They describe what the client will do, define how it will be done, and prescribe time frames for task completion. Objectives for Jason could include the following:

1. *Before he is discharged in 3 days, Jason will be able to list the signs and symptoms of high and low blood sugar.*

2. *By tomorrow, Jason will be able to test his blood for glucose with the equipment he will use at home.*

3. *By the day before discharge, Jason will be able to use a prescribed sliding scale to accurately draw up and inject insulin in the ordered doses at the ordered times.*

4. *Within a week after discharge, Jason will describe the benefits of controlling his blood sugar.*

Notice that the objectives are specific and measurable. We will be able to tell when Jason accomplishes each objective (Rankin & Stallings, 1996).

Also notice that the objectives do not all look alike. That is because they address three different **domains of learning** (Redman, 1997). Some objectives refer to things that people need to know. These are called *cognitive objectives*. In Jason's case, the first objective asks him to know the signs of hyperglycemia and hypoglycemia. *Psychomotor objectives* refer to skills or behaviors. Jason will need to manipulate equipment (a skill) to meet the next two objectives. The final objective addresses an attitude: We want Jason to verbalize a positive outlook on his abilities. This objective occurs in the *affective* domain.

Knowing the type of objective helps the nurse and client decide on teaching and learning methods. Jason may be able to learn the symptoms of hyperglycemia from a brochure, for instance, but he will need to practice drawing up insulin and in-

TABLE 9-5   DOMAINS OF LEARNING
....

DOMAIN	GOALS AND OBJECTIVES	TEACHING METHODS	APPLICATION CASE: GOAL IS TO ENCOURAGE BREAST-FEEDING IN PREGNANT WOMEN WHO ATTEND A LOW-INCOME CLINIC.
COGNITIVE SUBDOMAINS			
Knowledge (to know)	To state, to list, to define, to recall, to name, to repeat	Lecture, one-on-one instruction, programmed instruction, videos or audio tapes, reading materials, questions and answers	Display breast-feeding posters in prominent places around the clinic. Run a continuous video on breast-feeding in the waiting room. Leave brochures and printed materials in examination rooms. Plan a series of lectures at a convenient time for clients.
Comprehension (to understand)	To explain, to label, to describe, to interpret	Lecture, one-on-one instruction, programmed instruction, video program, reading materials, learning guides, study questions	Arrange face-to-face sessions during prenatal visits; ask if client has questions or concerns. Follow up educational activities by asking, "What difference could breast-feeding make for your baby?"
Application (to use)	To illustrate, to apply, to give examples	Demonstration, group discussion, simulation exercises, games, role-play, clinical practice	Demonstrate breast care and the process of breast-feeding using a simulation model or a video. Encourage partner participation in education.
Analysis (to identify elements)	To compare, to contrast, to differentiate, to debate, to question	Group discussion, games, group interaction, simulation exercises, role-play, case studies	Arrange small group sessions where women can discuss concerns about breast-feeding. Role-play issues that emerge from group discussions.
Synthesis (to use in new ways)	To assemble, to prepare, to create, to design, to formulate	Group projects, group discussion, simulation exercises, games, role-play, case studies	Invite women from the community who are successfully breast-feeding to discuss the process in small groups of pregnant women. Support breast-feeding efforts after delivery.
Evaluation (to judge)	To assess, to justify, to measure, to choose	Group discussion, guided imagery, role-play, self-evaluation worksheet	Ask women to share success stories related to breast-feeding. Provide questionnaire that helps client assess values and fears about breast-feeding; follow up with a one-on-one discussion.
Psychomotor (to perform)	To assemble, to demonstrate, to control, to manipulate	Demonstration, practice with supervision, independent practice, return demonstration, role-play, simulation, clinical experience	Demonstrate breast care and the process of breast-feeding using a simulation model or a video. Provide guidance and positive reinforcement to women after delivery as they initiate breast-feeding with newborn.
Affective (to feel)	To tolerate, to accept, to defend, to adopt, to appreciate, to value	Group discussion, group project, simulation exercises, games, role-play, life experience	Encourage client involvement. Reinforce positive statements about breast-feeding. Encourage attendance at group sessions where breast-feeding is discussed.

jecting himself to really learn those skills. You cannot learn to give an injection by reading about it! Table 9-5 provides an in-depth overview of the domains of learning and teaching methods appropriate to each domain.

The planning stage is not complete until the client agrees to the goals, objectives, and teaching methods. Although Jason's plan looks good on the surface, he may have a morbid fear of sticking himself. In that case, the objectives and plan would need to be changed to have someone in his household learn the "sticking" skills (injections and finger sticks), but Jason should be able to meet the other objectives and may eventually overcome his fears and learn the "sticking" skills himself.

Implementation

During implementation, the nurse and client use information from the assessment and planning stages to make decisions about learning activities. Learning activities must focus on the established objectives. Interventions are tailored to the client's needs and abilities. Teaching plans are then put into action, but this is not a static process. The nurse continually observes and asks for feedback to track progress. The nurse should discuss any problems with the client, modifying the plan as needs change. This is called *formative evaluation*: It helps the teacher adjust the format of the education as the teaching progresses. Box 9-1 provides some general pointers to guide teaching.

BOX 9-1 POINTERS FOR HEALTH EDUCATION

- Design teaching based on assessments of individual clients: needs, ability, knowledge base, learning styles, expectations, culture, language, readiness to learn, and so on.

- Develop educational objectives with input from the learner. Validate that the objectives are relevant to the learner's needs. Objectives serve as the basis for instruction and evaluation.

- Create a learning environment. It should be comfortable and free of distractions.

- Keep things simple.

- Focus on one issue at a time. Keep learning sessions short. Concentrate on outcomes that will be immediately obvious (e.g., feeling and looking better because of exercise rather than the more distant issue of preventing heart disease).

- Be sure written materials are appropriate. Keep sentences short. Use words a layperson can understand. Define medical words in simple terms. Use a font style and size that are easy to read. Use pictures and diagrams to clarify concepts.

- Be specific. "Lose weight," for instance, is not as effective as, "Lose 2 pounds this week."

- Avoid threatening messages that generate fear. Mild anxiety enhances learning, but high fear levels can lead to denial, tuning out the message, or inability to concentrate.

- Explain what you will be teaching and why it is important. This provides an "advance organizer" to keep session centered on the topic.

- Provide for success. Divide learning tasks into sequential learning units that start with easier concepts and build to more difficult ones. Encourage success at each level before progressing to more difficult tasks. This enhances self-efficacy and personal satisfaction.

- Use a variety of teaching methods. People learn in different ways, and a combination of methods reinforces learning. Varying methods also keeps people involved.

- Provide visual learning materials. Seeing as well as hearing enhances retention.

- Show the client what is expected. Model behaviors to demonstrate how things are done.

- Skills (both verbal and physical) require practice. (Examples: role-play communication skills, use a plastic model to teach self-catheterization techniques, use syringes to practice drawing up insulin.)

- Involve all the senses in practice sessions. This reinforces learning on several levels.

- Provide immediate feedback that praises or corrects specific details during practice sessions. Highlight successes and express honest confidence in the learner's abilities to accomplish learning objectives. If you have doubts about the learner's abilities, do not give false praise. Instead, reassess with the learner and develop a new teaching plan.

- Develop mechanisms for support. Include family and friends in education as possible and as acceptable to the client. Support groups that focus on specific issues have been shown to enhance learning while encouraging positive change and maintenance of newly developed behaviors.

- Discuss resources for further information and/or practice.

- Review major points of each learning session. Discuss plans for follow-up, reinforcement, and expansion of learning experience.

- Keep learners involved: Ask for feedback and evaluation during teaching and learning.

Source: Adapted from Byham, 1992; Damrosch, 1991; and Spradley & Allender, 1996.

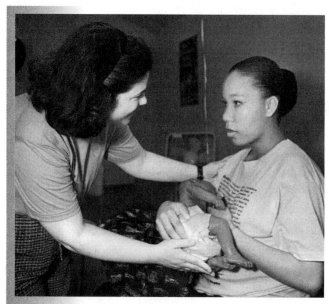

Nurse educating a teen mom about breast-feeding.

Evaluation

Evaluation is a process of gathering information to assess the extent to which learning objectives have been met—or not met. There are a number of ways to evaluate learning, but all evaluation methods should be based on the learning objectives. Objectives that are written with appropriate action verbs will tell you how to evaluate outcomes. An objective that says the learner will be able to list the steps in cardiopulmonary resuscitation (CPR), for instance, can be evaluated by asking her to write those steps on a piece of paper. If the objective states that the learner will be able to perform CPR, however, you will need to watch the technique on a mannequin. Learning can be evaluated through quizzes, direct observation, physiological measures (is the client's blood pressure lower?), client self-report and self-monitoring, or input from other health care team members (Redman, 1997).

The outcome of evaluation is a list of learning that has been accomplished as well as a list of those learning objectives that have not been met. *Summative evaluation* is a summary of what has occurred and is usually used as a summary of client accomplishments when the nurse is closing out a case. More often, formative evaluation is used. As with the nursing process, information from formative evaluation feeds back to the assessment phase, and the teaching process repeats itself with new objectives, plans, and interventions until the client and the nurse are satisfied with the final result (Rankin & Stallings, 1997).

Health Education in Communities

All nurses, regardless of work site or specialty, are expected to teach individuals and their families about health-related matters. Nurses who work in the community have additional opportunities to help people change behaviors for the improved health of aggregate populations. The following section describes teaching efforts that can occur in community settings, including individual, group, and community education.

Individuals, Families, and Groups

People live in groups, and the family is the most basic social group. For purposes of this discussion, the *family* is what the client says it is. For some, family members are related by blood or marriage. For others, family members include close social (and sometimes sexual) ties with people who are not otherwise related. Families may be supportive or not supportive. They may be healthy or unhealthy. They may be large and extended or small and nuclear. Some people have rejected or cannot identify a family; others have been rejected by their families. Regardless of family process or content, the individual is greatly influenced by this first social unit (see Chapters 9 and 11).

A *group*, on the other hand, is defined as people "with common goals interacting independently" (Rankin & Stallings, 1996, p. 202). Groups may come together for short periods to address one purpose (e.g., a bereavement support group) or may be more stable over time with larger purposes (e.g., a local unit of Alcoholics Anonymous). Families and groups are important entities for community health nurses to recognize. Families and groups may need direct education (e.g., the nurse teaches a parent group how to take an infant's temperature or how to recognize the signs of adolescent suicide), or they may need to be included as a support system for an individual client (e.g., the nurse includes family members in a discussion of safe food preparation for an immune-suppressed child). This chapter looks at two specific issues related to community education of individuals, families, and groups: discharge teaching and community-based teaching.

Discharge Teaching

Discharge teaching happens in formal inpatient and outpatient care settings, but it provides a basis for community care. Discharge teaching has become more complex in recent years because of changes in the way health care is provided. People are now discharged from acute care settings earlier, with less recuperation time. More procedures, including some that are quite complicated, are being done in outpatient settings. Hospitalization after delivery is usually less than 48 hours. All of these changes have led to people going home with more complex medications, treatments, pain, and anxiety. In addition, because the client spends less time in the formal care setting, there is less time for teaching. This is further complicated by the fact that teaching must often happen in the immediate aftermath of a procedure, a time when clients tend to be most anxious and least able to attend to educational messages (Hunt, 1997).

Nurses can overcome these barriers with careful assessment and planning. If possible, some teaching should take place in the clinic, home, or community before the acute event; preoperative education and prenatal classes are good examples of this. In addition, community resources need to be identified in advance: Is the family willing and able to provide care? Will home health services be required? Are there other options? Assessing these needs and establishing early contacts can ensure that the individual is well prepared. Bringing the needed supports (e.g., responsible family members or home care agencies) in early can decrease education time.

....

To quit smoking is easy. I've done it hundreds of times.
Mark Twain

....

....

Learning is what happens when what you thought would work doesn't.
Unknown

....

Education can then proceed through the teaching process as discussed earlier. Assessment should include a history of experiences that may influence this event, as well as individual and family coping mechanisms. Planning and implementation should be concise, clear, and supported by written information. Teaching should include demonstrations and return demonstrations for all treatments (e.g., dressing changes) and equipment (e.g., medication pumps). Follow-up telephone calls and referrals to community agencies for more intense follow-up should be scheduled (Hunt, 1997). The bottom line is that clients should not feel that they are on their own at the time of discharge. Ideally, they should feel secure in their own abilities to provide self-care. If this is not possible, clients should know how to arrange for the support they will need at home.

Community-Based Teaching

Discharge teaching provides information for clients who have been treated in a formal health care setting. More and more often, however, people need health education as a part of their daily lives. **Community-based teaching** can be complicated by a number of variables. The home setting itself can be difficult. The nurse will be on the client's "home turf," and there may be distractions from family members (especially if there are children in the house). In addition, teaching equipment will need to be brought into the house by the nurse, and the nurse may need to address learning needs for a wider range in individuals. Health education in the home must also be carefully coordinated among various care providers. To make matters even more difficult, all this must be done in a limited amount of time (Hunt, 1997). However, there are major advantages to teaching in the client's home:

- *The nurse can assess the client's environment and make changes in the teaching plan to compensate for problems and to take advantage of strengths.*
- *The family can be more easily involved.*
- *The client will usually be more comfortable in his or her own environment.*
- *The client will be learning in the environment in which he or she will be using new information to perform new skills and behaviors.*

Once again, application of the teaching process will help the nurse meet education goals. A most important step in community-based education is to keep the client and significant others involved in the entire process from assessment to evaluation. This helps the nurse address those issues of highest concern, establish trust within the family setting, and provide the basis for further education. Nurses serve as case managers in the community: They are the professionals who are responsible for coordinating information between the client and a variety of caregivers. In this process, nurses must cover objectives from each of the other care providers and integrate their orders with the needs of the client and family. To accomplish this complex task, nurses need to be aware of community resources so that they can make appropriate referrals. The result should be that community-based clients feel comfortable with their self-care (or family-care) status. Clients should move toward independent care or toward the knowledge that care will be maintained by trusted family members and/or professional providers (Hunt, 1997).

Community

Community health learning occurs when knowledge, attitudes, and/or behaviors change within an entire community. Over the past decade, major changes have been made in communities in areas such as seat belt use, limitations on smoking areas in public spaces, and decreased tolerance of drunk driving. All of these changes came about when individuals in communities stood up and demanded safer and more healthful environments. Changes such as these often require legislative action; at other times, a shift in the community norm is all that has to occur. Nurses have not often taken full advantage of their positions in communities to influence change, but they should. Education and political action are within the realm of what nurses should and can do to improve the health of communities and the individuals in those communities.

Communities consist of groups of people who identify membership in the community. These people share commonalties in language, tradition, ritual, and ceremony. They share values and norms and exert influence over each other. They have emotional connections, common needs, and a commitment to the community to meet those needs. Community may occur within a geographic location (as in a neighborhood or a town) or may be connected by something other than geography (as in ethnic or age-specific groups). Community is defined by all of these connections, so people who merely live in close proximity may not be a community (Israel, Checkoway, Schulz, & Zimmerman, 1994). An individual may have membership in more than one

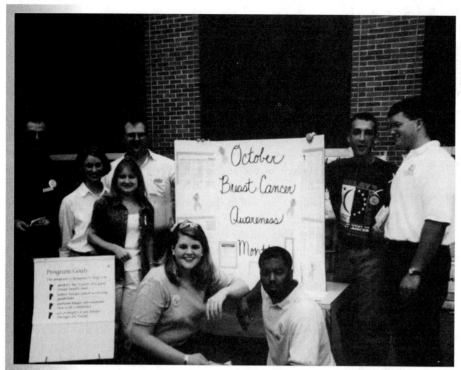

Breast cancer awareness education program for college students.

community and may have to deal with conflicting values from those communities. As you can see, a community has power that can affect behavior change. Although community support can be a powerful contribution to individual behavior change, lack of community support may doom an intervention to failure (Bigbee & Jansa, 1991). Table 9-6 gives a case study to illustrate the process of community education.

There are some things you learn best in calm, and some in storm.
Willa Cather

Community Assessment

As with individual health education, health education at the community level starts with community assessment, and as in individual education, the assessment needs to take into account the full spectrum of community variables. Individual behaviors take place within the context of community, and understanding this context can help nurses predict both barriers to and supports for behavior change (Israel, Checkoway, Schulz, & Zimmerman, 1994). The nurse needs a clear idea of what the community is: How do people in the community define *health* and *health care*? What is the norm for nutrition, elimination, exercise, sleep, sexuality, reproduction, and coping with stress? How is intellect supported? How does the community perceive itself? How are roles and relationships established and supported? What does the

community value? What ethnic and cultural identities exist in the community? What language(s) is(are) spoken? What ceremonies occur? What rituals are supported? How does the community share resources? Is there a sense of shared responsibility (Krozy, 1996)? Nurses can gather this information from community leaders, written histories and records, observations, consultations, and other community members.

Communities, like individuals, experience stressors. These stressors range from daily hassles (as in ongoing arguments from businesses that want to limit government controls) to chronic problems (e.g., homelessness or air pollution) to major events (e.g., the closing of an industry) to cataclysmic events (e.g., an earthquake or flood) (Israel, Checkoway, Schulz, & Zimmerman, 1994). Other community problems can include poverty, overpopulation, social injustice, lack of social organization, overcrowding (Krozy, 1996), a history of powerlessness, and tensions created by inequity and discrimination (Israel, Checkoway, Schulz, & Zimmerman, 1994). All of these contribute to community perceptions of powerlessness. Community empowerment, then, becomes a teaching strategy.

The illiterate of the 21st century will not be those who cannot read and write, but those who cannot learn, unlearn, and relearn.

Alvin Toffler

TABLE 9-6   COMMUNITY EDUCATION PROCESS CASE

Kris works as a school nurse at Center High School in a moderately-sized Midwest city. At a weekly team meeting, she tells her friend Sam, "I am so frustrated—we have five pregnant girls already this semester." Sam, who works at two middle schools, says, "You think that's bad? I have a case of chlamydia in a sixth grader!" Others add their comments until one says, "We clearly have a problem. What should we do?" The nurses decide to "do something about the risks of teen sexual activity." Because they already know the community well, the nurses decide to assess the problem by listing positive and negative community factors related to the problem of teen sexual activity.

ASSESSMENT	PLANNING	IMPLEMENTATION	EVALUATION
Positive factors: The community has a number of agencies that could be involved, including Planned Parenthood, Big Brothers/Big Sisters, the YMCA, churches, etc. Community schools have good reputations; most students graduate and many go to college. The state department of education supports a sex education curriculum based on harm reduction. School nurses have a ratio of 1:2,000 students. **Negative factors:** The school board (SB) supports and enforces an abstinence-only sex education curriculum as a result of pressure from a few vocal parents and one of the churches in the community. There are limited programs for students who are not succeeding in school and/or extracurricular activities. Most student come from families with working parents, and the majority have several hours of unsupervised time after school. Kris has had a number of students at her school tell her, "I want to get pregnant, it'd be cool." A survey of the nurses reveals 25 known teen pregnancies and 42 known cases of sexually transmitted diseases (STDs) in students over the past 24 months.	The nurses struggle with the question of what to do with the assessment information. After a long brainstorming session, they develop a plan. Each nurse will do the following: • Meet with his or her principal(s) to inform and educate about the problem • Attend the next two meetings of the SB and ask to have the topic of teen sexuality placed on the agenda • Encourage the use of the state's harm reduction curriculum • Volunteer to teach sexuality classes in the 5th to 12th grades • Visit 2 to 3 community organizations (including churches) to discuss the problem, ask for support, and volunteer assistance to develop after-school programs.	The nurses complete their assigned visits to the principals, SB, and local organizations. Each nurse reviews the state sex education curriculum and volunteers to teach classes at his or her assigned school(s).	**Summative evaluation:** All assignments are completed. **Formative evaluation:** All of the principals support the nurses' efforts. One principal asks about sexual abuse in students' family and peer relationships. The SB refuses to add the issue to the agenda. All of the nurses will teach sex education classes, but several principals and health teachers refuse to allow a harm reduction curriculum until approval by the SB. Two churches and the YMCA are interested in setting up sports, games, and homework assistance programs after school. Planned Parenthood wants to develop a peer education program to address pressures to have sex in order to be "cool." **Follow up:** The nurses reassess the situation and plan for the next steps. The nurses will do the following: • Set up in-services for the nurses to learn about teaching a harm reduction curriculum • Set up nurse counseling services for any student who wants to discuss issues privately; available to all students, but especially for students in abusive relationships • Continue attending SB meetings; encourage principals, teachers, and parents to add their support at those meetings • Collaborate with agencies as new programs are developed and encourage other agencies to consider developing their own programs.

The good news is that communities also provide support for behavior change. The nurse should assess those things that enhance opportunities for education and change. These might include the emotional support given to community members who are trying to effect change. In addition, established agencies and services may already be available to support change. Information dissemination systems may be in place, and respected community members may be willing to sway opinion toward change (Israel, Checkoway, Schulz, & Zimmerman, 1994).

Planning for the Community

The main point that needs to be made about community planning should be obvious: Planning requires community involvement (Andrade & Doria-Ortiz, 1995). Shared decision making leads to better acceptance of change, support for the process, and commitment to programs that emerge from the process (Foran & Campanelli, 1995). Involving large portions of the community in planning can be difficult, but it is necessary. Representation should be sought from government, business, service, health care, and religious entities as well as from the individuals who will be targeted by the plan. Input can be gathered in community meetings, focus groups, and interviews with key informants. Opposing views must be sought, acknowledged, and considered in any planning activity (Krozy, 1996). Planning can then progress to setting educational goals and selecting an appropriate theory base, taking into account the strengths and weaknesses of the community.

Common broad-based goals for community health education are to (1) help people change unhealthy, unsafe, or risky behaviors; (2) equalize access to health and support services; and (3) decrease the incidence of preventable conditions that have a negative impact on the community (Krozy, 1996). Goals and more specific objectives need to be established and agreed upon during the planning process. Consider using *Healthy People 2010* in this process. It delineates national goals for specific health issues targeted to at-risk populations (DHHS, 2000).

. . . .

You must learn from the mistakes of others. You can't possibly live long enough to make them all yourself.

Sam Levenson

. . . .

Foran and Campanelli (1995) identified the components of successful community health programs: They are flexible, they use ongoing evaluation to identify design problems as soon as possible, they use evaluation to guide change, they are valued by the community, and they evolve by incorporating new ideas and technologies as change occurs. Planners should understand all of these elements. And remember: Planning should develop teaching interventions as well as evaluation tools.

Implementing Community Plans

Andrade and Doria-Ortiz (1995) encourage an implementation process that helps a community meet its own needs. This requires empowerment of community organizations, adequate resources and services to meet the needs of at-risk community members, and sufficient resources in the health care system. They recognize that programs and services (especially those targeted to underserved populations) must be available, accessible, acceptable, and accountable. Programs that do not meet these criteria will not be used.

It is important to remember that community education and change are long-term processes—they do not happen overnight. Even after programs are established, there must be commitment to a continuing process of assessment, planning, implementation, and evaluation. Implementation will be enhanced if the process is participatory (members of the community are involved), cooperative, collaborative, empowering, and balanced. Hopefully, the process will promote group identification, reinforcing the idea of a shared fate and the need to look at more global aspects of health (Israel, Checkoway, Schulz, & Zimmerman, 1994).

The assessment and planning process will help nurses identify appropriate sites for community education. Where are the natural community networks? Are they centered around employment, recreational, religious, or commercial functions? Will organizations that are not viewed as health care agencies (e.g., schools and churches) get involved? Can early health-promotion programs be established in neighborhood elementary and middle schools? Are community colleges open to health education efforts? Will the justice system support health education for people who live in prisons, jails, and halfway houses? Establishing programs specific to people

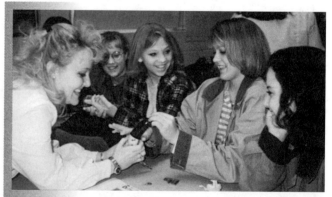

School nurse educating high school students about STDs.

> **A CONVERSATION WITH...**
>
> *On education:*
> *Education is less and less a preparation for life and more and more a part of it.*
> *Our species thinks in metaphors and learns through stories.*
> *Relying on competition as a way of motivating learning eventually subverts not only cooperation but also the willingness to learn.*
> —**Mary Catherine Bates**

who congregate in these sites can promote education in ways that target at-risk individuals (Andrade & Doria-Ortiz, 1995).

How health education is implemented also depends on assessment and planning. It helps to have a theoretical base (see Tables 9-2 and 9-3), knowing that some models are better for community intervention than others. Diffusion theory and social marketing theory, for example, were developed from community-focused research. The transtheoretical model also includes components of community action. Common teaching strategies for community intervention include lectures, small group work, facilitated discussions, demonstrations, printed and audiovisual materials, simulation exercises, guided imagery, and social marketing (Krozy, 1996). The important thing to remember is that the teaching strategy needs to match the learning objective (see Table 9-5) as well as the developmental level of the audience.

Evaluating Community Programs

As stated earlier, evaluation is an ongoing process in health education. Formal evaluation should be planned, and informal evaluation should be acknowledged and used in the process. Formative evaluation is used throughout the process. Summative evaluation occurs at a set point when goals are expected to have been met. Effective evaluation determines progress toward goals and identifies goals that have not yet been met. Data from evaluation are used to do the following:

- *Determine whether unmet goals are still a priority*
- *Plan interventions to address unmet goals*
- *Assess the impact of goals that have been achieved*
- *Assess evolving needs*
- *Establish new community goals and objectives*

The community health education process is much like the individual teaching process (it is cyclical and progressive in nature), but it is more complicated.

••••••••••••••••••••••••••••••

Self-love is the only weight-loss aid that really works in the long run.

Jenny Craig

••••••••••••••••••••••••••••••

Ethical Issues in Health Education

Health education on the surface seems like an appropriate and ethical thing to do. After all, how ethical would it be to withhold information that could relieve suffering, prevent pain, and avert disease? But health education has its own controversies. Some of these are discussed next; others will become obvious to you as you educate individuals and communities.

A major problem occurs when there are unexpected, negative consequences because of health education. These can be the result of erroneous, poorly planned, or improperly implemented education efforts (Guttman, Kegler, & McLeroy, 1996). For instance, let's say that you want to teach a group of people who are newly diagnosed with cancer that there is hope. You ask four or five people with cancer to speak to your group. Unfortunately, several of the presenters are dealing with anger and depression because of their disease, and they take this opportunity to share their pain and frustration with the health care system. At the end of the session, your audience is likely to be confused (at the least) or to feel complete despair (at the worst). They may lose confidence in the ability to survive cancer treatment; they may even decide to forego therapy altogether and "get it over with." Although this example is quite blatant, problems can occur even under ideal circumstances.

One of the primary concerns that nurses have to address is the fact that, in many ways, health education manipulates clients to change behaviors. Granted, the changes we seek (based on our assessment of the latest scientific evidence) are for the client's benefit, but we are nevertheless clearly trying to influence change (Redman, 1997). This may be difficult for nurses to accept. We have, after all, been taught to respect individual autonomy. Manipulation, no matter how subtle, is hard to justify. This is not a reason to stop teaching or to stop advocating for policies such as motorcycle helmet laws. Instead, it is something that each nurse must weigh carefully before, during, and after health education programs. It also helps to differentiate manipulation from information dissemination. Giving a pregnant adolescent information on options, including the whole spectrum of choices involved in either continuing or terminating her pregnancy, for instance, is information dissemination that she can use to make an informed decision. Encouraging her to have an abortion, to give the infant up for adoption, or to have the baby and raise it herself is manipulation, especially if she makes her "informed" decision based on a lack of complete information that the nurse has failed to share.

Another issue is science itself and the rate at which knowledge expands (Redman, 1997). We have all heard clients say, "This is so confusing. How am I supposed to know what I should be doing? Last night there was a story on the news about how exercise can cause joint deterioration and here you are telling me that I need to exercise more!" Nurses have an obligation to keep up with advances in health care, but even nurses get confused. This all adds to the complex nature of education and reinforces the need to be able to read and critique research (see the following research briefs for examples of studies about health education).

One of the real social issues in client education has to do with the growing gap between the classes (Guttman, Kegler, & McLeroy, 1996). People who are financially secure are better equipped to act on advice to improve their health. Those without economic resources, however, often see health behaviors (e.g., exercise and eating well) as things they simply cannot afford. Poverty affects peoples' health, which further decreases the ability to earn a living or to get ahead. Nurses need to recognize that poor health practices may be related to social and economic barriers as much as they are related to a lack of knowledge, motivation, or positive attitudes. When this is the case, social and community solutions need to be explored rather than falling into the trap of victim blaming (Marantz, 1990). How appropriate, for instance, is it to blame an alcoholic for her liver disease? What if she was raised in a house where alcohol was used to deal with stress? What if her life has been filled with loss, abuse, and trauma? And what if her only solace is to sink into an alcoholic daze? Is this situation her fault? Maybe. Maybe not. Is she beyond help? No, but help is not easy to give if you blame the

RESEARCH BRIEF

Miller, P., Wikoff, R., & Hiatt, A. (1992). Fishbein's model of reasoned action and compliance behaviors of hypertensive patients. Nursing Research, 41, *104–109.*

The authors of this study used the theory of reasoned action as a basis to examine medication compliance behaviors of 56 clients newly diagnosed as having hypertension. The purposes of the study were to (1) assess whether the constructs of reasoned action could be applied to clients with hypertension; (2) test whether intention was a sufficient predictor of behavior; and (3) test whether attitude, perceived beliefs of others, and motivation to comply were sufficient to determine intent. Demographic information and baseline physical data were collected during the first research visit. All subjects received extensive education about hypertension, medications, diet, smoking, exercise, and stress management. Six months later, subjects were asked to complete questionnaires that assessed attitude, perceived beliefs of others, motivation to comply, intention, and compliance behaviors related to diet, smoking, activity, stress, and medications.

Statistical analysis revealed that the model adequately predicted compliance to prescriptions for diet, smoking, activity, and stress, but not for medications. Compliance behavior was directly influenced by intention to comply. Intention, in turn, was influenced to varying degrees by attitude, motivation, and the perceived beliefs of others.

RESEARCH BRIEF

Swinburn, B. A., Walter, L. G., Arroll, B., Tilyard, M. W., & Russell, D. (1998). The green prescription study: A randomized controlled trial of written exercise advice provided by general practitioners. American Journal of Public Health, 88, *288–291.*

The purpose of this study was to determine whether a written prescription for exercise in addition to verbal advice to exercise would increase physical activity more than verbal advice alone. Four hundred fifty-six sedentary adults (251 with at least one medical condition related to inactivity) were all given the same verbal information about increasing physical activity. Subjects were then randomly assigned to a control group (which received verbal information only) or an experimental group (which received a written prescription for exercise as well as verbal information). Activity levels were assessed 6 weeks later by a questionnaire that quantified time spent exercising over the previous 2 weeks.

There was an increase in physical activity for both groups, indicating that discussing the need had a beneficial effect. However, greater increases in the number of people who exercised and the amount of time spent exercising were seen for those who received both verbal and written information. The authors concluded that clients could be positively influenced to exercise and that this influence was enhanced by the use of written, goal-oriented prescriptions.

client for her disability. Repetitious, ineffective teaching will not help the situation either.

A final ethical issue that deserves attention has to do with community and cultural norms (Guttman, Kegler, & McLeroy, 1996; Redman, 1997). We each bring cultural biases into our social interactions. This is true of nurses as well as of clients. In addition to all of their other cultures, nurses bring the culture of health care and scientific bias into every encounter. This makes it difficult for nurses to deal with situations in which, for example, we know that fat infants grow up into fat adults, but the pre-

dominant culture believes that only fat babies are healthy. Nurses cannot ignore these conflicting values. They must instead use creative problem solving to develop acceptable solutions on a number of different levels. This can be a messy process with many trials and only a few successes. The alternative is to try to force the culture of science on people who are not going to accept it no matter how hard you try. So why not take some chances? The outcome could be that new messages or teaching methods or solutions emerge, and that could be the best possible conclusion to a difficult situation.

HEALTHY PEOPLE 2010

OBJECTIVES RELATED TO HEALTH EDUCATION
Educational and Community-Based Programs
School Setting

7.2 Increase the proportion of middle, junior high, and senior high schools that provide comprehensive school health education to prevent health problems in the following areas: unintentional injury; violence; suicide; tobacco use and addiction; alcohol and other drug use; unintended pregnancy; HIV/AIDS and STD infection; unhealthy dietary patterns; inadequate physical activity; and environmental health.

7.3 Increase the proportion of college and university students who receive information from

their institution on each of the six priority health-risk behavior areas.

Health Care Setting

7.7 Increase the proportion of health care organizations that provide patient and family education.

7.8 Increase the proportion of patients who report that they are satisfied with the patient education they receive from their health care organization.

7.9 Increase the proportion of hospitals and managed care organizations that provide community disease prevention and health promotion activities that address the priority health needs identified by their community.

Source: DHHS, 2000.

CONCLUSION

Health education is an important intervention for nurses in all health care settings. The purpose of health education is to change behaviors and situations that put people at risk for injury, illness, disability, or death. It is a theory-based process that draws from learning theory as well as behavior change theory. The health education process is similar to the nursing process. It is appropriate in all clinical and community settings and can be applied to individuals, families, groups, and communities. Nurses must also be aware that health education poses some important ethical issues.

CRITICAL THINKING ACTIVITIES

1. Develop teaching plans for each of the following situations. Identify and use a theory base that can help guide the process. Discuss assessment, planning, implementation, and evaluation as a part of your process.

   - *Case 1:* Diane is a 48-year-old single mother who fractured her left wrist in a fall 3 weeks ago. The wrist was reduced in the hospital emergency room and set with a standard cast. Except for some pain and the need to modify a few of her activities, Diane has done well and feels that she will recover completely. Diane saw her nurse practitioner for a regular checkup 3 days ago. The nurse practitioner expressed concern about Diane's wrist and asked about the circumstances of the accident. When Diane described a situation that would not normally result in a fracture, the nurse practitioner ordered a scan to access bone density. The results show a 2.5% loss of bone mass. The nurse practitioner orders exercise and dietary changes. Diane and her provider agree to try these tactics for 6 months before considering medications. Diane's 14-year-old son lives with her. Her 20-year-old daughter recently married and moved out of state. The rest of Diane's family lives 350 miles away. She is the co-owner of a business that builds office complexes, and she typically works 10 to 12 hours a day. When you question her about her current diet and exercise routines, she shrugs and says, "To tell the truth, I'm way to busy to worry about those things. They just take up too much time."

   - *Case 2:* Janet, the nurse at Allen Elementary School, has documented 12 cases of head lice during the past week. Most of the affected students are from one third grade class, but two cases came from a second grade class and one each came from a fifth grade class and another third grade class.

- *Case 3:* The nursing home in Sheridan County has a respite care center where families can leave elderly clients between the hours of 7 AM and 7 PM. The program provides meals, organized activities, and nap facilities for 22 clients with various physical and cognitive disabilities. Families who use the service give positive feedback about improvements in their abilities to cope with the stresses of caring for elderly relatives in the home. Sheila is an 86-year-old woman with confusion and delusions who is a regular client. Over the past week, Fred, the nurse manager, has noticed bruises around Sheila's wrists. Fred asks Sheila's daughter about the bruises, and she replies, "Oh, I guess she gets those from the restraints. She's started wandering around the house at night. I'm worried that she might fall and break a hip, so I talked to some of the other families at our last group meeting and several of them suggested that I tie Mama into bed at night."

- *Case 4:* Community Care Center is a comprehensive outpatient health care facility that serves injection drug users. In addition to methadone treatment, the center provides counseling services, case management, first aid, and routine annual physical assessments. The physician who does the physicals is only in the center 2 days a week. She approaches Anita, the clinic nurse, and expresses concern about the amount of chlamydia that she has diagnosed recently. She asks Anita, "What do you think we can do about this?" Although Anita agrees that the pattern the physician describes is an important concern, she worries about the ethical issues that could occur if the clinic takes any action. What ethical issues could develop? How can Anita address those issues for the clinic staff, clients, and surrounding community?

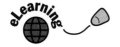

Explore Community Health Nursing on the web! To learn more about the topics in this chapter, access your exclusive web site:
http://communitynursing.jbpub.com

REFERENCES

Andrade, S. J., & Doria-Ortiz, C. (1995). *Nuestro bienestar*: A Mexican-American community-based definition of health promotion in the southwestern United States. *Drugs: Education, Prevention, and Policy, 2,* 129–145.

Bigbee, J. L., & Jansa, N. (1991). Strategies for promoting health protection. *Nursing Clinics of North America, 26,* 895–913.

Bradley-Springer, L. (1996). Patient education for behavior change: Help from the transtheoretical and harm reduction models. *Journal of the Association of Nurses in AIDS Care, 7*(Suppl.), 23–33.

Byham, W. C. (with Cox, J., & Shomo, K. H.). (1992). *Zapp! in education: How empowerment can improve the quality of instruction and student and teacher satisfaction.* New York: Fawcett Columbine.

Caplan, D. (1995). Smoking: Issues and interventions for occupational health nurses. *AAOHN Journal, 43,* 633–643.

Carter, W. B. (1990). Health behavior as a rational process: Theory of reasoned action and multiattribute utility theory. In K. Glanz, F. M. Lewis, & B. K. Rimer (Eds.), *Health behavior and health education: Theory, research, and practice* (pp. 63–91). San Francisco: Jossey-Bass.

Cates, Jr., W., & Hinman, A. (1992). AIDS and absolutism: The demand for perfection in prevention. *New England Journal of Medicine, 327,* 492–494.

Damrosch, S. (1991). General strategies for motivating people to change their behavior. *Nursing Clinics of North America, 26,* 833–843.

Department of Health and Human Services (DHHS). (2000). *Healthy people 2010: Conference edition.* Washington, DC: United States Government Printing Office.

Foran, M., & Campanelli, L. C. (1995). Health promotion communications system: A model for a dispersed population. *AAOHN Journal, 43,* 564–569.

Glanz, K., Lewis, F. M., & Rimer, B. K. (Eds.). (1990). *Health behavior and health education: Theory, research, and practice.* San Francisco: Jossey-Bass.

Guttman, N., Kegler, M., & McLeroy, K. R. (1996). Health promotion paradoxes, antimonies and conundrums. *Health Education Research, 11*(1), i–xiii.

Hunt, R. (1997).Teaching. In R. Hunt & E. L. Zurek (Eds.), *Introduction to community based nursing* (pp. 182–225). Philadelphia: Lippincott.

Israel, B. A., Checkoway, B., Schulz, A., & Zimmerman, M. (1994). Health education and community empowerment: Conceptualizing and measuring perceptions of individual, organizational, and community control. *Health Education Quarterly, 21,* 140–170.

Knowles, M. S. (1973). *The adult learner: A neglected species.* Houston, TX: Gulf Publishing.

Kreuter, M. W., & Strecher, V. J. (1996). Do tailored behavior change messages enhance the effectiveness of health risk appraisal? Results from a randomized trial. *Health Education Research, 11,* 97–105.

Krozy, R. E. (1996). Community health promotion: Assessment and intervention. In S. H. Rankin & K. D. Stallings (Eds.), *Patient education: Issues, principles, practices* (3rd ed., pp. 245–271). Philadelphia: Lippincott.

Marantz, P. R. (1990). Blaming the victim: The negative consequence of preventive medicine. *American Journal of Public Health, 80*(18), 186–187.

Miller, P., Wikoff, R., & Hiatt, A. (1992). Fishbein's model of reasoned action and compliance behavior of hypertensive patients. *Nursing Research, 41,* 104–109.

Mirotznik, J., Feldman, L., & Stein, R. (1995). The health belief model and adherence with a community center-based, supervised coronary heart disease program. *Journal of Community Health, 20,* 233–247.

Novelli, W. D. (1990). Applying social marketing to health promotion and disease prevention. In K. Glanz, F. M. Lewis, & B. K. Rimer (Eds.), *Health behavior and health education: Theory, research, and practice* (pp. 342–369). San Francisco: Jossey-Bass.

Orlandi, M. A., Landers, C., Weston, R., & Haley, N. (1990). Diffusion of health promotion innovations. In K. Glanz, F. M. Lewis, & B. K. Rimer (Eds.), *Health behavior and health education: Theory, research, and practice* (pp. 288–313). San Francisco: Jossey-Bass.

Palank, C. L. (1991). Determinants of health-promotive behavior: A review of current research. *Nursing Clinics of North America, 26,* 815–832.

Perry, C. L., Baranowski, T., & Parcel, G. S. (1990). How individuals, environments and health behavior interact: Social learning theory. In K. Glanz, F. M. Lewis, & B. K. Rimer (Eds.), *Health behavior and health education: Theory, research, and practice* (pp. 161–186). San Francisco: Jossey-Bass.

Prochaska, J. O., Redding, C. A., Harlow, L. L., Rossi, J. S., & Velicer, W. F. (1994). The transtheoretical model of change and HIV prevention: A review. *Health Education Quarterly, 21*(4), 471–486.

Rankin, S. H., & Stallings, K. D. (1996). *Patient education: Issues, principles, practices* (3rd ed.). Philadelphia: Lippincott.

Redman, B. K. (1997). *The practice of patient education.* St. Louis: Mosby.

Rosenstock, I. M. (1990). The health belief model: Explaining health behavior through expectancies. In K. Glanz, F. M. Lewis, & B. K. Rimer (Eds.), *Health behavior and health education: Theory, research, and practice* (pp. 39–62). San Francisco: Jossey-Bass.

Spellbring, A. M. (1991). Nursing's role in health promotion: An overview. *Nursing Clinics of North America, 26,* 805–814.

Spradley, B. W., & Allender, J. A. (1996). *Community health nursing: Concepts and practice* (4th ed.). Philadelphia: Lippincott.

Strang, J. (1992). Harm reduction for drug users: Exploring the dimensions of harm, their measurement, and strategies for reductions. *AIDS and Public Policy Journal, 7,* 145–152.

Strecher, V. J., Seijts, G. H., Kok, G. J., Latham, G. P., Glascow, R., DeVellis, B., Meertens, R. M., & Bulger, D. W. (1995). Goal setting as a strategy for health behavior change. *Health Education Quarterly, 22,* 190–200.

Swinburn, B. A., Walter, L. G., Arroll, B., Tilyard, M. W., & Russell, D. (1998). The green prescription study: A randomized controlled trial of written exercise advice provided by general practitioners. *American Journal of Public Health, 88,* 288–291.

10
Health Promotion and Wellness

Joan H. Baldwin and Cynthia O'Neill Conger

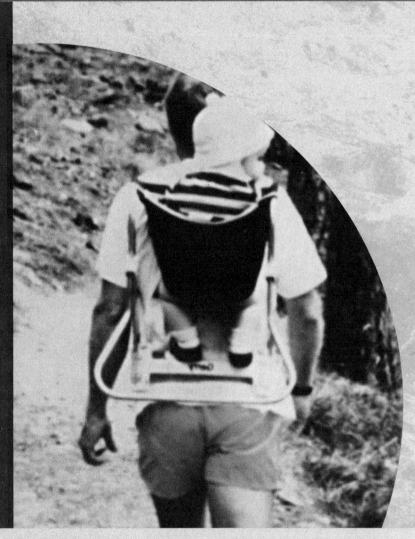

*All of the information about exercise, eating right, and how my body works
helped me change the physical me. The most important part is to understand
that it's not as much about the weight as it is about making the connection.
That means looking after yourself every day and putting forth your best effort
to love yourself enough to do what's best for you. . . . The biggest change I've
made is a spiritual one. It comes from the realization that taking care of my
body and my health is really one of the greatest kinds of love I can give myself. .
. . And there's no question I'm living a better life.*

Oprah Winfrey (Greene & Winfrey, 1996, p. 32)

QUESTIONS TO CONSIDER

After reading this chapter, answer the following questions:

1. What is the difference between health promotion and wellness?
2. What are levels of prevention?
3. What do health promotion and wellness look like?
4. What factors influence health promotion and wellness?
5. What are the different models for health promotion?
6. How can community health nurses use these models in the promotion of health in their clients?
7. How can a nurse use these concepts to promote self-health?

KEY TERMS

Health-promoting behaviors
Health promotion
High-level wellness

Levels of prevention
Personal health promotion

Professional health promotion
Wellness

Health promotion and **wellness** are important concepts throughout nursing education and practice in all settings. Nurses promote good health and wellness for themselves, their loved ones, and clients. Generally, the major steps to health and wellness include healthy eating, proper exercise, adequate sleep, and time to unwind and manage stress. Health promotion in this respect has always been a nursing focus. As the health care delivery system moves further into managed care, however, health promotion and wellness become still more important. Health promotion and disease prevention are the keys to managing health care costs. Promoting the health of individuals, families, populations, and communities is essential in nursing practice not only because it is the humane and ethical thing to do but also because of its practical and economic benefits.

It may be surprising to learn that there are several different definitions for the terms *health promotion* and *wellness*. There are definitions of health promotion and wellness for self, for other individuals, and even for populations and communities.

What do nurses really mean when they say they promote good health and wellness? There are many, many aspects of health promotion and wellness that will be important to know as a professional nurse. This chapter (1) briefly discusses basic concepts of health and health promotion as related to the concept of disease prevention, including definitions of *health promotion* and *wellness* as the terms are used in this chapter; (2) delineates factors influencing health promotion and wellness; (3) demonstrates some ways of looking at health promotion and wellness by discussing some models of health promotion, risk evaluation, and analysis tools, plus wellness guides that might be useful to know about to promote health and wellness; and (4) introduces two recent models of wellness.

Basic Concepts of Health and Health Promotion

How people generally define health may influence how they define health promotion (Baldwin, 1995; Green & Raeburn, 1990). For instance, if health is considered the absence of disease, the definition of health promotion would necessarily include the idea of disease prevention. However, if health is defined as a concept that expresses the positiveness of a full and joyful life, disease prevention is not a part of the definition. Edelman and Fain (1998) speak of this second characterization of health as "expanding consciousness, pattern or meaning recognition, personal transformation, and tentatively, self-actualization" (p. 9). One example is a woman living with a chronic disease such as diabetes, who still considers herself a healthy person; she may see herself being as far along toward self-actualization as she can be.

In 1983, Brubaker conducted a linguistic analysis of the term *health promotion* in nursing literature and found that it was rarely defined specifically and often used as though it had the same meaning as disease prevention. There continues to be debate about the definition of health promotion and whether the definition must necessarily include disease prevention.

Historically, health promotion as a concept has been linked with disease prevention. Clark and Leavell (1965) depicted three **levels of prevention**—primary, secondary, and tertiary—in a model; primary prevention includes health promotion as part of the model. When primary prevention methods are used, the basic premise of the model is that health-promotion activities "serve to further general health and well-being" (Clark & Leavell, 1965, p. 20). Because this is a model describing disease prevention factors, it leads one to connect health promotion with disease prevention. In this particular model, primary prevention methods include **health-promoting behaviors** that are designed to improve general health and well-being, with the emphasis being on preventing a disease in the first place. For instance, brushing teeth after meals is one step in preventing tooth decay, which would also be good for general health.

As early as 1965, Clark and Leavell noted that "health promotion is not applied for specific disease and as yet is not widely utilized" (p. 24). Identifying health-promoting strategies for secondary and tertiary prevention still seems to be a bit difficult today, but health-promoting activities are important in these levels as well. *Secondary prevention* refers to the early detection of disease and prevention of disease sequelae—"abnormal conditions resulting from a previous disease" (*Webster's Encyclopedic Dictionary*, 1996, p. 1747). A health-promotion action for a woman who has a diagnosis of fibrocystic breast disease would be to avoid caffeine. Poe and O'Neill (1997) determined that caffeine slows the process of the body's natural defenses, which normally results in the elimination of precancerous cells. Therefore, the potential for proliferation of abnormal cells is increased with caffeine ingestion. Tertiary prevention focuses on the minimization of loss of function as a result of disease. Health-promotion activities in tertiary prevention might include training for a competition by a diabetic skier who has only one leg. Good and reasonable physical fitness promotes health.

Today there are also reasons for using health-promotion strategies, behaviors, or actions without necessarily having to consider prevention of disease. Someone may choose certain health-promotion actions just because the actions make the person feel good or healthy. For example, many people like to walk or run several times a week and comment that if they don't walk or run, they don't have as much energy during the day. In this example, these people are not specifically concerned about preventing disease, they just want to feel as good as they can.

Selected Definitions of Health Promotion and Wellness

For the purposes of this chapter, health promotion has two definitions depending on if the nurse is applying health-promotion strategies to other people or if the nurse is promoting his or her own health. The definition of **professional health promotion** on behalf of others reflects the "organized actions or efforts that enhance, support, or promote the well-being or health of individuals, families, groups, communities, or societies" (Kulbok, Baldwin, Cox, & Duffy, 1997, p. 17). An example of this definition is when a school nurse teaches elementary school children the importance of washing hands to eliminate germs and dirt. The nurse first coats the children's hands with an invisible product that can be washed away with soap and water. After handwashing, a special light is shined on the children's hands; areas not carefully washed clean of the product glow green, demonstrating to the children that if hands are not carefully washed, "germs" may remain, much like the green, glowing product. Health education programs and physical education activities, to name two possibilities, are also examples of professional health promotion on behalf of others.

Personal health promotion reflects more emphasis on self-actualization and taking care of oneself. This definition identifies what motivates people "to attain and maintain their highest state of wellness, overall fitness, and self-actualization" (Baldwin, 1992, p. 10). For instance, the school nurse may recognize that walking daily for 30 minutes after work maintains physical fitness, dissipates work stress, and provides a sense of renewal and joy as she or he appreciates the spring flowers blooming.

What is the relationship between health promotion and wellness? As defined in this chapter, health promotion relates to behaviors or activities that result in wellness. Dunn (1959) describes **high-level wellness** as "an integrated method of functioning which is oriented toward maximizing the potential of which the individual is capable" (p. 447). The concept of high-level wellness is based on the assumption that every individual, regardless of personal challenges, has a potential for wellness within the limits placed by the challenge. In other words, high-level wellness is the highest level of well-being that a person can reach. To attain high-level wellness, there must be harmony in all aspects of a person's life. Box 10-1 lists two definitions of health promotion.

Health promotion and wellness, particularly when defined for one's own use, are closely related or even interrelated. In this chapter, *wellness* is a state of being; *health promotion* is how one gets there (Box 10-2). How one attains and maintains wellness is accomplished through various health-promoting behaviors. Examples of some health-promoting behaviors include (1) walking for at least 30 minutes 6 days a week, preferably with some intensity as though a bit late for an appointment (Bach, 1998); (2) eating foods that have omega-3 or monounsaturated fats, limiting daily total fat intake to less than 25% of total calories (Simopoulos, 1999); (3) adapting traditionally high-calorie or high-fat recipes to today's healthier levels (Jones, 1999); (4) meditating or visualizing to increase well-being (Cohen, 1998); and (5) learning how to relax (Cohen, 1998). Researchers today are

> ### BOX 10-1 KEY CONCEPTS: DEFINITIONS OF HEALTH PROMOTION
>
> Health promotion by professionals on behalf of others is *"organized actions or efforts that enhance, support, or promote the well-being or health of individuals, families, groups, communities, or societies"* (Kulbok, Baldwin, Cox, & Duffy, 1997, p. 17).
>
> Personal health promotion is *identification of what motivates people "to attain and maintain their highest state of wellness, overall fitness, and self-actualization"* (Baldwin, 1992, p. 10)

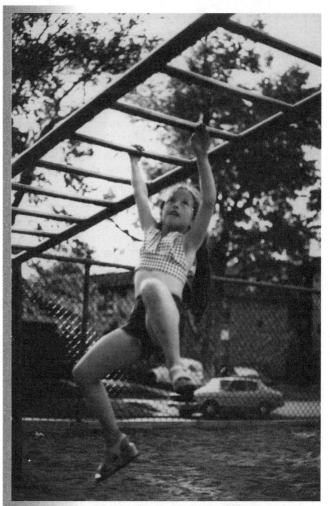

Children who are active earlier in life help decrease their risks for health problems as young adults.

BOX 10-2 DEFINITIONS OF WELLNESS, HEALTH-PROMOTING BEHAVIORS, AND THE INTERRELATIONSHIP BETWEEN HEALTH PROMOTION AND WELLNESS

High-level wellness is *"an integrated method of functioning which is oriented toward maximizing the potential of which the individual is capable"* (Dunn, 1959, p. 447).

Health-promoting behaviors are *"any actions or behaviors taken by individuals to improve or promote well-being or health"* (Kulbok, Baldwin, Cox, & Duffy, 1997, p. 17). These *"behaviors [are those] that enhance, support, encourage and/or promote a healthy state"* (Kulbok, Carter, Baldwin, Gilmartin, & Kirkwood, 1999).

The interrelationship of health promotion and wellness *can be represented by the idea that wellness is a state of being, and health promotion is how one gets there.*

emphasizing health-promoting activities such as these for individuals, families, populations, and communities to attain and maintain states of wellness (Cohen, 1998; Mandle & Castle, 1998; McCarthy & Mandle, 1998a, 1998b; Sandhu, 1998).

A person can be sick and be moving toward wellness using health-promoting actions or behaviors or can have a chronic disease and actually be experiencing high-level wellness. Remember, high-level wellness means "maximizing the potential of which the individual is capable" (Dunn, 1959, p. 447). So, if the diabetic woman mentioned earlier in this chapter is maintaining a healthy lifestyle, has no difficulty managing her diabetes, is happy, and feels well-balanced in her life, it could be said that the woman is likely to be experiencing high-level wellness. The woman is maximizing the potential of which she is capable.

The woman with diabetes is the one most likely to know what her maximum potential can be and how close she is to reaching it in her life. What high-level wellness is, using Dunn's (1959) definition, for any particular person is defined by that person and may change over time.

How can a 22-year-old student nurse who is in a car accident and becomes a paraplegic reach high-level wellness? According to the aforementioned definitions, the student nurse has a potential to be more or less well within the boundaries of the limits set by the condition. "Wellness is a bridge that takes people into realms far beyond treatment or therapy—into a domain of self-responsibility and self-empowerment" (Ryan & Travis, 1991, p. 3). The student nurse has choices. Relating to personal life, the student nurse has the choice to (1) do nothing about overcoming the physical, emotional, mental, and spiritual challenges of being a

paraplegic; (2) learn to use a wheelchair to go to classes and elsewhere; or (3) perhaps even go so far as to become a gold medalist in the ParaOlympics. Professionally, the student nurse can bend to the pressure of the barriers and drop out of the nursing program or fight the system to remain, making adjustments as necessary. There is no reason that a full, satisfying, professional nursing career should be out of reach for this student.

It is important to note that nurses do not define high-level wellness for clients, but rather they assist clients in identifying what they are capable of reaching to maximize their potential for high-level wellness. Remember what was noted earlier in the chapter: high-level wellness is the highest level of well-being *that clients can reach*. An overweight, heavy-smoking, heavy-drinking person may think, and even state, the belief that he or she is healthy, but given Dunn's definition, it is unlikely that the person is experiencing high-level wellness and maximizing his or her potential to the best of his or her abilities. It is relatively easy to apply this concept to individuals, but how does high-level wellness translate to communities?

Community Health Promotion and Wellness

Communities have potential for high-level wellness as well. Communities can be defined within geographic boundaries or as population groups with special needs or interests (Baldwin, Conger, Abegglen, & Hill, 1998). Communities usually have systems in place, such as planning commissions or committees, to identify what is high-level wellness for that group. For example, one element of wellness identified in the motto for Sandy City, Utah, is support for family values. One way the community supports family values is by promoting healthy family activities. Toward this end, the community master plan establishes a network of neighborhood parks that will be developed as neighborhoods expand. This process maximizes the potential of the community to reach what it has defined as high-level wellness.

Some community interventions that support wellness are relatively easy to identify by community members. Others, especially related to population wellness, are more difficult for communities to pinpoint. Nurses often collaborate with community groups to identify these strengths, assets, problems, and needs.

People with chronic and even terminal diseases may live their lives in such a healthy and balanced manner that high-level wellness might be attained, at least for a time. A person can use health-promotion behaviors and activities even if ill or diseased "to become an active participant in the healing process instead of a passive recipient" (Ryan & Travis, 1991, p.3).

Factors Influencing Health Promotion and Wellness

It is important to recognize that health care in the United States is finally experiencing a shift in focus from a rather one-sided emphasis on present and potential disease to a more balanced focus that includes an equal emphasis on health promotion, wellness, risk reduction, and disease prevention (Baldwin, Conger, Abegglen, & Hill, 1998). Educating clients, defined as individuals, families, populations, or communities, regarding their health requires information about health-promotion activities that the clients consider relevant to them. It is because of this shift in focus that we now are more strongly accentuating the importance of understanding the "why's" and "how-to's" of health promotion and wellness. Some of the factors influencing health promotion and wellness are the changes in societal expectations, shifting sands of the health care delivery system, U.S. government initiatives, public/private partnerships, and growing consumerism and emphasis on self-care.

Changes in Societal Expectations

Over the years, people in the United States have vacillated as to what good health and wellness are all about. Some cultures had lifestyles that encompassed running and athletic feats, such as hunting, that sustained life; other groups were much more sedentary. Types of foods eaten varied, and little attention was

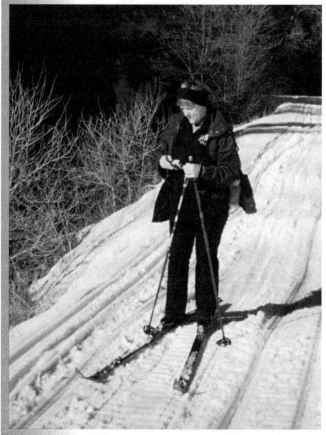

Vigorous exercise of large muscle groups lowers heart disease risks and promotes well-being in women.

paid to what foods were healthy or what foods were not; the important thing was being able to eat. Prior to the 1960s, the social system was such that the majority of people spent more time worrying about food, shelter, and safety (lower levels of Maslow's hierarchy) (Maslow, 1970) than self-actualization. The relationship of lifestyle and health had not been established scientifically. Health was primarily defined as the absence of disease, and health care delivery and research focused on controlling and trying to cure communicable diseases. The media played little or no role in sharing health-related information with the public other than reporting morbidity and mortality information.

Since the 1960s, societal expectations have changed. Increasing affluence has allowed the majority of society to move beyond a primary concern with food, shelter, and safety toward achieving self-esteem and self-actualization (Maslow, 1970). High-level wellness is a state of self-actualization, "maximizing the potential of which the individual is capable" (Dunn, 1959, p. 447). During the 1950s and 1960s, the leading causes of morbidity and mortality moved from communicable disease to chronic disease. With this shift, the health care profession had less success in controlling the causes of disease or in curing some of the diseases. Instead of cure, the focus became symptom management. It became more obvious that the method of control for chronic disease begins with health promotion and specific preventive measures. Since the mid-1960s, there has been a proliferation of research relating health promotion and wellness to lifestyle practices. This information has become so popular that the media has developed an interest in reporting health-promotion strategies. Today, experts on morning television programs regularly report the latest in health-related research and health-promotion strategies. With these societal changes in perception and the increasing costs of health care, pressure came to bear to look for the most cost-effective methods to deliver health care.

Shifting Sands of the Health Care Delivery System

The health care delivery system, as a fee-for-service system, focused on the treatment of illness rather than on health promotion and prevention of disease (Butterfield, 1993). However, research has demonstrated that the causes of most chronic illness are the practice of health-depleting behaviors *and* social and environmental barriers that limit the choices individuals, families, populations, and communities have relating to health-promoting activities. In addition, in a seminal article by McGinnis and Foege (1993), the chief preventable causes of death are translated to lifestyle choices and social influences. These causes include tobacco use; poor diet and activity patterns; alcohol consumption; exposure to environmental microbial or toxic agents; inappropriate use of firearms; promiscuous, unprotected sexual behaviors; motor vehicle accidents; illicit drug use; and socioeconomic barriers.

There are many social barriers that limit the choices clients have in relationship to health-promoting activities. Prime examples are those who live in inner cities or who live in rural or frontier areas. Food choices are limited by distance to full-service grocery stores and availability of transportation. The stores that are available tend to be small family-owned markets or gas station mini-marts. Both provide limited choice of foods at prices higher than full-service chain stores. In addition, gas station mini-marts may not sell produce but do sell high-fat, high-calorie convenience foods.

With the move to managed care and other community-based services for individuals and families and the realization that chronic illness and even death are grounded, for the most part, in lifestyle choices and social barriers, the focus of health care is changing. The principles of managed care require that health-promotion and disease-prevention activities be included in practice at both individual and population levels to prevent the costly occurrence of chronic disease and disability. For managed care organizations to realize profit, risk groups must be managed at both the individual and the aggregate levels (Baldwin, Conger, Abegglen, & Hill, 1998). Also, managed care organizations are becoming more involved in community activities such as community-based health centers, health fairs, Healthy Communities programs, and school-based clinics. Many managed care systems and other insurance companies encourage health-promotion education, activities, and behaviors for their members. In addition, industries have included wellness programs for employees, which may offer various types of reimbursement incentives, from lowering insurance premiums to giving bonuses to those members and employees who demonstrate health-promoting behaviors.

United States Government Initiatives

In the late 1970s, the Surgeon General of the United States, in a document titled *Healthy People*, reported to the nation about the expectations at that time regarding health promotion and disease prevention in this country (Baldwin, 1992, 1995; Kulbok & Baldwin, 1992; USPHS, 1979). The Surgeon General stated, "Let us make no mistake about the significance of this document, it represents an emerging consensus among scientists and the health community that the Nation's health strategy must be dramatically recast to emphasize the prevention of disease" (*Healthy People 2010*, 1998, p. 1).

In 1980, target outcomes, in the form of objectives for the year 1990, were given relating to the reduction of premature mortality in four age groups (*Laying the Foundation*, 1998). At that time, prevention of disease was the main thrust, with health-protection factors addressed and health promotion mentioned. Revised and updated objectives, written in 1990 for the year 2000 (*Healthy People 2000: National Health Promotion and Disease Prevention Objectives*), changed the order of health priorities.

Health promotion became the first consideration in the list of three important factors: health promotion, health protection, and preventive services (Baldwin, 1992; Kulbok & Baldwin, 1992). In 1998, the document *Healthy People 2010 Objectives: Draft for Public Comment* (DHHS) was published to elicit public and professional input into the developed national objectives for the year 2010.

Nurses must be involved at all levels of policy development. They have been members of task forces developing the components of each *Healthy People* document, and with the availability of the Internet, nurses had opportunity to give input and feedback on the *Healthy People 2010* development.

The document provides a wonderful opportunity for nursing students to assess populations within their local regions related to progress toward one or more of the objectives. At Brigham Young University College of Nursing, beginning nursing students write a scholarly paper that is based on *Healthy People 2010* objectives. The students have 1 year, through several nursing courses, to complete the assignment. Students pick a topic such as immunizations or maternal-child issues, conduct a literature review, consider nursing implications, and assess what is being done in the local community for the population of interest. Recommendations are made as to additional approaches that might be taken, and these are shared with community agencies (personal communication, J. Abegglen, May 5, 1999).

Public/Private Partnerships

Through a cooperative agreement between the American Public Health Association (APHA) and the Centers for Disease Control and Prevention (CDC), a major collaborative process resulted in another document, *Healthy Communities 2000 Model Standards: Guidelines for Community Attainment of the Year 2000 National Health Objectives* (APHA, 1991). The approach and document are considered valuable resources for communities wanting to explore and develop local health-promotion standards (*Model Standards*, 1998). The APHA built on the *Healthy People 2000* objectives, developing step-by-step criteria for each objective. Each objective had a measurable "goal" attached to it. For instance, the objective to reduce coronary heart disease deaths might have a measurable goal to reduce x amount of these deaths per 100,000 people by some specific date. These guidelines for adapting measurable criteria to the national objectives have been adapted and used by leaders, including nurses and other health care professionals in many states, counties, regions, cities, and even some neighborhoods, who wish to facilitate more healthful lifestyles for the populations they serve.

The Healthy Cities program originated in 1985 with a presentation at an international meeting in Canada. The theme of the presentation was that health is the result of much more than medical care; people are healthy when they live in nurturing environments and are involved in the life of their community

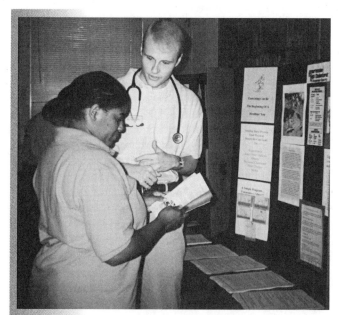

Education is a critical aspect of health promotion intervention. Health fairs are effective ways to share wellness information with large numbers of people.

(Duhl, 1986). A recent publication, *Healthy People in Healthy Communities: A Guide for Community Leaders* (DHHS, 1998), links healthy cities with healthy people to create a healthy community in a guide to how other cities and communities developed and implemented their healthy community initiatives.

There have been numerous partnerships and group efforts in which nurses have collaborated with Healthy Cities and Communities projects throughout the country. Flynn and other community health nurses began "Healthy Indiana," which was an early forerunner of ensuing Healthy Cities and Communities programs (Flynn, 1991). Other examples include work with homeless populations (Greiner & Berry, 1992; Moore, Neff, Smith, & Weber, 1999) and nurse managed care centers (Drapo & Woods, 1992). The growth of community nursing organizations demonstrates how nurses believe our focus should be on partnering and collaborating with communities and special populations in health-promoting efforts. Nurse educators and local public health nursing directors continue to forge collaborative bonds with cities, communities, and target population groups in developing community/population health-promotion needs and assets assessments (Baldwin, 1995).

The following is an example of nursing student involvement with community-level health promotion interventions. The Brigham Young University College of Nursing in Provo, Utah, offers a community/population assessment elective course to both nursing undergraduate students and university honor students. Various city and county health departments and local communities have requested assistance in assessing the needs of

key population groups. For example, the members of the Healthy Taylorsville Project requested the class's help in assessing the needs and viewpoints of the youth of the community. The college students collaborated with the school superintendent, principals, teachers, counselors, and junior and senior high school students. They produced a document outlining the needs of the youth and their suggestions and ideas about health-promotion strategies for the city of Taylorsville (Browning, Huls, Rather, & Stout, 1997). One example of the Taylorsville youths' suggestions was to place stoplights at two of the busiest streets in the growing city so that students could safely cross those streets to get to and from school. The document will be a major guide toward anticipated changes for many of the needs stated by the youth (personal communication, J. I. Morgan, Director of Administrative Services, Taylorsville, Utah, March 1998).

Growing Consumerism and Emphasis on Self-Care

Since the late 1960s, consumers of health care have increasingly demanded information relating to their health care and to items that promote health. In the past, consumers almost complacently

RESEARCH BRIEF

Jette, A. M., Lachman, M., Giorgetti, M. M., Assmann, S. F., Harris, B. A., Levenson, C., Wernick, M., & Krebs, D. (1999). Exercise—It's never too late: The Strong-for-Life program. American Journal of Public Health, 89(1), 66–72.

The authors of a randomized controlled trial compared the outcomes of a home exercise program taught to 107 older persons (with a mean age of 75.4) with a control group of 108 people (with a mean age of 75.6) who did not receive the home exercise program training until after the study was completed. The Strong-for-Life program was based on a video of several exercise methods demonstrated by an exercise expert. Simple movements, those an older person might perform in daily functions, such as rotating wrist joints and reaching across the body, were incorporated into the exercises. Some exercises were done while sitting; others included short walking routines.

Striking results were noted regarding strength improvements. There is promise in using videos in home exercise programs designed for older people; the benefits of this type of health-promoting, cost-efficient exercise that can be done in the privacy of the home are appealing to the growing population of the elderly, as well as having health and cost benefits for the nation.

accepted what physicians and others in control of health care systems told them regarding their health care. Over the last 30 years, consumers have become better educated and more proactive in demanding their rights and insisting that health care professionals be accountable for their actions. Evidence can be seen in the proliferation of satisfaction surveys, opinion polls, and litigation, as well as in the nature of advertising. Information related to dietary management, such as lowering the fat content in recipes, and exercise activities that claim to be health promoting are seen throughout the media. People are requesting more information on labels in order to discern whether the item contains anything that might be non-health promoting, especially something that might trigger an allergy or be too high in fat content. The health-promotion aspects of education have become a major focus for all age and ethnic groups.

Who is responsible for health? There is an expanding awareness that consumers must bear the responsibility for their own health. How can consumers do this? Self-care is the answer. Self-care is defined as those "activities initiated or performed by an individual, family, or community to achieve, maintain, or promote maximum health" (Steiger & Lipson, 1985, p. 12). Orem defines self-care as "the production of actions directed to self or to the environment in order to regulate one's functioning in the interest of one's life, integrated functioning, and well-being" (Orem, 1985, p. 31).

The impetus for the current interest in self-care began anew in the late 1970s and early 1980s. The U.S. Department of Health and Human Services (DHHS, 1982) published a document titled *Forward Plan for Health 1977-1981*. It seems remarkable to consider today, that for the first time ever, the authors of this report boldly suggested that lifestyle and psychosocial factors had a great impact on morbidity and mortality. A number of health-promotion elements such as nutrition, exercise, and fitness were mentioned.

In addition to the emphasis placed by government documents at that time, the popular press also supported the notion. In his book *Megatrends*, Naisbitt (1982, p. 131) forecast that self-care emphasizing health-promotion strategies would move health care out of the medical-institutional illness model into an era of self-responsibility for health and wellness.

The demand for self-care is currently coming from people themselves, private insurance carriers, managed care organizations, employers, and communities. In the past, individuals would never consider questioning the diagnoses or orders of their physicians. Insurance carriers now insist that there be at least two health care professionals' opinions before major surgery.

In addition, consumers are demanding information about complementary treatment options in addition to allopathic treatments suggested by physicians. Insurance and managed care companies are providing self-care books that assist subscribers to self-diagnose and self-treat simple illnesses and injuries, as well as provide tips on health-promoting activities for all members of the family. Incentives include managed care organizations paying bonuses to members for smoking cessation, weight loss, and

other health-promoting activities that move the members toward high-level wellness. At the workplace, large companies implement organizational wellness programs that assist employees to maximize personal wellness. Research has shown that an employee experiencing high-level wellness uses fewer sick days and is more productive on the job (National Institute for Occupational Safety and Health, 1996; DHHS, 1998). At home or from a local library or other community establishment, clients can access numerous Internet sites on any subject relating to self-care.

Self-care and consumerism are processes that assist people to know about health-promoting items and activities. At the population and community levels, the Healthy Cities and Communities program depends heavily on people within communities to identify problems and assets and engage in problem solving and self-care to correct problems and promote maximal community wellness. The success of the *Healthy People 2010* objectives for the nation is equally dependent on client education in health-promotion and self-care strategies as well as policy changes to improve social conditions allowing for the context within which personal choices about health are made. To make informed health-promoting decisions, appropriate and correct health-promotion information must be available to clients, as well as to legislators who make the policies.

Models of Health Promotion and Wellness

Numerous models of health promotion and wellness might be useful guides to assessing and promoting health and wellness in communities, populations, families, and individuals. Many models have been constructed to explain, assess, plan, or evaluate health-promotion education programs, states of health, wellness, and illness, and preventive measures.

As early as 1952, researchers expressed the need for a model to help explain and predict why certain at-risk populations took preventive actions and others did not, even when there was very little or nothing being charged for the preventive services (Rosenstock, 1974). The first popular model developed was the health belief model (Becker, 1974; Hochbaum, 1958; Padilla & Bulcavage, 1991; Rosentock, 1974). In this model, "the individual's weighing of the positive and negative valences of the threats of illness was emphasized" (Baldwin, 1992, p. 27). How the individual perceived his or her susceptibility to an illness and what might be the perceived benefits and barriers to doing something about preventing the illness were important factors in the health belief model. Even when the individual decided it was in his or her best interest to take some action to prevent the illness, there needed to be a trigger or cue to action to motivate the person to carry out the action (Baldwin, 1992; Rosenstock, 1974).

Several other models have been developed that might be useful to the nurse of today. As researchers continue the quest to predict and explain what factors contributed to health-promoting and health-protecting behaviors, the multidimensionality of the process became clearer. Further developments of the predictors of preventive health behavior originating in the health belief model were instigated in later models. Cognitive factors such as clients' definitions of health and perceptions about health behaviors, including benefits, barriers, and control, were seen as important to clients' health-promoting behaviors. Modifying factors, ranging from demographic, biological, behavioral, and interpersonal to environmental, including access to care, as well as factors that might influence the initiating of health-promoting and health-protective behaviors, were explored. Many of these multidimensional factors can be seen in the health-promotion models constructed in the 1980s and early 1990s (Palank, 1991; Pender, 1987; Simmons, 1990) and in health hazard risk evaluation and appraisal tools and wellness guides, which began appearing in the early 1970s and 1980s.

Health hazard risk evaluation and appraisal tools are commonly designed in survey questionnaire form to provide quantitative data elicited from clients' responses regarding lifestyle and health habits. Questions regarding activities of daily living ranging from personal health habits, such as, "How often do you brush your teeth?" "In what way and how often do you exercise?" and "Are you sexually active?" to questions regarding seat belt use and consumption of caffeine products are often asked. Often, information is required regarding family and personal medical histories and various demographic data. The information from these questionnaires can then be compared with known national and local health statistics to make predictions and health-promotion recommendations regarding morbidity and mortality risks for the clients. Wellness guides are generally in a question and answer form, designed to appeal to consumers who may have a common health or wellness question or concern.

In the late 1980s, the *Guide to Clinical Preventive Services* (U.S. Preventive Services Task Force, 1989) was developed, and in 1995, a second edition was published to help guide primary care health professionals providing preventive services. These tools and guides are used by physicians' and nurse practitioners' offices, hospitals, health departments, managed care systems, and other agencies to assist health care professionals counseling clients about reducing potential risks and increasing health-promoting behaviors. Models, tools, and guides continue to be designed to help explore factors involved in health promotion and wellness decision making for individuals, families, populations, and communities.

Two recent models are described to demonstrate how these techniques might be used to assess and facilitate wellness interventions: (1) holistic wellness: self-inventory of personal wellness using the medicine wheel (McDonald, 1997) and (2) the 4+ model of wellness (Baldwin & Baldwin, 1998). These models are similar in some respects to earlier models and tools in the assessment of multidimensional variables impacting health and wellness, but they differ somewhat in the approaches. Both of these models may be used with any ethnic population, as may several of the earlier models. The holistic wellness model allows clients to identify aspects that determine wellness and to define what well

RESEARCH BRIEF

Neuhauser, L., Schwab, M., Syme, S. L., Bieber, M., & Obarski, S. K. (1998). Community participation in health promotion: evaluation of the California Wellness Guide. Health Promotion International, 13(3), 211–222.

Short-term outcomes for participants using the California Wellness Guide were described and evaluated, using interviews from three population-based samples of women involved in the Women, Infants, and Children Supplemental Nutrition Program (WIC). From the pretesting stage to the end of the study at 8 months, the participants demonstrated significantly improved attitudes and knowledge regarding wellness information compared with the nonparticipants. Findings indicated that a wellness guide, such as the California Wellness Guide, which evolved from in-depth community involvement and contained many common health care topics, can raise the knowledge level and improve health-promotion and wellness behaviors of participants. This, in turn, could add immeasurably to the nation's health-promotion benefits.

and unhealthy states are for them. The 4+ model of wellness also encourages client participation in the assessment of wellness and adds two other dimensions: the consideration of what might be the sources of nurture and depletion for a client and how the nurse might facilitate interventions with the client, focusing on those sources of nurture and depletion to promote health and wellness.

Holistic Wellness: Self-Inventory of Personal Wellness Using the Medicine Wheel

The medicine wheel is a sacred symbol that is common to almost all Native American tribes (Four Worlds Development Project, 1985, p. 9). Ivan McDonald, a member of the Blackfeet tribe and health educator for Indian Health Services in Browning, Montana, developed the holistic wellness model using the medicine wheel as a basis (see the figure on p. 226). Although the descriptors for this model are specific to the values and beliefs of the Blackfeet culture of Native Americans, the wheel can be used to assess wellness for any person of any culture. The descriptors of "healthy" states and "unhealthy" states for the spokes of the wheel should reflect the individuality of the person.

The holistic wellness model is grounded in the Native American understanding of existence. The medicine wheel, as a representation of this understanding, is depicted as a circle that comprises the four sacred directions. Each direction represents not only one of the basic elements necessary for survival, but also a human element.

The East is symbolic of the sun and fire and of one's own creative spirit. The South represents water and one's emotions. The

RESEARCH BRIEF

Segal, L., Dalton, A. C., & Richardson, J. (1998). Cost-effectiveness of the primary prevention of non-insulin dependent diabetes mellitus. Health Promotion International, 13(1), 197–209.

A cost-effective analysis research study of intervention programs for the prevention of non–insulin-dependent diabetes mellitus (NIDDM) reported in international literature in recent years was undertaken. Epidemiological and clinical evidence pointed to weight loss, exercise, and fitness, plus appropriate nutrition, as health-promotion interventions leading to prevention of NIDDM. The research questions were aimed at whether preventing NIDDM was cost-effective in comparison with other potential resource use and if any NIDDM health-promotion programs were more cost-effective than other programs. Various media programs, such as the use of videos, and programs geared to overweight men compared most favorably in the study. NIDDM not only is a prevalent chronic disease today, but is also increasing in prevalence throughout the world, and many of the high-risk target populations are American Indian and Alaskan Native. Among the major risk factors for NIDDM is ethnicity.

HOLISTIC WELLNESS: SELF-INVENTORY OF PERSONAL WELLNESS USING THE MEDICINE WHEEL.

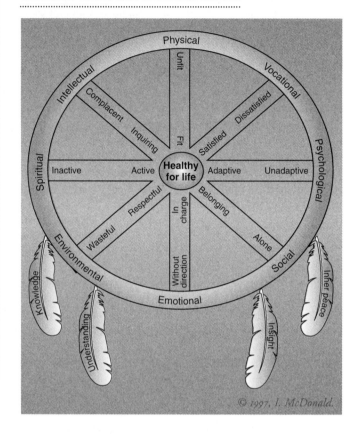

© 1997, I. McDonald.

West is the place of Mother Earth and one's intuition—the place of magic and dreams. The North represents air and minds filled with wisdom as one learns about the mystery of life.

Holistic wellness defines health in terms of the whole person, not only in terms of physical illness. The model represents how Native American people understand health as a balance within the person and between the person and everything around him or her—physical, vocational, psychological, social, emotional, environmental, spiritual, and intellectual. It focuses on optimal health, prevention of disease, and positive mental and emotional states (personal communication, I. McDonald, April 1998).

The spokes of the medicine wheel radiate from a center circle that represents wellness or "Healthy for Life." The spokes contain dimensions of the specific wellness (as the Physical Wellness spoke has the dimensions of unfit and fit), with the more positive part of the dimension being closest to the center Healthy for Life circle in preceding figure. The spokes are defined as follows:

- Physical wellness: *maintenance of your body in good condition by eating right, exercising regularly, avoiding harmful habits, and making informed, responsible decisions about your health*
- Vocational wellness: *enjoyment of what you are doing to earn a living and/or to contribute to society*
- Psychological wellness: *maintenance of mental health or the ability to think reasonably clearly and to avoid wildly distorting reality*

- Social wellness: *ability to perform the expectations of social roles effectively, comfortably, and without harming others*
- Emotional wellness: *understanding emotions and knowing how to cope with problems that arise in everyday life; ability to endure stress*
- Environmental wellness: *personal and global risks to health, socioeconomic status, education, and various other environmental factors that affect health, such as noise pollution, radiation, air pollution, and water pollution*
- Spiritual wellness: *a state of balance and harmony with yourself and others; includes trust, integrity, principles, ethics, the purpose or drive in life, basic survival instincts, feelings of selflessness, degree of pleasure-seeking qualities, commitment to some higher process or being, and the ability to believe in concepts that are not subject to a "state of the art" explanation*
- Intellectual wellness: *having a mind open to new ideas; covers such activities as speaking, writing, analyzing, critical thinking, and judgment*

The eagle feathers at the bottom of the wheel represent the progression of personal development: knowledge, understanding, insight, and inner peace. Each element is a higher level than the one before. However, the element before must occur before one can aspire to the next level. The progression of the feathers is similar to the progression for each dimension reflected in the spokes of the wheel. As the client develops inwardly toward Healthy for Life, there is progress from knowledge to inner peace.

The holistic wellness model includes social and environmental aspects as they relate to a person's wellness. From the perspectives of many cultures, a person's wellness depends on social relationships and harmony with the environment. For example, for some societies in Australia and Mexico, physical illness can be caused by breaches of social norm. Although this is not necessarily a common idea in many Western societies, from the worldview of most cultures, personal illness or wellness may be a result of social and environmental interactions.

How to Use the Holistic Wellness Model

The nurse could use the holistic wellness model as an excellent visual depiction of a client's self-defined wellness state. The model can be used by health professionals to help clients in both assessing what the client's values are relating to the eight dimensions and determining how well he or she is functioning within each dimension. It is important to note, though, that if one dimension becomes the focus of changing behaviors, other dimensions may suffer from lack of attention. Therefore, facilitating interventions through the use of this model requires that the nurse and client together consider how to strengthen all of the dimensions as equally as possible. In addition, the holistic wellness model is handy for quick evaluations of progress. It is also important to understand that the balance may shift depending on circumstances and that as symbolized by the medicine wheel, there is constant motion.

Several examples of how to intervene and facilitate the client's considering a more healthful lifestyle using health-promoting behaviors include the following: (1) If the client considers himself or herself to be on the unfit dimension of the Physical spoke, discuss ways for the client to become more fit. What does the client like to do in the way of exercise, and what can the client physically and realistically do? If walking is difficult for an elderly person, perhaps suggest starting with moving every possible body joint two or three times during a television or radio commercial or a rest while reading. (2) If the client believes he or she is inactive on the Spiritual spoke, review what spirituality means to the client and see if he or she can discover ways to become more active in that realm. (3) If the client sees that he or she is without direction on the Emotional spoke, address things that might be done by the client to make him or her feel more in charge of life. The major issue here is what the client believe he or she can realistically do to develop health-promoting behaviors that will lead to the client being more healthy for life.

At a community level, the model could be applied by changing the names on the outer ring of the medicine wheel. For example, things such as public transportation, community pride, health care services, and so on could substitute for the physical,

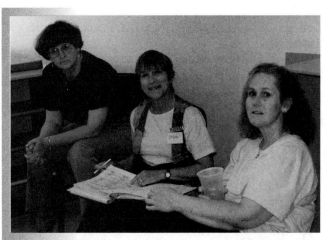

Dr. Joan H. Baldwin, chapter author (center), works with nurse practitioner students in a wellness program on a Ute Indian reservation.

spiritual, and psychological elements. The spokes would translate similarly. For instance, public transportation might be present (meaning all possible modes of transportation are available) to absent (meaning there is no public transportation in the community). The feather could be redefined as knowledge to data, understanding to information, insight to creative solutions, and inner peace to harmony of factors.

The 4+ Model of Wellness

The 4+ model of wellness (Baldwin & Baldwin, 1998) is designed to assist critical thinking about things that might negatively deplete or positively nurture wellness in a client. There are two layers, much like transparent plastic overlays, to this model: (1) the four domains of inner self and (2) the outer systems. When layer 2 is placed over layer 1, the total 4+ model of wellness appears.

The 4+ model of wellness begins with the inner self layer, depicting a sphere containing the four domains of inner self (see the following figure) of the client. The client might be oneself, another individual, a family, population, or community. The four domains of inner self are intellectual, physical, emotional, and spiritual (or spirit).

This portion of the 4+ model of wellness appears simple but is really quite complex. The intellectual component of the inner self relates to how the client thinks. The physical is how the client moves and senses things and includes all of the client's physiological (or inner workings, as in the case of a community as client) aspects. How a client feels anger, excitement, and so on is reflected in the emotional aspect, and the spiritual denotes the fire that drives the engine that connects one to others and to a higher power. The spiritual domain also includes the capacity to give love. Thus, the spiritual domain within each of us seems to have more than one role. This domain is likely to be the most

THE 4+ MODEL OF WELLNESS: THE FOUR DOMAINS OF INNER SELF.

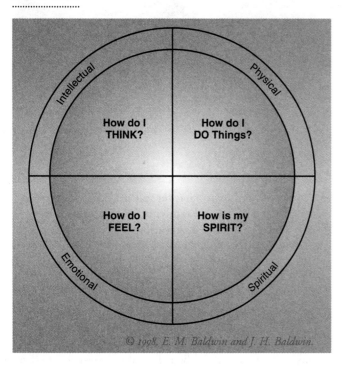

© 1998, E. M. Baldwin and J. H. Baldwin.

THE 4+ MODEL OF WELLNESS: THE OUTER SYSTEMS.

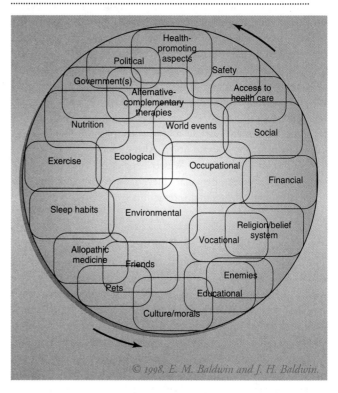

© 1998, E. M. Baldwin and J. H. Baldwin.

THE 4+ MODEL OF WELLNESS: THE FOUR DOMAINS OF INNER SELF PLUS THE OUTER SYSTEMS.

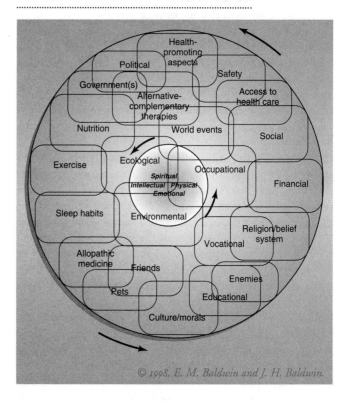

© 1998, E. M. Baldwin and J. H. Baldwin.

complex and sometimes difficult to understand, although it is one of the most important to consider.

Achieving a holistic and harmonious state within the inner self is one part of the model. For example, think of the four domains of inner self as a tire. When all four of the domains—intellectual, physical, emotional, and spiritual—are "pumped up," the tire is rounded and rolls along evenly. This is what is meant by a holistic and harmonious state. This healthy state of harmony is further affected by interconnectedness and interaction with systems outside the inner self, which are depicted in the second overlay—the outer systems (see the figures to the right)—as facets of another sphere surrounding the sphere of the four domains of inner self. The outer systems portion of this model is similar to the tool known as an *Ecomap,* which was discussed in Chapter 2.

All of the elements of the outer systems sphere interact and interconnect with each other and all the four domains of inner self. Imagine the two spheres constantly rotating about each other so that all components of each sphere interact with other elements within their own sphere and with each other at some time. The preceding figure depicts the idea of layering the spheres—the 4+ model of wellness: the four domains of inner self plus the outer systems.

Think of the total model as a client system, one system with many moving components. Using the 4+ model of wellness, the nurse can look for things that might be depleting the elements of the inner self rather than nurturing the elements toward harmony. By working with the client to consider things that might deplete

BOX 10-3 THE 4+ MODEL OF WELLNESS: SELECTED SOURCES OF NURTURE AND DEPLETION

INTELLECTUAL

Sources of Nurture
- Books/intellectual media activities
- Observation/contemplation
- Experience/critical thinking
- Knowledge building more knowledge
- Practicing "brain work," that is, children's play and games; children learn this way and so do adults
- Planning for the future

Sources of Depletion
- Brainwashing—imposed conditioned responses
- Mind-numbing repetition
- Boredom
- Noise
- Interruption
- Stresses/stressors
- Codependent behavior encouraged by a perpetrator—can lead to posttraumatic stress syndrome

EMOTIONAL
Sources of Nurture
- Relief from stress
- Accomplishments
- Winning
- Physical well-being, exercise, diet
- Rest/relaxation
- Meditation/biofeedback, etc.
- Ability to "vent" appropriately

Sources of Depletion
- Physical illness
- Weak intelligence (inability to solve a problem)
- Isolation/noise/threats

Source: Baldwin & Baldwin, 1998.

PHYSICAL
Sources of Nurture
- Appropriate nutrition
- Outdoor/indoor activities/exercise
- Rest/relaxation
- Physical "work"
- Biofeedback/complementary health therapies, etc.
- Appropriate physiological workings
- Physical therapy

Sources of Depletion
- Disease/illness/prepathogenesis
- Toxins/environmental hazards
- Drug/substance abuse
- Poor nutrition/diet
- Lack of sleep
- Noise
- Stress/stressors/allergies
- Excessive exercise/exertion
- Trauma

SPIRITUAL
Sources of Nurture
- Giving love/connecting with others
- Being of service/loving animals
- Beauty/music/art
- Quiet/peace, meditation/prayer
- Physical exercise/cheering
- Being loved/hugs and pat-pats
- Intellectual stimulus/creating

Sources of Depletion
- Too much demand for support of others
- Failure to experience connectedness, love, belonging

any one or all of the four domains and thinking of ways to strengthen those things that nurture the client, the nurse and client may be able to identify health-promoting actions for the client. Selected sources of nurture and depletion are listed in Box 10-3.

General observations
Strength in any domain, if not in excess, can nurture the other three domains. Also, depletion of any domain weakens and drains the other three domains.

Spiritual domain

On first consideration, the emotional and spiritual domains may appear similar, but in this model, these areas are quite different from each other. In this model, *spiritual* means the spirit or fire one has within. Excessive emotional highs may deplete the spirit. Of importance in this model is that *spiritual* does not mean religion or religious. Religion is actually a piece of the outer system that impacts the inner self. Parts of a religion may indeed nurture the spirit, but sometimes, as in the case of overzealousness, depletion of the spirit may occur.

Observations about excesses

Excessive striving in any area can be destructive in all four domains. An illustration would be someone who exercises to an extreme, to the detriment of personal relationships with others.

Excessive pain can be a depleting factor. For example, it is hard to think when you are suffering severe pain. One kind of severe pain is depression. Severely depressed people become so immobilized in several of the domains that they cannot move themselves toward strength in any of the areas through simple exercise or nutrition or even interaction with loving people. Serious disease or weakness (which can cause excessive physiological and other problems) can deplete several domains and can be a major factor in the client suffering a downward spiral to total collapse and death.

Any excesses or "lacks" within any of the four domains throws the inner self sphere extremely "off balance or out of harmony." Think of the inner self sphere as being a tire; the difference in pressure on any portion of the tire will throw the tire off balance. People in various cultures speak of the tremendous importance of balance or harmony in a person's life.

Contemporary researchers and authors are proposing that changing and growing systems do not necessarily seek total equilibrium, that constant change alters the state of harmony or balance continuously (Coveney & Highfield, 1990; Prigogine & Stengers, 1984; Wheatley, 1994). This might explain how the assessment of a client on one day may be far different from a similar assessment another day or even later in the same day. This is why it is important to observe the client over time—to get a broader picture of what might be occurring within that client system. There does not have to be "equilibrium" to have balance or harmony; in fact, a well-functioning system is always in a state of nonequilibrium because it constantly and inevitably changes focus. A system that is flexible and open can constantly move, changing and adjusting to regain harmony or a state as close to harmony as possible (Wheatley, 1994).

How to Use the 4+ Model of Wellness with Individuals, Families, Populations, and Communities

The nurse should begin by assessing the four domains of inner self for oneself or a client. Then, the components of the outer systems, which encircle and move around the four domains of the inner self sphere, must be considered. By using the total 4+ model of wellness to assess the interactions and interconnectedness of the elements in the outer systems to all aspects of the inner self, the nurse will be able to critically assess and analyze much about himself or herself or others. The nurse and the client may be able to determine which factors to work on strengthening or nurturing and which factors might be diminished or deleted to "pump up" the client system's wellness. Remember that the client can be a family, group, population, or community, as well as an individual.

Individuals

Consider a grossly overweight, older man as an individual client. The client has been prescribed a diet that is nutritionally sound and, if followed, should help him lose weight. The client could be thinking he is trying to follow his prescribed diet, and he is perplexed about not being successful in losing weight. The nurse could explore with the client as many aspects as possible of his four domains of inner self, as well as the outer system components, to begin to figure out what interventions might facilitate health-promoting behaviors for this client. After working with the client to assess what might be sources of nurture and depletion for each of his four domains, the nurse (and, in some difficult cases, a team of health care professionals), along with the client, would develop a wellness plan. Ideally, finding ways to nurture the client's four domains and considering how the depleting sources could be diminished would constitute the initial part of the plan. For example, there might be work environment stressors (sources of depletion), such as the fact that donuts

RESEARCH BRIEF

Jorgenson, J. (1997). Therapeutic use of companion animals in health care. Image: The Journal of Nursing Scholarship, *29(3), 249–254.*

An exploration of the research in several disciplines related to the use of animals for therapy in health care demonstrated applicability of the findings to enhance health-promoting nursing interventions for clients. A selective historical tour of the literature regarding the human-animal bond and its therapeutic effect in health care is a segue to more recent research on the subject. Considerations about the pros and cons of having animals interact with hospitalized clients are developed. The link between the benefits of stress reduction and positive psychoneuroimmunology changes in clients as a result of human-animal bonding therapies emerges as the strongest health promotion possibility for the use of this animal-assisted therapy.

and other sweet, high-fat, and high-calorie foods are encouraged at break time at the workplace, which makes adhering to the prescribed diet difficult. Brainstorming with the client about how he might discuss his need to be on the prescribed diet with his supervisor and how difficult it has been to not eat the donuts when they are in full view could be one step in the process.

There will be some sources of nurture that the client could also strengthen. A source of nurture might be that the man has a dog as a pet. Possibly the man and his dog could work with children in a day-care center for developmentally disabled children. There have been many research articles relating the health-promoting aspects of the human-animal bond (Edney, 1992; National Institutes of Health, 1987). In addition, the process of connecting older people with younger people has many nurturing benefits (Piper, 1999). A service opportunity such as this could possibly nurture all four of the client's domains, and certainly would nurture the children who are the recipients of this service (and maybe the dog, who might enjoy being with children).

Another important factor to remember when working with any client is that the client's goals or priorities in life may not be the same as what you might consider his, her, or its (in the case of a family, population, or community) goals or priorities "should" be. This is equally important to remember when establishing things that nurture or deplete a client. These also are factors in why clients do not always do what a health care professional tells them to do. Too often, if clients choose not to do what the health care professional says, or cannot do something for some valid reason, health care professionals indicate that the clients are "noncompliant" or cannot figure out why clients do not do what is "good" for them. These episodes sometimes create ethical concerns, especially concerning whose needs are being met. Building trust, rapport, and respect with clients often encourages the clients, in due time, to follow health care professionals' suggestions for health-promoting behaviors.

Families

Using the 4+ model of wellness when assessing more than one individual becomes more complex than assessing an individual. Consider a family as a large client system comprised of several smaller systems, or individual family members. Look for sources of nurture for the family. These sources might include things such as being broad-minded, being creative, having good problem-solving skills, being flexible, having family members who are interconnected with each other and the outer systems of the family, sharing spirituality, and being appropriately nurturing of the family's spirit and the spirits of others. A family that has developed these characteristics and continues to derive nurture from

them among others demonstrates a fair amount of harmony, health, and wellness. In the family Case Study that follows, look for potential sources of nurture and depletion in the various family clients.

Populations and Communities

Now, think about how the 4+ model of wellness might be used to examine a population or a community. If a family is a client system, then a population or a community can also be a client system; individuals within the population and individuals and target (or at-risk) populations within a community are the smaller systems within the larger client system of population or community. Remember that your own goals, values, and priorities are not necessarily those of populations or communities. These client systems also have their own goals, values, and priorities that can create ethical dilemmas for the nurse.

Sources of nurture for populations and communities may be similar to those for a family. As the client system becomes larger (as with more than one individual), the sources of nurture also become broader in many cases. Freedom from harassment, threats, or violence could be added to any level of client system sources of nurture but seems to be often pertinent to an at-risk or target population or community. Sources of depletion for a population could be the reverse of the sources of nurture. For instance, an at-risk population of unwed pregnant teenagers might be depleted by harassment, ridicule, or shunning by others with extreme moral views against unmarried young women being sexually active. The target population and community Case Study on p. 233 describes some of the things a nurse needs to consider when using the 4+ model of wellness.

• •

You have noticed that everything an Indian does is in a circle, and that is because the Power of the World always works in circles, and everything tries to be round. . . . The Sky is round, and I have heard that the earth is round like a ball, and so are all the stars. The wind, in its greatest power, whirls. Birds make their nests in circles, for theirs is the same religion as ours. . . . Even the seasons form a great circle in their changing, and always come back again to where they were. The life of a man is a circle from childhood, and so it is in everything where power moves.

Black Elk
Oglala Sioux Holy Man, 1863–1950

• •

CASE STUDY

How Everything Affects Everything— A Saga of One Man's Life and the Negative Influences on Him and the Families Involved

Sam had a difficult childhood. His mother left the family when Sam was about 3 or 4 years old. His father probably was devastated, but Sam was too young to understand all that had happened. Sam's paternal grandparents raised Sam, because Sam's father had to work long hours to even begin to make enough money to sustain himself, much less Sam. Sam's grandfather was strict and sometimes abusive to Sam's grandmother. No one in the family seemed to recognize that Sam believed that he was responsible in some way for his mother's leaving.

As Sam grew older, he became angry that his mother had left him, although he seemed to appreciate the fact that his grandparents took reasonable care of him. He was certain his father had no real love for him. Sam was a fairly bright young boy and did well in school. Sometime in the his teens, Sam began experimenting with marijuana. He managed to graduate from high school and began doing manual labor and odd jobs. He still lived with his grandparents.

Sam had several girlfriends over the next few years. The girls and many of his friends were younger than he was by several years. Sam was always the "leader" of the group. He and his friends abused alcohol and began taking many other kinds of "street drugs." Sam verbally abused his friends and girlfriends by telling them they were "stupid" and so on. Eventually, he married one of the young women. After a time, he was not only abusing her verbally, but also forcing her to start taking some of the drugs that he was taking.

Sam and his wife had a child. Amazingly, the child was healthy. As the child grew, Sam insisted on having the child by his side when Sam wanted the child to be there. Otherwise, Sam ignored the child. Sam said he "loved" the child, yet burdened the young child (then about 3 or 4 years of age) with Sam's concerns about money and Sam's belief that the child's mother was "no good." Sam also continued to have sexual liaisons

with other women. Sam's wife made several attempts to leave Sam, especially after some fairly severe beatings. The child often observed these situations. After several years of abuse, Sam's wife left him and took the child with her to live elsewhere. Sam threatened to find her and kill her if the child was not returned. After almost 2 years of legal interventions, Sam's wife won a divorce and legal physical custody of the child (meaning that the child would live with her, but that Sam might have some input into the raising of the child). Sam tolerated this process for a short time before he began verbally harassing and threatening his ex-wife on the phone.

There were several more months of harassment and the involvement of police and other legal interventions. When Sam was finally arrested for selling drugs and being intoxicated, among other things, the court agreed that Sam would be denied contact with his son.

1. Using the 4+ model of wellness, of Sam's four domains, how many were affected by his early life? by his high school adventures? by his adult life?

2. What additional information is needed in the scenario to assess Sam's wellness in the time before he went to jail? Consider what effect the outer systems components (e.g., social, vocational, environmental) may have had on Sam.

3. What sources of nurture and/or depletion are recognizable? Which of Sam's domains may have been affected, given the sources of nurture and/or depletion noted?

4. What health-promoting behaviors of Sam's family might have helped Sam during his early development? List Sam's family's possible sources of nurture and depletion.

5. While considering the 4+ model of wellness, what sources of nurture and/or depletion did the family of the ex-wife and child have? How might a nurse assist them to assess their own four quadrants individually and as a single-parent family?

6. How might a nurse help the ex-wife and child develop the health-promoting behaviors they might need individually and as a single-parent family?

7. Think about Sam's abuse of and involvement with substances. Consider his desire for drugs and Sam's early life and the life he was living as an adult. What view/attitudes might a nurse take as a logical and ethical approach toward Sam?

CASE STUDY

A Target Population Within a Community

The Teen Mothers' High School Program, which was located in one of the local high schools in the town of Urbansville, was used by more than 100 young, single women each year for 5 years. The City Council decided to participate in the formation of a community health-promotion program called "Healthy Urbansville." The council members wanted to improve the health-promoting aspects of their city. They called on leaders in the educational facilities in town, police/sheriff and fire departments, local business people, ecclesiastical representatives (e.g., of churches, temples, synagogues), and other local interested citizens, including representatives of the youth groups and senior citizens' centers, to be part of this community effort.

The city was fairly large and contained many community resource agencies and emergency funding processes to assist those in need. The city was located in an urban area of the western region of the country, with many parks and recreation areas. The city prided itself on the good relationships between its diverse populations, the cleanliness of the city, and the efforts toward appropriate city growth that had been in place for several years. There were several excellent libraries, theater and other media options, art and history museums, as well as restaurants of all kinds. Biomedical and complementary/integrative health therapies co-existed. There were churches of many different denominations readily accessible by most of the populations. Transportation opportunities were well distributed throughout the city, although there were continuing construction projects at various times throughout the dry seasons. There were, as in any large city, varying socioeconomic groups, including many homeless. Illicit drug dealing was being combated daily by the police and others, but it was
not out of hand. Violence was occasional, with robberies and burglaries being highest during the hotter months. Overall, the city considered itself a city with a future.

One of the major concerns of the Healthy Urbansville group that came forth after an in-depth community/population assessment process, which included the use of several surveys (plus the 4+ model of wellness), was that the rising numbers of teen pregnancies had a depleting effect on the community as a whole; families and resources within the community were hard hit. The age ranges of the teenage mothers was between 14 and 17; there were presently 1,000 young women in this age group, according to the most recent statistics. Statistically, teen pregnancies resulted in higher mortality rates than other age groupings. This concern became the main priority of the Healthy Urbansville group.

1. Using the 4+ model of wellness and given what this case study indicated, what assets (or sources of nurture) and what problems (sources of depletion) might exist in the community of Urbansville?

2. What might be the sources of nurture in the intellectual domain of the community? in the physical, emotional, and spiritual domains of the community?

3. Think of the teenage mothers in this community. What questions might you have regarding this target (at-risk) population? What are some of the sources of nurture (or assets) that might affect young women in the age group between 14 and 17 years of age? What are some of the potential sources of depletion (or problem areas) that might affect young women in this age group?

4. Given the sources of nurture (or assets) identified, what interventions might be made to strengthen these in the young women? What potential things might be done to diminish or delete the depleting sources (or problems)?

5. List several interventions for both the community and target population that could facilitate health-promoting behaviors for those clients, either individually or by working to diminish a source of community depletion.

CONCLUSION

This chapter contains a discussion of basic concepts of health and health promotion as related to disease prevention, including definitions of *health promotion* and *wellness* as the terms are used in this chapter; delineation of factors influencing health promotion and wellness; a brief summary of some ways of looking at health promotion and wellness by describing some models, guides, and tools involved in health protection, health promotion, wellness and risk evaluation, analysis, and reduction; and introduction of two recent models of wellness. Key concepts, case studies, research briefs, and critical thinking activities are presented to reinforce concepts and assist in "pushing the envelope" and expanding ideas for health-promotion interventions.

CRITICAL THINKING ACTIVITIES

1. Can a person who has been diagnosed with bipolar disorder and who is appropriately and successfully being managed with medications achieve high-level wellness?

2. Can a community experiencing a severe gang problem achieve high-level wellness? If so, how might this be done?

3. How might the Jedi Women (a community action group comprised of single, low-income mothers) define high-level wellness for their group? What activities might stimulate the group toward self-actualization?

4. What social barriers might keep clients from exploring health-promoting activities, including healthy eating, exercising, and so forth?

5. Why is it that lifestyle choices and social limitations and barriers exist? What situations might be lending themselves to building social barriers for clients?

6. Some community clients have noticeable limitations to their lifestyle choices, as noted in this chapter. Consider the clients in major cities, as well as in rural and/or frontier areas, in the United States 50 years ago. Compare the positives and negatives of their lifestyle choices at that time to similar people of today.

7. Discuss things a community or society could do to support an individual's self-care activities.

8. Describe how consumerism and self-care activities might encourage health-promotion and wellness behaviors.

9. Make a table with two columns. In the first, list self-care activities you engage in to nurture your wellness. In the second, list self-care activities you have not been doing but should. Plan interventions to include at least two new health-promoting behaviors in your daily life.

10. Identify two populations to which you belong. List five self-care practices these populations engage in for the benefit and nurture of their members.

11. How can communities engage in self-care?

12. Redefine the descriptors "unhealthy" and "well" for each of the spokes of the holistic wellness model as they fit from your or your client's cultural perspective.

13. Discuss the meaning of knowledge, understanding, insight, and inner peace, which are found on the eagle feathers on the bottom of the holistic wellness model, as they might fit your or your client's culture.

CRITICAL THINKING ACTIVITIES—CONT'D

14. With the client, evaluate the client's health at each spoke. Consider each spoke as having a weak or more negative dimension (e.g., on the physical spoke, unfit would be the weak dimension and fit would be the healthy dimension). Have the client place a dot on the spoke where the client thinks he or she is at the time on that spoke's dimension. The closer the client places the dot to the center of the wheel on any given spoke/dimension, the healthier the person considers himself or herself in regard to that dimension. Once a dot is placed on each spoke, the dots are connected to form a circle. The nurse and the client can visually evaluate whether the circle is balanced and where the weak dimensions are.

15. Discuss potential interventions and/or changes the client might decide to make to move himself or herself more toward the center of the holistic wellness wheel toward being "healthy for life."

16. For your own community, identify the system dimensions that would be important to assessing wellness.

17. Refer to Box 10-3. What other items could be added to the box to describe sources of nurture and sources of depletion for each of the four domains for an individual, a family, a population, or a community?

18. From Box 10-3, choose a source of nurture in one of the domains and describe how that source of nurture might affect another domain in a client.

19. How might an excess of any factor affect any (or all) of a client's domains?

20. If a person has a physical injury, which of the other domains besides the physical one might be affected? In what way(s)?

21. Consider a woman who is the sole support of several children and must also be the caregiver for an elderly, ill parent. What domains(s) in that person might be affected? How?

22. If that woman becomes totally depleted in several of her domains, how will the domains of the family she is caring for be affected? Describe.

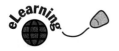

Explore Community Health Nursing on the web! To learn more about the topics in this chapter, access your exclusive web site:
http://communitynursing.jbpub.com

REFERENCES

American Public Health Association (APHA). (1991). *Healthy communities 2000 model standards: Guidelines for community attainment of the year 2000 national health objectives* (3rd ed.). Washington, DC: Author.

Bach, M. L. (1998). *ShapeWalking*. Los Angeles: Heel to Toe Fitness Walking.

Baldwin, E. M. & Baldwin, J. H. (1998). *4+ model of wellness*. Unpublished manuscript.

Baldwin, J. H. (1992). Moving towards harmony: Types and meanings of cues that prompt health-promoting decisions in women in the middle years. Doctoral dissertation, The Catholic University of America, Washington, DC. *UMI Dissertation Abstracts,* Order No. 9220772.

Baldwin, J. H. (1995). Are we implementing community health promotion in nursing? *Public Health Nursing, 12*(3), 159–164.

Baldwin, J. H., Conger, C. O., Abegglen, J. C., & Hill, E. M. (1998). Population-focused and community-based nursing—moving toward clarification of concepts. *Public Health Nursing, 15*(1), 12–18.

Becker, M. H. (Ed.). (1974). *The health belief model and personal health behavior*. Thorofare, NJ: Charles B. Slack.

Browning, B., Huls, J. Rather, R., & Stout, L. (1997). *Taylorsville youth assessment*. Unpublished manuscript. Provo, UT: Brigham Young University College of Nursing.

Brubaker, B. H. (1983, April). Health promotion: A linguistic analysis. *Advances in Nursing Science, 5,* 1–14.

Butterfield, P. G. (1993). Thinking upstream: Conceptualizing health from a population perspective. In J. M. Swanson & M. Albrecht (Eds.), *Community health nursing: Promoting the health of aggregates* (pp. 68–80). Philadelphia: W. B. Saunders.

Clark, E. G., & Leavell, H. R. (1953; 1965). Levels of application of preventive medicine. In H. R. Leavell & E. G. Clark (Eds.), *Preventive medicine for the doctor in his community: An epidemiologic approach* (3rd ed., pp. 14–38). New York: McGraw-Hill.

Cohen, J. (1998). Holistic health strategies. In C. L. Edelman & C. L. Mandle (Eds.), *Health promotion throughout the lifespan* (4th ed., pp. 333–356). St. Louis: Mosby.

Coveney, P., & Highfield, R. (1990). *The arrow of time: A voyage through science to solve time's greatest mystery.* New York: Fawcett Columbine.

Department of Health and Human Services (DHHS). (1982). *Forward plan for health 1977-1981.* Washington, DC: U.S. Government Printing Office.

Department of Health and Human Services (DHHS). (1998). *Healthy people in healthy communities: A guide for community leaders.* Washington, DC: Office of Disease Prevention and Health Promotion.

Department of Health and Human Services (DHHS). (1998). *Healthy people 2010 objectives: Draft for public comment.* Washington, DC: U.S. Government Printing Office.

Drapo, P. J., & Woods, E. (1992). Preparing community health nurses for the real world: Power, politics, and poverty. In *1991 Papers: State of the art in community health nursing education, research, and practice* (pp. 47–51). Lexington, KY: ACHNE.

Duhl L. J. (1986). *Health planning and social change.* New York: Human Sciences Press.

Dunn, H. L.(1959). High-level wellness for man and society. *American Journal of Public Health, 49,* 789.

Dunn, H. L.(1980). *High level wellness.* Thorofare, NJ: Charles B. Slack.

Edelman, C. L., & Fain, J. A. (1998). Health defined: Objectives for promotion & prevention. In C. L. Edleman & C. L. Mandle (Eds.), *Health promotion throughout the lifespan* (4th ed., pp. 3–24). St. Louis: Mosby.

Edney, A. T. B. (1992). Companion animals and human health. *Veterinary Record, 130*(4), 285–287.

Flynn, B. C. & Rider, M. S. (1991). Healthy cities Indiana: Mainstreaming community health in the United States. *American Journal of Public Health, 81,* 510–511.

Four Worlds Development Project. (1984). *The sacred tree.* Twin Lakes, WI: Lotus Light Publications.

Greene, B., & Winfrey, O. (1996). *Make the connection: Ten steps to a better body—and a better life.* New York: Hyperion.

Green, L. W., & Raeburn, J. (1990). Contemporary developments in health promotion: Definitions and challenges. In N. Bracht (Ed.), *Health promotion at the community level* (pp. 19–44). Newbury Park, CA: Sage Publications.

Greiner, P. A., & Berry, R. D. (1992). Student-faculty partnerships in a nurse-managed clinic for the homeless. In *1991 Papers: State of the art in community health nursing education, research, and practice* (pp. 67–69). Lexington, KY: ACHNE.

Healthy People 2010 (1998): http://web.health.gov/healthypeople/2010fctsht.html.

Hochbaum, G. M. (1958). *Public participation in medical screening programs: A socio-psychological study.* (Publication No. 572). Bethesda, MD: Public Health Service.

Jette, A. M., Lachman, M., Giorgetti, M. M., Assmann, S. F., Harris, B. A., Levenson, C., Wernick, M., & Krebs, D. (1999). Exercise—It's never too late: The strong-for-life program. *American Journal of Public Health, 89*(1), 66–72.

Jones, J. (1999). *Jeanne Jones' homestyle cooking made healthy.* Red Oak, IA: Rodale Press.

Laying the foundation for Healthy People 2010—The first year of consultation. (1998): http://web.health.gov/healthypeople/2010article.htm.

Kulbok, P. A, & Baldwin, J. H. (1992). From preventive health behavior to health promotion: Advancing a positive construct of health. *Advances in Nursing Science, 14*(4), 50–64.

Kulbok, P. A., Baldwin, J. H., Cox, C. L., & Duffy, R. (1997). Advancing discourse on health promotion: Beyond mainstream thinking. *Advances in Nursing Science, 20*(1), 13–21.

Kulbok, P. A., Carter, K. F., Baldwin, J. H., Gilmartin, M. J., & Kirkwood, B. (1999). The multidimensional health behavior inventory. *Journal of Nursing Measurement, 7*(2), 177–195.

Laffrey, S. C., & Kulbok, P. A. (1999). An integrative model for holistic community nursing. *Journal of Holistic Nursing, 17*(1), 88–103.

Mandle, C. L., & Castle, J. E. (1998). Health promotion & the individual. In C. L. Edleman and C. L. Mandle (Eds.), *Health promotion throughout the lifespan* (4th ed., pp. 119–143). St. Louis: Mosby.

Maslow, A. W. (1970). *Motivation and personality.* New York: Harper & Row.

McCarthy, N. C., & Mandle, C. L. (1998a). Health promotion & the family. In C. L. Edleman & C. L. Mandle (Eds.), *Health promotion throughout the lifespan* (4th ed., pp. 144–170). St. Louis: Mosby.

McCarthy, N. C., & Mandle, C. L. (1998b). Health promotion & the community. In C. L. Edleman & C. L. Mandle (Eds.), *Health promotion throughout the lifespan* (4th ed., pp. 171–192). St. Louis: Mosby.

McDonald, I. (1997). *Holistic wellness: Self inventory of personal wellness utilizing the medicine wheel.* Unpublished manuscript.

McGinnis, J. M., & Foege, W. H. (1993). Actual causes of death in the United States. *Journal of the American Medical Association, 270*(18).

Model standards. (1998): www.apha.org/science/model/msmain.html.

Moore, V., Neff, D., Smith, G., & Weber, J. (1999). *The homeless in Utah County: Food & Care Coalition.* Unpublished manuscript. Provo, UT: Brigham Young University College of Nursing.

Naisbitt, J. (1982). *Megatrends.* New York: Warner Books.

National Institutes of Health. (1987). *The health benefits of pets.* (Publication No. 1988-216-107.) Washington, DC: U.S. Government Printing Office.

National Institute for Occupational Safety and Health (1996). *National Occupational Research Agenda.* (DHHS [NIOSH] Publication No. 96-115.) Washington, DC: U.S. Government Printing Office.

Neuhauser, L., Schwab, M., Syme, S. L., & Bieber, M. (1998). Community participation in health promotion: Evaluation of the California Wellness Guide. *Health Promotion International, 13*(3), 211–223.

Orem, D. E. (1985). *Nursing: Concepts of practice* (3rd ed.) New York: McGraw-Hill.

Padilla, G. V., & Bulcavage, L. M. (1991). Theories used in patient/health education. *Seminars in Oncological Nursing, 7*(2), 87–96.

Palank, C. L. (1991). Determinants of health-promotive behavior: A review of current research. *Nursing Clinics of North America, 26*(4), 815–832.

Pender, N. (1987). *Health promotion in nursing practice* (2nd ed.). East Norwalk, CT: Appleton & Lange.

Piper, M. (1999). *Another country: Navigating the emotional terrain of our elders.* Los Angeles: Riverhead Books.

Poe, B. S., & O'Neill, K. O. (1997). Caffeine modulates heat shock induced apoptosis in the human promyelocytic leukemia cell line HL-60. *Cancer Letters, 121,* 1–6.

Prigogine, I., & Stengers, I. (1984). *Order out of chaos.* New York: Bantam Books.

Rosenstock, I. M. (1974). Historical origins of the health belief model. In M. H. Becker (Ed.), *The health belief model and personal health behavior* (pp. 1–8). Thorofare, NJ: Charles B. Slack.

Ryan, R. S, & Travis, J. W. (1991). Introduction. In R. S. Ryan & J. W. Travis (Eds.), *Wellness: Small changes you can use to make a big difference* (p. 3). Berkeley, CA: Ten Speed Press.

Sandhu, G. K. (1998). Health promotion for the twenty-first century: Throughout the lifespan and throughout the world. In C. L. Edleman & C. L. Mandle (Eds.), *Health promotion throughout the lifespan* (4th ed., pp. 667–675). St. Louis: Mosby.

Segal, L., Dalton, A. C., & Richardson, J. (1998). Cost-effectiveness of the primary prevention of non-insulin dependent diabetes mellitus. *Health Promotion International, 13*(3), 197–211.

Simmons, S. J. (1990). The health-promoting self-care system model: Directions for nursing research and practice. *Journal of Advances in Nursing, 15*(10), 1162–1166.

Simopoulos, A. P. (1999). *The omega diet.* New York: HarperCollins.

Steiger, N. J., & Lipson, J. C. (1985). *Self-care nursing: Theory and practice.* Bowie, MD: Brady Communications.

United States Preventive Services Task Force. (1989). *A guide to clinical preventive services: An assessment of the effectiveness of 169 interventions.* Baltimore, MD: Williams & Wilkins.

United States Public Health Service (USPHS). (1979). *Healthy people: The surgeon general's report on health promotion and disease prevention.* (DHEW Publication No. 79-55071.) Washington, DC: U.S. Department of Health, Education, and Welfare.

United States Public Health Service (USPHS). (1980). *Promoting health/preventing disease: Objectives for the nation.* (DHHS Publication No. 0-349-256.) Washington, DC: Department of Health and Human Services.

United States Public Health Service (USPHS). (1989). *Promoting health/preventing disease: Year 2000 objectives for the nation.* Washington, DC: U.S. Department of Health and Human Services.

United States Public Health Service (USPHS). (1990). *Healthy people 2000: National health promotion and disease prevention objectives.* Washington, DC: U.S. Department of Health and Human Services.

Webster's Encyclopedic Unabridged Dictionary of the English Language. (1996). New York: Gramercy Books/Random House.

Wheatley, J. (1994). *Leadership and the new science: Learning about organization from an orderly universe.* San Francisco, CA: Berrett-Koehler.

11

Holistic and Complementary Health

Margaret A. Burkhardt

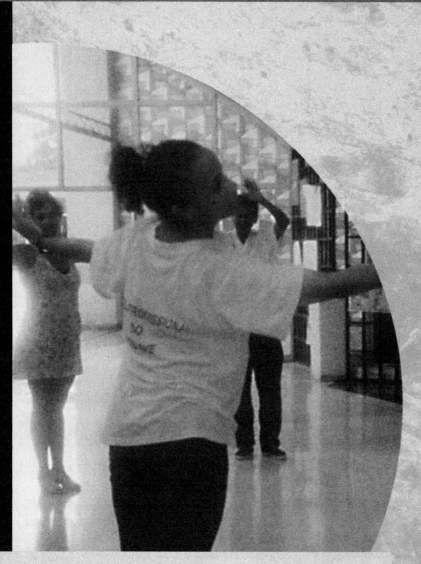

In recent years, health care professionals have become increasingly interested in therapies that lie outside the realm of conventional Western allopathic medicine. Many such therapies derive from folk wisdom, cultural perspectives, and healing practices of indigenous peoples and other ancient healing systems.

Chapter Focus

Holistic Framework

Historical Influences

Complementary Modalities: What Are They?

Complementary Health and Community Nursing Practice
  The Right to Choose
  Nursing Assessment

Potential Barriers to Use of Complementary Therapies

Integrating Complementary Therapies into Community Nursing Care
  Spirituality
  Music Therapy
  Imagery
  Herbal Therapies
  Touch Therapy

Questions to Consider

After reading this chapter, answer the following questions:

1. What is complementary health?
2. How does a nurse know when to choose a complementary intervention?
3. What are barriers to using complementary therapy?
4. What are some of the most common complementary therapies?
5. How does the community health nurse evaluate the effectiveness of complementary therapy?

Key Terms

Complementary health
Healing
Herbal therapies
Music therapy

Touch therapy
Office of Alternative Medicine (OAM)
Mind-body medicine

Health is wholeness, unfolding:
It is sharing, significantly, increasingly,
    in the varieties of human experience:
    physically, in the range of activities
        in which the human body can engage;
        not only aggression, but also conciliation,
        not only the proprieties, but also the singularities,
        not only to exhaustion, but also to the crest of vitality;
    sensually, in the possibilities of sensation;
        not confined to extremes:
            rage and excitement, passivity, suppression;
            not to pain:
            the pain of separation,
            the fear of aloneness;
        but knowing the quiet depths, the tenderness, the
            nuances flowing from tones, textures, odors,
            flavors;
            the joy of well-being, of union and reunion,
            the awesomeness of intimacy;
    culturally, socially, in the designs for living,
        across time and across the world:
        ways of talking, eating, dressing, pleasuring;
        ideas of beauty, of truth, of rightness.
It is growing in awareness:
    of sharing, significantly;
    of self;
    rising above existence, beyond time and space,
        the uniqueness of man.
And it is feeling good about it all, coming into Self-hood:
    expressing one's inner power,
    articulating one's reason-for-being,
    accepting one's sexuality,
        and interdependence:
        receiving and giving,
    holding on and letting go,
    following and guiding.
Toward wholeness:
    responding to the possibilities and limitations of human
        experience,
    reciprocating, resting, resurgent again;
    exploring, discovering
    opening, unfolding,
        from diffuseness toward coherence,
        simplicity toward complexity,
        disparity toward complementarity,
        vagueness toward decisiveness,
        confusion toward understanding,
        toward wholeness.

—Nancy Milio

More persons today are using alternative or unconventional therapies, either instead of allopathic modalities or combined with other
nonallopathic approaches. These approaches are often termed
complementary when they are used in addition to conventional
therapies. In this chapter, *complementary therapy* is used regardless
of the pattern of use, recognizing that health care providers need to
be open to exploring various approaches to health and healing to
support the best possible outcomes for clients.

RESEARCH BRIEF

Keegan, L. (1996). *Use of alternative therapies among Mexican Americans in the Texas Rio Grande Valley.* Journal of Holistic Nursing, 14(4), 277–294.

This descriptive study explored use of alternative
health practices among Mexican Americans in the
Texas Rio Grande Valley. A convenience sample of 213
subjects accessed through local clinics and hospitals
were surveyed using a one-page bilingual written
form designed to ascertain prevalence and use of alternative therapies, range of medical conditions for
which subjects were currently seeking care, and demographic characteristics of subjects. Findings indicated that 44% of respondents had used an alternative practice one or more times in the past year,
although 66% never reported the use of alternatives
to their biomedical practitioner. The alternative practices used included herbal medicine, prayer/spiritual
healing, massage, relaxation techniques, chiropractic,
curandero, megavitamins, imagery, energy healing,
acupuncture, biofeedback, hypnosis, and homeopathy.
The most commonly used alternative therapies were
herbal medicine, prayer/spiritual healing, massage,
relaxation techniques, chiropractic, and visits to a
Mexican folk healer (*curandero*).

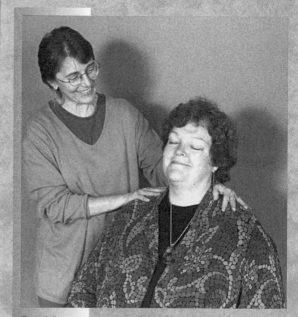

Dr. Margaret A. Burkhardt, chapter author, demonstrating healing touch with a client.

Nurses within the community need to be familiar with various healing modalities used by their clients and aware of complementary modalities that may promote health, enhance healing, or contribute to unhealthy outcomes with clients. This chapter discusses a holistic framework for the integration of complementary therapies into care, understanding of complementary modalities, and assessment processes and ethical issues regarding **complementary health**. Selected complementary modalities are discussed that can be incorporated into community nursing care.

. . . .

Care and love are the most universal, the most tremendous, and the most mysterious of cosmic forces; they comprise the primal and universal psychic energy.

Jean Watson

. . . .

Holistic Framework

A holistic understanding of life that appreciates that each person is a bio-psycho-social-spiritual unity provides a framework for inclusion of complementary modalities into nursing care. Within a holistic framework, nurses are attentive to *healing* as well as to *curing* (Burkhardt, 1985; Quinn, 1989). Curing is a process that attends to disordered physical or psychological parts of a person, with a focus on disease processes and restoration of the integrity of a specific component (usually physiological) of a person. The allopathic approach focuses on curing by combating disease with techniques that produce effects different from those produced by the disease (Dossey & Guzzetta, 2000).

Healing, on the other hand, acknowledges that disharmony in a whole person may be manifesting as disease or illness and seeks to understand the totality of the lived experience for a person, taking into account the personal response to and meaning of the apparent disease or illness process (Burkhardt & Nagai-Jacobson, 1997b). Healing requires a relationship between the caregiver and care receiver that acknowledges common humanity and connectedness. Physical, emotional, and spiritual concerns are addressed within the healing relationship. Healing may manifest as cure in one or more of the bio-psycho-emotional realms but can be present without a cure. Quinn (1989) aptly notes that, although diseases may be cured, people need healing. The desire to promote health, or the need for healing or curing, which is not being addressed by conventional approaches, often leads people to complementary modalities. Complementary or alternative therapies generally focus on body-mind-spirit integration through healing by an individual, healing between two individuals, or healing at a distance (Dossey & Guzzetta, 2000).

It is particularly important for nurses who work within the community to practice holistic nursing. Dealing with clients and families within their home environments enables nurses to appreciate cultural considerations in healing and to assess clients' use of

> **BOX 11-1 AMERICAN HOLISTIC NURSES' ASSOCIATION DESCRIPTION OF HOLISTIC NURSING**
>
> *Holistic nursing embraces all nursing practice that has healing the whole person as its goal. Holistic nursing recognizes that there are two views regarding holism: that holism involves studying and understanding the interrelationships of the bio-psycho-social-spiritual dimensions of the person, recognizing that the whole is greater than the sum of its parts; and that holism involves understanding the individual as an integrated whole interacting with and being acted on by both internal and external environments. Holistic nursing accepts both views, believing that the goals of nursing can be achieved within either framework.*
>
> *Holistic practice draws on nursing knowledge, theories, expertise, and intuition to guide nurses in becoming therapeutic partners with clients in strengthening the clients' responses to facilitate the healing process and achieve wholeness.*
>
> *Practicing holistic nursing requires nurses to integrate self-care in their own lives. Self-responsibility leads the nurse to a greater awareness of the interconnectedness of all individuals and their relationships to the human and global community, and permits nurses to use this awareness to facilitate healing.*
>
> Source: American Holistic Nurses' Association, 1994. Used with permission.

complementary modalities. Because holistic nursing has the healing of the whole person as its goal, nurses work in therapeutic partnership with clients and families to integrate those modalities that best facilitate the client's health and healing. Nurses also need to be aware of therapies that may be ineffective or cause potential harm when used alone or in combination with other modalities. The American Holistic Nurses' Association's description of holistic nursing presented in Box 11-1 provides a frame of reference for holistic nursing practice based on sound academic principles incorporating both the art and science of nursing.

Historical Influences

Before discussing complementary health care modalities, let's take a brief look at the process through which allopathic or biomedical care became the accepted "conventional" approach to health care in the United States. The United States is often referred to as a "melting pot" of persons from many different cultures, educational and socioeconomic backgrounds, and experiences. Health care practices have evolved (and continue to do so) from the healing traditions of both native peoples and those who have immigrated to this country. Before the mid-1800s, practitioners from various health care systems, including allopathy, naturopathy, homeopathy, and botanics, were acknowledged as legitimate healers in the United States. Micozzi (1996) notes that the history of contemporary biomedicine as a scientific paradigm was as much influenced by social history as by scientific laws. Allopathic biomedicine began to predominate by the mid-1800s and gained further prominence by the late 1800s through state licensing laws sponsored by and lobbied for by the American Medical Association.

Dossey and Swyers (1994) note that the prominence of biomedicine was shaped in part by two important developments. One development was in the realm of scientific discoveries, such as the identification of specific organisms as the cause of particular disease states and the identification of substances and vaccines that ward off the effect of pathogens, which greatly influenced the direction of biomedicine. The other was the 1910 release of Abraham Flexner's report titled *Medical Education in the United States and Canada*, which was influential in upgrading medical education programs, enabling medical schools with a stronger biomedical orientation to receive more financial backing from philanthropic foundations. This in turn prompted the stifling of medical schools teaching theories other than biomedical regarding the origin of illness and appropriate therapies. What was considered scientific was defined by biomedicine's "way of knowing," which emphasized that knowledge about the world requires empiricism (Micozzi, 1996). Other paradigms were either relegated to the "fringe" or subsumed into the biomedical paradigm. Although biomedicine gained power and prestige and became the gold standard for health care, small numbers of naturopathic, homeopathic, chiropractic, and practitioners of other healing systems continued to provide care.

Over the past several decades, however, health care consumers have become more active in seeking care outside the biomedical system. Some of the factors that may have contributed to this phenomenon include the following:

- *A shift away from infectious diseases as major causes of morbidity and mortality to health concerns that elude medical cure such as cancer, heart disease, hypertension, diabetes, and other chronic problems (Gordon, 1980)*
- *Increasingly depersonalized care and decreased personal control in health care decisions as a result of increased use of technology (Burkhardt & Nathaniel, 1998)*
- *A greater emphasis on self-care and personal responsibility for health*

- *A shrinking world that has allowed greater access to other cultures and their systems of healing*
- *Renewed appreciation that healing must address the whole body-mind-spirit person*

Although people have been using complementary therapies for years, the landmark study conducted by Eisenberg, Kessler, Foster, Norlock, Calkins, and Delbanco (1993) documented an unexpected frequency of use of these therapies and caused the medical establishment to take note. The results of this national telephone survey of 1,539 adults indicated that one in three Americans of all sociodemographic groups used complementary therapies, and of those who used these therapies, 72% did so without informing their conventional health care provider. This study also indicated that people tended to use complementary modalities for chronic rather than life-threatening conditions. To identify trends in alternative medicine use in the United States, Eisenberg, Rogers, Ettner, Appel, Wilkey, Van Rompay, and Kessler (1998) conducted another national telephone survey of 2,055 English-speaking adults in 1997 asking about their use of 16 therapies. The therapies included relaxation techniques, herbal medicine, massage, chiropractic, prayer or spiritual healing by others, megavitamins, self-help groups, imagery, commercial diet, folk remedies, lifestyle diet, energy healing, homeopathy, hypnosis, biofeedback, and acupuncture. Results of this survey indicated that alternative therapy use increased from 33.8% in 1990 to 42.1% in 1997. Use of herbal medicine, massage, megavitamins, self-help groups, folk remedies, energy healing, and homeopathy increased the most.

Keegan (1996) documented use of alternative therapies among Mexican Americans to be 44%, noting that 66% of this population never report the use of alternatives to conventional health care providers. Through a self-reporting survey of the use of complementary therapies among people in rural West Virginia, Burkhardt, Nathaniel, Nemeth-Pyles, and Boyd (1999) found that 83% of respondents (n545) used at least one of the 17 listed therapies within the past year. In this study, 41% of respondents reported that they never discuss these therapies with their health care provider and 34% only sometimes discuss these with their providers.

In response to growing awareness and use of complementary therapies, the National Institutes of Health (NIH) created the **Office of Alternative Medicine (OAM)** in 1992. The OAM was established to facilitate scientific and fair evaluation of complementary modalities that can contribute to the health and well-being of many people and reduce barriers to awareness and availability of promising complementary therapies. In 1998, the OAM was elevated to the National Center for Complementary and Alternative Medicine (NCCAM), one of the 25 institutes and centers of NIH. The NCCAM's mission is to conduct and support basic and applied research and training and to disseminate information on complementary and alternative medicine to practitioners and the public. The congressional mandate for the NCCAM provides for research training programs and a public information clearinghouse; however, the center is not a referral agency. The importance of research on and reliable information about complementary therapies is reflected in the increase in budget for the NCCAM from $2 million in 1993 to $50 million in 1999.

Complementary Modalities: What Are They?

Although the terms *alternative, complementary,* and *unconventional* are often used interchangeably in reference to nonbiomedical interventions, the term *complementary* best reflects the awareness that these therapies need to be considered adjuncts to, not replacements for, medical and surgical treatments. The definition of complementary modalities that was developed at the NIH/OAM Second Conference on Research Methodology in April 1995 notes that the broad domain of complementary and alternative medicine (CAM) encompasses all health systems, modalities, and practices other than those intrinsic to the politically dominant health system of a particular society or culture. CAM includes all practices and ideas self-defined by their users as preventing or treating illness or promoting health and well-being.

Each healing system (including biomedicine) has its own explanatory model that "summarizes the perceptions, assumptions, beliefs, theories, and facts that guide the logic of health care delivery" (Cassidy, 1996, p. 20). Some important distinctions between complementary and conventional medicine include differences in philosophical underpinnings, types of therapies offered, how therapies are administered, and interaction between practitioner and client (Cassidy, 1996; Dossey & Swyers, 1994). For example, in the biomedical model, the practitioner has traditionally been considered the authoritative expert who determines and designs care based on standardized treatments in which the client has variable involvement. With complementary systems, treatments are more often individualized and developed in collaboration with clients who are acknowledged as having responsibility for their own healing processes. Complementary systems generally appreciate that humans have natural built-in recuperative powers and often focus on therapies that enhance the client's natural healing processes. Unifying threads that are common to most complementary healing systems include emphasis on (1) one's relationships, sense of values, place in society, and sense of self; (2) the role of spiritual values and religion in health; (3) the impact on health of consciousness manifested through thoughts, feelings, attitudes, emotions, values, and perceived meanings; (4) diet, exercise, relaxation techniques, and modifications in lifestyle; and (5) utilization of whole foods and herbs rather than extracts (Dossey & Swyers, 1994). Many of these threads are common parts of nursing practice as well, and conventional medicine is beginning to pay more attention to them.

The NCCAM continues to use the seven fields of complementary and alternative health practice that were described in *Alternative Medicine: Expanding Medical Horizons* (National Institutes of Health, 1994) as the basis for the classification of alternative medical practices. The seven major categories of the classification each contain subcategories designated as *CAM*—practices that are not commonly used, accepted, or available in conventional medicine; *behavioral medicine*—practices that may fall within the domain of conventional medicine; or *overlapping*—practices that can be in either subcategory (NCCAM, 1999). The seven fields of practice with associated NCCAM classifications of alternative medicine practice are briefly summarized in the following section. Because the listing of specific modalities and therapies is updated and expanded on regularly, only a few selected examples are given for each category. The reader is encouraged to visit the NCCAM Web site for further information.

Diet, Nutrition, and Lifestyle Changes

This field focuses on the use of dietary and nutritional interventions in preventing illness, maintaining health, and reversing the effects of chronic disease. The rise in chronic illnesses related to diet has prompted a shift in nutritional research toward dealing with the effects of nutritional excess and away from eliminating nutritional deficiency. Evidence indicates that inadequate intake of some micronutrients may increase risks of problems such as coronary artery disease, cancers, and birth defects and that the required daily allowance for some minerals and vitamins may not be adequate to prevent chronic illnesses. Many alternative diets and dietary lifestyles that foster the inclusion of more fresh and freshly prepared fruits and vegetables, whole grains, and legumes may offer greater resistance to illness. For example, increased consumption of beans and lentils appears to decrease the risk of colon cancer (National Institutes of Health, 1994).

The NCCAM classifications *biologically based therapies* and *lifestyle and disease prevention* both relate to this field of practice. *Biologically based therapies*, which include naturally and biologically based products, may overlap with use of dietary supplements by conventional practitioners. The four subcategories are as follows:

1. Phytotherapy or herbalism: *plant-derived preparations used for therapeutic and preventative purposes, such as gingko biloba, echinacea, and green tea*

2. Special diet therapies: *dietary approaches used as alternative therapies for particular risk factors or for chronic disease in general, such as vegetarian, Pritikin, and macrobiotic*

3. Orthomolecular medicine: *products not covered in other categories that are used (usually in combinations and at high doses) as nutritional and food supplements for preventive or therapeutic purposes, such as ascorbic acid, co-enzyme Q10, and melatonin*

4. Pharmacological, biological, and instrumental interventions: *products and procedures applied in an unconventional manner, such as cartilage, enzyme therapies, iridology*

Lifestyle and disease prevention, which focuses on preventing illness, identifying and treating risk factors, and supporting healing, is concerned with integrative approaches for prevention and management of chronic conditions. The three subcategories are as follows:

1. Clinical preventive practices: *unconventional approaches, such as medical intuition and electrodermal diagnosis, used to screen for or prevent health-related concerns*

2. Lifestyle therapies: *changes or therapies based on unconventional systems of care or used in unconventional ways, such as dietary or behavioral changes, exercise, and addiction control*

3. Health promotion: *involves research on healing and the healing process, autoregulatory mechanisms, and factors affecting health promotion*

Mind-Body Control

This field focuses on the mind's capacity to affect the body and explores healing systems that make use of the interconnectedness of mind, body, and spirit. Most traditional healing systems acknowledge and incorporate the interconnectedness of mind-body-spirit, recognizing the power of each to affect the other. In the past 30 years, biomedicine has opened more to the awareness of the impact of the mind on the body, although exploring the role of spirituality in healing is still in its infancy. Mind-body-spirit interventions often enable clients to experience and express their illnesses in new and clearer ways and to explore the meaning aspects, which can have direct consequences on their health. Scientific exploration suggests that there is a complex interaction among the mind and neurological and immune systems (psychoneuroimmunology), which can be affected by interventions in this category.

The NCCAM classification of **mind-body medicine**, which involves psychological, social, behavioral, and spiritual approaches to health, relates to this field of practice. The four subcategories are as follows:

1. Mind-body systems: *whole systems that are used in combination with lifestyle or are part of traditional healing systems*

2. Mind-body methods: *specific modalities incorporating awareness of mind-body interaction in healing, such as yoga, t'ai chi, meditation, imagery,* **music therapy**, *and psychotherapy*

3. Religion and spirituality: *the nonbehavioral aspects of religion and spirituality that relate to biological function or clinical condition, such as nonlocality, confession, and spiritual healing*

4. Social and contextual factors: *interventions that are social, cultural, symbolic, or contextual in nature, such as caring-based approaches like holistic nursing, intuitive diagnosis, and community-based approaches like certain Native American rituals*

Alternative Systems of Practice

It is estimated that worldwide only 10% to 30% of human health care is delivered by conventional biomedically oriented practitioners. The remaining 70% to 90% of care varies from self-care according to folk principles to care sought within an organized health care system derived from traditions or practices that flow from paradigms of health and healing different from that of biomedicine. Some of these explanatory models have sound bases that have been developed, tested, and practiced over many more years than biomedicine. However, because they derive from a different worldview, the processes and modes of action of many of these modalities are not understood within the biomedical paradigm.

The NCCAM classification *alternative medical systems*, which addresses complete systems of theory and practice other than the Western biomedical approach, contains four categories:

1. Acupuncture and oriental medicine, *including herbal formulas, t'ai chi, and diet*

2. Traditional indigenous systems, *including Native American healing, Ayurvedic medicine, and traditional African healing*

3. Unconventional Western systems, *including homeopathy, environmental medicine, and Cayce-based systems*

4. Naturopathy, *including other natural systems and therapies*

Manual Healing

Touch or manipulation with the hands has been part of healing traditions as far back as one can explore. Although contemporary biomedical providers tend to be distanced from physical contact with clients because of attitudes of reliance on diagnostic equipment and tests, as well as legal and time constraints, at one time physicians' hands were considered their most important diagnostic and therapeutic tool. Manual healing methods derive from the understanding that dysfunction of one area of the body can affect the function of other discrete body parts. It is worth noting that osteopathic medicine was one of the earliest U.S. health care systems to use manual healing methods.

The NCCAM classification *manipulative and body-based systems* focuses on therapies and systems that are based on movement or manipulation of the body. The three subcategories are as follows:

1. Chiropractic medicine

2. Massage and body work, *including osteopathic manipulative therapy, Swedish massage, Chinese Tui Na massage and acupressure, and body psychotherapy*

3. Unconventional physical therapies, *including hydrotherapy, light and color therapies, and heat and electrotherapies*

Pharmacological/Biological Treatments

This includes any assortment of drugs, biological products, and vaccines not yet accepted by conventional medicine. Examples of some such products include cartilage products derived from sharks, chicken, and sheep, used for treating cancer; ethylene diamine tetraacetic acid (EDTA) chelation therapy, used for treating heart disease and preventing cancer; a liquid extract from mistletoe plants (iscador), used to treat tumors; and biologically guided chemotherapy.

The NCCAM classification *biologically based therapies*, which was discussed earlier, relates to this field of practice.

Bioelectromagnetic Applications

This is an emerging science studying how living organisms interact with electromagnetic fields. The understanding that electrical phenomena are found in all living organisms and that electrical currents in the body can produce magnetic fields extending outside the body is basic to this field of study. Exploration suggests that changes in the body's natural fields can produce physical and behavioral changes and that certain frequencies have specific effects on body tissues.

The NCCAM clarifications *biofield* and *bioelectromagnetics* relate to this field of practice. *Biofield* healing practices, which use subtle energy fields in and around the body for healing and health promotion, include healing touch, Reiki, therapeutic touch, and external Qi Gong. *Bioelectromagnetics* includes the unconventional use of electromagnetic fields for healing and health promotion.

Herbal Therapies

All cultures and healing traditions have included the use of plants and plant products. Many of today's drugs have herbal origins, and approximately 25% of drugs dispensed from pharmacies have at least one active ingredient derived from plants. According to the World Health Organization, an estimated 4 billion people (80% of the world's population) use **herbal therapies** for some aspect of primary care. Herbal therapies are a major component of indigenous healing traditions. Because of U.S. Food and Drug Administration regulations, herbal products can be marketed in the United States only as food supplements and can boast no specific health claims.

The NCCAM classification *biologically based therapies*, which was discussed earlier, relates to this field of practice. Aromatherapy is considered in this classification.

The national health goals of *Healthy People 2010: Increasing the Span of Healthy Life for Americans, Reducing Health Disparities among Americans, and Achieving Access to Preventive Services for all Americans* are designed to help bring the people of the United States to their full potential. The opportunities or objectives designated for achieving these goals relate to health promotion, health protection, and preventive services. Although the document does not address complementary modalities per se, many people use complementary therapies as part of their efforts to promote health and prevent illness. Most complementary modalities included in the classification system at the NCCAM relate to the goal of increasing the span of healthy life for people in this country. Appropriate use of complementary therapies and their practitioners may ultimately contribute to the goals of reducing health disparities. Because many complementary therapies focus on health promotion and illness prevention, appropriately integrating them into health care may promote access to preventive services for people in this country. Although research on the role of many complementary modalities in health promotion and prevention has expanded in recent years, more validation of the efficacy of these therapies is needed. Because health promotion strategies relate to individual lifestyle and choices, nurses need to be particularly aware of choices people make regarding the use of complementary therapies in dealing with health promotion and illness prevention.

Complementary Health and Community Nursing Practice

Community health nurses must remember that decisions about health care are based on more than scientific expertise. Health care choices are influenced by a person's values, culture, and spiritual and other beliefs; evaluation of risks, benefits, and economic considerations; and effects on lifestyle and role. All of these areas must be considered in deliberations about health care. Cassidy (1996) writes that "cultural relativity is pivotal to the study of alternative medicine, because each alternative system of medicine provides a different set of ideas about the body, disease, and medical reality" (p. 12). Community nurses need to be particularly attentive to the influence of culture because emotional, psychological, aesthetic, interpersonal, and other dimensions of health concerns differ across cultures and belief systems, impelling certain actions and constraining others (O'Connor, 1996). Our culture teaches us the meaning of health; how to be sick; and when, how, and from whom to seek care.

Community nurses must be aware of the values, goals, and beliefs of personal culture (their own and that of their clients), as well as the culture of the biomedical system and of other healing systems as they develop health care plans with clients. With this awareness, nurses can be more alert for potential conflicts and negative value judgments that may interfere with integrating complementary modalities into care. Consider, for example, a situation in which a nurse learns that her client with fibromyalgia is using herbs and vitamins recommended by a layperson who used kinesiology to determine what the client needed. Recognizing that the culture of the biomedical system would find this process unscientific alerts the nurse to potential negative value judgments from the client's biomedical practitioner regarding her choice and enables the nurse to consider ways to assist the client in integrating the different modalities. Clients are more likely to discuss their complementary health practices with nurses who approach them with an openness to exploring and including different modalities in care than they are with nurses who place judgments on such modalities.

The Right to Choose

Professional standards and codes of ethics direct nurses to respect each person and to value and support client autonomy. Basic to autonomy are the ability to determine personal goals, the ability to decide on a plan of action, and the freedom to act on one's choice. Consequently, the principle of client self-determination directs nurses to honor the right of persons to use modalities outside the realm of biomedicine in addressing their health care needs. When such choices are made, nurses may find it challenging to honor and respect the convictions derived from belief systems that underlie these choices, particularly when these beliefs are not understood or are contrary to their own. However, to deny such convictions in health care settings is "to deny the patient's very reality, sometimes risking serious psychological and emotional impact on patient and family alike, and always raising genuine ethical concerns about patient autonomy, provider beneficence, substituted judgment, and distributive justice" (O'Connor, 1996, p. 93). Attentiveness to client values and desires for treatment options require nurses to take seriously the client's need for healing as well as curing, and the contributions to health offered by other explanatory models. When nurses do not understand the other modality or question the efficacy or safety of the choice, they must explore these considerations with the client. A nonjudgmental approach that is respectful of differing values and beliefs and alert for ethnocentric bias on the part of the nurse enhances joint exploration (Burkhardt & Nathaniel, 1996).

Nursing Assessment

To have a broad picture of the many factors affecting a client's health and healing, nurses need to be aware of the various therapies being considered or used by clients. Community nurses need to develop the ability to incorporate discussion of complementary therapies into their nursing assessment in an open way, because clients may be hesitant to bring up the subject. Discussion may be prompted through open-ended questions such as "What do you do to take care of your health on your own?" "What other things have you tried (or thought about trying) for this health concern?" and "Sometimes people with your condition want to try other remedies, and I wonder if this is something that you have considered?" Another approach to opening a discussion of complementary therapies is to explore the use of specific modalities commonly used in your area with questions such as "Have you ever seen a (chiropractor, acupuncturist, herbalist, etc.) for that problem?" "Have you considered seeing the (*curandera*, medicine person, spiritual healer, etc.)?" or "Have you been using (special vitamins, a macrobiotic diet, herbal remedies, etc.) for your illness?"

Nurses must be knowledgeable about various modalities and therapies to effectively discuss their use with clients. Nurses need not subscribe to particular complementary therapies to effectively assess how clients use these therapies. Nor do nurses need to be practitioners of other modalities to discuss them with clients, any more than they need to be able to do surgery to discuss it. However, community nurses must be able to create an atmosphere that encourages a nonjudgmental assessment of all modalities being considered or used, with a goal of using whatever is beneficial for and will meet the needs of the client and family.

Community nurses should become familiar with and develop at least a talking knowledge of complementary therapies that may be commonly used in their communities to be better able to discuss their use with their clients. Many therapies work as an adjunct to biomedical interventions, some may interact in unhealthy ways with particular biomedical treatments, and the efficacy of many modalities is not fully known. When discussing choices with clients, nurses should draw on studies with which they are familiar in offering relevant information regarding particular therapies, allowing clinical and personal experience into the conversation in judicious ways, yet recognizing that the nurse never has all the pertinent information and that uncertainty is inherent in health choices (Hufford, 1996b). Based on their assessment and knowledge regarding particular therapies, nurses may find it appropriate to support or recommend some complementary modalities while discouraging the use of others.

Hufford (1996b) suggests that the client has major responsibility for obtaining information regarding complementary therapies and making health choices in this regard. However, nurses need to have some knowledge about risks and benefits associated with these therapies. For example, although garlic may assist in lowering cholesterol, large doses can cause irritation to the digestive tract, which may result in some bleeding. Nurses should encourage clients to explore the validity of claims made about particular therapies and assist them in doing so, especially if the nurse perceives the therapy to be potentially harmful for the client. However, complementary modalities should not be discounted merely because they are not understood within the Western biomedical framework. When clients are interested in complementary therapies, nurses should help determine whether risks are involved. When the potential for significant risks exists and the client is committed to using the therapy, the nursing goal is to minimize risks while maximizing treatment. If the client does not have as strong commitment to the complementary modality, nurses should encourage ongoing discussion of known risks and benefits related to various options (Hufford, 1996a). As part of their assessments, nurses need to determine the congruency between client and nursing goals regarding healing and curing; they also should review options considered viable by each as a means of meeting these goals. Maintaining an openness to working with traditional systems and their healers facilitates more effective and culturally congruent nursing and health care.

Potential Barriers to Use of Complementary Therapies

Professional integrity requires nurses to take an honest look at potential barriers that may limit availability of and access to complementary therapies for clients and that may hinder the research of complementary therapies. Dossey and Swyers (1994) suggest that barriers to use of complementary therapies can be structural in nature or can relate to regulatory, economic, and belief systems. Structural barriers include problems caused by a lack of common classification systems and definitions between biomedicine and complementary modalities, difficulty in obtaining original research on complementary therapies because they are not published in English in scientifically reviewed literature, and lack of understanding of culturally based explanatory models. For example, a family may wish to obtain more information about the efficacy of an herbal preparation that they heard may help with their mother's chronic illness, but the major research is published in Chinese. Regulatory and economic barriers include current federal mechanisms for regulating medical research, which do not favor the evaluation of many forms of complementary treatments; the cost of conducting the necessary laboratory and clinical trials of a product or procedure; and the existence of state medical practice acts that limit the practice of healing arts to holders of medical licenses. An example of this barrier is the limited access to naturopathic physicians because they are not licensed in most states.

Belief barriers include ideological skepticism flowing from comfort with the status quo, belief that high technology interventions are more effective, and attitudes that any modality other than biomedicine is unscientific. These barriers include attitudes of conventional practitioners that consider use of herbal preparations rather than medical intervention as a waste of money because they have not been "scientifically" studied, even when the client is experiencing benefit from the preparations. Although the work of the NCCAM and other organizations is helping reduce these barriers, nurses need to be alert for situations in which clients experience limited access to or availability of complementary modalities.

Power relationship between the nurse and client can present barriers to the client's use of complementary therapies. The nurse is in a role of power and authority derived from professional knowledge and skills. Persisting paternalistic attitudes within health care settings, which foster the dependent role for clients, may manifest as attitudes indicating that approaches to managing health concerns other than those proposed by the nurse are unacceptable and without sound basis. Consider, for example, a nurse who is very willing to support the physician's recommendation of surgery or strong narcotics for the management of severe pain but who is unwilling to discuss the client's interest in trying acupuncture, declaring that such approaches are unreliable. When nurses assume that a client's values and thought processes are the same as their own, they may believe that the only reasonable courses of action are those that they would choose. Such attitudes may prompt nurses to question the decision-making capacity of clients who choose complementary therapies in lieu of or in addition to conventional therapies or label them as noncompliant, both of which can present barriers to the client's use of therapies that may enhance the healing process.

Integrating Complementary Therapies into Community Nursing Care

As noted previously, holistic care should be the goal of all nursing practice. Although holistic care presumes attention to physical, mental, emotional, and spiritual concerns, many look upon spirituality as complementary therapy. The tendency to view body and spirit as separate and unrelated entities (which persists within contemporary health care settings) supports the view that physical concerns are the prime focus of biomedicine and that spirituality has little or no place in biomedical care. However, body-mind-spirit are inextricably intertwined, and spirituality cannot be separated from physical and emotional health.

This section briefly discusses ways of integrating spirituality and selected complementary modalities into nursing care. When considering integrating any modality into practice, nurses need to address two fundamental concerns: (1) safety—the potential side effects and risks for harm when the therapy is used alone or in combination with other therapies, and (2) efficacy—the therapy produces the effect that it is intended to produce. The examples of complementary modalities presented here are chosen because they can be particularly valuable nursing interventions that clearly fall within nursing's domain of practice. Educational programs are available through which nurses can become certified practitioners of many of these therapies. Although it is within nursing's domain of practice to address diet, nutrition, and lifestyle changes, nurses must recognize that when such modalities are considered complementary or alternative, they are based on nonorthodox systems of healing or are applied in unconventional ways. Nurses need to be aware that their clients are using these modalities, their reasons for using them, and potential risks and benefits.

The nursing role includes supporting that which promotes health and healing, advising caution where risks are involved, facilitating open communication about various options, and honoring the client's right to choose. Nurses can become knowledgeable about, and through training become, practitioners of alternative healing modalities such as acupuncture, oriental medicine, homeopathy, and Ayurvedic medicine. Some aspects of other healing systems may be easily integrated into nursing care, such as use of particular acupressure points for relief of headaches or nausea. However, nurses need to be aware of the scope of practice stated in their state's nurse practice act and incorporate only those modalities that are within their scope of nursing practice.

Spirituality

Spirituality is the essence of who one is, a unifying or animating force that permeates all of one's life and being. This essence is expressed in and through connectedness with one's self, with others, with nature, and with a God or a Life Force. Although one's spirituality and relationship with God or Life Force is often nurtured and expressed through one's religious beliefs and practices, for many, spirituality transcends the boundaries of religion. Spirituality is connected to values and is vital to the process of discovering meaning and purpose in life. Spiritual issues are core life issues that are often related to mystery, suffering, forgiveness, grace, hope, and love (Burkhardt & Nagai-Jacobson, 1997a, 2000).

The nursing assessment of spirituality requires attentive listening, the ability to be fully present with the client in this moment, and good communication skills. Assessment of spiritual concerns with clients includes exploration of issues of meaning and purpose; important values, beliefs, and practices; prayer or meditation styles; important relationships and their influence on the present circumstances; and desires for connection with religious groups or rituals. The process of assessment often is part of the intervention because merely providing the opportunity for clients to talk of their spiritual concerns enables them to become more aware of their spiritual journey and its impact on present life experiences. Because people often use story and metaphor in expressing their spirituality and spiritual concerns, nurses can approach spirituality by encouraging people to tell their stories. In this process, nurses can gain insight into those connections that support and inspire a client, relationships in need of healing, sources of strength, experiences that have given life meaning, and ways in which the person questions the meaning of life. Nurses can help clients attune to their spirituality by exploring and incorporating meaningful rituals into care such as sacred readings, drumming, and music; facilitating processes focused on mindfulness such as relaxation exercises, imagery, and paying attention to physical sensations; and fostering consideration of the place and meaning of prayer for clients and the ways they do or do not experience God or Life Force in their lives. Nurses need to be aware of their own spiritual perspectives to honor their own values and beliefs without imposing them on clients.

Prayer

The experience of prayer or some form of connecting to the "beyond" is fundamental to human life and experience. Dossey (1993, 1996, 1997, 1998) discusses the extensive evidence indicating that prayer and religious devotion are associated with health outcomes. He notes that research on intercessory prayer and distant intentionality indicate that open-ended, nondirective prayer such as "Thy will be done" or "Whatever is best for all concerned" is more efficacious than prayers for particular outcomes. He also reminds us that prayer does not require scientific evidence for validation. Prayer is an appropriate nursing intervention, whether the nurse prays for or with clients or arranges for clients to have the quiet and privacy needed for prayer or meditation. Nurses who include prayer as part of their client care need to remember that prayer has many forms and expressions and is culturally conditioned.

When nurses incorporate prayer for clients into their personal spiritual practices, they should not presume to know what the client needs; rather, they should express prayer in terms such as, "Whatever is for the client's highest good." Nurses who wish to pray with clients should do so with the client's permission and encourage clients to use their own forms and expressions of prayer. Very often, clients in health care institutions need nurses to help them make sacred space within daily routines in order to attend to their own prayer, either alone or with others.

Music Therapy

Music has been a vital part of all cultures and societies and has been linked with healing throughout history. Guzzetta (1997, 2000) notes that music therapy complements conventional therapies by providing clients with integrated body-mind experiences and by facilitating relaxation, self-healing, and active participation in health and recovery. Music can promote relaxation and can produce changes in emotions, behavior, and physiology. Music can be used alone or in conjunction with prayer, meditation, relaxation exercises, and guided imagery. Musical vibrations can help restore or maintain the body's regulatory function; can help reduce pain, anxiety, isolation, and psychophysiological stress; can enhance the immune system; and can facilitate development of self-awareness and help improve memory (Guzzetta, 1997, 2000).

Guzzetta reminds us that, when considering using music therapy with clients, nurses need to assess clients' music preferences, the importance of music in their lives, and the types of music that make them happy, sad, relaxed, tense, and so forth. Nurses must be aware that no one selection or type of music is best for all people or in all situations and that the client's mood and preferences determine the types of music used and the goals of each session. Nurses can introduce clients to music therapy, initially guide them through the process, and help them develop their own healing scripts and music libraries. Guzzetta (1997, 2000) offers guidelines for incorporating music therapy into clinical settings and provides a script that nurses can use with clients during a music therapy session. Research conducted through the music therapy program at the University of Miami indicated that music contributed to an increase in levels of melatonin and human growth hormone (leading to better sleep patterns and fewer aches and pains) in Alzheimer's clients and that the combined use of music and guided imagery in clinical trials contributed to lower liver enzymes in clients with chronic hepatitis B and lower levels of stress hormones in healthy persons (Simonton, Cohen, Kumar, McKinney, & Tims, 1997).

Imagery

Imagery is a way of using the imagination and connecting with the more subtle aspects of inner experiences that may involve all senses—vision, taste, smell, touch, and hearing. Images, which can be considered a bridge between conscious processing of information and physiological change, can be produced by conscious as well as subconscious acts and may precede or follow physiological change (Dossey, 1997; Schaub, 2000). Imagery enables access to our emotions and to our spiritual or higher self. Dossey (1997) describes several types of imagery: receptive, active, symbolic, process, correct biological, end-state, general healing, packaged, customized, and interactive guided imagery. Although nurses can use any type with clients to enhance their healing processes, they need to appreciate individual variations of images, colors, shapes, symbols, and meanings related to cultural diversity. Nurses can use imagery to help promote a sense of well-being with clients; encourage healthy behaviors; and help them modify their perceptions about their diseases, strengths, treatments, and healing capacities. Relaxation exercises are a form of imagery. An example of a situation in which imagery can be incorporated into nursing care is with bone or wound healing. Before the session, in terms the client can understand, the nurse describes the basic biological process involved in the healing. The imagery process begins with a relaxation exercise. While the client is in a relaxed state, the nurse instructs the client to imagine the natural process of healing that is occurring, helping the client by quietly describing the elements of the healing process, and ultimately imagining oneself as fully healed and back to normal activities. Many resources are available for nurses who wish to develop skills in integrating imagery into nursing care (Achterberg, Dossey, & Kolkmeier, 1994; Dossey, 1997; Schaub, 2000), including a nurses' certification program in interactive imagery sponsored by the American Holistic Nurses' Association and the Academy for Guided Imagery.

Herbal Therapies

Herbal and natural therapies, which have been used for healing in all cultures from before the time of written history, are becoming more common and are available in grocery stores and regular pharmacies. Although many natural and herbal preparations can enhance health and contribute to the prevention of disease, they are not necessarily safe just because they are natural (Duke, 1997; Murray, 1995). Because plants cannot be patented, little research has been done in the United States on plants as medicinal agents and there is a lack of standardization regarding the amount of the active ingredient of the plant that is in any particular herbal preparation (Murray, 1995). Although research on plants as medicinal agents is only in its infancy in this country, there is research to support the efficacy of many herbal and natural preparations (e.g., St. John's Wort and gingko biloba) that has been done in other countries (Murray & Pizzorno, 1998). Because many clients use herbs and other natural preparations, nurses need to become knowledgeable about common herbs, their uses, and potential interaction with pharmaceutical drugs. Nurses need to ask about use of herbal and natural preparations in the same way they include discussion of other medications. Of particular importance is advising clients who take herbal preparations to read labels and buy only those that have standardized extracts of the active herb. Students are encouraged to explore the many good references available that discuss the healing benefits, side effects, and interactions of various herbal and natural preparations.

Aromatherapy

Aromatherapy refers to the therapeutic use of the essential (concentrated) oils extracted from different parts of aromatic plants. The oils, which are widely available, may be applied to the body through massage, inhaled as mists, used as a compress, or mixed into an ointment. Although research on the health benefits of aromatherapy is in its infancy, use of this therapy shows promise in promoting relaxation; relieving stress, anxiety, pain, discomfort, insomnia, and restlessness; promoting wound healing; enhancing self-esteem; and stimulating immune function (Stevensen, 1995). Although aromatic oils have been used for varied purposes for centuries, recent years have seen a resurgence in the use of aromatherapy among lay people as well as nurses. Robins (1999) notes that aromatherapy is a safe therapy, with few adverse reactions reported in the literature, although its mechanisms of action and efficacy need further research. Robins suggests that nurses who wish to consider using aromatherapy as an adjunct in nursing practice should have some formal training, use caution when using these oils with people with very sensitive skin or severe respiratory disorders, and be aware that most of these oils should not be ingested.

Touch Therapy

Touch is essential for human survival and development. **Touch therapy** includes a broad range of hand techniques that a nurse can use on or near the body to support the client's movement toward balance, wholeness, and optimal functioning (Shames, 1997, 2000). Touch interventions used by nurses include both physical and energetic healing modalities such as therapeutic massage, therapeutic touch, healing touch, acupressure, shiatsu, and reflexology. Massage (particularly of the back) has long been considered an important nursing intervention used to promote relaxation, relieve muscle discomfort, and stimulate circulation. Many books and educational programs are available for nurses who want to expand their skills with therapeutic massage.

Therapeutic touch (TT), a noninvasive healing technique developed by a nurse, Dr. Delores Krieger (1979), involves touching with conscious intent to heal. In TT, the nurse works from a centered state using the natural sensitivity of the hands to assess the client's energy fields and treat imbalances. Healing touch (HT) (Hover-Kramer, Mentgen, & Scandrett-Hibdon, 1996) is a collection of energy-based healing techniques, which, like TT, are noninvasive. The HT practitioner also works from a centered state to assist in making energy available to clients through application of systemic and localized techniques. In addition to promoting relaxation, decreasing anxiety, and balancing energy, research suggests that these therapies can enhance immune functioning (Olson, Sneed, LaVia, Virella, Bonadonna, & Michel, 1997) and

> ## A CONVERSATION WITH...
>
> *In considering, re-considering Caring in the Community, perhaps a case can be made for Pure Caring, in that it is non-institutional, real-living situations, in the community where the most authentic, and yet demanding aspects of personal-professional caring become manifest. What the nurse offers first, by way of establishing relationship-centered care, is Self: by this I mean bring one's whole self into the present. It is from this professional and philosophical orientation that authentic caring can be witnessed and experienced at its finest.*
>
> **—Jean Watson, PhD, RN, FAAN, HNC**
> Distinguished Professor of Nursing,
> Endowed Chair in Caring Science,
> University of Colorado Health Sciences Center,
> Denver, Colorado
> September 29, 2000

promote wound healing (Wirth, 1992). Acupressure, shiatsu, and reflexology are systems that use the application of pressure (with fingers, thumbs, or a blunt instrument) to specific points along energy pathways (meridians) of the body (acupressure and shiatsu) or in the feet or hands (reflexology).

CONCLUSION

This chapter has discussed the use of complementary therapies within a holistic nursing frame of reference. Nurses must be aware that many people use complementary therapies in addition to biomedical interventions but often do not disclose this to their biomedical practitioners. Complementary modalities encompass all health systems, modalities, and practices other than those intrinsic to the politically dominant health system of a particular society or culture and include all practices and ideas self-defined by their users as preventing or treating illness or promoting health and well-being. Many complementary modalities are based in cultural healing practices, which derive from different explanatory models than that of biomedicine.

Nurses need to be attentive to client values and desires for treatment options, taking seriously the client's need for healing as well as curing and the contributions to health offered by other explanatory models. If nurses do not understand the other modality or question the efficacy or safety of the choice, they should explore these considerations with the client. Nurses need to be aware of the various therapies being considered or used by clients so that they are aware of the many factors affecting a client's health and healing. Community nurses need to develop the ability to incorporate discussion of complementary therapies into assessment in an open way and work toward integration of complementary therapies with conventional interventions. Holistic nursing care implies attentiveness to spiritual concerns as well as to physical and emotional concerns. Prayer, imagery, music therapy, and touch therapy are examples of complementary modalities that can be incorporated into health care with clients in the community

CRITICAL THINKING ACTIVITIES

1. Explore the history and current practice of a healing system other than biomedicine and interview a practitioner of that modality. Compare and contrast that healing system with biomedicine relative to explanatory model, preparation of practitioners, treatment modalities, and interaction with clients. Discuss the extent to which each system focuses on healing and curing.

2. Shauna is an outpatient oncology nurse who has cared for 53-year-old Marita during her 4 years of living with breast cancer. Marita has endured surgery and radiation and is currently undergoing another course of chemotherapy for recently discovered metastasis. Marita tells Shauna that she thinks the medical therapies are only making her sicker and that she has been doing a lot of reading about other ways of dealing with cancer. Marita says she is seriously considering discontinuing chemotherapy treatments and seeking healing through prayer and herbal remedies. She also indicates that she knows God can heal, but that if she is to die, she would rather die with dignity than be stuck in a hospital attached to machines. It is clear from what Marita says that she has thoughtfully considered the various options with their risks and benefits. Shauna tells the physician about Marita's plans; the physician exclaims that Marita is "out of her mind" and suggests that family members be enlisted to persuade Marita to continue with conventional interventions. What do you think of Marita's plan? What personal values are evident in Marita's decision? How do you think you would respond if you were in Marita's situation?

3. How can Shauna respond to Marita in a way that demonstrates respect for persons and supports her autonomy?

4. What perspective is reflected in the physician's response? How might the suggestion to enlist family assistance be considered coercion?

5. How do you think a holistic nurse would approach Marita and her care?

6. Talk with someone who uses a complementary health modality on a regular basis and discuss why they use the modality, the benefits of the modality, whether they discuss the therapy with biomedical practitioners, the cost, and how they pay for the modality.

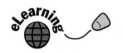

Explore Community Health Nursing on the web! To learn more about the topics in this chapter, access your exclusive web site:
http://communitynursing.jbpub.com

REFERENCES

Achterberg, J., Dossey, B. M., & Kolkmeier, L. (1994). *Rituals of healing*. New York: Bantam Books.

American Holistic Nurses' Association. (1994). http://www.ahna.org.

Burkhardt, M. A. (1985). Nursing, health and wholeness. *Journal of Holistic Nursing, 3*(1), 35–36.

Burkhardt, M. A., & Nagai-Jacobson, M. G. (1997a). Psychospiritual care: A shared journey embracing life and wholeness. *Bioethics Forum, 13*(4), 34–41.

Burkhardt, M. A., & Nagai-Jacobson, M. G. (1997b). Spirituality and healing. In B. M. Dossey (Ed.), *Core curriculum for holistic nursing* (pp. 42–51). Gaithersburg, MD: Aspen.

Burkhardt, M. A., & Nagai-Jacobson, M. G. (2000). Spirituality and health. In B. M. Dossey, L. Keegan, & C. E. Guzzetta (Eds.), *Holistic nursing practice* (3rd ed., pp. 89–119). Gaithersburg, MD: Aspen.

Burkhardt, M. A., & Nathaniel, A. K. (1996). Patient self-determination and complementary care. *Bioethics Forum, 12*, 24–30.

Burkhardt, M. A., & Nathaniel, A. K. (1998). *Ethics & issues in contemporary nursing*. Albany, NY: Delmar.

Burkhardt, M. A., Nathaniel, A. K., Nemeth-Pyles, M., & Boyd, J. (1999). *Utilization of complementary health practices among people in southern West Virginia*. Presentation at the 18th Annual American Holistic Nurses' Association Conference: Holistic Nursing, Heritage to Vision. Phoenix, AZ, June 16–20, 1999.

Cassidy, C. M. (1996). Cultural context of complementary and alternative medicine systems. In M. S. Micozzi (Ed.), *Fundamentals of complementary and alternative medicine*. New York: Churchill Livingstone.

Dossey, B. M. (1997). Imagery. In B. M. Dossey (Ed.), *Core curriculum for holistic nursing* (pp. 188–195). Gaithersburg, MD: Aspen.

Dossey, B. M., & Guzzetta, C. E. (2000). Holistic nursing practice. In B. M. Dossey, L. Keegan, & C. E. Guzzetta (Eds.), *Holistic nursing: A handbook for practice* (3rd ed.). Gaithersburg, MD: Aspen.

Dossey, L. (1993). *Healing words*. New York: HarperCollins.

Dossey, L. (1996). *Prayer is good medicine*. San Francisco: HarperCollins.

Dossey, L. (1997). The return of prayer. *Alternative Therapies in Health and Medicine, 3*, 10–17, 113–120.

Dossey, L. (1998). *Be careful what you pray for . . . you just might get it*. San Francisco: HarperCollins.

Dossey, L. & Swyers, J. P. (1994). Introduction. In National Institutes of Health, *Alternative medicine: Expanding medical horizons* (NIH Publication No. 94-066). Washington, DC: U.S. Government Printing Office.

Duke, J. A. (1997). *The green pharmacy*. Emmaus, PA: Rodale Press.

Eisenberg, D. M., Kessler, R. C., Foster, C., Norlock, F. E., Calkins, D. R., & Delbanco, T. L. (1993). Unconventional medicine in the United States. *New England Journal of Medicine, 328*, 246–252.

Eisenberg, D. M., Rogers, B. D., Ettner, S., Appel, S., Wilkey, S., Van Rompay, M., & Kessler, R. C. (1998). Trends in alternative medicine use in the United States, 1990-1997. *Journal of the American Medical Association, 280*(18), 1569–1575.

Gordon, J. S. (1980). The paradigm of holistic medicine. In A. Hastings (Ed.), *Health for the whole person*. Boulder, CO: Westview Press.

Guzzetta, C. E. (1997). Music therapy. In B. M. Dossey (Ed.), *Core curriculum for holistic nursing* (pp. 196–204). Gaithersburg, MD: Aspen.

Guzzetta, C. E. (2000). Music therapy. In B. M. Dossey, L. Keegan, & C. E. Guzzetta (Eds.), *Holistic nursing: A handbook for practice* (pp. 585–610). Gaithersburg, MD: Aspen.

Hover-Kramer, D., Mentgen, J., & Scandrett-Hibdon, S. (1996). *Healing touch: a resource for health care professionals*. Albany, NY: Delmar Publishers.

Hufford, D. J. (1996a). *Ethical dimensions of alternative medicine*. Presentation at the First Annual Alternative Therapies Symposium: Creating Integrated Healthcare. San Diego, January 18–21, 1996.

Hufford, D. J. (1996b). Informed consent and alternative medicine. *Alternative Therapies in Health and Medicine, 2*, 76–78.

Krieger, D. (1979). *The therapeutic touch*. Englewood Cliffs, NJ: Prentice Hall.

Micozzi, M. S. (1996). *Fundamentals of alternative and complementary medicine*. New York: Churchill Livingstone.

Murray, M. (1995). *The healing power of herbs* (2nd ed.). Rocklin, CA: Prima Publishing.

Murray, M. & Pizzorno, J. (1998). *The encyclopedia of natural medicine* (2nd ed.). Rocklin, CA: Prima Publishing.

National Institutes of Health. (1994). *Alternative medicine: Expanding medical horizons* (NIH Publication No. 94-066). Washington, DC: U.S. Government Printing Office.

O'Connor, B. B. (1996). Medical ethics and patient belief systems. *Alternative Therapies in Health and Medicine, 2*, 92–93.

Olson, M., Sneed, N., LaVia, M., Virella, G., Bonadonna, R., & Michel, Y. (1997). Stress-induced immunosuppression and therapeutic touch. *Alternative Therapies in Health and Medicine, 3*(2), 68–74.

Quinn, J. F. (1989). On healing, wholeness, and the haelan effect. *Nursing and Health Care, 10*, 553–556.

Robbins, J. L. W. (1999). The science and art of aromatherapy. *Journal of Holistic Nursing, 17*(1), 5–17.

Schaub, B. G. (2000). Imagery. In B. M. Dossey, L. Keegan, & C. E. Guzzetta (Eds.), *Holistic nursing: A handbook for practice* (pp. 539–584). Gaithersburg, MD: Aspen.

Shames, K. H. (1997). Touch. In B. M. Dossey (Ed.), *Core curriculum for holistic nursing* (pp. 205–210). Gaithersburg, MD: Aspen.

Shames, K. H. (2000). Touch. In B. M. Dossey, L. Keegan, & C. E. Guzzetta (Eds.), *Holistic nursing: A handbook for practice* (pp. 613–638). Gaithersburg, MD: Aspen.

Simonton, O. C., Cohen, D. Kumar, M., McKinney, C., & Tims, F. (1997). *Music as a healing force*. Presented at Second Annual Alternative Therapies Symposium: Creating Integrated Healthcare, Orlando, April 16–19, 1997.

Stevensen, C. J. (1996). Aromatherapy. In M. S. Micozzi (Ed.), *Fundamentals of alternative and complementary medicine* (pp. 137–148). New York: Churchill Livingstone.

Wirth, D. (1992). The effect of non-contact therapeutic touch on the healing rate of full thickness dermal wounds. *Subtle Energies, 1*, 1–20.

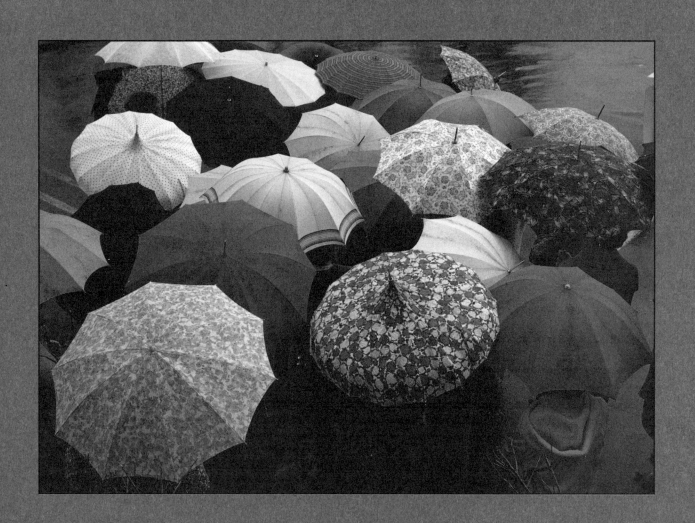

PART TWO

Diversity in Community–Based Nursing Roles

Community-based nursing may offer nurses more diversity than most any other specialty because of the focus on community based settings. Community-based nursing roles are unique in their diversity because of the nature of their implementation, not simply because of the setting where the care occurs. Community-based nursing has always embraced a variety of roles due to the diversity and complexity of public and community health problems. Because the focus of the care is on individual and family, community-based nurses are involved in prevention based nursing interventions and risk identification factors which influence health. Community-based nurses assist individuals and families in settings, such as schools and churches, and in the prevention of health problems through self-care and accountability. For example, a school nurse may administer immunizations to students in the school setting to prevent and control community disease in the community at large. Although the focus of these roles remains health promotion and protection, specialization such as occupational health nursing, disaster nursing, school nursing, home health, hospice, and the care of faith communities through health ministries have emerged as challenging career opportunities for community health nurses.

Unit IV

Diversity in Community Health Settings and Roles

Chapter 12

The Nurse's Role in Ambulatory Health Settings

Karen Saucier Lundy, Vicki Sutton, Barbara Foster

with contributions by: Fran Martin, Ann Brown, Bonnie Rogers, Emily Chandler, and Ruth Berry

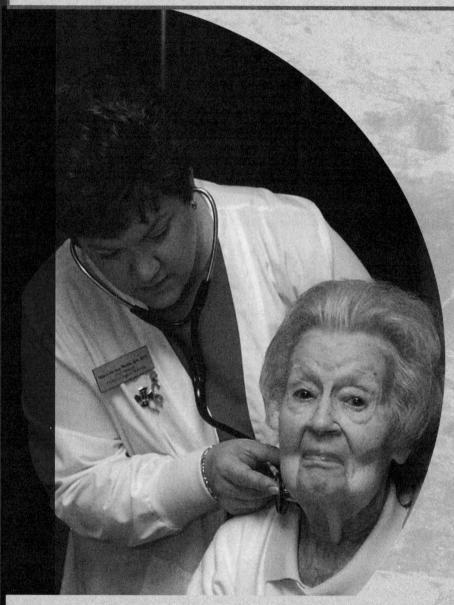

Hospitals are an intermediate stage of civilization. While devoting my life to hospital work I have come to the conclusion that hospitals are not the best place for the sick except for surgical cases.

Florence Nightingale, 1860

CHAPTER FOCUS

National League for Nursing Educational Competencies for Graduates of Associate Degree Nursing Programs (2000)

Office Nursing Practice
Professional Behaviors
Communication
Assessment
Clinical Decision-Making
Caring Interventions
Teaching and Learning
Collaboration
Managing Care
Education and Recommended Experience for Office Nurses

School Nursing
Professional Behaviors
Communication
Assessment
Clinical Decision-Making
Caring Interventions
Teaching and Learning
Collaboration
Managing Care
Education and Recommended Experience for School Health Nurses

Occupational Health
Occupational Health Nursing
Work-Related Risks
Professional Behavior
Communication
Assessment
Clinical Decision-Making
Caring Interventions
Teaching and Learning
Collaboration
Managing Care

Education and Experience Recommendations for Occupational Nursing

Professionalism in Occupational Health Nursing

Health Ministries and Parish Nursing
Professional Behavior
Communication, Assessment, and Collaboration
Clinical Decision-Making and Caring Interventions
Teaching, Learning, and Managing Care
Education and Recommended Experience for Parish Nurses

Missionary Nursing
Professional Behavior
Communication
Assessment and Collaboration
Clinical Decision-Making and Caring Interventions
Teaching and Learning
Managing Care
Education and Recommended Experience for Missionary Nurses

Correctional Health Nursing
Nursing Practice in Correctional Settings
Public's Health
Forensic Nursing: An Emerging Nursing Role

Shelter Nursing
NLN Competencies for Shelter Nursing
Abuse Shelters
Homeless Shelters
Disaster Shelters
Education and Recommended Experience for Shelter Nurses

Ambulatory Care Center Nursing
NLN Competencies for the Ambulatory Setting
Ambulatory Emergency/Trauma Centers
Ambulatory Surgery Centers
Education and Recommended Experience for Ambulatory Care Center Nurses

QUESTIONS TO CONSIDER

After reading this chapter, the student will be able to answer the following questions:

1. What are the National League for Nursing Educational Competencies for Graduates of Associate Degree Nursing Programs and how are they related to ambulatory health care?
2. What is ambulatory health care?
3. How have the settings in which nurses work changed in the past ten years with regards to hospital versus ambulatory settings?
4. What are the opportunities for community nurses in ambulatory health care settings?

KEY TERMS

Ambulatory care
Correctional nursing
Forensic nursing

Health ministry
National League for Nursing Educational Competencies

for Graduates of Associate Degree Nursing Programs
Occupational health nursing

Parish nursing
School nurse
Shelter nursing

Health care in the United States has been moving out of the hospital and into the community for more than two decades. As a result, nursing roles have changed to meet the demands of these diverse settings. The last survey conducted in 2000 by the Division of Nursing of the U.S. Department of Health and Human Services (USDHHS/HRSA/BHPD/DN, 2000), found that the majority of registered nurses still work in hospitals, although the percentage has continued to decline while ambulatory settings have continued to see an increase in the move to community-based health care. The reasons are varied and are covered in Chapter 2 (Health Care Systems). In summary, due to changes in funding of health care services by the federal government and other third party payers, the availability of advanced technology and knowledge, and consumer demands, allows more health care to be delivered out of the hospital in such settings as ambulatory care and surgical centers, school settings, occupational settings, and churches, just to name a few. The percentage of nurses who worked in a hospital setting in 2000 was 59%, down from 69% in 1984. The total number of nurses who were employed in community-based settings in 2000, including community-based nursing homes, jails and physician offices, was 36%, an increase of over 141% from 1984 (USDHHS/HRSA/BHPD/DN, 2000).

Ambulatory care refers to personal health care provided to individuals who are not patients in a health care institution and usually refers to any health care provided in non-institutional settings (Mezey and Lawrence, 1995). Procedures such as appendectomies and intravenous chemotherapy can now be safely delivered in homes, outpatient ambulatory care centers, and freestanding clinics. As health care has moved more and more into the community, the role of the nurse in these settings evolved to one that focuses on short term stays, health teaching and health promotion, and evaluation often done by phone or other forms of technology, such as telehealth and email. In other words, care is delivered more conveniently and with considerable savings for the system and the client with comparable, quality outcomes previously only obtained in inpatient settings. Nursing roles and interventions often vary considerably in similar ambulatory settings based on organizational or institutional policy, state practice organizational or institutional policy, and other regulatory requirements. The purpose of this chapter is to provide a general overview of the ambulatory practice settings and opportunities in the community with an emphasis on the **National League for Nursing (NLN) Educational Competencies for Graduates of Associate Degree Nursing Programs** (2000) as they apply to ambulatory care practice. Selected Healthy People 2010 objectives will be included as appropriate to the ambulatory setting.

National League for Nursing Educational Competencies for Graduates of Associate Degree Nursing Programs (2000)

As the primary national accrediting agency for Associate Degree Nursing, the NLN's mission is to "advance quality nursing education that prepares the nursing work force to meet the needs of diverse populations in an ever-changing healthcare environment." (National League for Nursing Educational Competencies for Graduates of Associate Degree Nursing Programs, 2000, p. ix). In 2000, the NLN invited the National Organization of Associate Degree Nursing (N-OADN) to join its efforts to establish updated competencies for ADN graduates. Changing community needs as well as changes in health care delivery during the past decade have already been discussed, and the NLN recognized that associate degree nursing program graduates must be prepared for these new settings. Historically, "associate degree nursing program graduates were prepared to provide direct client care to individuals with common recurring and/or predictable problems within a structured health care setting and with support from the full scope of nursing expertise" (NLN, 2000, p. 4). With the changing managed care, community-driven, health care environment, the revised competencies reflected the following changes in the health care system related to ambulatory health care:

- *Focus on wellness and health promotion*
- *Focus on management of chronic conditions*
- *Focus on consumer empowerment*
- *Shift of care into the community*
- *Aging population*
- *Increasing cultural diversity*
- *Emphasis on collaboration*

Considering these trends to be the new challenges for preparing associate degree nurses for the new century of increasing community-based care, core components of nursing practice began to emerge as new competencies were explored (NLN, 2000). The following eight components will be used to organize the chosen examples of ambulatory care in this chapter:

1. *Professional Behaviors These refer to a commitment to the profession of nursing as reflected by accountability for standards of practice, accountability for one's own actions and behaviors, and practicing nursing within legal, ethical and regulatory policies. Participating in continuing education, demonstrating a caring for others, and valuing the profession of nursing are also part of this component.*

2. *Communication* Communication in nursing is the effective interchange of information, both verbally and non-verbally and in technological forms as appropriate. This includes therapeutic communication, which is a goal directed toward positive outcomes and problem solving with clients as they cope with change.

3. *Assessment* Assessment is the collection, analysis, and synthesis of appropriate data for the purpose of developing a holistic baseline for the client. Multiple sources are used, such as interviewing, history taking, and an assessment of family and community support.

4. *Clinical Decision-Making* This component involves making accurate assessments using multiple methods to both access information and use the critical thinking process to formulate clinical judgments.

5. *Caring Interventions* Caring involves nursing behaviors that demonstrate compassion and "being" with the client, understanding the "here and now" of the client's situation, and nurturing and protecting in a holistic manner. Caring creates a positive, safe, and hopeful environment for the client.

6. *Teaching and Learning* Teaching and learning are a common care component of community-based nursing. As clients move toward autonomy, they should become more informed and self-assured about their ability to care for themselves. Health education takes many forms—from the Internet to phone calls to personal contact and group education. Evaluation of the effectiveness of the teaching that has taken place should always be included in the educational process.

7. *Collaboration* Collaboration is the involvement of others in the process of planning, problem solving, goal setting, and assumption of responsibility for outcomes. Members of the health team include a variety of professionals, the client's family, and community resources.

8. *Managing Care* Managing care is the efficient, effective use of human, physical, financial, and technological resources to meet client needs and support organizational outcomes. Such a process is accomplished through collaboration with others in the transition from one health care service to another at home or work.

Definitions and further details of these components can be found on the inside back cover of your text. Again, each of the roles presented will be discussed in relation to these core components.

Office Nursing Practice

The office or clinic nurse may be the most familiar roles in the community-based health care system. The nurse is often em-

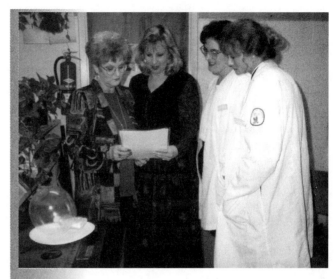

School nurses working with counselors and teachers.

ployed by a physician, a group of physicians, a nurse practitioner, or by a health maintenance organization. The office or clinic nurses may deliver direct care or assign certain duties to other personnel who work under their direction and supervision (McEwen, 1998).

Office nurses work in a variety of settings. For example, nurses may work in the office of a physician who practices family medicine or who specializes in areas such as obstetrics and gynecology, pediatrics, internal medicine, cardiology, dermatology, ophthalmology, surgery, or the like. Nurses may also work in the office or clinic of a nurse-practitioner whose health care focus may include family, adult, or pediatric health. Other nurses may work in the office of a health maintenance organization or in the clinic of a group of nurse midwives. Group practice is far more common today in the competitive managed care environment. Research has demonstrated that office nurses tend to stay in the same job longer than most other nurses, with an average of nine years (Chitty, 2001).

Professional Behaviors

The American Association of Office Nurses (AAON) is the national professional organization of office nurses. The AAON was organized in 1988, and its mission is "to enhance the delivery of effective patient care by providing continuing education in the field of office nursing, patient education and office management, and by promoting the professionalism and recognition of this specialized field of nursing". Members of AAON receive a special Office Edition of RN magazine, the official journal of AAON, and NEON (Nurses Exchange Office News), a quarterly newsletter (http://www.aaon.org/).

Communication

In order to develop a trusting, helping relationship with clients and families, therapeutic communication is an essential skill for office nurses. Therapeutic communication facilitates the accurate assessment of any real or potential problems and the development of an appropriate plan of nursing care. Successful and consistent physician-nurse communication is critical to positive outcomes for clients in the office setting. With advanced technology, the Internet and email have become common ways that nurses and physicians communicate with each other and other health professionals, access protocols and patient records, and communicate with clients in a timely manner. According to research, such technology has enabled physicians to access information on the client immediately with a reduction in paper work (Talsma and Jaffe, 2001).

Assessment

Assessment skills are also an essential competency for office nurses. Office nurses must have the ability to accurately assess both physical and psychosocial problems and appropriately record observations and data collection in accordance with the format required by the setting.

Clinical Decision-Making

Clients and the focus of healthcare may vary greatly and are determined by the area of practice. The job descriptions, tasks, and responsibilities of office nurses are determined by the setting and specialty of the medical practice. For example, functions of office nurses in a pediatrics medical practice may range from teaching parents about infant care, telephone follow-up for referrals to other health professionals (such as speech therapy) to the administration of immunizations. A nurse working in the office of an obstetrics practice may provide patient teaching and counseling, collect specimens, assist with diagnostic procedures, treatments, and provide follow-up of mothers who are noncompliant with care recommendations and who fail to make appointments. This follow up may take the form of phone calls or home visits. Critical decision making in the clinical area includes telephone triage, making decisions about the severity of patient complaints and referral to physician or other professional, explaining treatments and medication administration and side effects, interpreting lab data and explaining procedures. A common role that the office nurse plays is in the area of health education, breaking down complex topics and instructions into understandable terms after the physician has seen the patient.

Caring Interventions

Office nurses also use caring interventions to enhance the delivery of client care. Examples of caring interventions include comfort during procedures, listening, answering questions, teaching, making appointments and arrangements for any follow-up care, and supporting and encouraging the client as needed.

Teaching and Learning

Because of the limited time that physicians spend with clients in the office setting, the office nurse helps to ensure that instructions given by the physician or nurse practitioner are understood. Health education should focus on prevention and literature given to support the plan of care. Follow-up with clients assists the nurse in assessing the appropriateness of educational strategies. Referrals to media and web resources are becoming common educational resources and are especially useful in the ambulatory setting.

Collaboration

Collaboration with members of the health care team helps provide continuity of care for the client. Fragmented care may be reduced and/or prevented with collaboration with other agencies, other health professionals and resources. Collaboration with the client and/or family encourages compliance with the recommended therapy.

Managing Care

Office nurses may serve as formal or informal case managers for the needs of clients by coordinating the services required to meet client needs. Managing clients' care often requires the nurse to serve as liaison between and among members of various healthcare disciplines. In this way, primary, secondary, and tertiary health-care may be provided. Office nurses must be responsive to the needs of individual clients while providing quality health care in a cost-effective manner. Within a managed care environment, physicians and nurse practitioners are often pressured to see more clients during office hours, which gives them less time with clients. Because of these changes, the office nurse often has more responsibility doing procedures, teaching clients about treatment plans and following up with clients to make sure instructions are understood.

Education and Recommended Experience for Office Nurses

There are few formalized requirements for office nurse roles. Some nurse practitioners and physicians might prefer a year's experience in the hospital; others hire new RNs.

School Nursing

School nursing, which is a specialized focus of community health nursing, dates back to the early 1900s, when Lina Rogers was hired as the first school nurse in an effort to reduce high absentee rates in New York City Schools (Costante & Smith, 1997). Rogers, who was hired by the Board of Education, focused primarily on immunizing school children against communicable diseases and screening for potential physical problems that could impact the child's ability to learn, such as vision or hearing deficits. Her efforts so dramatically reduced absenteeism due to illness that additional school-based nurses were hired in the state of New York.

School nursing and the school nurse's role have evolved considerably since Rogers' time. The National Association of School

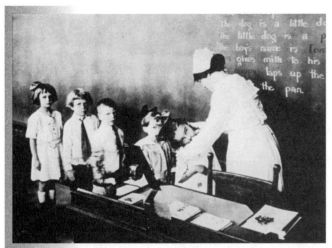

Early school nurses screened for hearing, vision, and orthopedic problems.

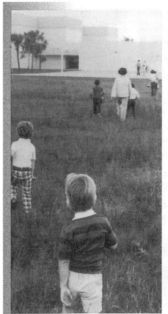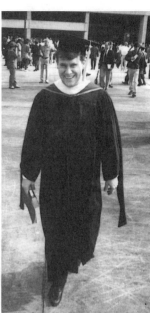

School health is important from entry into kindergarten through college graduation.

Nurses (NASN) defines **school nursing** as "a specialized practice of professional nursing that advances the well-being, academic success, and life long achievement of students." (Ward & Barney, 2002). The American Nurses' Association defines a **school nurse** as "a licensed, professional nurse whose practice focuses on the healthcare needs of clients in the larger school community" (American Nurses' Association, 1983). Today school nurses may be employees of individual school districts, where they provide for the healthcare needs of students and their families in one or more schools, or they may be part of a healthcare team working in partnership with a school or school district in a school-based health center (Dickson, 2001; Hacker & Wessel, 1998).

Whatever their method of employment, school nurses share the same goals, which are: (a) to ensure students' access to primary health care, (b) to provide a system for dealing with crisis medical situations, (c) to provide mandated screening and immunization monitoring, and (d) to provide a process for identification and resolution of students' healthcare needs that affect educational achievement (American Academy of Pediatrics, 2001).

Whether school-based or school-linked, the school nurse is an integral component of a school district's overall health program. The school nurse provides and manages children who are in need of acute, chronic, episodic, and emergency care; manages screening and immunization programs; provides health counseling; serves as an advocate for students with special needs; and helps to develop and coordinate early-intervention health education programs aimed at primary prevention (American Academy of Pediatrics, 2001).

Professional Behaviors

The goal of school nursing is to advance the well-being, academic success, and life-long achievement of students. School nurses

facilitate positive student response to normal development, promote health and safety, and intervene with actual and potential health problems. They actively engage and collaborate with others to build student and family capacity for adaptation, self management and care, self-advocacy and life-long learning, according to the National Association of School Nurses. Some school districts require that school nurses also be certified teachers. Professionalism reflects meeting the accepted standards for the school system of practice, including continuing education and maintaining competency. The 2001 American Nurses Association's Scope and Standards of Professional School Nursing Practice as written in collaboration with the National Association of School

• •

School nursing is a specialized practice of professional nursing that advances the well-being, academic success, and life-long achievement of students. To that end, school nurses facilitate positive student responses to normal development, promote health and safety, intervene with actual and potential health problems, provide case management services, and actively collaborate with others to build student and family capacity for adaptation, self management, self-advocacy, and learning (NASN, 1999).

• •

Nurses provides a framework for the professional expectations of nurses who serve the students in our nation's schools. In addition, it defines and clarifies the role of nursing within schools and the school community, as well as within the larger surrounding community, reflecting a public health focus in school nursing practice.

Communication

As a counselor and coordinator of services, the school nurse uses anticipatory guidance and effective communication skills to assist students and families in a variety of areas to promote a healthy lifestyle. The nurse must also focus on communication among all school personnel, including teachers and administrators, concerning student needs and any trends noted in the clinic that may affect learning. With the advent of the Internet, the school nurse can assist students with learning about health and disease and how students can be more accountable for their own health through knowledge.

Assessment

Many students have physical problems that, if not recognized and treated early, will negatively impact their ability to succeed in the classroom. The school nurse is instrumental in managing programs to identify these at-risk students, and, if necessary, collaborates with the child's parents, teachers, and appropriate health care professionals to arrange for further evaluation (Wold & Dagg, 2001). Screening programs typically managed by the school health nurse include vision, hearing, scoliosis, height, and weight. In each program, the nurse is involved with assessment, planning, implementation, and follow-up activities.

The school nurse also assesses the school environment for hazards, such as dangerous fumes from chemistry labs or wet floors in the cafeteria. The nurse must be ever vigilant about the school learning environment and its affect on health. Each can be a detriment to the other and, therefore, assessments must be

FYI

A survey of 1,546 school districts with an identifiable school health program showed that only 60% listed "nursing" as the major field of the person in charge of school nursing.

TABLE 12-1   **HEALTH SERVICES PROVIDED IN SCHOOLS**

TYPE OF SERVICE	% DISTRICTS OFFERING
Administration of first aid	98.7
Administration of medication	97.1
Screens (height/weight, sensory)	86.8
Abuse evaluation/follow-up	82.8
Emotional/behaviors	80.0
Monitoring of vital signs	77.7
Cleaning/changing of dressings	76.8
Health component of IEP	75.6
Case management	58.1
Nutritional counseling	57.5
Mental health counseling	56.2
Cardiovascular screenings	49.6
Complex nursing to at-risk students	49.6
Employee wellness	48.6
Fitness screenings	45.2
Urinary catheterizations	40.2
Health risk appraisals	35.7

Source: A Closer Look, 1995.

RESEARCH BRIEF

Swanson, N., & Leonard, B. (1994). Identifying potential dropouts through school health records. Journal of School Nursing, 10(2), 22–26, 46.

Lack of basic health information and lack of routine screening and follow-up of identified problems, in combination with poor attendance, seemed to be strong predictors of students at risk for dropping out of an inner-city high school in the Midwest. The mean number of visits to the health office for those who dropped out of school was less than it was for those who stayed in school ($p = < .001$).

conducted on a regularly scheduled basis with student, faculty, staff, and nurse involvement.

Clinical Decision-Making

As provider of care, the school nurse uses clinical decision-making skills to administer first aid and emergency care when needed. First aid usually consists of treating minor cuts, abrasions, sprains, or insect bites. Emergency care usually consists of stabilizing the student and arranging for transfer to a physician or nearby medical facility. The school nurse may be the one who notifies the parents. Following school district protocols and standard protocols, the school nurse also administers medications and treatments when prescribed. This function is especially important to the child with an acute or chronic illness. In addition, the school nurse must either provide safe and effective direct services to the student with special health needs or must facilitate the performance of special

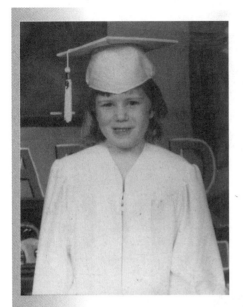

Children in kindergarten can often be screened early for health problems that can affect learning.

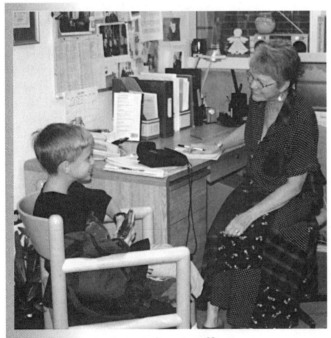

School nurse seeing student in office.

procedures, such as ventilator care, bladder catheterization, or tracheotomy suctioning, for the students who require them (American Academy of Pediatrics, 2001).

Caring Interventions

The school nurse may need to counsel a student or involve the family on a variety of sensitive issues including prevention of communicable and sexually transmitted diseases, pregnancy, alcohol or substance use, or family violence. This takes compassion, patience, and a sensitivity to the issues being discussed, as well as using critical decision-making skills.

Home visits may be required for the nurse to assess the family environment and to provide counseling and emotional support (Wold & Dagg, 2001). Many times the school nurse simply must be available for students who are experiencing "test pains" or stress related pressures and to provide comfort and therapeutic listening.

. . . .

You have brains in your head.
You have feet in your shoes.
You can steer yourself
Any direction you choose.

Dr. Seuss

. . . .

The school nurse has a unique role in providing health services for students with special needs. The school nurse also counsels the special needs child, his peers, and school personnel in an effort to enhance the child's acceptance in the school environment. This includes children with chronic illness and disabilities varying in severity. The school nurse must assess the student's health status, identify health problems that may create a barrier to their educational progress, and then develop a plan for managing the student's problems in the school setting. This plan is usually developed with

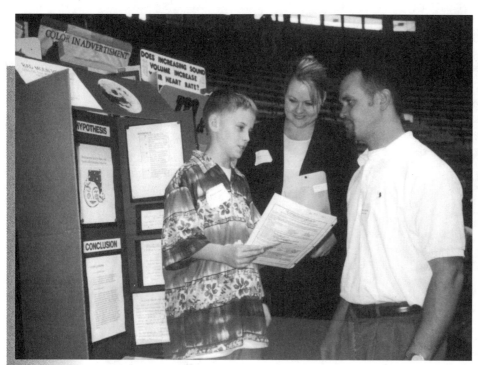

This school nurse is assisting a student with a science fair project.

the student, the parents or guardians, and the child's primary physician (American Academy of Pediatrics, 2001).

Teaching and Learning

The school nurse is in a unique position to work with other school personnel and health care professionals to develop education programs that can profoundly affect the health and lives not only of students and their families but also of the community at large. So many of the problems addressed in *Healthy People 2010* (DHHS, 2000) are problems that could be remedied or substantially reduced by early childhood intervention and prevention programs—programs that naturally fit into the learning environment that the educational system offers. Targeted problems that *Healthy People 2010* addresses include peer pressure; injury prevention; tobacco, alcohol, and drug use; nutrition; obesity and physical inactivity; sexually transmitted diseases; and unintended pregnancy (DHHS). The effectiveness of school-based education programs was described by the CDC (1999). It reported on one program that showed a 37% reduction in the onset of smoking among seventh grade students who had been enrolled in a program on the dangers of tobacco.

Students serviced by one of three school-based health centers in Mississippi have shown a dramatic increase in attendance and in test scores since the centers were established (Dickson, 2001). The centers not only provide primary care to students, but nurses have also begun talking to students about such issues as

how to prevent tooth decay, obesity, and malnutrition. Students with asthma and their parents have benefited from programs developed to educate them about treatment modalities and prevention of disease exacerbation. In the first five years of the health center's existence, one school district has seen attendance jump from 95.5% to 98.5%, while the number of second graders reading on grade level rose from 11% to 82% (Dickson, 2001). The superintendent of this school district gave much of the credit to the school nurses when he said, "If you have a boat with a hole and you're trying to get across the Mississippi River, you're not going to get across no matter how hard you try. The nurses plug up that hole." He further explained that trying to keep kids in school just "wasn't working until we got those nurses in school to get those kids healthy" (Dickson, 2001).

Collaboration

The school nurse is in a setting where the goals are not necessarily health-related but focused on educational outcomes. This is a challenge as the school nurse collaborates with others who may be unaware of the influence of health problems on learning (Martin and Brown, 1991). Many schools now use the team approach, with speech therapists, school psychologists, audiologists, psychometrists, and physical therapists to case manage students with identified problems affecting their learning. Through collaboration, the team can do much more than any one person, especially in the school environment, when health

SCHOOL NURSING ROLES.

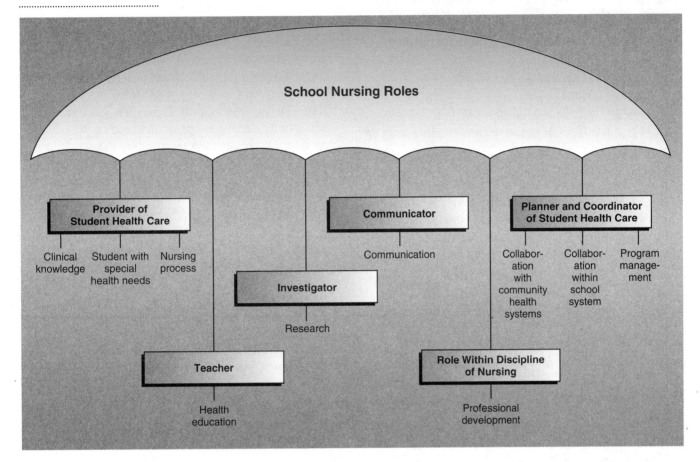

and learning must be constantly associated and justified with school administrators.

Managing Care

Laws in all states require basic childhood immunizations before a child can enroll in school. Although few schools provide actual immunizations to students, the school nurse monitors the immunization records of each student to ensure compliance with local policies and state regulations. The records must show either date of immunization or reason for exemption (e.g., religion or documented case). When deficiencies are noted, it is the nurse's responsibility to intervene according to district guidelines to ensure that the student complies. Depending on the school district, this may mean a simple notification to parents regarding the immunization deficiency or, with parental permission, administration of the vaccination at the school (Martin and Brown, 2001).

As school and healthcare personnel have become more aware of the importance of Hepatitis B immunizations, some states

have written and received grants to make the Hepatitis B vaccine available to all students in the state. The role of coordinating the Hepatitis B immunization programs on a county-wide basis rests with the school health nurse who must communicate the importance of the vaccine to students, parents, and the public, and then must coordinate the administration of the actual immunizations at regularly scheduled times throughout the year (Dickson, 2001).

CASE STUDY

A Day in the Life of a School Nurse

Pleasantville Elementary School, early September: The school nurse, Ms. Davis, RN, plans to do the first grade vision screening today, but first she will see the children who are waiting outside her clinic office door. First in line is Jason. Jason's mother wants him to be "checked out for chicken pox." Jason's cousin, Tommy, a second grader, now has chicken pox.

The school secretary knocks on the door. She has Mrs. Perez, who is visibly upset, and her three children with her. "We have a problem," says the secretary. "These children, ages 8, 6, and 5 years old, have not had any shots since their birth in Mexico. School policy will not allow me to register them. I told the mother that you could help them."

In the hallway sits 8-year-old Shelly Strong. Mr. Bullen, her teacher, is concerned because Shelly says she has asthma and needs a "breathing treatment." This is Mr. Bullen's first year to teach school. He is not sure what Shelly is talking about and says that he has never seen a breathing machine like the one Shelly brought to school in her backpack today.

Out in the hall, 9-year-old Steven (who is taking Ritalin for ADHD) and Hiram (who has a physical disability and uses crutches) are yelling and shoving each other. Both 9-year-olds have a history of poor anger control. Mr. Bullen assists Ms. Davis in breaking up the fist fight. Their teacher, Mrs. Adams, has become very frustrated with their behavior.

Ms. Davis seems to be in control of the situation. She has learned to be flexible with her schedule and to prioritize her nursing duties. Ms. Davis assesses Shelly's respiratory condition. Shelly has the signed papers from her mother and the physician giving permission for the inhalation treatment. The school nurse documents her condition and begins Shelly's treatment. She also records the time of treatment and the amount of albuterol as prescribed by her physician. She calls Mrs. Strong, Shelly's mother, at work and sets up an appointment for that afternoon to discuss Shelly's emer-

gency care plan for future asthma attacks. Ms. Davis informs Mr. Bullen of the meeting and requests his presence. She makes a note to schedule a staff in-service on asthma: its signs, symptoms, medications, and treatments.

Ms. Davis assesses Jason for chicken pox and finds him presently free of eruptions. She sends him back to class with an excuse, then records the office visit in a nurse's note for the day. She schedules herself to check Jason in 1 week, because he has been exposed to herpes zoster and has not had chicken pox.

Ms. Davis has not forgotten about the Perez family. She discusses the immunization schedule with the mother. She teaches her about the diseases covered by the immunizations, reviews their medical records and a brief medical history for each child, then prepares the correct immunizations for each one. Ms. Davis administers the immunizations and discusses possible side effects with the mother. Ms. Davis gives the mother and the school secretary the proper paperwork for the children to be registered in school that day.

Mrs. Perez speaks mostly Spanish. Ms. Davis has been taking Spanish night classes at a local college to communicate with the growing Spanish population in her area. Mrs. Perez requests information on applying for Medicaid. Ms. Davis sets up an appointment with the Medicaid office for Mrs. Perez to discuss this and draws a map for the mother. Ms. Davis asks if she can visit with her and the children at home to assess for other needs. The mother agrees.

Shelly's treatment has been completed. Ms. Davis assesses her respiratory condition and allows her to return to Mr. Bullen's class. Ms. Davis then schedules an appointment with Mrs. Adams (Steven and Hiram's teacher). She wants to share some resource materials on behavior management that are now available. Also, she wants to discuss Steven's medication dosage and classroom behavior. Ms. Davis then makes a referral to the school psychologist regarding the repeat incident between the two boys. She schedules time on her calendar for classroom education regarding children with disabilities in grades K–6. By 10 AM she is ready to begin calling on her first class for vision screening.

HEALTHY PEOPLE 2010

OBJECTIVES RELATED TO SCHOOL HEALTH

Disability and Secondary Conditions

6.9   Increase the proportion of children and youth with disabilities who spend at least 80% of their time in regular education programs.

Educational and Community-Based Programs

School Setting

7.1   Increase high school completion.

7.2   Increase the proportion of middle, junior high, and senior high schools that provide comprehensive school health education to prevent health problems in the following areas: violence; suicide; tobacco use and addiction, alcohol and other drug use; unintended pregnancy; HIV/AIDS and STD infection; unhealthy dietary patterns; inadequate physical activity; and environmental health.

7.3   Increase the proportion of college and university students who receive information from their institution on each of the six priority health-risk behavior areas.

7.4   Increase the proportion of the nation's elementary, middle, junior high, and senior high schools that have a nurse-to-student ratio of at least 1:750.

Injury and Violence Prevention

Unintentional Injury Prevention

15.31   Increase the proportion of public and private schools that require use of appropriate head, face, eye, and mouth protection for students participating in school-sponsored physical activities.

Violence and Abuse Prevention

15.39   Reduce weapon carrying by adolescents on school property.

Physical Activity and Fitness

Physical Activity in Children and Adolescents

22.8   Increase the proportion of the nation's public and private schools that require daily physical education for all students.

22.9   Increase the proportion of adolescents who participate in daily school physical education.

Tobacco Use

Exposure to Secondhand Smoke

27.11   Increase smoke-free and tobacco-free environments in schools, including all school facilities, property, vehicles, and school events.

Source: DHHS, 2000.

CASE STUDY

Teachers Challenge Ruling on Medical Procedure

Teachers at the Burkett Center for the Multi-handicapped in Birmingham, Alabama appealed a state ruling that forces them to perform medical procedures on their students. They argued that because they must handle complicated medical procedures for students in their classrooms, they were violating state nursing codes. They were also concerned that their liability insurance would not cover them if something went wrong. Among the procedures the teachers were required to perform were catheterization, tube feeding, suctioning, and certain blood tests.

The circuit court judge ruled that while they were in college they should have known they would have to perform medical procedures at work. He also said that the state nursing code exempts the "gratuitous nursing for the sick by friends or members of the family" and that due to the close nature of teacher and student work, the teachers are friends. The president of the county Federation of Teachers points out that if teachers are "friends" of the students, why do they have to get written permission to do such things as take them on field trips? If teachers are "friends," why are they paid employees? "Our teachers want to educate rather than medicate."

Source: Teachers Challenge Ruling on Medical Procedure, 1993.

. . . .

A clinician specializing in children would not have difficulty finding the kinds of mental and emotional disturbances present in a child preparing to murder. The masks of children are very transparent, though understandably not to busy or untrained parents and teachers who are emotionally invested in not seeing problems in the children they care for.

Peter Loffredo, New York Times, March 26, 1998
An editorial after the Jonesboro shooting

. . . .

The school nurse's responsibility is to be aware of school district policies and state laws that govern communicable diseases for which children cannot be immunized. These diseases include, but are not limited to, influenza, impetigo, pediculosis, infectious mononucleosis, and ringworm. The school nurse must understand when and how long a child with one of these diseases must be excluded from school and when that child may return to the classroom in order to avoid being a threat to other students. Most state boards of health issue guidelines to schools for those conditions, including when the student can return to school.

Education and Recommended Experience for School Health Nurses

A baccalaureate degree in nursing is recommended by the American Nurses' Association and the NASN as the entry level for practice as a school nurse, and many school districts require it. Throughout the United States, there are still many practicing school nurses who hold an Associate Degree or diploma as highest degree. Certification in pediatrics or as a school nurse is preferred by both the NASN and the ANA.

Occupational Health

Work is where we spend most of our time and is one of life's most worthwhile and rewarding experiences. Most of us as adults spend about one fourth to one half of our lives at work. Work is necessary for supporting our families, our communities, and our country. Although most workers never get hurt or find themselves damaged or injured from a hazard on the job, all types of work have some kind of health hazard associated with them.

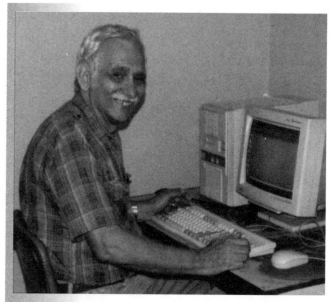

Computers in the workplace result in worker risks such as eye strain and carpel tunal syndrome.

These hazards can have short and long term affects on workers and cost the employer lost wages, retraining of new employees, and insurance costs. The community often loses a productive worker and his or her contribution to the local economy. If federal disability is awarded, such hazards and their consequences then become economic drains. Occupational health and occupational nursing then is a critical component of keeping employees and working environments safe and healthy, thus contributing to worker productivity and employer contributions to the nation's economy. There are 138 million workers in the United States (Bureau of Labor Statistics, 1999). Each day, an average of 1237 persons die from work-related diseases, and an additional 156 die from injuries on the job. Every five seconds a worker is injured.

....

It is neither wealth nor splendor but tranquility and occupation which gives happiness.

Thomas Jefferson

....

Occupational Health Nursing

Occupational health nursing was once called industrial nursing or industrial hygiene and began during the Industrial Revolution in England when Phillipa Fowerday was hired by the J and J and Coleman Company in 1878. Her work in the mustard company was critical. She provided both home care services to employees and their families and jobs in the clinic (Godfrey, 1978). In the United States, occupational health nursing began in the late 19th century when Ada Mayo Stewart was hired by the Vermont Marble Company. She visited sick employees in their homes, provided emergency care, taught healthy living habits, and taught mothers about child care. She also provided teaching lessons on health to school children. At the turn of the century, industrial health services flourished rapidly across the country as it became evident that nursing care could have a positive impact on worker productivity, decrease illness and injury, and reduce absenteeism. Although conditions were harsh and profit over people continued to be the prevailing value of employers, during the next several years consciousness about worker rights, including unions, began to emerge. After World War II, when more than 4,000 nurses were employed in industrial nursing, the American Association of Industrial Nurses was created in 1942. During the years that followed, occupational health and safety became public issues. In today's work environment, nurses who work in the delivery of occupational health services are called occupational health nurses. **Occupational health nursing** is the specialty practice that focuses on the promotion, prevention, and restoration of health within the context of a safe and healthy work environment (American Association of Occupational Health Nurses AOHN, 1999; Sitzman, 2002).

Work-Related Risks

Construction workers have the highest injury rate in private industry, while trucking and warehousing have the highest injury rates in the service sector. Mining injuries, while declining, still remain high. Nearly half of the farm injuries in the U.S. result in permanent, disabling conditions. Back injuries account for more than 40% of these injuries. Vision and hearing problems due to exposure to noise and chemical exposure are on the rise. Because of the long latency period between exposure and some of the long term effects, such as cancer and asbestosis, adequate numbers are not available to account for all industrial hazards contributing to these chronic, and often fatal, diseases. Workers in nuclear power plants have been concerned because of the long period of exposure resulting in diseases (Landels, 2002). In today's climate, bioterrorism has become an occupational threat. There is an immediate need for occupational disaster plans and strategies to cope with bioterrorism in workplaces. Dealing with bioterrorism requires occupational nurses to become familiar with the various types of organisms and chemicals used in bioterrorism and to develop a plan of action for the work environment (Saslazar and Kelman, 2002).

FYI

Back injuries are the most prevalent and most costly injury in the occupation of nursing.

FYI

With 879 fatalities, truck drivers suffered more workplace deaths in 1998 than any other profession.

Source: National Safety Council, 1999.

FYI

Women are more likely to be murdered at work than to die in a traffic accident. Of the 482 women killed on the job in 1998, 34% were murdered.

Source: National Safety Council, 1999.

The eight groups of occupational disease/injuries as priorities of NORA (DHHS, 1996) are

- *Allergic and irritant dermatitis*
- *Asthma and chronic obstructive pulmonary disease*
- *Fertility and pregnancy abnormalities*
- *Hearing loss*
- *Infectious diseases*
- *Low back disorders*
- *Musculoskeletal disorders of upper extremities*
- *Traumatic injuries (fatal and non-fatal)*

The professional society in occupational health nursing is the American Association of Occupational Health Nurses (AAOHN). AAOHN does the following:

- *Promotes the health and safety of workers*
- *Defines the scope of practice and sets the standards of occupational health nursing practice*
- *Develops the* Code of Ethics *for occupational health nurses with interpretive statements*
- *Promotes and provides continuing education in the specialty*
- *Advances the profession through supporting research*
- *Responds to and influences public policy issues related to occupational health and safety*

(AAOHN, 1999)

The official journal is the *AAOHN Journal.*

TABLE 12-2   LAWS WHICH AFFECT OCCUPATIONAL HEALTH

- **Americans with Disabilities Act of 1990 (ADA)**

  This law is intended to prevent discrimination against persons with disabilities. Under Title I of the Act, persons with disabilities are entitled to equal employment opportunities with regard to their disabilities.

- **The Family Medical Leave Act**

  This act requires employers with 50 or more employees to provide a maximum of 12 weeks unpaid job related leave in a 12 month period to employees with family health issues.

- **Workman's Compensation**

  The workers compensation system in each state and in the District of Columbia is designed to cover monetary loss as a result of work-related injuries, including salary, medical, hospital, or funeral expenses and dependent support in cases of occupational death.

Professional Behaviors

The American Association of Occupational Health Nurses (AAOHN) specifies the focus of the occupational health nurses as one who provides health care services to worker populations with an emphasis on promotion, protection, and restoration of workers' health within a healthy work environment. The occupational nurse is often the only health professional in the occupational setting and usually practices more independently than other nurses in the community. The occupational health nurse is often faced with making decisions that can decrease productivity for the organization by limiting unsafe work practices or recommending recovery time for workers. Many decisions made by the nurse can affect the profitability of the organization.

RESEARCH BRIEF

Conrad, K. M., Furner, S. E., & Qian, Y. (1999). Occupational hazard exposure and at risk drinking. American Association of Occupational Health Nurses Journal, *47(1), 9–16.*

This research study examined associations between workers' reported exposure to occupational hazards and their risk for alcohol use. The sample was drawn from the National Health Interview Survey (NHIS) and included 15,907 working adults. *Occupational hazard exposures* were defined as chemical or biological substances, physical hazards, injury risk, and mental stress. *At-risk drinking* was defined as binge drinking and driving while drinking. Of the workers in the sample, 60% reported exposure to one or more occupational hazards, 31% of the sample reported binge drinking, and 15% drove after drinking too much. In a multivariate analysis that controlled the background of the subjects, workers who reported occupational hazard exposure were 1.2 to 1.4 times more likely to engage in binge drinking than workers without exposures. Similar results were found for drinking and driving and occupational exposure. All multivariate statistical analyses were significant. Findings suggest that workers who perceive themselves as being at risk for occupational hazards are at greater risk for binge drinking and driving after drinking. Occupational nurses can lead workplace initiatives to reduce occupational risk exposures and, at the same time, reduce risks for workers at risk for alcohol consumption.

BOX 12-2 AAOHN *CODE OF ETHICS*

- The occupational health nurse provides health care in the work environment with regard for human dignity and client rights, unrestricted by considerations of social or economic status, personal attributes, or the nature of the health status.

- The occupational health nurse promotes collaboration with other health professionals and community health agencies to meet the health needs of the workforce.

- The occupational health nurse maintains individual competence in health nursing practice, based on scientific knowledge, and recognizes and accepts responsibility for individual judgments and actions, while complying with appropriate laws and regulations (local, state, and federal) that have an impact on the delivery of occupational health services.

- The occupational health nurse participates, as appropriate, in activities such as research that contribute to the ongoing development of the profession's body of knowledge while protecting the rights of subjects.

- The occupational health nurse strives to safeguard an employee's right to privacy by protecting confidential information and releasing information only upon written consent of the employee or as required or permitted by law.

- The occupational health nurse strives to provide quality care and to safeguard clients from unethical and illegal actions.

- The occupational health nurse, licensed to provide health care services, accepts obligations to society as a professional and responsible member of the community.

Source: AAOHN, 1996.

FYI

Labor Day—Why Do We Celebrate It?

Labor Day is associated with the beginning of school and is usually celebrated with barbecues and picnics. We rarely remember that Labor Day was created as a way for us to remember the tremendous labor struggles to improve worker conditions in the United States. In the 19th century, workers often worked 16-hour days, 6 and 7 days a week. Children were commonly used as a labor resource. Injuries were common, thousands of workers died, "caught in the grinding machinery of our growing industries" (p. 1319). In the labor market of today, despite improvements, workers continue to die in the workplace, while many more are injured, sometimes for life. We should remember all workers, past and present, on Labor Day. The authors encourage us to remember the "historical toll in lives and limbs that workers have paid to provide us with our modern prosperity . . . the continuing toil is far too high and workers have died and continue to die in order to produce our wealth" (p. 1320). They deserve to be remembered and honored on Labor Day.

Source: Rosner & Markowitz, 1999.

BOX 12-3 ELEMENTS OF A WORKSITE ASSESSMENT

- The work, work processes, and related hazards, products, exposures
- Work environment (e.g., cleanliness, clutter, ventilation, noise, temperature, lighting, safety signs, wash disposal mechanisms)
- Worker population characteristics
- Staffing and personnel
- Corporate culture and philosophy
- Written policies/procedures for occupational health care
- Safety committee (frequency, interdisciplinary, measurements, recommendations)
- Occupational health and safety programs/services and types of occupational health visits
- Types and expenditures for medical/workers' compensation claims
- Most common illnesses/injuries
- Health-promotion/education programs
- Regulatory compliance with OSHA standards

Communication

In the occupational setting, the nurse often works with non-health professionals and must use appropriate non-technical terms when communicating with workers and administrators. Worker trust must be established, and good rapport is critical with both workers and administration. Translation of lab results and diagnostic tests that include ramifications for the work environment are common communication tasks for the occupational health nurse.

Assessment

The occupational health nurse conducts routine physical exams, immunization assessments, and screening programs to assess for potential health problems of the workers. Included in the assessment component is an evaluation of the work environment, which often takes the form of a routine "walk through" of the work area to identify risks and hazards for the specific worker population. The occupational health nurse must be familiar with the specific risks associated with the worker population so that assessment is appropriate and efficiently implemented.

BOX 12-4 INTERDISCIPLINARY FIELDS OF PRACTICE SPECIFIC TO OCCUPATIONAL HEALTH

OCCUPATIONAL MEDICINE

The assessment, maintenance, restoration, and improvement of the health of the worker through the principles of preventative medicine, and promotion of worker health and productivity

INDUSTRIAL HYGIENE

The science devoted to the anticipation, recognition, evaluation, and control of environmental factors and stresses associated with work and work operations

SAFETY

The design and implementation of strategies aimed at preventing and controlling workplace exposures that result in unnecessary injuries or death

ERGONOMICS

The study of humans at work and the evaluation of the stresses that occur in the work environment and the ability of people to cope with these stresses so that the job demands are matched with human capabilities

---

TABLE 12-3	NONFATAL OCCUPATIONAL INJURY INCIDENCE RATES IN THE UNITED STATES BY INDUSTRY, PRIVATE SECTOR

WORK-RELATED NONFATAL INJURIES (PER 100 FULL-TIME WORKERS)

Construction	12.9
Agriculture	11.0
Manufacturing	10.8
Transportation/public utilities	8.8
Wholesale/retail trade	8.2
Mining	7.0
Services	6.8
Finance, insurance, realty	2.7
AVERAGE	8.3

Source: Bureau of Labor Statistics, U.S. Department of Labor, 1993.

TABLE 12-4	NEW CASES OF REPORTED OCCUPATIONAL ILLNESS IN THE UNITED STATES, BY CATEGORY OF ILLNESS, PRIVATE SECTOR

CATEGORY OF ILLNESS	NUMBER*	PERCENTAGE
Disorders associated with repeated trauma	459,300	61
Skin diseases or disorders	120,800	16
Disorders caused by physical agents	37,400	5
Respiratory conditions caused by toxic agents	36,900	5
Poisoning	13,400	2
Dust diseases of the lung	4,800	1
All other occupational illnesses	759,400	100

*Excludes farms with fewer than 11 employees.
Source: Bureau of Labor Statistics, U.S. Department of Labor, 1993.

Clinical Decision-Making

The occupational nurse uses multiple methods to access information for base assessment as described above, as well as analyzing and integrating knowledge about the specific risks associated with the environment in which he or she works. Evidence-based practice is encouraged in order to more effectively implement justified interventions for the worker.

Caring Interventions

The occupational nurse must possess good interpersonal skills to assure that complex health and safety information are conveyed, understood, and respected by workers and administrators. Compassion for the worker is critical since work can be a major stressor as well as an important means of survival for workers and their families. Illness and injury can create fear and insecurity in the worker and lead to more serious consequences. Therefore nurses remain sensitive to the way in which they relate to their clients.

Teaching and Learning

Much of the nurse role in an occupational setting involves teaching appropriate safety measures in the work environment and healthy lifestyle management, as well as educating management about the need for a healthy workforce.

Collaboration

The occupational health nurse often acts as a consultant on health matters, immunization and communicable disease control and immunization campaigns, and works with management to reduce risks. The nurse in this setting must also assist management in complying with legal regulations of OSHA and other health policies related to maintaining a safe worker environment. Collaboration with nonhealth professionals is common, thus requiring the nurse to translate health information into lay terms.

TABLE 12-5	CIVILIAN LABOR FORCE, UNITED STATES, BY INDUSTRY

INDUSTRY	WORKFORCE SIZE (IN MILLIONS)
Agriculture	3.1
Mining	0.7
Construction	7.2
Manufacturing	19.6
Transportation and public utilities	8.5
Wholesale and retail trade	24.8
Finance, insurance, real estate	8.0
Services	41.8
Public administration	5.8
TOTAL	119.3*

*Because of rounding, the sum of the components does not add up to the total. Source: Bureau of Labor Statistics, U.S. Department of Labor, 1994.

BOX 12-5 CATEGORIES OF WORK-RELATED HAZARDS

Biological/infectious hazards: *infectious/biological agents, such as bacteria, viruses, fungi, or parasites, that may be transmitted via contact with infected clients or contaminated body secretions/fluids to other individuals*

Chemical hazards: *various forms of chemicals, including medications, solutions, gases, vapors, aerosols, and particulate matter, that are potentially toxic or irritating to the body system*

Environmental/mechanical hazards: *factors encountered in the work environment that cause or potentiate accidents, injuries, strain, or discomfort (e.g., unsafe/inadequate equipment or lifting devices, slippery floors, work station deficiencies)*

Physical hazards: *agents within the work environment, such as radiation, electricity, extreme temperatures, and noise, that can cause tissue trauma*

Psychosocial hazards: *factors and situations encountered or associated with one's job or work environment that create or potentiate stress, emotional strain, and/or interpersonal problems*

Source: Rogers, 1994.

TABLE 12-6	LABOR FORCE BY JOB

OCCUPATIONAL CATEGORY	NUMBER OF WORKERS (IN MILLIONS)
Executive, administrative, and managerial workers	15.4
Professional workers	16.9
Technicians and related support workers	4.0
Sales workers	14.2
Administrative support workers, including clerical workers	18.6
Precision production, craft, and repair workers	13.3
Operators, fabricators, and laborers	17.0
Service workers	16.5
Farming, forestry, and fishing industry workers	3.3
TOTAL	119.3*

*Because of rounding, the sum of the components does not add up to the total. Source: Bureau of Labor Statistics, U.S. Department of Labor, 1994.

Managing Care

The occupational health nurse is very involved in the coordination of policy related to legal requirements, such as workman's compensations, family leave, smoking restrictions, and referrals for lifestyle health problems. Stress related to workload and family obligations can spill over into the work place and should be addressed as a work-related hazard. The occupational health nurse must stay especially current on legal issues and rights related to workers as well as the accountability of the nurse dealing with such issues (D'Arruda, 2002).

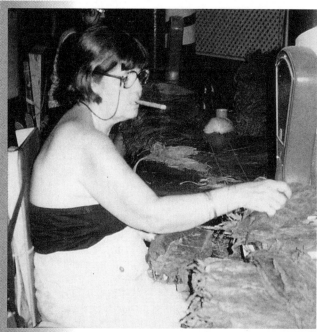

Woman working in a cigar factory.

Education and Recommended Experience for Occupational Nurses

The majority of occupational health nurses received their basic nursing education in associate degree and diploma programs. Ideally, a baccalaureate degree is recommended for occupational health nurses because of the complexity of the role and the autonomy of practice. The AAOHN recommends a minimum of two years professional nursing experience in some form of ambulatory or emergency setting before starting in occupational health. Certification in occupational health is desirable and available through the AAOHN.

BOX 12-6 AMERICAN ASSOCIATION OF OCCUPATIONAL HEALTH NURSES STANDARDS OF OCCUPATIONAL AND ENVIRONMENTAL HEALTH NURSING PRACTICE*

STANDARD I

Assessment

The occupational health nurse systematically assesses the health status of the client, workforce, and environment.

STANDARD II

Diagnosis

The occupational health nurse analyzes health data of the individual, workforce, and environment collected to formulate diagnoses for intervention planning.

STANDARD III

Outcome Identification

The occupational health nurse identifies a specific expected outcomes plan based on diagnosis.

STANDARD IV

Planning

The occupational health nurse develops a goal-directed plan of care that is comprehensive and that formulates interventions for each level of prevention and for therapeutic modalities to achieve desired outcomes.

STANDARD V

Implementation

The occupational health nurse implements interventions to promote health, prevent illness and injury, and facilitate rehabilitation, guided by the plan of care.

STANDARD VI

Evaluation

The occupational health nurse, reflecting best practice standards, systematically and continuously evaluates responses to interventions and progress toward the achievement of desired outcomes.

STANDARD VII

Resource Management

Based on corporate goals and objectives, number of clients, clients' health needs, specific health hazards, and associated costs, the occupational health nurse collaborates with management to provide resources that support an occupational health program that meets the needs of the workforce.

STANDARD VIII
Professional Development
To enhance professional growth and maintain professional competency, the occupational health nurse assumes responsibility for professional development and continuing education. Overall evaluation is accomplished through ongoing self-evaluation and analysis of data from quality improvement/assurance mechanisms.

STANDARD IX
Collaboration
To promote employee health and safety, and a safe and healthful work environment, and to provide effective and efficient health care services, the occupational health nurse collaborates with employees, management, other health care providers, professionals, and community representatives in assessing, planning, implementing, and evaluating care and services.

STANDARD X
Research
Through essential research, the occupational health nurse is committed to and contributes to the scientific base in occupational health nursing to improve and advance the practice and uses research findings in practice.

STANDARD XI
Ethics
As a client advocate for accessible, equitable, and quality health care services, including a safe and healthful work environment, the occupational health nurse uses an ethical framework, which provides parameters for ethical judgments, as a guide for decision making in practice.

*Note: This reflects only the category headings. Refer to source for entire document.
Source: AAOHN, 1999.*

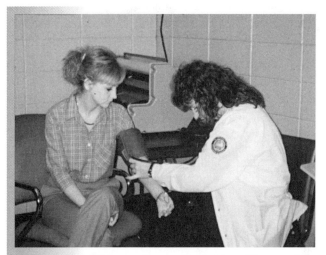

The nurse conducts assessments in the office setting.

Health Ministries and Parish Nursing

Health ministry is a concept that encompasses spirituality and the activities that may be carried out by a specific faith community to meet the needs of a community or a specified population, such as the homeless, elderly, women, children, and persons with disabilities. The professional discipline of nursing incorporates the physical, emotional, cultural, and spiritual domains of practice and involves collaboration among a variety of healthcare dis-

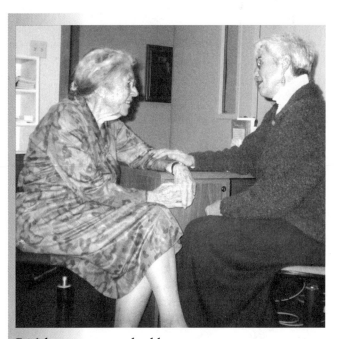

Parish nurse counsels elder woman.

CASE STUDY

A Health Fair—Medicines and More

"Medicines and More" was the result of interest expressed on the part of members of the Wellness Committee of Second Presbyterian Church, Lexington, Kentucky. Comments from a retired health professional and from an older adult caregiver noted that they were concerned about numerous conversations and observations regarding confusion with medications. Quickly, the committee's discussion included stories of inquiries regarding multiple names for medicines, complex over-the-counter preparations, duplicate medicines for the same ailment, values and dangers of herbal preparations, problems eating or not eating food with medicines, medication errors indicating the need for reinforcement of emergency assistance, and others.

Members decided a fair would reach many people quickly. Although a major target was the older population, the committee believed that the information was valuable for members of all ages, for families as well as for individuals who were living alone. Because members already gathered on Sunday mornings for educational and worship services, and because many elderly persons regularly participated in the monthly "Retirees Lunch," it was decided to plan the event to coincide with established habits. The committee further decided that because they wanted to provide information applicable for all ages and for the total congregation, they would schedule the fair during and following the Retirees Lunch in a room adjacent to the dining room. Families and those members not participating in the lunch were guided directly to the fair location following worship service. Retirees would be the special fair participants after lunch.

After agreeing on a number of objectives, the members listed tasks and eagerly offered to take responsibility for the many jobs. These jobs included marketing and publicity, obtaining resources, volunteering for hosting the various exhibits, taking blood pressure readings, greeting community presenters, and monitoring flow on the day of the fair.

The parish nurse contacted the local health department nutritionist and the university's college of pharmacy. A pharmacy brown-bag event was very popular, and the nutritionist provided helpful information regarding food-medicine interaction, supplements, and herbal preparations. Committee members contacted a local hospital's home care agency for information on Lifeline emergency calling. The senior nursing student contacted the local police department for 911 guidelines, supplied various phones for demonstration and practice, and obtained literature and posters at the State Pamphlet Library. In collaboration with the parish nurse, a County Cooperative Extension "Look-a-Likes" display was updated. Children and adults were able to view models and a brochure depicting potentially dangerous and confusing foods, medicines, and household products.

To encourage participation at all exhibits, and to obtain evaluation data, members who completed surveys were eligible to win loaves of whole-wheat variety breads. The committee reviewed the evaluations within two weeks, reported the results and extended thanks to planners and attendees in the congregation's newsletter, and gained information for planning future programs regarding nutrition and exercise.

Effective and enjoyable health fairs can be simpler or more elaborate than the one described. The community presenters gained a new resource for their information. Both the pharmacists and the nutritionist expressed that they had never envisioned the benefits of providing health information in a faith community setting, and the county's extension agency appreciated help in renewing their display and obtaining feedback for additional outreach options. Collaborating with these professionals and their agencies created new partnerships with mutual benefits. Planning fairs to promote healthy behaviors is encouraged by Dillon and Sternas (1997).

(Contributed by Chandler and Berry, 2001)

HEALTHY PEOPLE 2010

OBJECTIVES RELATED TO OCCUPATIONAL SAFETY AND HEALTH

Occupational Safety and Health

20.1 Reduce deaths from work-related injuries.

20.2 Reduce work-related injuries resulting in medical treatment, lost time from work, or restricted work activity.

20.3 Reduce the rate of injury and illness cases involving days away from work due to overexertion or repetitive motion.

20.4 Reduce Pneumoconiosis deaths.

20.5 Reduce deaths from work-related homicides.

20.6 Reduce work-related assault.

20.7 Reduce the number of persons who have elevated blood lead concentrations from work exposures.

20.8 Reduce occupational skin diseases or disorders among full-time workers.

20.9 Increase the proportion of worksites employing 50 or more persons that provide programs to prevent or reduce employee stress.

20.10 Reduce occupational needlestick injuries among health care workers.

20.11 Reduce new cases of work-related noise-induced hearing loss.

Source: DHHS, 2000.

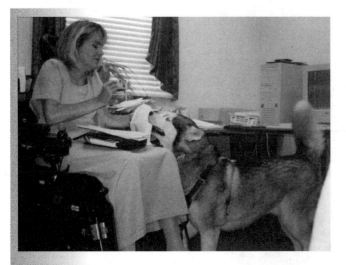

Accommodation in the workplace for persons with disabilities can be successfully implemented with assistive animals.

ciplines. According to Chandler and Berry (2001, p. 984) "Communities of faith seek ways to continue a tradition of service, often to those who need it most. The commitment is to health and wholeness for self and others. Participation in advocacy, health education, promotion, and illness prevention are intrinsically linked to spiritual health."

Historically, nursing has included the provision of care, assistance, and advocacy for those in need, particularly those who are disadvantaged or underserved. Because of numerous trends in society, health ministries are being recognized as a viable option in community health and community-based health care. For example, the increasing life expectancy, combined with a growing geriatric population plagued by multiple chronic illnesses creates a healthcare environment conducive to a growing need for health ministries. The community-based nursing role also requires collaboration among various community members and leaders in order to be successful and accepted. Health ministry activities provide a means of reaching out to those who have physical as well as spiritual needs (Chandler and Berry, 2001).

Parish nursing is a relatively new model of health care delivery, yet it is based on the historical context of nursing in which religious congregations provided care for the sick. The spiritual dimension of care is central to the practice of parish nursing. Parish nursing programs are supported by many different denominations (Solari-Twadell and McDermott, 1999). Parish nurses may work as unpaid volunteers or they may be paid for nursing care by the sponsoring organization. Best estimates place at least 2000 parish nurses serving congregations throughout the United States. The nurses are in faith communities that include Christian, Muslim, and Jewish gatherings. Parish nurses are then key players in health ministries of faith communities (Chandler and Berry, 2001). The concept of modern-day parish nursing is attributed to Lutheran congregations guided by Lutheran Hospital in Chicago. Parish nursing is a relatively new role in the community, although the roots of spiritual and physical care of clients by church workers go back several centuries.

Professional Behaviors

The goal of parish nursing is the enhancement of quality of life for all members of the congregation. In 1998, the American Nurses Association (ANA) adopted the *Scope and Standards of Parish Nursing*, prepared by the Health Ministries Association, Inc. Basic preparation courses recommended for the parish nurse consist of at least 30 hours of course work in parish nursing (Chandler and Berry, 2001).

RESEARCH BRIEF

Fehring, R. J., Miller, J. F., & Shaw, C. (1997). Spiritual well being, religiosity, hope, depression, and other mood states in elderly people coping with cancer. Oncology Nursing Forum, 24(4): 663–671.

One hundred elderly people with a diagnosis of cancer were administered measures to determine the relationships between spiritual well-being, religiosity, hope, depression, and other mood states. Each person was administered an intrinsic and extrinsic religiosity index, a spiritual well-being scale, the Miller hope scale, and the Profile of Mood States scale. A consistent positive correlation was found among intrinsic religiosity, spiritual well-being, hope, and positive mood states. Significantly higher levels of hope and positive moods existed in elderly patients with high levels of intrinsic religiosity and spiritual well-being.

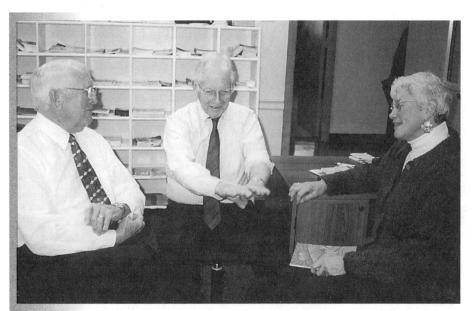

Counseling church members between church services.

Communication, Assessment, and Collaboration

Therapeutic communication skills are an essential competency of parish nursing, allowing nurses to establish helping, trusting client relationships. Communication skills also enable parish nurses to interact and collaborate with individuals, families, congregations, community contacts, and other health care professionals. Assessments of congregations are initiated by parish nurses, often using survey forms and questionnaires to determine and prioritize the needs of members.

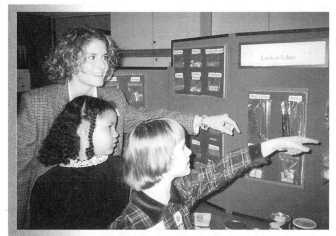

Health fair at church provides opportunities for the nurse to discuss drug use with children.

Clinical Decision-Making and Caring Interventions

Parish nurses may apply nursing research and outcome management in various ways. For example, the services of parish nurses may include providing personal health counseling and health education, teaching personal lifestyle management skills, initiating and facilitating referrals to congregations and/or community resources, all while integrating faith and health. Parish nurses can become involved in nursing research by first identifying problem areas through the process of "assets mapping" of the church , then collecting, analyzing, interpreting, and applying the data to the practice of parish nursing. Various caring interventions and parish nursing activities must be implemented in order to provide these services (Cerroto, 1998). For example, parish nurses may establish support programs, provide stress management or CPR classes, screen for diabetes or high blood pressure, and hold health fairs. The parish nurse should tailor the interventions to meet unique needs of the congregation (Chandler and Berry, 2001).

RESEARCH BRIEF

Oman, D. & Reed, D.(1998). Religion and mortality among the community-dwelling elderly. American Journal of Public Health, 88(10), 1469–1475.

This study of 1,931 older residents of Marin County, California analyzed the association between attending religious services and all cause mortality over a 5-year period, looking at six confounding factors: demographics, health status, physical functioning, health habits, social functioning, and support and psychological state. Persons who attended religious services had lower mortality rates than those who did not, and religious attendance tended to be slightly more protective coupled with high social support. This study lends support to the existence of a "protective effect" of religious attendance on health. A broad implication is the potential benefit of partnerships between religious organizations and health promotion efforts.

Teaching, Learning, and Managing Care

Parish nurses understand the importance of life-long learning. The International Parish Nurse Resource Center and the annual "Westberg Symposium" provide educational opportunities and networking benefits. As managers of care, parish nurses must have spiritual maturity, practical professional experience, competent communication and negotiation skills, and a commitment to personal holistic health. Parish nurses must also have the ability to practice independently and must have leadership, organizational, clinical, counseling, and teaching skills. A recent example of a successful Parish Nursing Collaboration Model in a Health Ministry program in Texas involved teaching nurses within the church attempting to lead the church congregation to healthier lives (Pattillo, M.M., Chesley, D. Castles, P. and R. Sutter, 2002). Strengths of the congregation are assessed and utilized. Congregational and community partnerships are vital to the success of parish nursing, resulting in the likelihood of wide-reaching health ministry activities (Chandler and Berry, 2001).

Education and Experience Recommendations for Parish Nurses

No specific educational or clinical requirements have been established, although it is recommended that parish nurses participate in 30 hours of work with a mentor.

CASE STUDY

Polluted indoor air has become increasingly recognized as a potential public health problem. As an occupational health nurse, you have been asked to assess a small company with 75 workers who manufacture plant food. The workers have complained of headache, eye and throat irritations, and fatigue. Upon assessment, you find the company housed in a 30-year-old building with inconsistent maintenance. The ventilation system is old and has had cooling problems. The workers complain of incon-sistent heating and cooling and "stuffiness." You find a greater-than-expected incidence of asthma, worker sick days, and headaches requiring neurologist care.

1. What are some likely contributing factors to worker illness?

2. What should the nurse suggest that the owner do next in determining the contributing causes to the worker health problems?

3. What role could the occupational health nurse play in the prevention of future problems in this work environment?

Say what is easily forgotten.
Do what is easily overlooked.
Think what is everlasting.

Hugh Prather, *Spiritual Notes to Myself.*
Berkeley: Conari Press (1998).

Missionary Nursing

A discussion of health ministries and parish nursing would be incomplete without reviewing the role of missionary nurses. In the United States, the number of nurses who serve or work as missionary nurses continues to increase yearly. Exact figures are unavailable because these nurses may serve or work on a private, local, state, national, or international level. Another reason that exact numbers are unavailable is to protect the safety of missionary nurses. Their lives are at risk due to religious beliefs as well as unstable political situations.

Many of the major denominations in the United States have nurses who serve or work as missionary nurses. Examples of denominations in the United States that have missionary nurses are: the International Mission Board of the Southern Baptist Convention; Presbyterian Church in America; the General Board of Global Ministries; and The United Methodist Church.

Some missionary nurses may serve or work as short-term or part-time missionary nurses, for a period of weeks or months, while working full time in other nursing roles (e.g., hospital staff, office nurse, or nursing education). Many short-term or part-time missionary nurses routinely participate in mission trips to areas of the United States or to areas abroad (e.g., Mexico, Honduras, the Ukraine) where underprivileged and underserved populations are in dire need of food, clothes, medicine, and healthcare. Missionary teams travel to these areas to meet the specific needs of clients and communities. Missionary teams may include various combinations of nursing, medical, surgical, dental, and lay people. Each mission trip is as unique as the clients and communities to which it ministers. Interpreters are used, as needed, in order to overcome language and cultural barriers. Often, healthcare clinics are set up in churches, schools, or outside under makeshift canopies. Many of these clinics are primitive; others may be equipped with some modern technology, if electricity is available. Missionary teams may provide health care and also assist with the building of churches, houses, and schools.

Other missionary nurses may be career missionary nurses, working for years or even a lifetime in this capacity. Missionary nurses may work as a "home missionary" in the United States or as a "foreign missionary" in countries outside of the United States. Career, or full-time, missionary nurses who work abroad become totally immersed in the culture of the people they serve and learn to speak the native language fluently. Many of the foreign countries are impoverished, war-torn, and desperate for physical, nursing, medical, and spiritual attention. Some countries are considered unsafe and resistant to the outside interventions.

Missionary nurses focus on meeting the physical, spiritual, and emotional needs of clients. Missionary nurses often report that serving and working in this role provides almost indescribable personal fulfillment and job satisfaction. Most consider missionary nursing a "calling." Many describe missionary nursing as "pure nursing" (i.e., unencumbered by mounds of paperwork). Nursing schools are seeing an increase in the number of students who seek to become a nurse in order to serve or work as a missionary nurse. Many nursing students receive credit for clinical hours by participating in mission trips. Missionary nursing is based on the principles and philosophy of community health nursing and community-based nursing practice.

Professional Behavior

The needs of clients and communities vary greatly, depending on the location, culture, economy, type of government, and access to affordable health care. Missionary nurses must be committed to serving and ministering to the various needs of clients and communities within diverse cultures and populations. The primary purpose of missionary nursing is to meet the spiritual, physical, and emotional needs of persons throughout the world.

Communication

Communication skills and therapeutic communication are essential to the role of missionary nurses. Often, different languages and cultures are barriers to communication. Missionary nurses must be caring, patient, compassionate, and committed to providing culturally appropriate care.

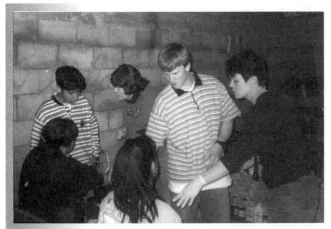

Chapter author Barbara Jo Foster, far right, on mission trip to Mexico.

Assessment and Collaboration

Missionary nurses routinely assess the needs of clients and communities. Specific needs are then prioritized. Collaboration among fellow members of the missionary team and individuals or groups within the community enables missionary nurses to plan ways to meet specific needs. Goals may be set in order to meet the needs of clients and communities on subsequent mission trips.

Clinical Decision-Making and Caring Interventions

Missionary nurses may apply nursing research and outcome management in various ways. For example, the specific needs of various populations and diverse cultures may be compared on private, local, state, national, and international levels. Data may be analyzed and utilized to meet the unique needs of each culture and population group. Various caring interventions and missionary nursing activities may be implemented to provide needed services. Caring interventions of missionary nurses require concern, compassion, patience, and commitment.

Teaching and Learning

Missionary nurses must strive to learn all they can about the culture of the populations and communities they serve. Teaching is also an important component of missionary nursing. For example, in some countries cholera may be a constant threat to the health of a community, so missionary nurses may teach ways to prevent cholera. Language and cultural barriers are frequently encountered and must be overcome in order to enable nurses to establish helping, trusting relationships.

Managing Care

Missionary nurses may formally or informally manage the care of clients and communities from diverse cultures. Managing care requires spiritual maturity, therapeutic communication and negotiation skills, and a personal commitment to the overall health and well-being of clients and communities. Missionary nurses pay particular attention to the spiritual needs of clients. Whenever possible, basic needs, such as food, water, clothing, and housing are provided.

Education and Recommended Experience for Missionary Nurses

There are relatively few requirements for missionary nurses, except for specialty training and requirements set by the religious organization. Due to the autonomy, risk, and unpredictability of missionary nursing, however, mastery of a second language and experience in clinical nursing are preferred. The missionary nurse must obtain skills necessary to practice nursing in the selected foreign country and follow the regulations of the host country.

. . . .

"They must be true Nurses to be true Missionaries."
Florence Nightingale
1892

. . . .

Correctional Health Nursing
Nursing Practice in Correctional Settings

The role of the community health nurse in correctional settings is relatively new. Healthcare for this population has unique challenges for the nurse in this specialized legal setting. The basis of correctional healthcare is providing primary care for inmates from the time of entry into the system, through transfers to other facilities, and to final release from custody back to the community

A Day in the Life of a Prison Nurse

Miriam Cabana, RN, MSN

The nurse supervisor turned on to the blacktop road that ribboned through the 22,000-acre southern prison. As the expansive horizon of flat delta land passed on her short drive to the prison hospital, she recalled the conversation with her husband earlier in the day. He was the warden of the prison and had mused that the full moon usually means some form of violence would erupt within the prison units and that it was an "ideal" time for an escape attempt. She knew he was diligent in his efforts to protect the community as well as to maintain a safe environment for those incarcerated, which often included protecting them from violence inflicted on each other; and he shared her strong opinion about society's obligation to provide inmates with access to safe, competent healthcare. At the very least, there would be more physical altercations among the inmates or increased somatic complaints screened by phone from the emergency department. She instinctively knew her evening shift would be busy. Oh, for the days in her nursing career that the "full moon" myths were associated only with increased birth rates!

The transition between shifts for both nursing and security personnel was smooth. Predictably, several inmates remained in the large holding room with barred windows and doors, waiting their turn to see the physician. They were the last clients of the scheduled sick call. Once their assessment, diagnostic tests, or treatments were completed, the hospital correctional officers assigned to transportation would return them in handcuffs and a secured van to their respective housing units. The phone rang constantly and required the nursing supervisor and a second RN to screen the calls from officers in the housing units who reported the inmate complaints, requests for medications, refills, accidents, or any unusual behavior or symptoms observed by the officers. The nurses made the decision that required assessment in the emergency room, and two hospital officers would pick up the inmate and bring him to the hospital. The LPN and two EMTs assisted the physician. Finally, at around 8 PM, the nurs-

ing supervisor realized that the phone calls were becoming less frequent. She always felt like she was playing Russian roulette, hoping she and her staff asked the right questions or were receiving accurate replies for accurate phone assessments.

The loud ring from the "red" emergency phone jarred everyone into a state of readiness. The phone was connected to the warden's office, the central security office, and the hospital emergency department, so that all key personnel were alerted with the dialing of a single number. The ominous sound always meant an emergency of some description. As nursing and security staff gathered at the doorway to listen, the nursing supervisor quickly picked up the receiver. The excitable, stuttering voice on the other end was barely intelligible. It was obvious the officer was in trouble and had to be coaxed by the security chief to report the housing unit number. The nursing supervisor had heard the word "stabbing" and the unit number. Suddenly she heard the quivering male voice on the other end cry out, "Oh my God, he's gonna kill all of us!" before the line went dead. She immediately dispatched one of the two life-support ambulances. The second ambulance was on its way to another far-flung maximum security housing unit so the RN, a former critical care unit nurse, could assess an inmate complaining of severe chest pain. The supervisor instructed the transportation officer and RN to report to the scene of the stabbing as soon as the assessment was completed unless the inmate required further monitoring in the emergency department. She and the remaining nursing and security personnel then put into action the plan they had developed as a team shortly after her arrival. The two major trauma rooms and the staff were ready to receive victims of violence within minutes after the departure of the ambulance. The physician on call was on her way to the hospital to await their arrival.

The radio was crackling with orders and the relaying of information from security. The ambulance crew was unable to enter the housing unit until the violent rampage had been quelled and the drug-crazed inmate had been subdued by the E-squad, officers who received continuous training in confronting violence within the prison and searching for escaped felons. She could hear and feel the palpable fear and chaos; the number of victims could not be immediately determined and could not be reached because the perpetrator wielded a homemade knife, daring the officers to come near him or the victims. She had never been so close to violence. The ambulance crew described the horror of the scene to her as they arrived with the first victim removed from the unit: a young male with multiple stab wounds to the chest. A second physician was called for assistance because two other victims were reportedly arriving. She and the physician worked quickly to start IVs, insert chest tubes, and stabilize the first victim for transport to a hospital intensive care unit 30 miles away. The second victim arrived with cardiopulmonary resuscitation (CPR) in progress; he had been stabbed in the back repeatedly, then literally picked up and flipped over and stabbed in the face, chest, and abdomen. Each time his chest was compressed, blood gushed from the multiple wounds, which totaled more than 50. After a grueling hour, the inmate, in his early twenties, was pronounced dead. She had never seen so much blood. Linens were soaked with the warm, moist liquid that continued to drip from the sides of the stretcher on which the inmate lay, and one could not avoid the pools of blood on the floor.

She silently wondered what could provoke such a hideous act of violence. She choked back the tears of anger, fear, and bewilderment. There were no family or friends to mourn or to console, since the family would be notified by phone. Her past experiences and education had not prepared her for the little value placed on life within prison and the potential for raw violence within human beings. She gently covered him with a clean sheet as she remembered her husband's frequent rebuttal to her complaints about late-night phone calls from inmates' parents: Everybody here is some mother's baby.

She entered the corridor and knew the pounding of her heart could be heard over the din of the animated conversations between officers and healthcare personnel. She managed to assign staff to transport the first victim to the hospital and to prepare the body of the deceased victim for the funeral home before she retreated into the quiet conference room. She could not control the violent shaking of her entire body or the feeling of revulsion that manifested as an overwhelming nausea. She knew what she had to do, but for the first time since she had become a nurse, she doubted her ability to be nonjudgmental. How could she provide care for someone who had committed such a senseless act of violence? The respect for the individuality of clients and human worth had been the foundation of her 20-year nursing career, yet, for the first time, she questioned her own ability to follow these beliefs. She also had to confront her paralyzing fear for the safety of her family as well as her own safety in her world of nursing. Finally she was able to leave the conference room and enter the noisy clinical area. Still shaking, she took a deep breath and picked up the chart of the next client to be assessed: the inmate who had stabbed the first two clients and had brought violence into her world that night.

(Earley, 1999). Nurses in correctional facilities provide healthcare to populations incarcerated in jails, prisons, juvenile detention facilities, and similar settings. Ages range from youths to aged adults. Women, although representing a small minority of the incarcerated population, make up a growing number of persons in correctional facilities (ANA, 1995).

Although often not fully realized by the general population, the existence of healthcare in correctional facilities is based on the Eighth Amendment of the U.S. Constitution, which prohibits "cruel and unusual punishment" of those convicted of crimes. Furthermore, as a public health concern, correctional institutions are reservoirs of physical and mental illness, which constantly spill back into the community. Appropriate treatment must be provided, with a focus on prevention of transmission of communicable diseases. The health of the general community is affected as the inmate population continues to increase.

The consequences of untreated illness in the system are not just for the inmate or even just to the correctional system. These are public health problems that require effective management and close collaboration between correctional health and the public health system (Conklin, Lincoln, & Flanigan, 1998).

Incarcerated populations have greater health risks than the general population for communicable disease, especially HIV and tuberculosis, violence-associated risks, decreased educational levels, substance abuse, and poverty. Not only do inmates have higher risks for many of these health problems upon admission, but environmental conditions within the correctional facility and behaviors associated with incarceration lend themselves to the spread of communicable diseases. The nurse in the correctional setting can provide interventions aimed at interrupting the chain of contagion and can educate the inmates about self-care and protection from these risks. Inmate education is an essential function of **correctional nursing.** The goals are for inmates to remain healthy while incarcerated and to return to the community properly educated about remaining free of communicable diseases, as well as to prevent others from becoming infected. Peer education groups have been an effective strategy in the correctional system (Conklin, Lincoln, & Flanigan, 1998).

The first standards for nursing practice in correctional settings, the *ANA Scope and Standards of Nursing Practice in Correctional Facilities*, were developed and approved by the ANA in 1985 and revised in 1995. These standards address the scope of nursing practice in correctional settings as well as standards of care and standards of professional performance (ANA, 1995).

. . . .

Prisons do not exist in a vacuum: they are part of a political, social, economic, and moral order.

James B. Jacobs, 1977

. . . .

Forensic Nursing: An Emerging Nursing Role[1]

Forensic nursing, although relatively new in the United States, has been a recognized subspecialty of nursing in other parts of the world for several years. Forensic nursing derives its role and functions from the gap that exists between criminal justice/law enforcement and health care for victims of crime.

In 1992, a group of nurses, most of whom were sexual assault nurse examiners (SANEs), met in Minneapolis, Minnesota. As a result of this meeting, it was decided that nurses involved in an array of roles that interacted with the criminal justice system would operate under the "umbrella" of forensic nursing. Another result of the Minneapolis meeting was the formation of the International Association of Forensic Nursing.

In 1996, the ANA recognized forensic nursing as a subspecialty in nursing practice. This was significant because it enabled and allowed the practitioners to define the scope of practice and determine standards of practice and care. The *ANA Scope and Standards of Forensic Nursing Practice* were approved and published in 1997. A major function of forensic nursing, especially in cases of interpersonal violence (i.e., rape assault), is the assessment and documentation of injury and the appropriate collection, packaging, and storage of physical and biological evidence. Forensic nurses can be found functioning in rape crisis centers, emergency departments, and nursing homes. In some regions of the United States, forensic nurses are coroners and death investigators assisting the police with homicide cases and cases of unexplained death.

The Memphis Sexual Assault Resource Center came in to existence in the mid-1970s. It was one of the first programs of its type in the United States. In those early years the client population consisted mainly of adult women. Later, changes in

―――――――――

[1]This section on forensic nursing was authored by Margaret M. Aiken, PhD, RN, Sexual Assault Nurse Examiner (SANE), Memphis Sexual Assault Resource Center, Memphis, Tennessee.

BOX 12-7 LEVELS OF PREVENTION ACTIVITIES IN CORRECTIONAL FACILITIES

PRIMARY PREVENTION	SECONDARY PREVENTION	TERTIARY PREVENTION
Stress reduction education	Treatment of infections	Injury rehabilitation
Prenatal care	Trauma care for injuries	Diabetes foot care
Immunizations	Screening for suicide risk	Stroke rehabilitation
Violence prevention	Disaster and emergency care	

child abuse law precipitated an exponential increase in the number of children evaluated. In the late 1990s, services were expanded to the collection of biological evidence from those suspected of crimes (sexual offenses, homicide, and driving under the influence [DUI]).

Shelter Nursing

Another focus of community-based health nursing is **shelter nursing**. Shelters are facilities established to assist people who for one reason or another have found themselves to be homeless. While some shelters simply provide a place to get out of the weather, other shelters offer a wide range of services often specializing in the concerns of specific populations such as the homeless, victims of abuse, or runaway youth.

Shelters are usually run by a combination of paid professionals and volunteer staff, including psychologists, nurses, lawyers, and others. Shelters may be sponsored by churches, community governments, and a variety of social agencies and are designed to provide services to people who often suffer from various problems (Townsend, 2000). There is really no such thing as a typical shelter. Shelters are housed in warehouses, churches, government buildings, and single-family homes that have been converted to supervised residences (Carson, 2000). The location of many shelters is kept secret in order to protect the safety of the residents.

NLN Competencies for Shelter Nursing

The community health nurse, as provider of care, manager of care, and member of the nursing discipline, is in a unique position to help meet the needs of those people for whom shelters are their lifeline—the difference between life and death. It is essential that the shelter nurse exhibit the following competencies when working with all persons who enter a shelter in search of help and hope.

1. *Professional Behaviors. Professional behaviors essential to the shelter nurse would include crisis intervention and counseling; health promotion and maintenance; screening and evaluation; provision of a therapeutic environment; assisting clients with self-care activities; administering and monitoring treatment regimens; health teaching; and outreach activities, including home visits and community action (Townsend, 2000).*

2. *Assessment. Shelter nurses must be able to accurately assess the needs of the population for whom they provide care. Depending on the type of shelter, nurses will care for clients with a multitude of physical needs ranging from bruises and broken bones to pneumonia, STDs, AIDS, substance abuse, tuberculosis, and dysentery. Too often, however, it is*

the client's spiritual and mental needs that are harder to assess. Shelter clients often suffer from mental illness, depression, anger, guilt, poor coping mechanisms, a multitude of stressors, and low self-esteem.

3. *Communication and Collaboration. Shelter nurses must be able to use therapeutic communication skills to develop a trusting relationship with their clients. It is the shelter nurse who is in the best position to let the shelter client know that his or her feelings of anger and despair are normal and that others have experienced these same emotions in similar situations (Townsend, 2000). Through collaboration with the healthcare team, the nurse works with the client in individual and group settings in an effort to develop coping skills that will serve as a stable base upon which the client can begin to build a future.*

4. *Caring Interventions. One of the most important tasks of the shelter nurse is simply to care for the shelter client. This starts with being nonjudgmental. It probably goes without saying that none of the shelter clients desire to be at the station in life in which they find themselves when they come to the shelter. Among the caring behaviors the shelter nurse must exhibit are listening, providing feedback, helping the client to recognize available choices, and accepting and supporting the client in whatever he or she chooses to do.*

5. *Teaching and Learning. One of the most beneficial things shelter nurses can do is to teach their clients about the availability of resources in the community (Townsend, 2000). In addition to not having a place to live, shelter clients often lack the knowledge and skills that will help them to leave the shelter and function on their own. Clients may need assistance with completing paperwork to get federal or local assistance that will enable them to find a permanent home. They may need training or education to get a job, and many of the mentally ill lack the knowledge as to how to get the medications that will treat their mental illness.*

   The shelter nurse may need to teach parenting skills, methods of building self-esteem, and alternative coping mechanisms to many of the shelter's clients. The mentally ill often need information about their medications in order to promote compliance. This includes when and how to take their medications as well as ways to reduce troublesome side effects. Some clients need assistance with hygiene as well as how to socially interact with others.

6. *Managing Care. Nurses often serve as case managers for a selected group of clients who have been seen in shelters (Townsend, 2000). As case manager, the nurse coordinates services that are required to meet the needs of the client. This is done in an effort to prevent avoidable episodes of illness, physical and mental, among these at-risk clients. Responsibilities include negotiating with many health care*

providers to obtain whatever services are needed by the client. This coordination of services by the shelter nurse is done in an effort to optimize client functioning and problem solving, improve work and socialization skills, promote leisure-time activities, and enhance the overall independence of the individual (Townsend 2000).

7. *Clinical Decision-Making.* The shelter nurse is often in an autonomous role requiring critical thinking skills involving the use of assessment data, including history, which is often incomplete. Decisions have to be made based on available information and must focus on present acute problems while planning for uncertain future living conditions. Much of the clinical decision-making activities of the shelter nurse focus on the "here and now" of prioritizing problems and addressing pressing needs. If time allows and clients return or stay in the shelter, the nurse can then begin making long-term goals to assist the client with decisions about finding a more stable living environment and to increase knowledge about self care and self respect. Research that utilizes clinical pathways is often helpful once the client's problems have been identified, including evaluation of care and response of client (Hitchcock, Schubert and Thomas, 1999).

Abuse Shelters

Most cities in the United States now have shelters, or "safe houses," where women can go to obtain protection for themselves and their children. Most battered women who reside in shelters have experienced multiple traumatic events with some even suffering from post-traumatic stress disorder (Humphreys, Lee, Neylan, & Marmar, 2001). Shelters not only provide a haven of safety to the abused and battered woman, they provide health care, counseling, a milieu to express the intense emotions she may be experiencing, and a wealth of support including financial, social, and spiritual (Humphreys, et al., Townsend, 2000).

Homeless Shelters

In the United States, the homeless population is "among the poorest of the poor" (Zuvekas & Hill, 2000, p. 153) and consists not just of adult men and women but also a countless number of children (Huang & Menke, 2001). A large segment of this population faces potential barriers to work as many have serious mental and physical disabilities, and others have single or multiple drug addictions (Hatton, 2001). In addition to meeting the medical and mental health problems of the homeless, shelters provide a safe, supportive environment for individuals who simply have no other place to go. While a small percentage of the homeless use the resources available to improve their lives, others become dependent on the provisions that the shelter offers (Townsend, 2000).

Disaster Shelters

When major flooding, tornadoes, landslides, and earthquakes strike, thousands of families are often displaced from their homes. For some families, displacement may be on a short-term basis. For others, their home and all their belongings are gone. The greatest immediate need usually reported by most disaster victims is shelter (Daley, Karpati, & Sheik, 2001). This need is closely followed by food and hygiene requirements. Disaster victims include the young and the very old as well as those who are ill and those who are pregnant. Because of this, there is also a great demand in shelters for medications along with medical and nursing care (Daley, et al.).

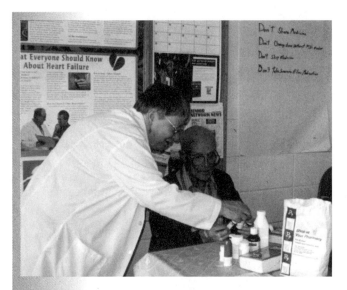

Nurse in homeless shelter counsels elder man about medications.

Education and Recommended Experience for Shelter Nurses

There are relatively few requirements for shelter nurses, except for specialty training such as disaster certification for disaster shelters. Experience in clinical nursing is preferred due to the autonomy and unpredictability of shelter nursing.

Ambulatory Care Center Nursing

Perhaps one of the most innovative and dramatic changes in community-based healthcare is in the diversity in care delivered in ambulatory care centers, from ambulatory surgical centers to ambulatory oncology care settings. These freestanding centers provide acute care to walk-in (ambulatory) clients without the custodial feel of traditional hospital care.

A Day in the Life of a Nurse Who Faces Violence: Sexual Assault Nurse Examiner (SANE)

Margaret M. Aiken, PhD, RN

It was 10 PM, Thursday night. As the SANE readied herself for bed, she checked to see where her pager, keys, and her clothes were. She climbed into bed and pulled the covers up around her chin. She was exhausted. Her last thought as she drifted off to sleep was, *As tired as I am, they will probably have me out the whole damn night.* Like a knife, the pager's sound cut through the stillness of the night. She jerked herself from sleep into an upright position. She fumbled for the bedside light, toppling a glass of water to the floor as she did so. She pressed the reset button on the pager to reveal the source of the call. It was the police dispatcher calling her. By rote, she dialed the number imprinted in her brain by repetitions over 12 years.

"Communications, Smith."

"Hi! This is Donna Anthony with Rape Crisis."

"Hi Donna. They have a car in route to the center with a victim. Their ETA is approximately 2:30."

"Thanks. I will be there at about the same time."

Donna had slept in her underwear and a pair of sweats, so she had only to pull on a T-shirt, put on shoes and socks, brush her teeth and hair, and leave. It was about a 20-minute drive to the center. As she drove down the street in the quiet night, she wondered just how many times she had moved through this scenario. There was always the thought, *I wonder if this will happen to me sometime when I am called out like this. What prevents it from happening?* The drive to the center was so practiced and automatic that it was not uncommon to reminisce and engage in fantasy: *I wonder what this victim will be like. A street person? A child? An addict? Or a regular person like me? One could argue the "regular" person thing. What kind of nut is cruising the streets in the middle of the night when they could be snug in bed? I wonder which detective will be with the victim. Will it be a sympathetic one? Whoops, I almost drove right past the place. I really must pay better attention.*

As she pulled into the lot she noticed that the police car was already there. She greeted the officer, inquiring whether he had been waiting long. The officer introduced her to the victim, Anne Smithridge, who was a retired employee from one of the local banks. They went through all the rituals to gain entrance into the building and the suite of offices. Once they got inside, Donna made coffee, offered some to Ms. Smithridge and to the detective, and poured herself a large cup, thinking, *Please God, help me wake up.* Ms. Smithridge was escorted to the examining room, where she would be interviewed and examined. This woman was in her sixties, lived alone in a single family home. A man had broken into her home to rob her and then had forced her to have sex as an apparent afterthought. Donna interviewed her, examined her, collected evidence, and filled out the many forms required. She offered emotional support throughout the process. Donna was surprised at how "together" this woman was in view of what had happened. It took approximately one hour to complete the entire process. Donna's good work in assessment and evidence collection had contributed to the conviction of many perpetrators.

Before leaving the center, Donna called the dispatcher to see if there were any more "calls." Hearing that there were none, she informed the dispatcher that she was going home. All three left the center at the same time. As she drove home, again on "automatic pilot," she began thinking about the scores of assaulted women she had seen over the years. Each time she left the center, she made a concerted effort to forget the case. She feared that if she were to keep all the information in her active memory, she would lose her sense of balance.

The victims/survivors of rape whom she best remembered were probably those touched by either humor or horror, which likely does a disservice to all those who are abused and defiled and go unnoticed in a blur of the many. She arrived home. Wearily, she crept into the house, which was still dark. She went to the back of the house to her bedroom and again readied herself for bed, checking for the location of pager, keys, and so on. As she climbed into bed, she was reminded of the spilled water as she stepped in the puddle in her sock feet. She pulled off the socks and then padded into the bathroom to get a towel. She simply threw the towel in the pooled water, said "the hell with it," and slid between the sheets. It was now 4:30 AM

and all was well (she hoped). Donna now had to ready herself for the day at her regular full-time job at the clinic. It would be a long day, but she would make it. People often ask her why she continues in this stressful job. She invariably responds that no matter what, she feels that she does a "good thing." As she drifted off to sleep, she clicked off all the things she had to do before leaving home for her "real job." In terms of time, it would be tight, but she would make it. Indeed, it had been quite a night in the life of a SANE!

These alternative sites for acute care have been very successful because of their efficiency, cost effectiveness, and high degree of client satisfaction. They can provide faster service with less paperwork and administrative time involvement. These ambulatory care centers are smaller in size than hospitals, employ fewer people and have less technical equipment, which keeps prices down.

NLN Competincies for the Ambulatory Setting

1. *Professional Behaviors.* The American Academy of Ambulatory Care Nursing provides standards and guidelines for ambulatory centers in the community. Because of the brevity of client contact in these centers, nurses must be focused and well-educated as professionals caring for persons who are frightened, stressed, and are quickly discharged.

2. *Communication.* The amount of time that the ambulatory care center nurse stays with clients in these centers is short. Therefore, communication is of special significance to clients and their families and other health professionals. Focused and precise, nurses in these settings should communicate with deliberate yet compassionate purpose due to the short length of time with the clients.

3. *Assessment.* The ambulatory health center nurse conducts assessments, serves as an assistant to physicians as either a scrub or circulating nurse for surgical procedures, and takes histories during admission. Assessment after procedures is especially important at surgical centers because the collected data assists the physician in making the decision to discharge the client.

4. *Clinical Decision-Making.* The ambulatory center nurse makes quick decisions based on well-thought through clinical assessments and uses multiple interventions depending on the setting and diagnosis. The ambulatory center nurse analyzes data and integrates knowledge about the specific risks associated with the illness or procedure and takes appropriate action.

5. *Caring Interventions.* The nurse in the ambulatory care center must possess good interpersonal skills in which complex health and safety information can be conveyed in an understandable and concise manner to clients and their families and in a respectful way to workers and administration. Compassion for the client and the family is critical since they are aware that they will only be under medical supervision and care for a short time. Nurses must promote self-care and confidence in the client's ability to follow through with post-discharge instructions.

6. *Teaching and Learning.* Much of the nurse role in an ambulatory care setting involves teaching discharge measures and often includes follow-up the next day to evaluate the health status of the client after services.

7. *Collaboration.* The nurse in the ambulatory care setting collaborates with other health professionals to share and manage critical information about the client before, during, and after procedures. The team approach provides the client with comprehensive care so that upon discharge, successful healing is more likely.

8. *Managing Care. The ambulatory care center nurse manages quick turnaround for clients with acute illnesses, which requires excellent organizational skills and a knowledge of critical information related to the specific illness or injury. Evaluation using outcome measurement can provide vital information about how to make the system work more efficiently while maintaining quality (Williams, 1993).*

Ambulatory Emergency/Trauma Centers

These centers, often referred to as "urgent care, urgicare, or walk-ins" do not perform major surgeries, and most are in urban areas and shopping centers. Usually they are in close proximity to full-service hospitals when clients need additional care. As a relatively new resource for immediate care, ambulatory emergency centers are staffed by physicians, usually family practitioners or internists, registered nurses, licensed practical nurses, lab technicians, diagnostic technicians, and clerks. Ambulatory care centers try to generate consumer satisfaction by being convenient, cost effective, and caring. They do this by providing the four "As." They are: affable, available, accessible, and affordable. These centers are often open seven days a week from 12-16 hours a day. Treat minor illnesses, such as upper respiratory tract illnesses, impetigo, diarrhea, dehydration, urinary tract infections, asthma, and cellulites. Many also treat more serious symptoms and illness such as chest pain, back pain, seizures, and anaphylaxis. Pregnancy tests are offered, suturing of lacerations, casting and splinting of fractures, treatment of wounds, burns, and eye injuries. These centers offer limited diagnostic services, such as routine radio logic services, complete blood cell count, bacteriology, electrolytes, and toxicology tests. The majority of clients are adults, although most centers treat children as

well. Return visits can be arranged, but most are referred back to their family physician or a specialist (Seidel, J, Henderson, D. and Lewis, J., 1991).

Ambulatory Surgery Centers

Ambulatory surgery refers to a surgical process in which clients have surgery, recover, and are discharged home the same day. Because of advances in anesthesia, surgical techniques, and a desire for convenience, these centers have grown significantly in the past ten years. Cost containment is a major factor in the proliferation in same-day surgical centers. Approximately 65% of all surgical procedures are now performed safely on an ambulatory basis without compromising the quality of care (Atkinson and Fortunato, 1995). Surgical procedures generally do not exceed 90 minutes in length and do not require more than four hours recovery time. Each center has emergency equipment and trained personnel, including registered nurses. Pharmacy services are also available. Laboratory and radiological services may be performed on site or by referral to nearby facilities.

Education and Recommended Experience for Ambulatory Care Center Nurses

There are no special educational requirements for RNs practicing in ambulatory care centers. Many of these centers prefer RNs to have one year of emergency room experience, operating room, or post-anesthesia care. Certification in operating room nursing or in post-anesthesia care would be preferred in ambulatory surgical centers.

CONCLUSION

Many nursing students today will choose to work outside the hospital in ambulatory health care settings. For over twenty years, A.D.N. nursing roles have changed to meet the demands of these diverse settings. Although the majority of registered nurses still work in hospitals, predictions are that ambulatory and community-based care will continue to increase due to changes in technology, health care costs, managed care and consumer preference, among many other factors. This chapter has covered selected settings and CHN role options available in community-based ambulatory health care based on the National League for Nursing Educational Competencies for Graduates of Associate Degree Nursing Programs.

CRITICAL THINKING ACTIVITIES

1. Juan, a 10-year-old boy, has spina bifida and hydrocephalus. As a result, he has limited bowel function, wears a brace for severe curvature of the spine, and uses a wheelchair for mobility. In addition, Juan has only one kidney and wears a urine collection bag under his clothing. This appliance requires frequent emptying during the school day. He takes several medications to prevent infection and promote waste elimination. Juan lives in a single-parent family with his mother and two brothers. His extended family of aunts, uncles, and cousins is 200 miles away in another state. As a community health nurse, discuss four health outcomes that you and his family would plan for Juan's care. Give the rationale for each one.

2. Danielle, a 15-year-old student, recently learned that she is 3 months' pregnant. When she informed her mother, Danielle was "thrown out" of the house and is now staying with her 28-year-old boyfriend. Danielle has been absent from school four times in the last two weeks. Select nursing interventions at the primary, secondary, and tertiary levels for Danielle. Include holistic interventions.

3. The next time you go to a fast-food restaurant, observe the potential for occupational hazards in the workers who serve your food. Are there prevention strategies that could prevent those hazards?

4. Ask one of the staff members at your nursing school about workplace hazards in the office. Ask him or her to describe what the most prevalent injury or illness associated with his or her work is. What could be done to prevent this risk?

5. Investigate your nurses association's position on workplace violence in health care. How can nurses protect themselves from this occupational hazard?

6. Identify a health problem in your home community that could be addressed by building a potential partnership with a local faith community.

   • In what ways could a faith community address the problem to enhance public sector efforts?

   • What kind of partnerships could be forged with the faith community to enhance their contribution?

   • What are the steps that need to be taken to initiate a plan?

   • How will your own faith experience influence your participation?

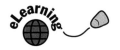 Explore Community Health Nursing on the web! To learn more about the topics in this chapter, access your exclusive web site:
http://communitynursing.jbpub.com

REFERENCES

A closer look: A report of selected findings from the National School Health Survey, 1993–94 (1995). Denver: Office of School Health, University of Colorado Health Sciences Center.

American Academy of Pediatrics. (2001). "The role of the school nurse in providing school health services." *Pediatrics, 108*, 1231–1232.

American Association of Occupational Health Nurses (AAOHN). (1996). *Standards of occupational health nursing practice.* Atlanta, GA: AAOHN.

American Association of Occupational Health Nurses (AAOHN). (1999). *Code of Ethics.* Atlanta, GA: AAOHN.

American Nurses' Association (ANA). (1995). *Scope and standards of nursing practice in correctional facilities.* Washington, DC: Author.

American Nurses' Association (ANA). (1995). *Scope and standards of school nursing.* Washington, DC: Author.

Atkinson, L. J. and Fortunato, N. H. (1995). *Ambulatory surgery.* In L. J. Atkinson and N. H. Fortunato. *Berry and Kohn's Operating Room Technique.* St. Louis, MO: Mosby Year Book, pp. 833–839.

Bureau of Labor Statistics (1994). *Employment projections: 1994.* Washington, D.C., US Department of Labor.

Bureau of Labor Statistics (1999). *Employment projections: 1999.* Washington, D.C., US Department of Labor.

Carson, V. B. (2000). *Mental health nursing: The nurse-patient journey* (2nd ed.) Philadelphia, PA: W.B. Saunders Company.

Centers for Disease Control and Prevention (CDC). (1997). *Youth risk behavior surveillance system.* Atlanta: U.S. Government Printing Office.

Chandler, E. and Berry, R.D. "Health ministries: Health and faith communities." In Lundy and Janes (Ed.), *Community Health Nursing: Caring for the Public's Health.* Sudbury, MA: Jones and Bartlett Publishers.

Chitty, K. C. (2001). *Professional nursing: Concepts and challenges* (3rd Ed). Philadelphia, PA: W.B. Saunders Company.

Conklin, T., Lincoln, T., and Flanigan, T. (1998). "A public health model to connect correctional health care with communities." *American Journal of Public Health* 88(8), 1249–1251.

Costante, C. & Smith, E. (1997). "Beyond band aids: School health nurses as program developers and coordinators." *Journal of School Health, 67*, 291–292.

D'Arruda, K.A. (2002). "Business law: Fundamentals for the occupational health nurse." *AAOHN journal: Official journal of the American Association of Occupational Health Nurses,* May; 50(5), pp. 234–241.

Daley, W. R., Karpati, A., & Sheik, M. (2001). "Needs assessment of the displaced population following the August 1999 earthquake in Turkey." *Disasters, 25*(1), 67–75.

Department of Health and Human Services (DHHS). (2000). *Healthy People 2010: Conference Edition.* Washington, DC: U.S. Government Printing Office.

Dickson, B. (2001). "MNA's efforts reap benefits for Mississippi's children." *Mississippi-RN, 63*(2), 16–17.

Earley, J. (1999, Spring, Summer). "Nursing behind bars." *Minority Nurse,* pp. 22–23.

Godfrey, H. (1978). "One hundred years of industrial nursing." *Nursing Times,* Nov. 30, 615–621.

Hacker, K. & Wessel, G. (1998). "School-based health centers and school nurses: Cementing the collaboration." *Journal of School Health, 68*, 409–415.

Hatton, D. C. (2001). "Homeless women and children's access to health care: A paradox." *Journal of Community Health Nursing, 18*, 25–35.

Hitchcock, J. E., Schubert, P. E., & Thomas, S. A. (1999). *Community health nursing: Caring in action.* Albany, NY: Delmar.

Huang, C. Y. & Menke, E. M. (2001). "School-aged homeless sheltered children's stressors and coping behaviors." *Journal of Pediatric Nursing, 16*, 102–109.

Humphreys, J., Lee, K., Neylan, T., & Marmar, C. (2001). "Psychological and physical distress of sheltered battered women." *Health Care Women International, 22*, 401–414.

Landels, M. (2002). "Day in the life: An occupational health nurse at a nuclear power station." *Nursing Times.* March 98(12), pp. 65.

McEwen, M. (1998). *Community-Based Nursing.* Philadelphia, PA: W.B. Saunders.

Mezey, A. P and Lawrence, R. S. (1995). "Ambulatory care." In A. R. Kovner (Ed.). *Jonas's Health Care Delivery in the United States* (5th Edition). New York: Springer Publishing Co, pp. 122–161.

National League for Nursing (NLN)/Council of Associate Degree Nursing Competencies Task Force. (2000). *Educational Competencies for Graduates of Associate Degree Nursing Programs,* Sudbury, MA: Jones and Bartlett Publishers.

Pattillo, M.S., Chesley, D., Castles, P, and Sutter, R. (2002). "Faith community nursing: Parish nursing/health ministry collaboration model in central Texas." *Family and Community Health* 25:3; 41–51.

Rosner, D. and Markowitz, W. (1999). "Labor Day and the war on workers." *American Journal of Public Health*, September, 89(9), 1319–1321.

Salazar, M and Kelman, B. "Planning for biological disasters: Occupational nurses as 'first responders'." *AAOHN*, April; 50(4), pp. 174–181.

Seidel, J.S., Henderson, D.P., and Lewis, J. B. (1991). "Emergency medical services and the pediatric patient: Resources of Ambulatory Care Centers." *Pediatrics, 88*(2) August.

Shelly, J. A. & Miller, A.B. (1999). *Called to care: A Christian theology of nursing.* Downers Grove, IL: InterVarsity Press.

Sitzman, K. (2002). "Group wellness in the workplace." *AAOHN journal: Official journal of the American Association of Occupational Health Nurses* April; 50(4), pp. 200.

Talsma, J. and Jaffe, G.(2001). "How will the doctors' office evolve in the digital age?" *Ophthalmology Times, 26*(2), pp. 10–13.

Townsend, M. C. (2000). *Psychiatric mental health nursing: Concepts of care* (3rd ed.) Philadelphia, PA: W. B. Saunders.

United States Department of Health and Human Services/Health Resources and Service Administration/Bureau of Health Professions/Division of Nursing (USDHHS/HRSA/BHPD/DN) (2000). *The Registered Nurse Population: Findings from the National Sample Survey of Registered Nurses,* March, 2000. Rockville, MD: Government Printing Office.

Ward, S. & Barney, V. (2002). "Know your school nurse: Information is available about school nurses and what they do." *Arkansas Nursing News, 19*(1) 29.

Williams, S. J. (1993). "Ambulatory health care services." In S. J. Williams and P.R. Torrens (Eds.). *Introduction to Health Services* (4th Edition). Albany, NY: Delmar Publisher, pp. 108–133.

Wold, S. J., & Dagg, N. V. (2001). "School nursing: A framework for practice." *Journal of School Health, 71*, 401–405.

Zuvekas, S. H. & Hill, S. C. (2000). "Income and employment among homeless people: The role of mental health, health and substance abuse." *Journal of Mental Health Policy.*

Chapter 13
The Home Visit
Karen Saucier Lundy

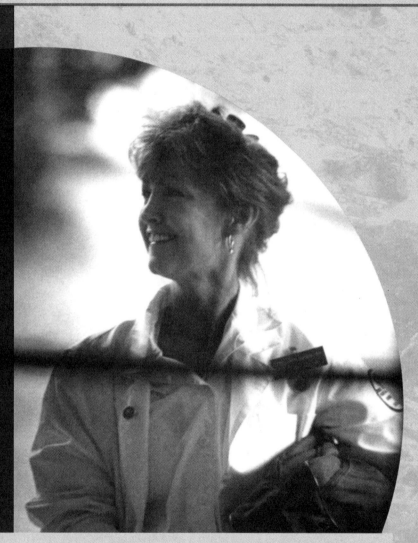

Historically, homes were the earliest practice settings for community health nurses. Clients were seldom in hospitals, but recovered from illness at home and learned about disease prevention and treatment at home; as always, nurses reached out to them through the home visit.

QUESTIONS TO CONSIDER

After reading this chapter, answer the following questions:
1. What is home health visiting?
2. How is a home visit conducted?
3. What are the stages of a home visit?
4. What are the advantages and challenges of a home visit?
5. How effective are home visits in improving health for populations?

KEY TERMS

Behavioral distractions
Environmental distractions

Nurse-initiated distractions
Visiting nurse

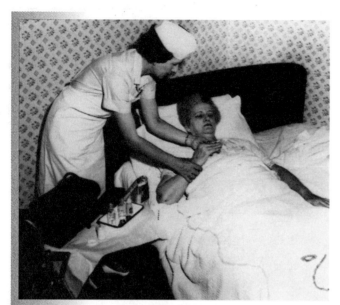

The acceleration of home health nursing came during the 1960s, when Medicare approved home health visits for reimbursement.

Community health nursing roles during the latter part of the 19th century and throughout the 20th century have always had the home as a common setting for practice. One specialized role that emerged was that of the **visiting nurse**, organized by visiting nurse associations funded by philanthropic donations. Physi-

cians often made home visits as well. Box 13-1 identifies milestones in the historical development of health care at home.

The evolution of home care in the United States resulted from social, economic, technological, demographic, and political forces that continue to shape our health care delivery system (NAHC, 2001). By the end of World War II, the physician shortage and the continued explosion of medical technology in the hospital brought many physicians into hospitals, and physician home visiting became a thing of the past (Hafkenschiel, 1990). By the early 1960s, home care was primarily provided by public health and visiting nurses, who assessed clients, provided the necessary services, and managed the therapeutic plan of care. Public health nurses focused on prevention and education; visiting nurses provided sick care in the home. By 1963, according to the National Association for Home Care (NAHC 2001), the number of home health agencies, primarily private philanthropic organizations, had grown to 1,100. The services involved a variety of professional disciplines, including skilled nursing. Nurses who make home visits today are employed by a variety of agencies, and roles can encompass elements of the visiting nurse (sickness care) and public health nurse (health promotion, case finding, disease prevention, and education). However, in the current reimbursement driven health care system, most nurses who visit clients at home tend to specialize in home health services, with an emphasis on illness care and posthospital follow-up, or public health services, which deliver care in the home for prevention and health education. The role of the home care nurse is increasingly more important as a specialty within community-based health care. Home health nurses may be

BOX 13-1 MILESTONES IN THE HISTORY OF HEALTH CARE AT HOME

1800–1900	Most individual care was given at home. Sources of care varied but most care was provided by small, mostly voluntary philanthropically financed organizations.
	Visiting nurses were viewed as the solution to warding off infectious diseases of the poor and immigrants that threatened urban life.
1877	Precursor of modern home health nursing, visiting nursing, was first established in the United States by the women's branch of the New York City Mission.
	First home health nurse, Frances Root, visited the sick poor for the New York City Mission. Root graduated in the first nursing class of Bellevue Hospital in 1874.
1912	The American Red Cross established a rural visiting nurse service for the "sick country person" nationwide. Following the war, the need was so tremendous that the Red Cross could not keep up with the chapter's demands for nurses.
	Three thousand visiting nurses were working on behalf of 810 associations and agencies.
	Metropolitan Life Insurance made visiting nurse services available to 90% of its 10.5 million policyholders in the United States and Canada, creating the first nationwide system of insurance payment for home-based care.
1920s	Marked distinction between public health nurses, with a focus on health promotion and prevention, and visiting nurses, with an emphasis on bedside care for the sick occurred during this era.

BOX 13-1 MILESTONES IN THE HISTORY OF HEALTH CARE AT HOME—CONT'D

1947	Montefiore Hospital in the Bronx, New York, started the first hospital-based home care program, offering medical nursing and social services to its clients.
1965	Medicare legislation was enacted to meet the home care needs for the elderly. Approximately 1,275 organizations were initially certified and were limited to nonprofit home care agencies and health departments.
	Medicaid, a state medical assistance program for the poor, was established. Services were expanded to include therapists, aides, homemakers, social workers, and nutritionists.
	The Older Americans Act was initiated to help maintain and support older persons in their homes and communities. Home care entered its current period of rapid growth.
1967	Medicare certified agencies reached 1,753. Home health expenditures amounted to less than 1% of the total Medicare budget.
1970s	Health policy providers saw home care as a cost-containment measure and as an alternative to institutional care.
	Consumers expressed great acceptance for home care when available as an alternative to institutional care.
1973	Home health Medicare benefits were extended to the younger disabled population.
1980	Medicare-certified agencies reached 2,924.
	The percentage of Medicare clients discharged to home health care increased from 9.1% in 1981 to 17.9% in 1985.
	Government expense on home-based services totaled $4.5 billion, while an estimated 2–4 times this amount was spent by families for privately purchased home-based care.
1981	Proprietary agencies were admitted to the Medicare program.
1982	The National Association for Home Care (NAHC) was founded.
1983	Medicare added hospice benefits.
	Diagnosis-related groups (DRGs) and the prospective payment system (PPS) implemented by the federal government results in shorter hospitalization incentives and the discharge of sicker clients to the home setting.
1986	The growth of Medicare-certified home care agencies leveled off at around 5,900 as a result of increasing Medicare requirements and unreliable payment policies.
1987	Approximately 2.5% of the U.S. population received home care services.
	A coalition of U.S. congressmen, consumer groups, and the NAHC filed a lawsuit against the Health Care Finance Administration that resulted in a rewrite of the Medicare home care payment policies. This rewrite allowed the program for the first time to provide beneficiaries with the level and type of services that Congress originally intended.
1997	The Federal Bureau of Labor Statistics declared home care as the fastest growing segment of health care and the second fastest growing industry.
	An estimated 20,215 home care organizations provide service to more than 7 million Americans with acute, long-term, or terminal health conditions.
	Congress passed the Balanced Budget Act (BBA) of 1997, which resulted from the rapid growth of the home care industry and the increasing concern and incidence of fraud and abuse in health care; an interim payment system (IPS) for home health services was created as a new reimbursement mechanism.
1998	The BBA of 1997 took effect. This change in the reimbursement mechanism for home care services resulted in sweeping changes. Home care agencies were reimbursed by the Medicare program by an aggregate per beneficiary payment limit. This was an interim step toward a prospective payment system similar to the DRG system used in the acute care setting.
2000	Prospective payment system (PPS) implemented.

employed by home health agencies, hospices, hospitals, public health departments, or clinics. Public health nurses may see clients at home through the auspices of the state health department, a local hospital, or a rural clinic. In this chapter, the home visit as a practice environment is described in the context of the emerging community-based health care system. Home health nursing and hospice as specialities in community-based care will follow in Chapter 14.

The Home Visiting Process

One has only to look around any local hospital to see that it would seem to be much more efficient for clients to come to the nurse and other health care providers, where resources are plentiful. Certainly, one of the primary reasons that hospitals were first developed in the Middle Ages was so that caregivers could see more clients and watch them throughout the day and night. Yet there are very good reasons for seeing clients in their own homes. Box 13-2 lists common purposes of home visiting; Box 13-3 details the stages of the home visit, with information about the sequential steps in the home visiting process; and Box 13-4 provides information about differences between the home setting and the acute care setting. Box 13-5 provides hints on communicating effectively in the home setting.

Advantages of Home Visits

····························

Besides nursing the patient, she shows them in their own homes how they can call in official sanitary help to make their own

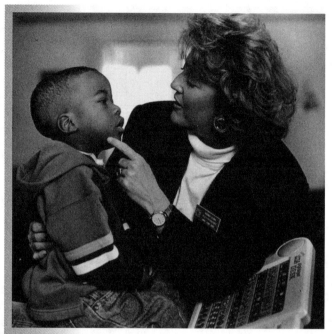

Home visits take an average of 45 to 60 minutes to complete depending on purpose of visit.

poor room healthy, how they can improve appliances, how their homes may not be broken up.

Florence Nightingale, 1890

····························

BOX 13-2 PURPOSES OF HOME VISITS

CASEFINDING

- Public health and protection
- Abuse, neglect cases
- Communicable disease
- School-related health conditions

ILLNESS PREVENTION
AND HEALTH PROMOTION

- Prenatal and well baby care
- Child development
- Elder care

CARE OF THE SICK
AND TERMINALLY ILL

- Home health
- Hospice

Community health nursing is holistic. Seeing clients in the artificial and controlled environment of a hospital reveals little to the nurse about the family's health influences and ability to carry out the plan of care (Allen, 1991). In the home, the nurse gets the complete picture, including environmental factors that affect health, social and psychological influences, relationships between and among family members, and the interaction of the client with family and social networks. In a hospital, clients are separated from the context of their everyday lives: health care providers control their every movement (including self-regulated body functions), they wear institutional clothes, and care is organized around physician and nurse schedules. Such separation of clients from the context of their lives makes it easier for nurses in the hospital to focus only on the biomedical aspects of disease (Liaschenko, 1994). This is not the case in the home, where illness is but one aspect of the totality of the client's living experience (Coffman, 1997). Hazards and resources are quickly evident and allow a more realistic plan of care to be established, which promotes the achievement of mutually set health strategies and goals. In addition, on a home

BOX 13-3 FROM BEGINNING TO END . . . CONDUCTING A SUCCESSFUL HOME VISIT

PREVISIT/PLANNING STAGE

- Determine which clients need to be seen.
- Prioritize the scheduled visits based on client need, distance between visits, laboratory work, and coordination with other professionals and physician.
- Review the chart, orders, client diagnosis, goals of care, and reasons for the home visit.
- Telephone the client for validation of scheduled visit; ask client about specific needs, such as supplies, and any special hazards, such as pets or environmental concerns; caregiver schedule.
- Secure directions to the home.
- Conduct inventory of bag, needed equipment and supplies for clients, and educational materials.
- Review safety considerations, such as timing of visit, environmental assessment.

IMPLEMENTING THE VISIT

- Initiate the visit: introduction and identification of nurse to client, brief social phase to establish rapport.
- Practice appropriate hygienic practices before client assessment.
- Review plans for visit with client.
- Determine expectations of client regarding home visits.
- Conduct assessment: environment, client, medication, nutrition, functional abilities and limitations, psychosocial issues, and evaluation of previous visit intervention effectiveness.
- Modify the plan of care based on client need and situational dictates.
- Perform nursing interventions.
- Deal with distractions: environmental, behavioral, and nurse initiated.

EVALUATING THE VISIT

- Evaluate effectiveness of interventions based on established short-term (response during visit) and long-term outcome criteria (effects of intervention at subsequent visits or other client contact).
- Evaluate as to primary, secondary, tertiary interventions.
- Evaluate conduct of visit: availability of appropriate supplies, preparation of nurse for visit.

DOCUMENTATION

- Document based on established outcome criteria and agency requirements.
- Validate diagnoses and additional health needs based on visit.
- Evaluate goals and objectives.
- Review actions taken, response of client, and outcome of interventions (short and long term).
- Record both objective (nurse-based) and subjective (client-based) data.
- As appropriate, use federal agency reimbursement guidelines, such as Medicare, for progress documentation and certification/recertification requirements.

TERMINATION

- Termination begins with the first visit as nurse prepares the client for time-limited nature of home visiting.
- Review goal attainment with client/family and make recommendations and referrals as necessary for continued health care issues.
- Develop strategies for appropriate closure with clients who die, refuse visits, or are terminated because of nonreimburseable services.

visit, the nurse can see firsthand how well the client can perform self-care and can make a more accurate evaluation of medical and nursing interventions. Such information can provide the nurse with valuable indicators in the evaluation of the effects of therapeutic interventions, as compared with the limited time and artificial constraints of the clinic or hospital environment (Liepert, 1996). There is a distinct advantage to the client when care is provided in the home.

For example, rather than having to obtain transportation to a health care facility. Transportation can be an obstacle for many clients, including those who do not have access to a private car or mass transit, are unable to drive, or are confined to their homes. Another advantage is that clients are able to exercise more autonomy on their own turf, which allows the nurse to promote a sense of empowerment in the client and family (Ruetter & Ford, 1996). The client becomes part of the interdisciplinary team, rather than

BOX 13-4 CHALLENGES IN HOME SETTINGS

Control belongs to the client because care is being provided in his/her home.

A feeling of isolation and lack of support often results from the nature of the home setting.

There are no nurses or other team members in the next room to confirm an assessment or to distinguish an abnormal finding.

The home environment and family support system are unpredictable and not always conducive to optimal care.

Dealing with multiproblem families is difficult emotionally for the nurse, especially in the home setting where family dynamics and interactions are more intense and visible.

Difficulty in communicating with the various team members can be a stressor.

The volume of documentation required can be difficult as a result of the variety and demands of various funding sources and standards.

Frustrations with the system are a common concern. There is often difficulty explaining Medicare or Medicaid's ever-changing requirements to clients and families, as well as to other providers.

Complex case loads that encompass all age groups with diverse problems are common in home care. The skills and knowledge required are broad, requiring the nurse to become a strong generalist.

Concern for personal safety is an issue as violence has increased in all delivery settings.

a dependent, passive recipient of care. As such, effective community health nurses can use this as a way to increase the client's ability for self-care and enhance the sense of accomplishment in meeting health goals for self and family.

Home visits often take place over long periods, which afford the nurse ample opportunities for developing the authentic trust relationship necessary for a true collaborative partnership to develop between nurse and client. A result is that clients are often more willing to share sensitive and more intimate issues in the home setting, which allows the nurse to gain insight into complex interpersonal influences (Stulginsky, 1993a, 1993b).

Home Call: Mother and Child

There's so little here: one table,
not laden, one blind
shut. One bulb
hung straight down. One woman,
not well (that look
of someone who won't talk
because they've been beaten
so the bruises don't show), and one
boy, dancing over, no
diaper, eager for the coin
of candy you lay in his
hand. He leans into your
yellow dress, reaching up,
a tendril attaching, lifting
out of the dark, unfurling
his last leaf. She watches him
watch you,
you with a house
she imagines half glass, where light
pours in, and everything
is already paid for: your
dress, the shine of health you wear
as though you own it, the look
of wealth, and (this too is
visible) the knowhow
to make the right phone calls,
calls to those, who, when you call,
will do what you say, pay
what you tell them, when
and to whom. You, she imagines,
who have at least two
of everything, you lift her son
to your yellow breast, that
well lighted place, where the air's
clean, and you don't
hate yourself, waiting in line
to pay for a sack of potatoes
you can't afford, She watches him
cling to you, she waits to see
what you will do; you who
have things, you who can
do things, you who can do
what you choose to, you
who can do something for them,
if you choose to, a little something
or nothing.

by Marilyn Krysl
Source: Krysl, M., *Midwife and other poems on caring.*
New York: National League for Nursing, pp. 11–12.

Knowing in Nursing

I stepped outside of myself so that I could know
So that I could know the meaning of the earth
Its green springs and quiet winter nights.
So that I could know the depths
of the great, blue ocean
A place from which we all came.

CASE STUDY

A community health nurse is following a child with high blood lead levels. During a follow-up visit to the clinic, the mother was distracted and kept looking at her watch while the nurse explained how important it was to keep the child from coming in contact with leaded paint. The child failed to keep an appointment with a university clinic for a chelation treatment. The community health nurse could not reach the mother because the phone had been disconnected. On a home visit, the nurse found out that the father had been injured while working at his car repair service shop, located on the same lot as their mobile home. He had taken a temporary job while he recovered from the back injury, on an "as-needed" basis for a local garage, and used his own tow truck for jobs. He was on call 24

hours a day. Because of his business, many old cars were all over the yard, explaining a potential source for the lead poisoning in the child. Also, his injury had kept him from repairing the family car, so the only transportation was the tow truck.

1. Identify three of the most serious health threats in this family.

2. Identify two nursing goals for this family.

3. What is the first action you would take on the first home visit?

4. What further information would be important to know about these family members?

5. Name two strengths of this family.

I stepped outside of myself so that I could know
that there was more than the moon,
and the sun, and the stars...
And that when I looked upon the earth
so that I could know the meaning of life and
appreciate its continuance in death.

I stepped outside of myself so that I could know
how to raise my arms in loving, caring ways
And say to those who would listen
Let me share myself with you and all that I know...

by Robyn Rice, RN, MSN

Effectiveness of Home Visits

Research from a variety of studies indicates that successful home visiting programs have resulted in improved health outcomes. But how effective are home visits, such as those that are preventive in nature, in the long run? In a recent research study, prenatal and early childhood home visits by nurses reduced subsequent antisocial behavior and experimentation with drugs in adolescents born into high-risk families. The study, which evaluated the effects of home visits by nurses over the course of 15 years to low-income, unmarried women, found long-term

RESEARCH BRIEF

Twohy, K. M., & Rief, L. (1997). What do public health nurses really do during prenatal home appointments? Public Health Nursing, 14(6), 324–331.

This research study used a descriptive design to identify and describe the nursing interventions and activities used by public health nurses in home-based delivery of care to high-risk prenatal clients. Fourteen home appointments by nine public health nurses were audio taped, transcribed, and coded using the Nursing Interventions Classification (NIC) as the coding scheme. Seven interventions accounted for nearly 83% of the nursing care during the home visits. Those seven interventions were active listening, childbirth preparation, family integrity promotion (childbearing), parent education (childbearing family), prenatal care, self-esteem enhancement, and support system enhancement. Weak relationships were found between the interventions

and the written care plan, the interventions identified in the coded transcriptions, and the chart documentation of the events of the home visit. Many interventions or activities were not part of the written nursing care plan. Implications are for further study to clarify what constitutes a nursing intervention, to clarify the need to formalize psychosocial activities as nursing actions, and to examine the usefulness of the nursing care plan. Because the nursing care plan should give direction to care, it should be relevant to care and consulted before and updated after each home visit. Further research needs to be conducted regarding the actual use of the nursing care plan and for what purpose it is written.

benefits that included fewer episodes of children running away from home, arrests and convictions, and drug abuse when compared with similar groups of women who received prenatal and well-child care in a clinic. The adolescent children of these mothers also had fewer sexual partners and smoked and drank less (Olds & Kitzman, 1993).

Other research has revealed that successful home visiting programs should be broad in focus (e.g., improved pregnancy outcome versus hypertension management during pregnancy), which may contribute the most lasting effects in health status. Also, home visits that occur over time and in greater frequency accomplish more in terms of improved health status for the clients than single visits (Barkauskas, 1983). Home visiting to targeted high-risk groups who have complex and multiple needs have been linked with more significant changes in health status than those at medium or low risk (Byrd, 1998; Deal, 1994; Olds & Kitzman, 1993). Numerous studies have demonstrated that home visiting by nurses to pregnant and postpartum women and their infants reduces risk factors that result in preterm births, abuse and neglect, and maternal health problems. In addition, home visits improve healthy behaviors and are cost-effective (Gomby, Larson, Lewit, & Behrman, 1993; Olds, 1992; Olds, Henderson, Phelps, Kitzman, & Hanks, 1993).

. . . .

Hospitals are an intermediate stage of civilization. While devoting my life to hospital work I have come to the conclusion that hospitals are not the best place for the poor sick except for surgical cases.

Florence Nightingale, 1860

. . . .

Home health visits have been linked with fewer hospital readmissions, fewer emergency department visits, and cost savings when compared with acute care. A study of clients with congestive heart failure who were visited by home health nurses linked fewer hospital admissions, from 3.2 admissions per year to 1.2 admissions per year, with home health visits. The length of stay decreased from 26 days per year to 6 days per year (Kornowski, Zeeli, Averbuch, & Finkelstein, 1995).

Schoen and Anderson (1998), in their extensive review of the effectiveness of home visiting programs, found that the most successful programs have the following elements:

- *A focus on families in greater need of services rather than universal programs*
- *Interventions that begin in pregnancy and continue through the second to fifth years of life*

- *Flexibility and family specificity regarding duration and frequency of visits, according to the family's need and risk level*
- *Active promotion of positive health-related behaviors*
- *Use of a broad, multiproblem focus to address the full complement of family needs*
- *Assistance to family with reduction of stress by improving social and physical environment*
- *Use of nurses and professionals specifically trained in home visiting*

Challenges of Home Visits

Ironically, many of the aspects of home visiting that make it more advantageous for the nurse and client than the hospital environment also contribute to the challenges of home visiting. Because the nurse is more independent and less tied to the physical constraints of the agency, professional isolation can be a problem, especially for a novice nurse. In the clinic or hospital, help or consultation with other professionals is only a few steps away. For the home visiting nurse, that becomes more difficult and can be a source of considerable anxiety. With advanced technology, such as laptop computers, pagers, and cellular phones, the nurse must use different strategies for connecting with other professionals.

The intimacy of the home visit can create boundary issues for the nurse and the client. For example, the boundary between professional distance and social intimacy because of the informality of the home is a constant challenge for the community health nurse. Certainly, there is a certain amount of socialization that occurs in all home visits as the nurse maintains therapeutic rapport and extends courtesy to her client hosts. Nurses also may find themselves disclosing more about themselves than they would in a hospital setting. Such self-disclosure must be monitored carefully so that the client-nurse relationship remains therapeutic. For example, a nurse's concern about her own child's illness might be mentioned in casual comments and then become a significant source of anxiety for the elder client who becomes overly worried about the child's well-being.

The nurse must also deal with the challenge that providing care may actually increase a person's feelings of vulnerability, simply by being seen at home by a nurse. The client may perceive that by accepting the nurse's help, his or her own ability to give self-care is inadequate. In their ethnographic study, Magilvy, Brown, and Dydyn (1988) found that home health clients often expressed concerns about relying on a home health nurse as a sign of vulnerability. They expressed a need to maintain their independence and mobility and saw the nurse as a reminder of their dependency or reliance on outside help. Therefore, the nurse must constantly promote the collaborative nature of the

BOX 13-5 SECRETS OF PROFESSIONAL CONVERSATION: THE HOME VISIT

1. *Break the ice with a warm topic.* Try opening with a cliché such as the weather, pets, sports, children, yard flowers, garden, or any subject that interests *most* people. This often establishes an initial conversational bond that helps make the transition to other more sensitive topics easier. Example: "How has all this rain lately affected your garden?" or while pointing to pictures in home, ask "Are these your children?"

2. *If you are extremely uncomfortable or have a sense of unidentified anxiety, explore possible source with the client.* Often, nurses can sense nonverbal conflict in the home, with the client, or with the family. By acknowledging that this is valuable information can be elicited from the client. Example: "Things seem a little unsettled today. Do you want to talk about anything before we get started with your assessment?"

3. *Pick up the pace by asking open-ended questions.* This forces discussion because questions can't be answered with a simple yes or no. Answers will be longer so you will be able to notice other things that are being said to keep the conversation going. Example: "Why do you like living out in the country? What do you think about the new road going through town? What if . . . ?"

4. *Show sincere interest.* Listening is a skill that must be practiced daily. This means make good eye contact. When the client is speaking, our tendency is to spend that time planning what we will say next. This is not only discourteous and nontherapeutic, but causes us to miss important information. Flatter your client/family with sincere comments: All people crave appreciation. Make sure you *individualize* compliments with details, such as commenting on how much more energetic your client is or noting that a young mother is attending to her new baby's cries very well. Listening is an excellent way to demonstrate your respect for your client! Example: Instead of rehearsing your next line, focus on your *genuine* response to what he/she is saying. Challenge yourself to come up with questions about the points the person has raised.

5. *Develop a broad outlook.* Avoid using the word *I* too often. Watch the great conversationalists—Oprah Winfrey, Jane Pauley, Barbara Walters,

Katie Couric, or Larry King—they seldom mention themselves, know a little bit about a lot of subjects, and demonstrate a curiosity about a broad range of topics. Example: Read the local newspaper daily and try to listen to at least one news show every other day. This ensures that you will expand your consciousness about community and national issues that concern your clients. Read a variety of opinions about a wide range of issues. Challenge yourself to think about things in new ways.

6. *Avoid judging others in advance (i.e., "prejudice").* Try to suspend judgment about your client. Coming to conclusions about people before you have even entered their homes, based on what you have read in their chart or know about their income, shuts down your curiosity and prevents you from learning what you need to know about their health status. Example: In a home visit with a new mother who consistently misses clinic appointments, keep an open mind and ask her about other aspects of her life. Listen to her accounts of how her life has changed since giving birth.

7. *Quote your client when possible.* A very flattering and confirming strategy to promote your client's self-confidence is to use actual quotes from previous conversations (either from the same visit or previous visits, which means you have to really listen!) to illustrate health information. Example: "Since you mentioned last visit that you felt a 'bit better when I am able to cook my own breakfast,' I think that taking care of yourself as much as possible really makes a difference."

8. *End a conversation gracefully.* Breaking away from a conversation in the home can often be more difficult than starting one. After we "connect" with someone, most of us are hesitant to interrupt when you need to move on to other topics or to end the visit. The reality is that there will eventually come a point in any conversation when you will have to end it. Prepare when you enter the home to end the conversation. Example: Prepare an exit early on in a polite and friendly way. "I have so enjoyed our visit, but I must get going in order to see my other clients," or, "I see from the clock that it is near lunch and I know you must be hungry."

Source: Adapted from King, L. (1994). How to talk to anyone, anytime, anywhere: The secrets of good conversation. *New York: Crown.*

client-nurse relationship and frequently praise the client for efforts to improve health, no matter how small or insignificant the changes might be. Nurses accustomed to using "take charge" skills such as are rewarded in the hospital often find that they may lead to failure in the home setting (Coffman, 1997; Liaschenko, 1994).

In the home setting, the client has the right to self-determination and can reject or accept the therapeutic interventions offered by the nurse. This important aspect of autonomy cannot be overemphasized when in the client's home. The nurse must remember that true collaboration means that the nurse and client set goals, develop strategies, and evaluate outcomes of care together, no matter how difficult that may be for the nurse who has been taught that "the nurse always knows best" (Zerwekh, 1997). For example, a prenatal client may refuse to stop smoking during pregnancy, expressing to the nurse that she is too nervous because her mother-in-law has moved in with the family. The nurse may be able to provide the client with assistance in reducing the number of cigarettes smoked per day.

Successive approximations in the attainment of client goals means that progress is measured in small increments, rather than in the dramatic turnaround of the acute care setting (Stulginsky, 1993a). For many nurses, this is perhaps the most difficult challenge of all, especially for nurses who have primary experience in the hospital specialty units, such as the trauma department or intensive care unit. The community health nurse cannot solve all of the client's problems during home visiting, nor should such attempts be made. Only those health problems that are amenable to therapeutic nursing interventions and that are mutually agreed on by the client and nurse should be the focus during home visits. For example, the client with diabetes may not be able to eliminate sugar from her coffee and tea but over time has discontinued using sugar with her cereal.

Another challenge that often emerges is when the nurse faces the immediate pressing demands of the family and a different, preset agenda determined by the agency, usually as a result of funding source policy (Cowley, 1995). Usually, the funding source states a specified number of visits or a specified time frame for the care (e.g., 60 days). The dilemma occurs for the community nurse when the client needs additional care but not specifically at the skilled level. The client may express the need for more assistance in learning to exercise with the artificial hip appliance. The nurse could refer the client to local support groups and community senior centers that offer specialized exercise classes. Community health nurses may be some of the most creative nurses out there as they struggle to find myriad ways of meeting client needs when conventional reimbursement sources end. Consulting with other team members and using support groups provide resources and support in these complex and frustrating situations, which are becoming all too common in the managed care arena.

Distractions in the Home Environment

Conducting a visit in the home, as compared with the nurse-controlled environment of the hospital, is unique in that the nurse must compete with many distractions. Although the distractions that nurses encounter on home visits may seem on the surface negative and interfere with the plan of care, Pruitt, Keller, and Hale (1987) contend that distractions can also provide valuable information about the client's world. Distractions can generally be classified as environmental, behavioral, or nurse-initiated.

Environmental distractions take the form of excessive stimuli, such as television and radio, children playing and making noise, phone calls, traffic, or construction noise. Other environmental sources of distraction may come from crowded or cluttered living conditions; the nurse almost always faces less than ideal living conditions on home visits. Nurses have their own picture of what an ideal living environment should look like, and such values influence the way distractions affect assessment and interventions. For example, the nurse may find a cluttered home a sign of a client's depression or disinterest in a healthy environment. By remaining open to other explanations, the nurse may discover that the client feels comforted by the various objects, furniture, and photos. How we "clutter" our homes has much to do with what is important to us—and to our clients—and thus this can be a valuable way for us to learn about the client's values. How we "use" our space, no matter how large or how small, reflects our values and lifestyles (Pruitt, Keller, & Hale, 1987). Noticing how the furniture is arranged, the number and kinds of photographs around the home, and the kinds of objects displayed can help nurses understand a client's family circle and ties as well as those things that bring the client joy. The "doggie smell" and dog hair throughout the house may be what makes an elderly woman's house a home. Elders often have cluttered homes because they have accumulated the memories and possessions of a lifetime; they also may place furniture close together to make it easier to hear conversations. The nurse learns to minimize distractions, for example, by asking to turn down or "mute" the television or avoiding visiting when the client is most likely to be watching favorite television programs. If interruptions become a problem, observing how the client reacts can provide the nurse with clues to how much of a threat the distraction is to the client's health (Pruitt, Keller, & Hale, 1987). One solution in visiting a pregnant women with a 3-year-old who may be distracting her is to have the child draw a picture for the nurse. Such a strategy can provide the nurse with ample time to perform assessment tasks with the mother. In a multiperson household where privacy is premium, often retreating to a back room or even outside to a porch is all that is necessary for a few moments of distraction-free assessment time. Balancing courtesy with objectives for the visit becomes a skill that requires tact, humor, and creativity.

Another distraction is **behavioral distraction**. The client may exhibit behaviors that distract the nurse from the plan of care and goals of the home visit. Clients may avoid talking about health problems for a variety of reasons and may instead engage in social communication. Clients may have very real concerns that are not consistent with what the nurse sees as priority problems (Pruitt, Keller, & Hale, 1987). By examining such avoidance, the nurse may find that these concerns should be addressed first. For example, a nurse who is seeing an older woman with diabetes may find that the client refuses to discuss her daily blood sugars, but instead wants to talk about an auto accident that occurred the night before near the client's home. Upon closer examination, the nurse finds that the accident has claimed the life of an elderly woman only casually known to the client, and the client then remarks, "It isn't too much longer that I will be able to drive, and then what will I do?" The client was exposing her feelings of vulnerability about losing her mobility and independence. Other behaviors that may hinder the goals of the home visit include blocking or silence in response to inquiries related to health status. The nurse must use appropriate therapeutic communication techniques, as well as exhibit patience, to provide optimal comfort for the client in the home environment.

Nurse-initiated distractions can evolve from prejudices, fears, preoccupation with the tasks of home visiting, and reactions to lifestyles and living conditions different from the nurse's own. This "baggage" that all nurses carry with them on home visits should be carefully acknowledged and examined to prevent negative effects on nurse-client interactions. Nurses may fear home visiting because of safety concerns, concerns over being alone without colleagues for support and consultation, and fears of being rejected by the client. Practicing nursing in the uncontrolled environment of a client's home can threaten even the most secure nurse in terms of autonomy and control. Other distractions that are common are talking on the phone with the home office or other health care professionals or making arrangements for other clients while in the client's home. The nurse must be aware of how such distractions influence the nurse-client relationship. While in the home, the client should remain the focus as much as possible. By being preoccupied with staying on schedule, tasks, and documentation of the visit, the effectiveness of home visiting can be seriously threatened.

The nurse may also become frustrated with clients who are labeled as noncompliant or seem to have contributed in some way to their health problems, such as emphysema in a smoker or liver cancer in an alcoholic. Understanding that these feelings are shared at one time or another by most nurses can be the first step to prevent effects on care. Talking with colleagues and having open dialog with other professionals in similar settings can help nurses understand not only the source of these distractions but helpful ways that others have used to minimize their effects on client care (Pruitt, Keller, & Hale, 1987).

CONCLUSION

The origins of home visiting began with organized health care. Visiting families and clients in the home can provide the community health nurse with more realistic expectations of the family's needs and more appropriate interventions. Advantages and disadvantages of home visiting should be considered when choosing this setting for community-based nursing care.

CRITICAL THINKING ACTIVITIES

1. Read the poem *Home Call: Mother and Child* by Marilyn Krysl on p. 300.
   - How does the mother perceive the nurse in terms of power?
   - Do the status differences in the nurse and the mother affect the outcome of this home visit as intervention?
   - How could the nurse be culturally sensitive in this situation while educating the mother about appropriate child care?
   - How is power represented in this poem?
   - Identify one appropriate nursing intervention in the described home visit.

2. The following questions are common ones that student nurses ask about home visiting. As you read this chapter, reflect on your own responses to the questions.
   - What do clients in the home think of student nurses caring for them, especially if an instructor is not present?
   - What if the client or family member asks me a question that I don't know?
   - What will I be expected to do as far as skills in the home setting?
   - What about safety issues?
   - What do I do if a client "codes" while I am there?
   - Are there specific legal implications that I should be aware of in the home setting?

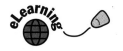 Explore Community Health Nursing on the web! To learn more about the topics in this chapter, access your exclusive web site:
http://communitynursing.jbpub.com

REFERENCES

Allen, C. E. (1991). Holistic concepts and the professionalization of public health nursing. *Public Health Nursing, 8*(2), 74–80.

Barkauskas, V. H. (1983). Effectiveness of public health nurse home visits to primarous mothers and their infants. *American Journal of Public Health 73*(5), 573–580.

Byrd, M. E. (1998). Long-term maternal-child home visiting. *Public Health Nursing, 15*(4), 235–242.

Coffman, S. (1997). Home-care nurses as strangers in the family. *Western Journal of Nursing Research, 19*(1), 82–96.

Cowley, S. (1995). In health visiting: A routine visit is one that has passed. *Journal of Advanced Nursing, 22,* 276–284.

Deal, L. W. (1994). The effectiveness of community health nursing interventions: A literature review. *Public Health Nursing, 11,* 315–323.

Gomby, D. S., Larson, J. D., Lewit, J., & Behrman, R. (1993). Home visiting analysis and recommendations. *The Future of Children, 3,* 6–22.

Kornowski, R., Zeeli, D., Averbuch, M., & Finkelstein, A. (1995). Intensive home care surveillance prevents hospitalization and improved morbidity rates among elderly patients with congestive heart failure. *American Heart Journal, 4,* 762–766.

Liaschenko, J. (1994). The moral geography of home care. *Advances in Nursing Science, 17,* 16–26.

Liepert, B. D. (1996). The value of community health nursing: A phenomenological study of the perceptions of the community health nurses. *Public Health Nursing, 13,* 50–57.

Magilvy, J. K., Brown, N. J., & Dydyn, J. (1988). The experience of home health care: Perceptions of older adults. *Public Health Nursing, 5*(3), 140–145.

National Association of Home Care (NAHC). (2000 and 2001). *Basic statistics about home care.* Washington, DC: Author.

Olds, D. L. (1992). Home visitation program for pregnant women and parents of young children. *American Journal of Diseases of Children, 146,* 704–708.

Olds, D. L., Henderson, C. R., Phelps, C., Kitzman, H., & Hanks, C. (1993). Effect of prenatal and infancy nurse home visitation on government spending. *Medical Care, 31,* 155–174.

Olds, D. L., & Kitzman, H. (1993). Review of research on home visiting for pregnant women and parents of young children. *The Future of Children, 3*(3), 53–92.

Pruitt, R. H., Keller, L. S., & Hale, S. L. (1987). Mastering the distractions that mar home visits. *Nursing and Health Care, 8,* 344–347.

Ruetter, L. I., & Ford, J. S. (1996). Perceptions of public health nursing: Views from the field. *Journal of Advanced Nursing, 24,* 7–15.

Schoen, S., & Anderson, S. (1998). The role of home visitation programs in improving health outcomes for children and families. *Pediatrics, 101*(3), 486–490.

Stulginsky, M. M. (1993a). Nurses' home health experience. Part 1: The practice setting. *Nursing and Health Care, 14,* 402–407.

Stulginsky, M. M. (1993b). Nurses home health experience. Part 2: The unique demands of home visits. *Nursing and Health Care, 14,* 476–485.

Zerwekh, J. V. (1997, Spring). Making the connection during home visits: Narratives of expert nurses. *International Journal of Human Caring, 1*(1), 325–333.

Chapter 14
Home Health and Hospice Nursing

Karen B. Utterback, Karen Saucier Lundy, Debra K. Lance, and Mary E. Stainton

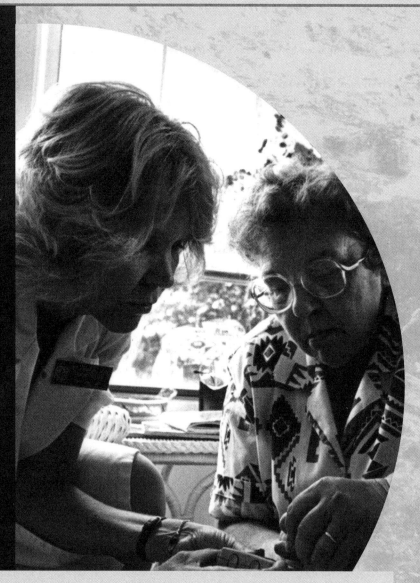

Home health care was established in the latter part of the 19th century, as nursing schools began graduating more and better trained professional nurses. Influencing this movement to home care was the explosion of scientific knowledge about microorganism transmission and communicable disease and the accompanying advancement in technology.

QUESTIONS TO CONSIDER

After reading this chapter, answer the following questions:

1. What factors have contributed to the increased growth in home health care in the past 30 years?
2. What is a typical home health client like as far as diagnosis and age?
3. What are common reimbursement sources for home health services?
4. How does home health nursing differ from other health care settings?
5. How are technologies being used in home care?
6. What is hospice, and how does it differ from home health?
7. What is the future of home care nursing?

KEY TERMS

Capitated rate
Conditions of participation (COP)
Disease state management (DSM)
Fee-for-service rate
Home health care
Home health care nurses

Home health care nursing
Hospice
Informal caregivers
Palliative care
Plan of care
Skilled nurse visits (SNVs)

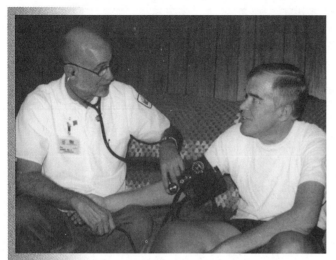

Home health nurse Jim Jones, RN, conducts a physical assessment.

Home Health Nursing

Home health care refers to the delivery of health services in the home setting for purposes of restoring or maintaining the health of individuals and families. Managed care and technological advances and research have all contributed to the movement from the hospital to the home as a diverse and dynamic service delivery setting for care (NAHC, 2000). Providing home care services to some 7.6 million individuals who require health care, **home health care nursing** is the choice for many community health nurses who are attracted by the autonomy, flexibility, and challenge of caring for persons in their own home. Home health care nursing, according to the American Nurses Association (ANA, 1999), is a synthesis of community health nursing and selected technical skills from other nursing specialties. It involves the same primary preventive focus with home health clients and the secondary and tertiary prevention foci on the care of individuals in collaboration with the family and caregivers. **Home health care nurses** provide care to a broad spectrum of ages and clinical diagnoses (Rice, 1996).

Home health care should be holistic and focused on the individual client, integrating family, caregivers, and environmental and community resources to promote optimal health for the client confined to the home. See Boxes 14-1 and 14-2 for a look at a typical home health nurse's day and client load.

Annual expenditures for home health care were close to $33.1 million for 1999. Almost any care that can now be provided in the hospital can also take place in the home, which has created numerous practice opportunities for home health nurses. Home care services are provided to persons with acute care needs, long-term health conditions, permanent disabilities, or terminal illnesses (NAHC, 2000).

According to the Department of Health and Human Services, home health care is that component of the continuum of comprehensive health care whereby health services are provided to individuals and families in their places of residence for the purpose of promoting, maintaining, or restoring health, or of maximizing the level of independence while minimizing the effects of disability and illness, including terminal illness (Warhola, 1980). The appropriate services to meet the needs of the individual client and family are planned, coordinated, and made available by providers organized for the delivery of home care through the use of employed staff, contractual arrangements, or a combination of the two patterns.

Changes in the health care system and advances in technology and information challenge nurses to redefine the terms *home* and *care* (Frantz, 1997). Clarke and Cody (1994) challenged nurses to rethink the central concepts of nursing: person, environment, health, and nursing. In the home, boundaries between nurse and family as caregivers become blurred, each providing essential care to the client. The home has long been considered the private domain of the family—it is increasingly becoming the "employment setting" for the home health nurse, where nurse and client needs intersect. In the hospital, there are often dramatic changes from illness to health; in the community home setting, the changes are subtle as a chronic disease state emerges as the dominant mode of health and illness. The physician remains the center authority in the hospital; in the home, autonomy of the family and client are vital and requires a collaborative effort between caregivers and health providers.

• •

My view you know is that the ultimate destination is the nursing of the sick in their own home. I look to the abolition of all hospitals . . . but no use to talk about the year 2000.
                                        Florence Nightingale, 1867

• •

Standards of Home Health Nursing

The ANA has endorsed the Standards of Home Health Nursing as the basis for home health nursing practice; these standards are found in Box 14-3. These standards, similar to other nursing practice standards, use the nursing process and identify two levels of nursing practice—the generalist and the specialist—to detail the role and function of the home health nurse. Generalist roles include direct care provider, educator, resource manager, collaborator, and supervisor of ancillary personnel. The nurse as specialist has a master's degree and serves as consultant, administrator, researcher, and clinical specialist. The nurse in the specialist role may develop and evaluate agency policy, perform staff development, and be responsible for organizing and managing interdisciplinary

BOX 14-1 SUMMARY DESCRIPTION OF CLIENTS IN SAMPLE HOME HEALTH DAILY NURSING SCHEDULE

On each skilled nursing visit:

1. Wash hands.
2. Set up equipment, including laptop computer.
3. Obtain complete assessment with review of systems. DOCUMENT.
4. Contact physician with assessment results, if indicated. DOCUMENT.
5. Ask the client or caregiver to recall previous instruction, making corrections if needed. DOCUMENT.
6. Perform procedures; wash hands. Note response to care. DOCUMENT.
7. Instruct client/caregiver from plan of care. Note response to instruction. Review as needed. DOCUMENT.
8. Schedule next visit with the client/caregiver.
9. Clean equipment; wash hands.

Ms. Lottie AAA. Hx: 74 y/o with a longstanding history of osteoarthritis, using a walker for mobility in her small rural home. She has a recent diagnosis of type II DM. The physician has requested daily SNVs to instruct her in blood glucose monitoring, diabetic diet, and medication regimen after the initiation of an oral hypoglycemic agent. She lives alone but receives assistance from her many children and grandchildren in the community.

Mr. Ali BBB. Hx: 81 y/o with CHF for several years and is particularly forgetful since the death of his wife last year. His physician has requested SNVs because he has had two recent hospitalizations with exacerbations of his disease. Although he lives alone, his daughter drops by each morning at 09:00 to offer help. The nursing visit is set so that instruction can be given to both.

Mr. Carlo CCC. Hx: 26 y/o with paraplegia and development of a stage II sacral ulcer. He has a roommate who helps with shopping and some activities of daily living. He previously spent most of his day in the wheelchair but has begun to take rest periods midmorning, midafternoon, and early evening. He is pleased with the air cushion for his wheelchair and the gel overlay for his bed.

Ms. Helaria DDD. Hx: 78 y/o with recent onset of idiopathic HTN. She lives with her elderly husband and a very active dog, Maggie. Her children have hired a caregiver for ADLs and housekeeping. The physician has ordered BP assessments 2–3 times a week for 3 weeks to assess the effects of her new medication, quinapril HCl. Systolic pressure at 160 or greater and diastolic pressure at 94 or greater are to be reported. One dosage adjustment has been made, and she has been normotensive on the last two visits. Visit times are varied to give the physician an across the day view.

Mr. Paul EEE. Hx: 34 y/o with congenital lower extremity malformation, type I DM, and open wounds on both lower limbs. He helps his elderly father with financial matters and record keeping. The client meticulously records his wound progress and e-mails any concerns to the nurse and physician. He provides wound care to the areas he can reach, and the nurse performs care to the area outside his reach. He is well educated about his health conditions. He depends on home health aides for most of his personal care. A supervised home health aide visit is planned.

Key for Abbreviations: ADLs, *activities of daily living;* BP, *blood pressure;* CHF, *congestive heart failure;* DM, *diabetes mellitus;* HTN, *hypertension;* Hx, *history;* SNVs, *skilled nursing visits;* y/o, *year old.*

Contributed by: Jim Jones, RN, C, Case Manager Home Health Nurse, South Mississippi Home Health, Hattiesburg, Mississippi.

staffing services. The ANA offers certification in home health nursing through the American Nurses Credentialing Center. Certification as a generalist in home health requires the following:

- *Active RN (registered nurse) license in the United States*
- *Baccalaureate or higher degree in nursing*
- *A minimum of 2 years of practice as an RN*

- *A minimum of 2,000 hours of practice as an RN in home health nursing during the past 2 years*
- *Current practice as an RN in a home health nursing setting for a minimum of 8 hours per week*

The nurse in home health nursing must have excellent critical thinking and decision-making skills. In the home health set-

BOX 14-2 SAMPLE HOME HEALTH DAILY NURSING SCHEDULE*

◆ 07:00   Get ready for the day:

➤ **Check laptop and ensure that the nightly transfer of schedule and patient information completed successfully.**

[The laptop stores the vital scheduling information and the patients' electronic medical record and crucial teaching tools to assist the clinician in carrying out the specific plan of care or care path for the patient.] If so, unplug and pack up the laptop for the day. If the transfer did not complete successfully, this message will be present on the laptop and the process must be attempted again. If problems continue, contact the helpdesk at the office for assistance.

➤ **Call office, check overnight voice mail for any last-minute messages.**

[Night on-call nurses may have taken calls that require schedule change, such as notification that a patient had entered the hospital for care.]

➤ **Organize client visits by priority.**

[Some patient's require a timed visit due to needed lab studies or the presence of a caregiver to receive instruction.]

➤ **Check nursing bag and automobile to see that all needed supplies are available for assessment and procedures.**

◆ 07:30   Turn on pager and cell phone, grab the lunch cooler. You need to travel about 30 minutes to the outlying community to see your first two clients.

◆ 08:00   Arrive at Ms. Lottie AAA. Ms. AAA is now testing her blood glucose with minimal prompting. She is praised for her performance and correct entry of the WNL results. Her meal plans for the day are reviewed, and suggestions are made. Instruction on signs and symptoms of hyperglycemia/hypoglycemia is given with handouts of this in pictorial and text form. She is reminded to fast for tomorrow's visit. The visit has lasted an hour and you will travel back toward town to see your next client.

◆ 09:15   Arrive at Mr. Ali BBB. His daughter greets you at the door with his daily wt. record and the information that he has gained 3 pounds overnight. He is SOB, resp. 34, pulse is 100, BP is 150/92 mm Hg, temp. 98.3°F. His 14:00 dose of furosemide is in the mediplanner for the past 2 days. Ausc. of his lung fields, posterior, indicate fine crackles in the lower lobes bilaterally, and the

mid lobe on the right. Physician contact is made, and furosemide is given IV as ordered. He admits to forgetting medications that don't come at meal times. Instruction is given to move the 14:00 dose to noon, and his daughter will call after lunch as a reminder on medications. Signs and symptoms that require contact with the nurse/physician are reiterated. Now vital signs indicate resp. at 26, pulse 92, and BP 132/84. He has voided twice. Arrangements are made to return later in the afternoon for reassessment. A call is placed to the office to move an afternoon visit to tomorrow and the other patient is notified. You have spent an hour and 15 minutes here and now you travel back into town for your remaining clients.

◆ 10:50   Arrive at Mr. Carlo CCC. You arrive at his home 15 minutes after the scheduled time with sincere apologies. The old dressing is removed, and the wound is gently cleaned with normal saline. The 0.5-cm measurement reveals that healing is rapidly occurring. Skin preps are applied to the intact skin, a hydrocolloid dressing is placed, and the edges are secured with tape. You continue discharge planning because the wound is nearly healed. A review of pressure relief measures and self-inspection using a mirror are discussed. He is eager to return to a more regular routine, and you encourage his plans. His roommate offers coffee, which you graciously decline. Your 40-minute visit is ended with travel a short distance to the next client.

◆ 11:40   Arrive at Ms. Helaria DDD. Maggie, an energetic poodle, has loudly announced your arrival, and she meets you at the door before the bell is rung. You are led to the bedroom for her positional BP checks, but extracting Maggie from Ms. Helaria's lap is a problem. This accomplished, you find her sitting BP is 138/82, standing BP is 128/80, and supine BP is 144/88. She denies headache, dizziness, back pain, fatigue, dry mouth, or GI upset. She is still unclear about taking the medication because she feels "just fine." You repeat the silent threat of HTN, and the need to take her medication as ordered. She agrees and promises to call if any side effects are noted. At 12:10 you are ready to travel toward the next client, with a pull over for lunch.

◆ 12:15   After your fruit and cheese, you check your voice mail for any messages that may affect your afternoon travel.

◆ 12:50   Arrive at Mr. Paul EEE. The door is open when you arrive, and he calls out to "come on back." The aide has arrived just before you and is performing his routine care. You check the aide worksheet and note that the POC isn't being followed. You provide the needed supervision and document your findings. Before care

BOX 14-2 SAMPLE HOME HEALTH DAILY
NURSING SCHEDULE*—CONT'D

can begin, a trip back to the car is needed to bring in sterile syringes. His self wound care is observed along with the wound characteristics noted. The distal wound is irrigated with $\frac{1}{2}$ H$_2$O$_2$/$\frac{1}{2}$ normal saline using an 18-gauge blunt needle. The wound is rinsed with normal saline, and packed with NS moistened gauze packing, covered with gauze sponges, and wrapped with roll gauze. Tape is applied to secure the dressing. Your pager goes off and requires a brief call to one of the clients with medication instruction. Your visit, with interruptions, has lasted an hour and 10 minutes.

◆ 14:15   Arrive at Mr. Ali BBB. He reports voiding several times since you left. You note that there is no apparent SOB, resp. is 22, pulse is 80, BP is 132/82, and temp. is 98.8°F. His lungs have only faint scattered crackles in the bases. Instruction is given again regarding which high potassium foods to include in his diet. He has several bananas on hand and eats one while you talk. His daughter is called at home and reminded to call the agency if signs and symptoms indicate a fluid increase. This visit is over after 30 minutes, and you leave to return to the office.

◆ 15:05   Arrive at the office. Attend scheduled in-service training and competency testing at office. Submit notes, verbal order, and check voice mail for tomorrow's assignments and schedule. Load supplies, and return any calls. Make a note in your daily planner about the in-service on laptop use in the home for next Wednesday. Check the on call schedule and leave a report for the night nurse should Mr. BBB call with continuing problems.

◆ 15:30   GO HOME. (Your own!)
Plug laptop into phone jack and electrical outlet to recharge and be available for the automated data transfer set to occur during the night.

Key for Abbreviations: Ausc., *auscultation;* BP, *blood pressure;* GI, *gastrointestinal;* H$_2$O$_2$, hydrogen peroxide; HTN, hypertension; IV, intravenous; NS, normal saline; POC, plan of care; resp., respirations; SOB, shortness of breath; temp., temperature; WNL, within normal limits; wt., weight;

Refer to corresponding Box 14-1 for a summary description of each client.
Contributed by: Jim Jones, RN, BEd, Case Manager Home Health Nurse, South Mississippi Home Health, Hattiesburg, Mississippi.

ting, the nurse practices autonomously and without the support of a peer group. In addition, giving care in the home of the client necessitates a sensitivity for the client's environment and culture to a much greater degree than other practice settings. Current advances in technology and pharmacology have resulted in the need for the home care nurse to be increasingly more competent in infusion therapies and complex wound therapies.

The Medicare Era

With the enactment of Medicare in 1965, significant growth and change throughout the U.S. health care system created a broad spectrum of health services for the elderly population. Medicare made home care services, primarily **skilled nursing visits (SNVs)** and curative or restorative therapy, available for all persons older than 65. These services were extended to the disabled population in 1973, and hospice services were added in 1983. **Hospice** services provide **palliative care** and supportive social, emotional, and spiritual services to the terminally ill and their families (NAHC, 1999). There were 7,152 Medicare-certified agencies in the United States in 2000 that provided home health services (NAHC, 2001). The total national expenditure for health care was approximately $1.311 billion in 2000, with a slowing down of growth for an average annual growth rate of

5.3%. The slowed growth trend is attributed to the influence of managed care and an overall low inflation rate for the economy. Approximately 62% of total personal care, which is a subset of health care as goods and services used by individuals, went to hospitals and physicians, whereas only 3% was spent on home care (NAHC, 2001). Medicare is the largest single payer of health care services in the home.

Certainly, one of the primary benefits of health care in the home is that it is significantly less expensive than in the hospital. Home health care can reduce per client expenditures, as well as reduce the number and length of hospitalization episodes. For example, an average Medicare charge on a per-day basis for hospital care in 2000 was $2753 compared with $421 for a skilled nursing facility and only $100 for a home health charge per visit (NAHC, 2001).

More than half the clients who receive home health care are older than 65, and the amount of home health they use tends to increase with age. Approximately 40% of the clients have one or more functional limitations. The most common single diagnostic category for home health services is for diabetes. Diseases and conditions associated with the circulatory system are next, including hypertension and heart failure. These diagnoses are followed in frequency by chronic ulcers of the skin and osteoarthritis. The services focus on assisting the client to reach or maintain an optimal state of health,

BOX 14-3 ANA STANDARDS OF HOME HEALTH NURSING PRACTICE

STANDARD I: ORGANIZATION OF HOME HEALTH SERVICES

All home health services are planned, organized, and directed by a master's-prepared professional nurse with experience in community health and administration.

STANDARD II: THEORY

The nurse applies theoretical concepts as a basis for decisions in practice.

STANDARD III: DATA COLLECTION

The nurse continuously collects and records data that are comprehensive, accurate, and systematic.

STANDARD IV: DIAGNOSIS

The nurse uses health assessment data to determine nursing diagnoses.

STANDARD V: PLANNING

The nurse develops care plans that establish goals. The care plan is based on nursing diagnoses and incorporates therapeutic, preventive, and rehabilitative nursing actions.

STANDARD VI: INTERVENTION

The nurse, guided by the care plan, intervenes to provide comfort; to restore, improve, promote health; to prevent complications and sequelae of illness; and to effect rehabilitation.

STANDARD VII: EVALUATION

The nurse continually evaluates the client's and family's responses to interventions to determine progress toward goal attainment and to revise the database, nursing diagnoses, and plan of care.

STANDARD VIII: CONTINUITY OF CARE

The nurse is responsible for the client's appropriate and uninterrupted care along the health care continuum and therefore uses discharge planning, case management, and coordination of community resources.

STANDARD IX: INTERDISCIPLINARY COLLABORATION

The nurse initiates and maintains a liaison relationship with all appropriate health care providers to assure that all efforts effectively complement one another.

STANDARD X: PROFESSIONAL DEVELOPMENT

The nurse assumes responsibility for professional development and contributes to the professional growth of others.

STANDARD XI: RESEARCH

The nurse participates in research activities that contribute to the profession's continuing development of knowledge of home health care.

STANDARD XII: ETHICS

The nurse uses the code for nurses established by the American Nurses Association as a guide for ethical decision making in practice.

Source: ANA, 1999.

independence, and comfort in their home setting. Box 14-4 lists the most common diseases and disorders seen in the home health client.

Persons who most need home health care require assistance in activities of daily living (National Institute on Disability and Rehabilitation Research, 1996). **Informal caregivers**, such as family members, friends, and others who provide services on an unpaid basis, provide the bulk of home care with guidance and support from home health professionals.

The provision of care in the client's place of residence contributes to the unique nature of this part of the health care delivery system. Home care represents a cost-effective and satisfying means of meeting the client's health care needs (Shamansky, 1988). Many factors have contributed significantly to the growth of the home care industry in recent years, including the aging of the population, advances in technology, shorter inpatient hospital stays, and the increasing availability of outpatient services. According to Maraldo (1989, p. 303), "Home care is most suited

BOX 14-4 TOP 10 MOST COMMON DIAGNOSIS-RELATED GROUPS REFERRED TO HOME HEALTH CARE FOLLOWING HOSPITALIZATION

1. Major joint and limb reattachment procedure of lower extremities
2. Heart failure and shock
3. Cerebrovascular disorders, excluding transient ischemic attacks
4. Simple pneumonia and pleurisy, with complications and/or co-morbidity
5. Chronic obstructive pulmonary disease
6. Major small and large bowel procedures with complications and/or co-morbidity
7. Hip and femur procedures, excluding major joints
8. Coronary bypass with cardiac catheterization
9. Circulatory disorders with acute myocardial infarction and cardiovascular complication
10. Nutritional and miscellaneous metabolic disorders

Source: Prospective Payment Assessment Commission Report to Congress. (1996, June). ProPac analysis of MedPAR and home health claims data from the Health Care Financing Administration. Washington, DC: U.S. Government Printing Office.

BOX 14-5 SAMPLE ROLE DESCRIPTION OF A STAFF HOME HEALTH NURSE

- Establish effective relationships with the client, family, and other health professionals.
- Collaborate with other health professionals and providers in evaluating the client's response to the plan of care.
- Develop a discharge plan with the client and the caregivers as well as the other health professionals.
- Use principles of teaching and learning to educate clients and caregivers in the knowledge and skills that promote self-care and prevention or control of disease progression or disability.
- Participate with clients, their caregivers, and other health professionals in decision making that reflects knowledge of care that is ethical, legal, and informed.
- Identify and discuss ethical conflicts and act as advocate for the client regarding confidentiality and informed consent.

Source: South Mississippi Home Health Agency. (1999). Hattiesburg, Mississippi, staff registered nurse job description. Hattiesburg, MS: Author.

to become the centerpiece of a new health care delivery system, because survey after survey demonstrates that consumers prefer home care to other types of care." Many complex therapies previously administered only in hospital intensive care units are now safe and available in the home setting. Intravenous (IV) therapy has become common in the home setting, infusing antibiotics, chemotherapy, analgesics, total parenteral nutrition (TPN), and blood products (Sheldon & Bender, 1994). Pediatric hospitalizations have dropped by 46% in the years 1971 to 1993 as more procedures and treatments have been done outpatient and in the home. Pediatric postoperative recovery often occurs in the home (Dougherty, 1998). The ability to provide sophisticated pain control and other comfort measures to the terminally ill, along with an increased understanding and recognition of the importance of preserving dignity in the dying process, have contributed to the growth of hospice services. Often, with the provision of an intermittent skilled service along with the assistance of the home health aide for personal care and exercise therapy, the client is able to remain in the comforts of his or her own home rather than requiring institutional care (Milone-Nuzzo, 1998). (See Box 14-5.)

Types of Home Health Agencies

Home health agency structures vary depending on the type of organization and corporate structure. These differences impact the entity's obligations to local, state, and federal law and regulations. The structure also determines the agency's tax obligation. Agencies are classified as official, nonprofit, proprietary, and institution-based. Box 14-6 describes the various classifications of agencies.

Official agencies are publicly funded units in state or local health departments and supported by taxes. These agencies provide home health services through legislative statutes. Home health services when offered through official agencies may be provided by community health nurses who also function in various other roles, such as in health promotion and communicable disease prevention. Medicare, Medicaid, and private insurance companies reimburse for home health services. Such reimbursement formulas are often complex. Because of the proliferation of private agencies as well as reevaluation of priorities for public health for disease prevention, most public health services that provide home health are located in underserved and isolated areas.

Nonprofit home health agencies are made up of voluntary agencies, as well as private, nonprofit agencies. Voluntary agencies are supported by charities such as United Way or private endowments. The earliest Visiting Nurse Associations are examples

BOX 14-6 HOME HEALTH AGENCY CLASSIFICATIONS

Public/Governmental Agencies: *A public or governmental agency is an agency operated by a state or local government. Examples are state-operated health departments and county hospitals.*

Nonprofit Agencies: *A private, nongovernmental agency exempt from federal income tax. These agencies are often supported, in part, by private contributions or other philanthropic sources, such as foundations. Examples include Visiting Nurse Associations and Easter Seal Societies, as well as nonprofit hospitals.*

Proprietary Agencies: *A private, profit-making agency or profit-making hospitals.*

Institution-Based Agencies: *An institution-based agency can be propriety, nonprofit, official, or voluntary and operates within the organizational structure of a hospital or HMO. The nature of the home health agency will be dictated by the type of hospital structure.*

Source: *Home Health Agency (HHA). (1998). Med-Manual 2180. Citations and Description, State Operations Manual (HCFA Publication No. 7).* Washington, DC: U.S. Government Printing Office.

of voluntary agencies. This type of agency is privately owned and exempt from federal income tax. These agencies do not receive any state or local tax revenues. Certain nonprofit hospitals may also have home health agencies as part of their community services. These types of agencies are usually governed by boards of directors composed of representatives from the community from which they serve. With the increase in numbers of for-profit private agencies, the numbers of these agencies have declined in recent years. Service is provided by the client's need for home health rather than by ability to pay.

Proprietary agencies include private, profit-making agencies or profit-making hospitals. These agencies receive the largest percentage of their revenue through third-party payers. Because of a highly competitive, managed care market, many proprietary agencies are now part of national health care organizational chains managed through corporate headquarters. Another trend is the development of alliances among home health care agencies and other agencies that become contracting partners in networks. Proprietary agencies make up approximately 40% of all Medicare-certified agencies.

Institution-based agencies emerged in the 1970s as hospitals began providing a greater emphasis on continuity of care. As the high cost of hospitalization and movement with diagnosis-related groups (DRGs) led to earlier discharges, hospitals developed their own home health agencies with their inpatient population as the major source of referrals to home health. Clients have the advantage of staying within the same system and enjoy greater ease of movement between and among services. These agencies are second only to proprietary agencies in total number of Medicare-certified agencies in the United States, making up around 30% of agencies.

Home Health Care Documentation

Before the advent of Medicare and federal reimbursement of home health services, home health care was paid for by clients, primarily through donations and philanthropic organizations. Today, Medicare and Medicaid make up the principal funding sources for home health. Part A (hospital insurance) and Part B (supplemental medical insurance) of Medicare include coverage for home health services. Because Medicare and Medicaid together finance more than 75% of home health services, the discussion of financing and documentation of care is directed primarily toward meeting Medicare requirements. Medicaid, as a state-administered program, provides a range of home care benefits that vary widely from state to state. Private, third-party health insurance also provides some reimbursement for home health services.

Because of the reimbursement policies of the Medicare program, accurate and appropriate documentation by the home health nurse is critical for current and future reimbursement of the agency and maintenance of certification of the agency. Documentation activities affect home health to a much greater degree than in perhaps any other setting (Rice, 1996). Documentation requirements are defined in the Medicare Condition of Participation (COP). These documentation requirements have a direct impact on reimbursement for the home health agency. Basically, documentation requirements for home health care are among the most stringent of any health care settings. Each professional note of documentation must demonstrate a skilled level of care and must be inclusive of all care rendered. The professional nurse is responsible for documenting the supervision of the licensed practice nurse (LPN) as well as the home health aide.

As Lovejoy (1997) states, "Because visits and supplies translate to costs, nurses enter the front-line of margin producing responsibility when moving from hospital or other settings to home care" (p. 12).

Disease state management (DSM) is an emerging approach to population disease managed care that considers all elements of home health care in an integrated fashion, rather than each one separately as in present outcome management (Schaffer & Behrendt, 1998). Clinical pathways are outcome driven with specific time frames of expected courses of recovery. The home health nurse participates in controlling the timing and coordination of the practice patterns to achieve the desired outcome set for the client. Because multiple providers and team members from different practice settings are involved, they each share in the responsibility and accountability of outcomes.

DSM provides a standardization of approach to clients within a population defined by a particular disease they all have in common (Hickey, 1998). Disease management improves the health of certain client populations while cutting the costs to the health care delivery system. Although DSM is not managed care, it is associated with managed care as an effective way to reduce total costs of care. DSM has been most effective when applied to chronic disease management. Many managed plans are implementing DSM, which standardizes care in all settings, including the home.

Martin (1998) provides this example of how DSM works. Consider the population of diabetics and the role played by the examination of feet. Diabetes is an expensive disease, and amputations are common, costly outcomes of poorly managed diabetes. The question for a facility might be asked: "Do we have more diabetic amputations in our home health agency than the national average?" A benchmark, such as a state or national statistic, is always used as the basis for DSM. If the answer is yes, an examination begins with a review of all clients with diabetes in that agency. Data from the electronic clinical records, which are housed within the agency's database, are analyzed to determine how clients with diabetes are cared for, from the physician to the home health nurse to the family caregiver to the client himself or herself. Through such an analysis, it is discovered that observation of the feet, while widely known to be a part of the assessment of a diabetic, has not been consistently examined by all caregivers. Research directs this intervention, based on the knowledge that routine observation of the feet provides opportunity to not only detect early signs of poor circulation, but gives the client a chance to learn what to look for in a self-examination. If the caregivers conduct these assessments, along with the home health client, fewer amputations should occur. A new policy is implemented: "At every client encounter, examine the feet of diabetic clients and at that time, teach them to do the exam themselves." This policy is shared with everyone who has any contact with the client. A year later, amputation rates are again examined. A predicable change should have occurred: There should be a decline in the amputation rate. This example shows that other populations with chronic conditions, such as asthma, hypertension, and sinusitis, can benefit from the application of DSM (Hickey, 1998).

The challenges of DSM are related to the expense of implementing such an approach. When DSM is applied to a population, there will be additional time and visits on the front end, client education programs will be necessary and additional staff may need to be hired to manage the information system. Clients are managed by protocol and are given the information they (and their caregivers) need in a standardized format at every encounter. Support is provided so that clients can manage their chronic disease. All members of the health care team must be involved, from the pharmacist to the social worker. There is a heavy emphasis on teaching clients why, when, and how to take medications and how to manage the plan of care. Community organizations, such as the American Lung Association, are used for support and educational resources.

Clinical practice guidelines are now available for the most commonly seen chronic diseases in the population (Schwartz, 1997). Disease management programs will continue to grow in the future as outcomes research and database integration provide a continuum of care from hospital to home (Remington, 1997). See Box 14-7 for DSM concepts and guidelines. See Box 14-8 for proper documentation language.

BOX 14-7 DISEASE STATE MANAGEMENT CONCEPTS

COORDINATION OF PRIMARY AND SPECIALTY CARE

1. Referrals are coordinated from one provider to another.
2. Client is treated by the most appropriate caregiver in the most appropriate setting.

PRACTICE GUIDELINES

1. Optimal approach to client care is established.
2. Providers are educated to follow the established practice guidelines given the clients' individual needs.
3. Client care and cost-effective treatment are enhanced.
4. Clients achieve optimal outcomes.

CLIENT EDUCATION AND EMPOWERMENT

1. Clients are educated in appropriate self-care.
2. Health awareness is increased, and complications are decreased.

PREVENTIVE CARE AND WELLNESS

1. Individuals at risk for a given disease are targeted.
2. Individuals are taught wellness and prevention strategies.
3. Future complications and costs are minimized.

BOX 14-8 CHOOSING THE RIGHT WORDS: DOCUMENTATION AND LANGUAGE IN HOME HEALTH NURSING

KEY WORDS TO USE

Unstable	Does not comprehend
Deteriorating	New problem
Change in	Leaving
Improving	Remaining at
Taught	Deterioration in
Assessed	Complains of
Instructed	Needs assistance with
Observed	Unable to perform
Evaluated	Specific limitations
Comprehends	Remains

WORDS TO AVOID

No change	Reinforced
Doing well	Chronic
No problems	Reviewed
No complaints	Reinstructed
Condition stable	Monitored
(unless at discharge)	Generalized weakness
Appears	

Source: North Mississippi Medical Center Home Health. (1999). Tupelo, MS.

Financing and Payment Systems for Home Health Services

Medicare

The federal government, through the Health Care Finance Administration (HCFA), contracts with regional insurance companies or fiscal intermediaries to provide reimbursement for home care services. To qualify for Medicare benefits for their client population, home health agencies must follow the federal regulatory requirements called **conditions of participation** (**COP**). The COP for home health agencies and hospice services define the requirements that an agency must meet to participate in the Medicare program. The COPs are detailed and prescriptive. Requirements related to organizational structure, clients' rights, and the covered disciplines, which include skilled nursing, physical therapy, speech therapy, occupational therapy, home health aides, and medical social services, are all specified in the COP. The COP also address the specific skilled services that each of these disciplines can provide, training requirements for aides, and other requirements that the agency must abide by to become

an approved provider of Medicare home care or hospice services. The standards set forth in the COP not only stipulate what agencies must do to qualify for Medicare but also form the basis for evaluation of the quality of the services provided. Each agency must incorporate these requirements in their policies and procedures. The home health agency must follow these policies and procedures with absolute compliance to the regulations to ensure Medicare payment of episode of care.

Under the current Medicare program, home health services are paid for either on a fee for service or on an episode of care basis. The Medicare Program defines an episode of care as being 60 days in length. Payment for the 60 day episode of care is determined by the results of the Outcomes and Assessment Information Set (OASIS). The OASIS is an assessment dataset that groups patients into one of 80 groups for payment purposes and the dataset is used to determine patient outcomes of care. The dataset is completed at specific time points throughout the patient's course of home health care. There are a number of circumstances that would result in the payment rate for the episode being prorated for the agency. An example of this would be a patient that required 4 or less visits in a 60 day episode.

As previously discussed, documentation requirements and record-keeping standards must be adhered to strictly and are primary responsibilities of the home health care nurse. This is required to ensure coverage for the care rendered. The visit and progress notes completed by the direct care staff are essential to justifying the need for the services rendered. Each visit made by the agency must be considered "reasonable and necessary" to the plan of treatment established by the physician in order for Medicare to consider the service to be covered. The fiscal intermediaries for Medicare are responsible for reviewing a portion of the agency's clinical documentation on an ongoing basis. This is done to ascertain that the services provided by the agency were appropriately ordered by the physician, were reasonable and necessary, and met the qualifying and coverage criteria for payment.

Agencies are responsible for filing detailed cost reports. These cost reports identify expenses made by the agency in providing direct care of the client, which include the number of complete and prorated episodes of care, the number of visits made per discipline, the number of Medicare clients, and indirect care such as administration and other overhead expenses. This cost report is used to determine the future rate setting and payment levels for the Medicare Home Health Program.

The COPs require that the client meet several qualifying criteria to receive covered services by the Medicare program. These qualifying criteria for home health services are that the client be (1) under the care of a physician, (2) essentially confined to the home, and (3) require skilled services of a registered nurse, physical therapist, or speech pathologist on an intermittent basis. See Box 14-9 for general questions that can guide the nurse in the documentation of homebound status.

The physician must certify that the client is essentially homebound and establish an individual plan of care (POC) for

BOX 14-9 GENERAL QUESTIONS TO GUIDE THE NURSE IN DOCUMENTATION OF HOMEBOUND STATUS

- How often does the client leave home for social reasons?
- How long does he or she stay gone?
- How taxing or difficult is it for the client to leave home?
- What kind of assistive devices are used when the client leaves home?

Source: Denise Pugh, RN, MSN, North Mississippi Medical Center Home Health, Tupelo, MS.

BOX 14-10 SUMMARY OF MEDICARE CRITERIA FOR HOME HEALTH CLIENTS

QUALIFYING CRITERIA FOR A MEDICARE BENEFICIARY TO RECEIVE HOME HEALTH SERVICES

- Essentially confined to the home
- Under a plan of care established by a physician
- In need of intermittent skilled nursing, physical, or speech therapy

COVERED SERVICES FOR HOME HEALTH

- Skilled nursing
- Physical therapy
- Speech therapy
- Occupational therapy
- Home health aide
- Medical social services

QUALIFYING CRITERIA FOR A MEDICARE BENEFICIARY TO RECEIVE HOSPICE SERVICES

- A life expectancy of 6 months or less
- Seeking palliative treatment only

HOSPICE INTERDISCIPLINARY TEAM

- Registered nurse
- Physician
- Pastoral/counselor
- Medical social services

the client. The POC is established by the physician in collaboration with the home health team and must be updated as changes occur in the client's condition, or at least every 60 days. The nurse plays a key role in establishing the POC for both home care and hospice. The nurse collaborates with the physician and with other health team members to establish the appropriate POC for the client. The POC is based on the client's health history and a current comprehensive assessment of the client's physical, psychological, social, and spiritual needs inclusive of the OASIS dataset. The nurse's knowledge of the resources available in the community is very important to establish the plan that will optimally meet the client's needs. Box 14-10 summarizes the concepts of Medicare criteria for home health clients.

Medicaid

Medicaid is authorized by Title XIX of the Social Security Act and provides health services to low-income persons. As a source of reimbursement for home health services, Medicaid is federally aided but state operated and state administered. Each state determines program eligibility, benefits covered, and the rates of payment for providers. Clinical guidelines for Medicaid reimbursement basically follow those of the Medicare program. Medicaid covers

FYI

How is home health paid for?
- *Medicare*
- *Medicaid*
- *Private insurance*
- *Payment by individual or "out of pocket"*

home health services, including skilled and unskilled services. If a client qualifies for both Medicare and Medicaid, Medicare is generally the primary reimbursement source. A comparison of Medicare and Medicaid benefits are detailed in Table 14-1.

Private Insurance

For a growing number of home health clients, private insurance as a third-party payer in the private sector provides reimbursement for home health care services. Three major types of organizations provide this type of reimbursement: indemnity insurance companies that pay a percentage of billed charges, nonprofit

TABLE 14-1	A COMPARISON OF MEDICARE AND MEDICAID IN HOME HEALTH REIMBURSEMENT
MEDICARE (TITLE XVIII)	**MEDICAID (TITLE XIX)**
Age 65 and older or disabled	Income-based eligibility
Homebound status	Homebound status not always required
Intermittent service	Intermittent service
Skilled service	Skilled service not always required
Restorative services	Custodial and maintenance services
Physician certification required	Physician certification required
Medical, therapy, or social service	State option: medical, therapist, or social service
Provides rental and purchase payments	Provides purchase payments
Reimbursement: "reasonable cost"	Reimbursement: maximum allowed, determined by state

Blue Cross and Blue Shield, and health maintenance organizations (HMOs). As more managed care networks emerge as reimbursement mechanisms, HMOs are growing in number and scope in comprehensive health care services. The services provided in the private sector vary by payer, but most often, the documentation and clinical guidelines follow Medicare standards for reimbursement (MacLaren, 1994).

Payment by Individual

Individuals who do not have health insurance, those who do not meet their insurance coverage requirements, or those who do not qualify for federal assistance may pay the established charges by the agency or be allowed to pay on a sliding scale based on income. Clients who no longer qualify for Medicare or Medicaid may also desire home health care services and continue to pay after certification has expired. Each agency has its own policies concerning both payments by individual and medically indigent care, which may be provided at no charge.

Quality Assurance and Public Accountability

Regulation and Licensure

In addition to Medicare requirements, most states require that home health and hospice agencies be licensed to operate within their state. Agencies operating in states that require licensure must abide by the state's minimum standards for licensure, in addition to the regulations included in the COPs. The HCFA, under the direction of the Department of Health and Human Services, contracts with state licensing and certification authorities to provide survey and audit services for the purposes of certifying home care agencies to participate in the Medicare program. Surveys are performed at regular intervals, and at least every 3 years to insure compliance with state licensure requirements and continued certification to participate in the Medicare and Medicaid programs. These surveys may be conducted more often for

new providers or providers that had deficiencies on their previous evaluations. These surveys involve record reviews, staff and client interviews, and home visits. The purpose of the survey process is to ascertain that all regulations are being met in providing home care services to the Medicare and Medicaid beneficiaries. State authorities are responsible for responding to and investigating any complaints lodged against the agency and initiating any action indicated through the appropriate regulatory body.

Accreditation

Accreditation of agencies is another aspect of quality assurance, but unlike state licensure, it is not required for Medicare or Medicaid participation. Accreditation is a demonstration of a commitment to providing a high standard of excellence in the delivery of care. Some third-party payers, such as managed care networks or insurance companies, may require accreditation. To meet the stringent standards of accreditation, an agency must demonstrate team effort from all involved in the delivery of care (Lovejoy, 1997). There are three nationally recognized organizations which provide voluntary accreditation for home health agencies: The Joint Commission's Home Care Accreditation Program (JCHCA); The Community Health Accreditation Program (CHAP), a subsidiary of the National League for Nursing (NLN); and the National Home Caring Council.

Managed Care and Home Health

Managed care has become the dominant pattern of organizational reimbursement in the United States. As a result, most persons in the United States with private health insurance are in some type of managed care arrangement or network. A majority of states are in some form of Medicaid managed care program (Children's Defense Fund, 1998). Managed care will influence nursing practice as agencies respond to strong incentives to lower costs. As has been discussed, nursing interventions and their ef-

CASE STUDY

Mrs. Ollie Mae Thompson is a 68-year-old woman. Her referral diagnosis is congestive heart failure. She was discharged from Baxterville General Hospital after a 5-day stay. She lives with her 75-year-old sister in a two-bedroom house in a small rural community. Upon arrival at the home, the health nurse finds Mrs. Thompson lying in bed. Her sister is watching television in the living room. During the visit, Mrs. Thompson relates the history of her illness. About a month ago, she noticed swelling in her feet and legs and extreme shortness of breath while picking tomatoes from her garden. She had to rest after picking only a small bucket of tomatoes. She also noticed that she had to stop midway between the house and the mailbox to catch her breath. Mrs. Thompson recalled that she had to use two or more pillows in order to breathe easy enough to sleep. She began awakening during the night with shortness of breath and had to sit up in the bedside chair to "get her breath back again" before going back to sleep. She also reported getting up several times a night to urinate, which was a change in her usual habits. She grew increasingly more concerned about herself when she became so fatigued that she neglected her garden crops.

The nurse, when conducting a medication review, found that Mrs. Thompson had been taking digoxin following a myocardial infarction 9 months earlier. Immediately before the present symptoms began, Mrs. Thompson has discontinued taking the digoxin because "I felt fine and didn't think I needed it anymore."

Mrs. Thompson's present medications are as follows: digoxin 0.25 mg/day, furosemide (Lasix) 40 mg/day, and KCl 20% tsp per day in juice. She re-ports that she is taking the "heart pill" but has stopped the "fluid pill" because it makes her have to urinate frequently and getting up makes her dizzy. She took the "other liquid" for about 2 days but has since quit taking it "because it makes the juice taste funny." Since discharge from the hospital, she has required assistance with self-care and is using a wheelchair for most ambulation. She spends much of her day in bed, because "I feel so weak, I can't stand for very long." Her physician told her to "cut down on her salt," and she was given a diet sheet in the hospital, which she misplaced before reading it. She has a return appointment to see her physician in 2 weeks.

Her breakfast today consisted of two fried eggs, two pork sausage patties, two slices of toast with butter and jelly, and two cups of regular coffee. She is complaining of shortness of breath and is expressing frustration that "I will never be able to grow my own vegetables again." Her legs are extremely swollen with 3+ pitting edema; they are cool to the touch. She does not have socks on. She reports that she is concerned about her sister's "back problems" and that she fears relying on her too much for care such as bathing and ambulating. Her vital signs are as follows: blood pressure, 140/90 mm Hg; pulse, 54 beats/min; and respiratory rate, 24 breaths/min.

1. Based on the preceding information, is Mrs. Thompson homebound?

2. Identify two nursing goals for Mrs. Thompson.

3. What action would you take regarding Mrs. Thompson's physical findings?

4. Identify one nursing goal related to Mrs. Thompson's caregiver.

5. What further information would you want about Mrs. Thompson?

fectiveness will be measured against client outcomes and client satisfaction of care. Home health nurses will continue to focus on the family as caregiver, with a greater emphasis on teaching the family/caregiver more effective ways of caring for the client. With increasing responsibilities resting with the caregiver, more efficient use of the nurses' time can occur resulting in shorter illness episodes. All home health nurses must be effective case managers to ensure that the highest quality care is delivered in the shortest time possible (Peters & Eigsti, 1991).

The Balanced Budget Act of 1997 mandated that the HCFA be prepared to implement a prospective payment system (PPS) for home health by federal fiscal year 2000. The prospective payment system for home health is similar to the methodology used for hospitals since 1981 and for skilled nursing facilities beginning in 1998. In 1981, hospital reimbursement by the Medicare program changed from a cost-based reimbursement system to a prospective payment system using DRGs as the basis for reimbursement. Skilled nursing facility reimbursement is a prospective rate varied by a "case-mix adjuster." This case-mix adjuster is determined from information collected in a standardized data collection tool designed to measure clients' need for additional care and services. Case-mix adjustment in the home health setting

RESEARCH BRIEF

Ettinger, B. (1998). Disease management: Maintaining skeletal health among postmenopausal women. American Journal of Managed Care, 4(3), 387–396.

Although disease management is often considered oriented toward treatment, the emerging paradigm for prevention of osteoporotic fractures in postmenopausal women is changing. Conventional wisdom backed by previous research has considered menopausal women to have little opportunity for building bone resulting from calcium loss of aging. With diagnostic procedures, such as bone densitometry, and recently developed drugs, such as biphosphonates and deselective estrogen receptor modulators, there is increasing optimism that bone mass can be regained. Even when treatment is begun in women in their 60s and 70s, fractures can be prevented through increased bone building interventions. Implications for home health nurses are to educate older women about the use of such pharmacological agents, weight-bearing exercises, calcium intake, and the need for bone density screening tests.

A CONVERSATION WITH...

You have to be prepared for anything in home health. Home health nurses use the nursing process just like other nurses; one difference is that they begin the assessment when they pull into the driveway or yard. The nurse may see a 2-month-old for an evaluation for failure to thrive at 8:00 AM, a 10-year-old for post-appendectomy nonhealing surgical wound care at 9:30 AM, and a 101-year-old for catheter care at 10:45 AM. I believe that more than any other nursing care, the art and science of nursing must hold hands in home health. You must know how to administer a high-powered antibiotic IV, know the science and possess the skill it calls for to do it properly. And at the same time, the home health nurse must use the art of caring when a client hammers a nail into his wall for you to hang that IV on when the medical equipment company fails to deliver the IV pole on time. The true art is to use the client's nail and tell him how important he is in the delivery of his care.

—Ilene Purvis Bloxsom, RN, BSN,
Home Health Nurse

is accomplished in a similar manner using the OASIS dataset. Managed health care plans, such as HMOs, preferred provider organizations (PPOs), and networks, are providing home care services as part of their health plans at an increasing rate.

Managed care plans generally reimburse home health agencies based on a fee-for-service or capitated rate methodology. A **fee-for-service rate** is generally based on a per visit or hourly rate for each discipline. A **capitated rate** is generally awarded based on a population or group of "lives" for which the agency is paid a "per member per month" rate. Reimbursement of this nature requires that the agency make an estimation of the anticipated needs of the population to determine if the arrangement is financially feasible.

As the focus in managed care shifts to outcomes of care, research linking outcomes to care delivery has resulted in Medicare's OASIS: Standardized Outcome and Assessment Information Set for Home Health Care. Shaughnessy (1996) developed the OASIS instrument as a data set with the following categories of items: demographics and client history, living arrangements, supportive assistance, body systems, activities of daily living/independent activities of daily living (ADL/IADL), medications, equipment management, and emergent care. Data are collected upon admission to the home health agency, at a specified time during care, and upon discharge of home health services. OASIS is used to measure outcomes of care based on the home health interventions provided. The instrument is mandated by Medicare and is the condition of participation for certified home health agencies. These data are being used by the

HCFA to provide information about the population of Medicare and Medicaid clients receiving home health care and their clinical outcomes.

Interdisciplinary Team Approach in Home Health

Collaboration is mandatory in home health nursing. Medicare requires an interdisciplinary team approach in order for agencies to be Medicare certified. A collaborative approach is clearly evident in the definitions and standards of home health nursing. Collaboration is necessary to ensure the continuity of care as the client moves from hospital to home. *Discharge* has traditionally referred to the client's exit from the hospital to the home; in today's fluid health care system, clients are transitioned in and out of different realms of agency service necessitating complex professional referrals. To be in legal compliance with federal regulatory statutes, the physician must certify the plan of treatment for the client. In most instances, it becomes the responsibility of other team members to evaluate the client's status and response to treatment and then, with the physician, modify the plan of treatment accordingly. The nurse serves as manager or coordinator of care for this interdisciplinary team effort. To function in this role, the nurse must have a clear understanding of the roles of the other team members, and a working knowledge of community resources. Traditionally, the roles and functions of the home care nurse have been that of direct care provider, educator, and case manager or coordinator of care. Direct care activities or skills include assessments, performing procedures and treatments, and client and family teaching. Indirect care includes ancillary personnel supervision, referrals, consultation, and team conferences. The nurse assesses and identifies the problems and needs. Referrals to other disciplines and community agencies may be needed and this care is coordinated by the nurse under the direction of the physician. For example, if a nurse identifies a home health client who is having financial difficulty with out-of-pocket deductibles for necessary equipment, a referral to a social worker would be appropriate.

Within an interdisciplinary model, the unit of care should be the family, and nursing care is designed and provided within the context of the community in which the client lives. The home care nurse cares for clients across the life span with multiple medical diagnoses and responses to illness. Health promotion and disease prevention are the focus of care (Brown, 1998). The nurse develops a POC under the direction of a physician with the assistance of a multidisciplinary team, which becomes the home health care team and may include social workers, therapists, chaplains, nutritionists, and others as appropriate. The client also participates in developing their plan of care, and evaluating, along with the team, the outcomes of care. The nurse and team members plan their visit schedule around client preferences, other discipline visits, physician appointments, and geographic areas. Appropriate planning by all disciplines before the visit is essential. This includes laboratory work or any supplies needed along with the activities of the visit that center around the goals set for the client in the previously established POC. Some agencies have care maps or critical paths that define the day-to-day activities and outcomes to be met during each visit. Others use goals established on admission and modify them as appropriate. Detailed descriptions of member roles of the home health care interdisciplinary team can be found in Box 14-11.

Role of Family Caregivers in Home Health

As community health nurses have long been aware, home health nurses contribute less to the well-being of a home health client

---

BOX 14-11 MEMBERS OF THE HOME HEALTH CARE INTERDISCIPLINARY TEAM

- *Home health nurse* is the traditional provider of care in the home. Home health nurses provide skilled nursing services and coordinate care within the interdisciplinary team.

- *Physician* refers clients for home care services and approves the plan of care.

- *Home health aides* provide personal care that includes activities such as bathing, shaving, and skin and nail care. The home health aide also performs basic tasks that include things such as emptying urinary drainage bags, taking vital signs, assisting with ambulation and performing exercises assigned, and light homemaking activities such as preparing a meal, changing linens, cleaning room, and laundry.

- *Physical therapists* provide evaluation of the client's rehabilitation needs and potential, which may include areas such as range of motion, strength, balance and coordination, gait analysis, muscle tone, pain, endurance, equipment needs, and home safety. The physical therapist then develops and implements the treatment plan that includes teaching the client and family the home therapy regime and establishing a maintenance therapy program.

- *Speech therapists* provide services related to the evaluation of rehabilitation needs and potential in clients with speech and language disorders and swallowing disorders. The speech therapist develops and implements a restorative treatment program involving the client and family.

- *Occupational therapists* focus on evaluation and treatment of the client's upper extremities by assisting to restore muscle strength and mobility for functional skills. The program established is designed to restore physical function and sensory-integrative function or develop compensatory techniques. Vocational and prevocational assessment and training, as well as design and fitting of orthotic and self-help devices, are also provided by the occupational therapist.

- *Medical social workers* provide assessment of the social and emotional factors related to the client's illness and plan of treatment. This includes assessment of the relationship of the client's medical/nursing requirements to the home situation, financial resources, and community resources. The medical social worker may provide counseling for the client related to areas such as depression, addictions, reaction/adjustment to illness, and strengthening family support systems. Counseling for the client's family may be necessary to treat the client's illness/injury in resolving family problems that are obstructing or preventing the client's treatment.

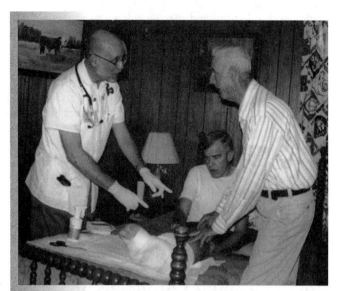

Home health nurses work with the family caregiver to implement the plan of care.

than the more significant influence of family caregivers. Informal caregiving provided by family caregivers is an integral part of our health care system. Among people 45 and older, approximately 2 in 5 report some experience with long-term care in their families. As the population ages, the demand for informal, family caregivers will escalate over the next 30 years (ANA, 1995). Home health clients would be unable to stay in their homes even to be the recipient of home health nursing care were it not for the family members and other caregivers who dedicate themselves to their care. Community health nurses have traditionally been family-oriented when conducting home visits. One only has to look at our legacy of Lillian Wald and the Henry Street nurses to see the foundation of family-oriented care. Only when the family becomes recognized as the unit of service within the context of the larger community can significant, long-lasting change occur. With the ever-present influence of Medicare and other funding sources, nurses often focus their care efforts on providing only those services that are reimbursable in the home setting (Kenyon, Smith, Hefty, Bell, McNeil, & Maraus, 1990). The individual ill client has steadily become the focus in home care, with the family and other caregivers fading to a contextual backdrop (Bradley, 1996).

Recent research has revealed that the family caregivers of home health clients often have unmet health needs and that the role of caregiver is associated with high stress and increased illness when compared with similar populations. The role is often unpaid and associated with isolation and selfless dedication to the health of the home health client (Levine, 1999). Quite often, these caregivers are the only other adult in the home and, as such, have little choice about being the one responsible for the

household and ill client. Many studies report that family caregivers tend to be female and themselves in late adulthood (see Bull, 1990; Pruchno & Potashnik, 1989; Kiecolt-Glaser, Glaser, Shuttleworth, Dyer, Ogrocki, & Speicher, 1987). The community health nurse must strive to consider these caregivers in the assessment of the environment and resources, because if the family caregiver has unmet health needs, eventually his or her caretaking abilities will be affected. Zelwesky and Deitrick (1987, p. 77) go so far as to state, "Accurate needs assessment of the client and his or her family may prevent family burn-out, extend caregiving abilities, conserve family resources, and delay or prevent institutionalization." In her 1996 study, Bradley contends that although prevention activities are not covered by Medicare in home health, "We depend on the family care giver to provide needed care to many of our clients. If the care givers become ill, their caregiving ability decreases. The likelihood of our losing the original home health client to nursing home care or hospitalization increases when we do not promote the family care giver's health" (p. 287). So although not a financial gain in the short term, there may be significant long-term financial benefits in caring for the ones who care for our clients day in and day out. The home health nurse must assess the role of the family caregiver in the context of how well the client functions in the home environment (Levine, 1999). Supporting the caregiver may mean little more than listening carefully to his or her needs regarding personal health status and providing suggestions for health promotion and time management apart from the client. Support groups for caregivers can also provide valuable resources that ultimately strengthen the care provided to the client. The home health nurse has many opportunities to praise the caregiver and remind him or her of the need to pay attention to self for the sake of the client. Day-care programs and respite care can provide needed breaks for the family caregiver and should be encouraged by the home health nurse. As the need for informal caregiving increases in the future, home health nurses will need to become more involved in the promotion of local, state, and national health care policy development related to the support of family caregivers as a health care resource (ANA, 1995).

Legal and Ethical Issues in Home Health

Home health nurses are confronted with legal and ethical issues related to nursing practice daily. Complex family situations create daily dilemmas for the home health nurse, such as questions regarding caretaking abilities of the family caregivers, financial constraints, and respect for autonomous decision-making with the vulnerable client. In the home, nurses are often caring for clients over a long period, as compared with the acute care setting, and as a result, they face boundary issues related to processionals and self-responsibility for care.

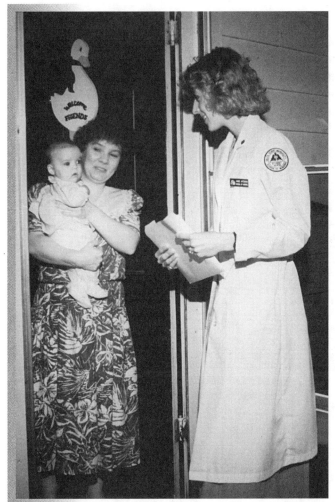

Home health nurses see a variety of clients with diverse health care needs.

One source of ethical dilemma in health care is in providing necessary nursing care for identified client needs when financial coverage is no longer available. Agency policy may include options for temporary services or the nurse must assist the client and family in making alternative plans for care. Clients noncompliance with the treatment plan are constant, and ethical issues related to use of resources can be sources of significant ethical conflict. Reporting abusive, neglectful, and unsafe conditions, care, or practices may often be necessary as a legal and ethical mandatory practice. Knowing a client's rights and responsibilities, as well as the rights and limitations of the home health care nurse, is a critical component of home health care nursing practice. Referral to social work, support groups, and appropriate agencies are often the appropriate response. Lovejoy (1997) recommends the creation of agency support groups for home health care nurses and other professionals. A support group can provide

needed discussion and conflict resolution in the environment of shared experiences with others. Lovejoy (1997) makes the following recommendations in the creation of an efficient support group in home health:

- *A clinical nurse specialist should facilitate and coordinate the support group. This clinical nurse specialist should have experience in leading support groups and ideally should have experience in the field as a home health staff nurse.*
- *Support group meetings should not be mandatory. Nurses should be encouraged to attend meetings but never required to attend.*
- *Support groups should have a mix of new and experienced nurses. All other health professionals should be encouraged to be a part of the group as well.*

The support group should be sponsored by the agency, be a part of the formal organizational structure, and have rules and bylaws as appropriate. If the group is informal, minimal rules should relate to frequency of meetings, commitment of members, confidentiality issues, and termination of membership.

An effective support group should help make members feel better about themselves and their abilities and more at ease in the complex home environment. One unexpected benefit of the support group in home health agencies is that members often are able to see co-workers in a new light and learn to trust them as resources. Home care is often a lonely profession without the benefit of working closely with colleagues on a daily basis. The support group, along with modern telecommunication strategies, can bridge the isolation of "nursing on the road" (Lovejoy, 1997).

Home Care Bill of Rights

Medicare-certified agencies are required to provide home health clients with a written bill of rights before the initiation of service. Each home health client is required to be informed of his or her right for health care treatment, and this must be documented in the client's permanent record. To assist home health provider agencies with this requirement, the National Association of Home Care has developed a Home Care Bill of Rights. This document provides the client with details of what can be expected from home care agencies in the delivery of their care. Agencies often use a modified form of the NAHC Bill of Rights.

Advance Medical Directives

Home health nurses must also be involved in the requirements for informed decision-making as specified in the Home Care Bill of Rights related to treatment options and refusal when the client is unable to make decisions and communicate those decisions to the health care provider. The advance medical directive is a document that describes client intent and wishes regarding various types of medical treatment in selected situations. Medical directives were developed in the early part of the 1990s in response to increased

Home Health Bill of Rights.

SOUTH MISSISSIPPI HOME HEALTH, INC.
BILL OF RIGHTS & RESPONSIBILITIES

Each patient referred to South Mississippi Home Health, Inc. (henceforth referred to as SMHH) has the right to be informed in writing of his or her rights and responsibilities prior to care being rendered. The patient's family or guardian may exercise the patient's rights when the patient has been judged incompetent. SMHH has an obligation to protect and promote the rights of their patients.

Quality of Care

Patients have the right:
- to have a relationship with SMHH that is based on honesty, ethical standards of conduct, and compliance with state and federal laws;
- to be assured of service without regard to age, race, religious preference, sex, marital status, national origin, handicapping condition or whether or not he has executed an advance directive;
- to expect kindness, consideration, and respect;
- to discuss problems regarding services by calling locally _____;
- to voice a formal complaint with SMHH by calling Corporate headquarters at _____, and requesting the Patient Rights Coordinator;
  - to know about the disposition of such complaints;
  - to voice their grievances without fear of discrimination or reprisal; and
- to know the state's home health hotline;
- the purpose of the hotline is to receive complaints or questions about home health agencies.

Decision Making

Patients have the right:
- to be notified in writing of the care that is to be furnished and the proposed frequency of the visits;
- to participate in the planning of the care and in any changes;
- to accept or refuse services or request a change in home health care provider without fear of reprisal or discrimination;
- to make advance directives concerning his care; and
- to refuse to participate in experimental research.

Privacy

Patients have the right:
- to expect confidentiality; and
- to expect SMHH to release information only as required by law or authorized by the patient.

Financial Information

Patients have the right:
- to be informed of the extent to which payment may be expected from Medicare, Medicaid or any other payer known to SMHH;
- to be informed of the charges that will not be covered by Medicare;
- to be informed of the charges for which the patient may be liable;
- to be notified of any changes in the above, orally and in writing, within thirty working days.

South Mississippi Home Health Policy:

South Mississippi Home Health, Inc. nurses, aides and therapists are CPR certified. It is the policy of this company that, in the event of a cardiac arrest and in the absence of a Do Not Resuscitate order from your physician, CPR efforts will be initiated.

SMHH will comply with a patient's advance directives in providing care, to the extent allowed by State law. However, SMHH respects the right of our employees not to implement your advance directive due to personal convictions. In this case, SMHH will make every effort to comply with your advance directive or transfer you to another provider. SMHH may discharge or refer the patient to another source of care if the patient's inability or refusal to comply with the plan of care compromises SMHH's commitment to quality care.

Patients have the right:
- to know SMHH policies which apply to his/her conduct.
  A patient and/or his family shall be responsible for:
  a. cooperation with SMHH staff in the plan of care.
  b. providing SMHH personnel with accurate information as to the symptoms and condition as well as compliance with the prescribed plan of care.
- to be given notice of the reason for transfer or discharge from SMHH, which may be any of the following:
  a. Goals have been met.
  b. Requires a different level of care.
  c. Refuses the continuation of care.
  d. Ill will on the part of the patient and/or family toward SMHH.
  e. Danger to SMHH staff.
  f. Noncompliance with Bill of Rights and Responsibilities.
  g. Noncompliance with Patient Account Policies.
  h. Unsigned physician's Plan of Care.

technology in the treatment of acute and chronic illnesses and the increased awareness by the consumer population of the need to make informed decisions regarding treatment options and the refusal of medical interventions. There are two types of advance medical directives: living wills and health care proxies, also known as *durable power of attorney.* Either type of directive specifically addresses the client's desire for health care or refusal in the event of becoming incapacitated and unable to make decisions. The living will documents a client's decision to decline life-prolonging interventions if that client becomes terminally ill. A health care proxy, or durable power of attorney, specifies the name of a person who will make health care decisions if the client becomes incapacitated and cannot make them. The client maintains the right to change any of these documents at any time. Each state differs in laws and regulation in the implementation of advance directives, and the home health nurse must remain informed to such statutes.

RESEARCH BRIEF

Anderson, M., Pena, R., & Helms, L. (1998). Home care utilization by congestive heart failure patients: A pilot study. Public Health Nursing, 15(2), 146–162.

This study was conducted to determine norms of resource utilization for clients with congestive heart failure (CHF) who are admitted and discharged from a not-for-profit home health agency (HHA). Forty agency records were retrospectively reviewed using the resource utilization inventory to collect the characteristics and resource utilization of the sample group. The CHF clients were older than most home care clients and had chronic health problems. Because of these chronic health problems, more than half the study population had caregivers so that the clients could remain in their own homes. Most clients clearly demonstrated the need for skilled nursing or home health aide visits after being hospitalized for an acute CHF episode. Less than half the study group was discharged from the HHA as improved and often were discharged to another health care facility. These results provide a beginning direction for profiling the CHF client's consumption of resources for setting prospective payment reimbursement rates. Home health care costs have increased more than any other health care service covered by Medicare, and new payment methods are being considered. A prospective payment system would replace the per visit rate paid to home care agencies by Medicare. To remain viable under a new payment system, HHAs will need information about resource utilization of various diagnoses in order to demonstrate effective client care.

Information and Technology in Home Health

Communication and Data Management

Home health care nurses depend on the use of information technology in clinical practice. There is continued demand for and improvement in the information systems available for use in the home. Chapter 8 provides a detailed look at how technology is changing the way client care is being delivered in all settings. As health care becomes more mobile, remote points of access within a safe and secure infrastructure will become the norm (Nugent, 1999). Computerized records and care planning tools, such as critical pathways, are helping the home care nurses achieve greater time and client management. Many home health nurses now practice almost exclusively from home and use laptop computers to document visits. Although working from home does not allow for the camaraderie of team communication that occurs in other settings, it does provide many nurses with more work flexibility (Neal, 1997). With tools to manage this information, many health care organizations have decision-support systems that would benefit the management of client care in the home by issuing reminders, offering a menu of options, or linking the nurse to important educational tools and information needed. As improvements in health networks continue, the nurse can access test results from the laboratory, and information from other providers involved in the coordination of care in the home. Electronic commerce may replace traditional home health methods of communicating with partners in health care, especially as disease management programs continue to grow. Security programs within the organization should protect the confidentiality of individually identifiable health care information. This includes training, security audits, and policies regarding access to different types of information.

Health care information systems of the twenty-first century should guide quality improvement efforts, improve the coordination of care, advance evidence-based health care practice, and support continued research. Because the health care industry is so fragmented, it will be important to work toward data sharing as is common now in so many nonhealth industries. Although all health care organizations collect information, it is uncommon for this to be brought together in a way that can shed light on how variations in the process of care affect outcomes. Information on the experiences and perspectives of clients and the health care team can now be collected with available computer systems. Information on health care outcomes is becoming standard practice in most home care settings (The President's Advisory Commission on Consumer Protection and Quality in the Health Care Industry, 1998).

Delivery of Care

Home care nursing must redefine the assessment parameters that are critical to be performed in person and those that can be done

RESEARCH BRIEF

Jerant, A.F., Schlachta L., Epperly, T.D., Barnes-Camp, J. (1998). Back to the future: The telemedicine house call. *Family Practice Management, 5,* 18–22, 25–26, 28.

The Center for Total Access at the Department of Defense Southeast Telemedicine Testbed at Fort Gordon, Augusta, Georgia, in clinical partnership with Eisenhower Army Medical Center and its regional hospitals, has ongoing research trials of telenursing applications. Telenursing is the use of telemedicine technology to deliver nursing care. The word *telemedicine* comes from the Latin word *tele*, meaning "distance," and *mederi*, meaning "healing." Telenurses "visit" clients at home using telemedicine technology developed by the Eisenhower Army Medical Center, the Georgia Institute of Technology, and the Medical College of Georgia. A real-time connection over the local cable network allows audio and video contact and measurement of physiological parameters in the client's home. The system, called the Electronic Housecall, includes blood pressure cuff, oxygen saturation monitor, temperature probe, three-lead electrocardiogram monitor, and stethoscope. Clients with common chronic conditions, such as diabetes, heart disease, asthma, and chronic obstructive pulmonary disease, are the target population for study. Findings are that these frequent electronic home visits result in fewer expensive emergency department encounters and inpatient admissions. Home telenursing enables closer monitoring so that problems are identified and acted on before they escalate into crises.

through technology such as telenursing. We must also redefine "touch." Do we touch a client physically, as in palpation, or do we also use the term generically, in that we can touch a client with a few therapeutic words over the phone, television, or computer (Frantz, 1997)? The home care nurse can now deliver care and information through a lens, a screen, or a telephone into the home. Home telenursing can never replace in-person home health care; however, the appropriate mix of in-person and electronic visitation, along with the appropriate level of providers to accomplish both, will provide better and more holistic care for the home client and family. Telenursing technology can assist the home care nurse in managing the plan of care remotely to capture vital signs and teach clients and their families self-care management.

Laptop-based medical management systems have been used in the home setting for monitoring wound care and linking the home health nurses to physician consultation. This allows the physician consultants to view client wounds from a live video image. The traditional method in the home requires the nurse to take Polaroid photographs of wounds and forward them to physicians for review. Using the telemedicine system, visiting nurses dial the physician, forward the image in real time, and decisions regarding treatment protocols are exchanged between the providers and client (Kincade, 1997).

As home telemedicine and telenursing systems mature, physical therapy can be administered, nutrition counseling conducted, and occupational therapy supervised. As computer ownership and use in the home become as common as television use, e-mail can be used to communicate with clients and clients can report directly to health care providers. Successful programs have used e-mail to remind clients about medication dosing and educational information for postsurgery clients on a daily basis (Jerant, 1999). Client access to the Internet is becoming more common. Such systems will allow nurses aides to conduct physical home visits and be supervised by nurses at an agency or at home (Schlachta, 1996). The home care industry will use these technologies to track client outcomes, reduce service redundancy, and supplement care provided by visiting nurses and other disciplines.

RESEARCH BRIEF

Johnson, B., Wheeler, L., & Deuser, J. (1997). Kaiser Permanente Medical Center's Pilot Tele-home health project. *Telemed Today, 5, 16–18.*

The home health department at Kaiser Permanente Medical Center in Sacramento, California, followed 100 clients who had chronic obstructive pulmonary disease, cardiac disease, stroke, and wounds requiring regular nursing care with home telemedicine visits by nurses, while another 100 clients received traditional home visits in person and occasional phone calls. Telemedicine units, which work via phone lines and were approved by the U.S. Food and Drug Administration (FDA), provide interactive video conferencing as well as heart and breathing sounds monitoring with an integrated electronic stethoscope. The home units cost approximately $5,000, while the central monitoring station costs approximately $7,500. Client satisfaction with telemedicine visits and the in-person home visits were both rated high, with no difference in the two groups. Care delivery cost savings of 33% to 50% were estimated for the telemedicine group.

Healing a person does not always mean curing a disease.
Dr. Dame Cicely Saunders,
founder of St Christopher Hospice in London

Hospice Care in the Home

Hospice services for the terminally ill became covered expenses under Medicare in 1983. Hospice nursing provides palliative nursing care for terminally ill clients and their families, with an emphasis on physical, psychosocial, emotional, and spiritual needs. Palliative care is comfort-oriented care and refers to interventions that alleviate or lessen the severity of disease or illness without curing it. The goal of the hospice program for home care is to improve the quality of life for people who are no longer able to benefit from curative interventions, with an emphasis on treating the symptoms of the disease to promote comfort. The word *hospice* comes from Latin *hospitium*, meaning "guesthouse." Hospice is holistic in nature and views dying as a normal part of living. Through hospice care in the home, the client can live in dignity and comfort in the context of home and family. Hospice care is primarily provided at home, although facilities also exist that provide these services in an inpatient setting while still offering support for families in a homelike environment. Clients in long-term care facilities can also receive hospice services with the facility considered by Medicare as the place of residence of the client (Brooks, 1997). Medicare can pay for bereavement counseling for as long as a year after the loved one's death. Clients who most often benefit from hospice care and are most commonly seen in hospice care are individuals with cancer, acquired immunodeficiency syndrome (AIDS), end-stage lung or heart disease, and those with chronic diseases. Many HMOs and insurance companies also cover hospice services for their clients. Thirty-six states now offer hospice coverage under their Medicaid programs. Although each hospice service has individual policies concerning payment for care, a common principle of hospice care is to offer services based on a need rather than the ability to pay. For this reason, hospice services may often rely more than other home health services on grants and voluntary donations (Hospice Foundation of America, 1999).

For hospice services, the physician must certify that the client has a life expectancy that would normally be expected to be 6 months or less and is seeking palliative treatment only. Hospice clients must be recertified every 60 days. Clients and family are encouraged to be involved in all decisions about caregiving and medical interventions. Admission to a hospice should not be viewed as a failure of other therapies. Rather, a more holistic approach would suggest that previous treatments had become inappropriate and referral to a hospice as movement into another model of more appropriate therapy for terminal care (Hospice Foundation of America, 1999).

FYI

In 1998, hospices served nearly 540,000 clients throughout the United States.

Source: National Hospice Association, 1999.

The nurse has traditionally cared for the dying and the bereaved, whether on the battlefield or in the trauma unit or in the home—so how is hospice different? Hospice emerged as an organized movement in England with the founding of the first hospice at St. Christopher in London in 1950 by Dr. Dame Cicely Saunders. Dr. Saunders defined hospice care as "hospice is not a place to go to die, but rather a concept of care based on the promise that when medical science can no longer add days to life, more life will be added to each day." She inspired the hospice movement in the United States with the first home care hospice services founded by Florence Wald in 1974 in Connecticut (Box 14-12).

The hospice movement was strongly influenced by the research of Dr. Elisabeth Kubler-Ross, who conceptualized death as the final stage of growth as contrasted with the prevailing fear of death and the dying process as failure on the part of the medical system (Kubler-Ross, 1969, 1975). Over the past 30 years, with the prolongation of life, advanced technology, and a growing recognition that dying and terminally ill clients require a special kind of care, hospice as a community health nursing specialty has grown. Thousands of persons with life-limiting diseases have relied on hospice services for comfort,

BOX 14-12 FLORENCE WALD, RN, FOUNDER OF U.S. HOSPICE HOME CARE

Florence Wald introduced America to the hospice tradition by founding the first home care hospice program in the United States in New Haven, Connecticut, in 1974. Ms. Wald, at age 81, was inducted into the National Women's Hall of Fame in July 1998 in recognition of her work to bring care for the terminally ill through palliative and psychological care. Wald believed that although medical science has given doctors new ways to understand and control disease, "their focus on the patient as a human being was being eroded."

Source: Associated Press. (1998, July 14). Wald among inductees in Women's Hall of Fame.

dignity, and compassion at the end of life. Medicare hospice care for the terminally ill in the home generally cost significantly less than care for clients in the standard Medicare program. Reasons include less technology used in the care of the client and family and friends provide most of the day care at home. Although hospice care does not provide 24-hour-a-day care in the home, hospice staff members are usually on call 24 hours a day. Volunteers make up an integral part of hospice care and are required to be a part of Medicare-certified hospice service. Inpatient respite care is available for the family, which provides family caregivers periodic relief. A written POC is also required. Medicare mandates that four core services be provided directly by the hospice: nursing, medical, social work, and counseling (Wilson, 1993). Services provided by hospice are as follows:

- *Nursing service on an intermittent basis*
- *Physician services*
- *Drugs for pain relief*
- *Physical, occupational, and speech therapy*
- *Home health aides*
- *Medical supplies*
- *Spiritual and pastoral services*
- *Continuous care during a crisis*
- *Bereavement services for the family, up to a year following death*

Hospice provides coordinated services for the family of the client with a terminal illness. Hospice, as a specialized kind of home health care, is designed to provide comfort and support to clients and families in the final stages of terminal illness. Goals center on providing care in which clients can spend their last days with dignity, at home or in a homelike setting, surrounded by family members and loved ones. Comfort involves physical and spiritual comfort and emotional support of the client, family, and caregivers (Waters, 1996). See Box 14-13 for a sample agency hospice philosophy.

. . . .

I look up in the night sky. Is anything more certain that in all those vast times and spaces, if I were allowed to search them, I should nowhere find her face, her voice, her touch? She died. She is dead. Is the word so difficult to learn?

C. S. Lewis

. . . .

Hospice Care for Children

Although hospice services have traditionally been associated with adults, recognition has grown among health care professionals that children with terminal illnesses can also benefit from hospice care (Martinson, 1993). The epidemic of children with AIDS has prompted the development of pediatric hospice services for children with life-limiting illnesses (Oleske &

> ### BOX 14-13 HOSPICE PHILOSOPHY: ONE AGENCY'S COMMITMENT
>
> *Hospice affirms life. Hospice exists to provide support and care for persons in the last phases of incurable disease so that they might live as fully and comfortably as possible. Hospice recognizes dying as a normal process whether or not resulting from a disease. Hospice exists in the hope and belief that, through appropriate care and the promotion of a caring community sensitive to their needs, clients and families may be free to attain a degree of mental and spiritual preparation for death that is satisfactory to them.*
>
> *North Mississippi Medical Center Home Health Services. (1999). Hospice Philosophy.*

Czarniecki, 1999). The first hospice home for children, The Helen House, was established in 1982 in the United Kingdom. By 1993, only 1% of U.S. hospice clients were children. Palliative care for children with terminal diseases, such as AIDS and cancer, can ensure the child's comfort through the course of their illness. Oleske and Czarniecki (1999) advocate that children with a life-limiting illnesses, regardless of diagnosis, socioeconomic

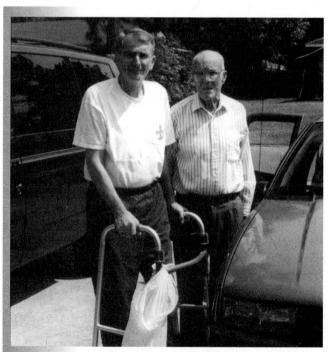

When visiting clients with disabilities, family members are included in the plan of care in order to promote independence and autonomy.

status, or geographic location, should receive a continuum of palliative care and have access to hospice services that enhance life and ease the burden of dying. They contend that "children should know, in an age appropriate way, that death is near but that it will not be painful, not faced alone, but rather in the company of those they love" (Oleske & Czarniecki, 1999, p. 1291). Opportunities for hospice nursing with children will most likely increase in the future.

Nurses who work in hospice care have specialized training in grief and bereavement management. Although spiritual care has been a major component of nursing practice since its inception, nurses are often uncomfortable with spiritual components related to death (Brant, 1998). Hospice nurses must be especially comfortable in their skills related to the spiritual needs of their clients. Holistic nursing care for the hospice client means assessing for suffering in the spiritual realm, because the total person is incomplete without such consideration. Providing spiritual care does not mean that hospice nurses must hold the same beliefs of those for whom they care (Brant, 1998). Hospice nurses who provide palliative care approach clients with a nonjudgmental, listening ear. Nurses provide spiritual care by assisting clients in their final days in their search for meaning of past, present, and future events. They attempt to make sense of their life experiences and nurses, in the holistic tradition, must be involved in this healing aspect of this last stage of life.

Nurses as team members in hospice care are often the ones with the prolonged, close contact with clients and family members and as such can provide comprehensive information about the well-being of the family and caregivers to the physician and other members of the hospice team.

Ethical issues have special considerations for hospice workers. Working with families during a family member's imminent death brings challenges related to professional boundaries, family responsibilities, and complex decisions about care. The threat of legalized suicide is of concern to all nurses but is an especially significant issue in the field of hospice nursing. Legalized suicide and euthanasia practices threaten the natural cycle of dying and the final stage of growth (Brant, 1998). Providing appropriate, holistic, and comforting end of life care, as larger numbers of the baby boom generation age, will continue to emerge as critical professional issues for home health nurses who specialize in hospice care (Brant, 1998).

....

Hospice does not speed up nor slow down the dying process. It does not prolong life and it does not hasten death.
                                    National Hospice Foundation

....

Other future issues for hospice nursing care include the expansion of community-based residential hospice care facilities, which include respite care, home care, acute inpatient care, and expanded bereavement counseling for families. With the grow-ing number of elders, adults with AIDS, and children with prolonged terminal illnesses, hospice services will be challenged to provide myriad home- and community-based services for families caring for the terminally ill. Humane care for the dying strains families who are already overburdened with dual career demands and child care. Such facilities can provide nurse managed, holistic care for the terminally ill in a noninstitutional, natural environment more conducive in the promotion of health in the final stage of life (Barant, 1998; Wilson, 1993).

....

We need to continue to educate nurses in the art of palliative care, emphasizing holistic care that encompasses the mind, body and spirit. Total suffering encompasses all three of these components, and end-of-life care must include the same. We can instill hope that goes beyond the grave.
                              Jeannine M. Brant, RN, MS, AOCN,
                                  oncology clinical nurse specialist
                  Saint Vincent Hospital and Health Center, Billings, Montana

....

....

Life Goes On
I felt like a rainbow covered with dirt in this room.
I couldn't bear seeing
my uncle and aunt washed
with sad feelings.
My grandpa's hand had no life to it.
Though life went on and the
trees kept swaying.
I wondered what would life
be like without his hand to
cross my hair.
My rainbow just did not shine that day.
The wind took over everything.
I love the wind.
It changed everything in that room.
It made me feel like a hundred
butterflies had flown from his
chest.
His stuck together lips and
hard breathing harmed me.
I couldn't stand there.
Water was pulled from my eyes.
Our hands parted and I
kissed him and walked into
reality.
                              Alexandra Zacharias, age 10,
                  on the occasion of the death of her grandfather
                  Source: *The Educational Forum, 55*(3), Spring, 1991.

....

The Future of Health Care in the Home

As the home health industry continues to evolve, the home care nurse will require advanced clinical skills in community health nursing, as well as an understanding of data management and information technology systems. Knowledge of case management concepts to reach positive clinical and financial outcomes by using resources more effectively will be required. Case managers within home care will have clinical nursing expertise and a sense of measuring nursing impact on specific client populations, such as those with heart disease or cancer. These case managers will be increasingly required in home health nursing practice to possess problem-solving and decision-making skills that require negotiation, and a strong sense of client collaboration. Principles of managed care and practicing in coalitions are important skills for all health care workers, but especially for those who work in the home health field (Frantz, 1997). The opportunity for professional growth in home care nursing is endless. A challenge to provide clients and their caregivers the best of home care continues to be a challenge with the myriad changes in health care today. Growth in information systems and decision-making tech-

nology are offering business solutions to home health care. These advances enhance the practice of home care nursing by offering additional resources to manage client care to achieve quantifiable positive health outcomes.

Advanced practice nurses and nurse specialists will become required roles on the interdisciplinary team that offer direction, education, and support (Nemcek & Egan, 1997). As advanced practice nurses assume service privileges in acute care facilities, it is expected that they will eventually demand the ability to discharge clients to home health. Home health nurses will be increasingly accountable for not only client outcomes but will be called on to use business skills, such as cost-benefit analysis, to objectively support the total cost of care. The planning for care based on expected outcomes and participating in policy-making decisions that involve nursing practice will be an expectation of all staff home health nurses (Blaha, 1998).

Conclusion

In a managed care environment where the most efficient and effective delivery setting is chosen, nurses will find the home setting a likely practice environment. Community health nursing will continue to include the home as a viable and attractive setting for practice in sickness and in health. See Box 14-14 for some nurses' thoughts about being home health nurses.

BOX 14-14 THOUGHTS ON BEING A HOME HEALTH NURSE . . . FROM THE FIELD

"Probably the best part of the job is being on your own and being able to spend quality time with clients who really believe you can help them."

"There have been so many good memories and experiences—all of my clients are very special, they are like family. I really get to know them, their families, their fears, and their dreams. Home health is very rewarding."

"After working for many years in intensive care, I had grown weary of less and less time getting to know my patients as I was getting better and better at managing the machines that really cared for them. In home health, each day I am doing exactly what I went into nursing for—helping people feel better, using the skills I have worked so hard to develop."

"One of the more memorable home visits was the time the client's pigs got out of the pen and the physical therapist and I had to chase the pigs before we could attend to the client's needs."

CRITICAL THINKING ACTIVITIES

1. Home health care is one of the fastest growing nursing roles in health care today. Managed care has created incentives for hospitals to limit acute care episodes and client admissions. Clients continue to be discharged earlier than ever after surgery, childbirth, and acute episodes of chronic diseases. More and more "high-tech" health care can be replicated in the home, such as chemotherapy, IV therapy, and assisted ventilation. With this likely to continue as all health agencies struggle to contain costs, consider the following opinions about home health nursing. Respond to each statement and document your agreement or disagreement with the opinion.

   • Home health nursing is more accurately described as "hospital care at home."

   • Home health nursing is a new emerging specialty in preventive acute care and is not really a community health role or a hospital role.

   • Home health nurses are generalists who can provide health promotion services to well clients, such as newly discharged mothers and babies, as well as newly discharged post–heart transplant clients with complex intravenous immuno-suppressive drug therapy.

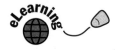 Explore Community Health Nursing on the web! To learn more about the topics in this chapter, access your exclusive web site: http://communitynursing.jbpub.com

REFERENCES

American Nurses Association (ANA). (1999). *Standards of home health nursing practice*. Washington, DC: Author.

American Nurses Association (ANA). (1995). *Position statement: Informal caregiving*. Washington, DC: Author.

Anderson, M., Pena, R., & Helms, L. (1998). Home care utilization by congestive heart failure patients: A pilot study. *Public Health Nursing* 15(2), 146–162.

Blaha, A. (1997). The current and future national voice for home healthcare nursing. *Home Healthcare Nurse, 15*(12), 873.

Bradley, P. J. (1996). Home healthcare nurses should regain their family focus. *Home Healthcare Nurse, 14*(4), 281–288.

Brant, J. (1998). The art of palliative care: Living with hope, dying with dignity. *Oncology Nursing Forum, 25*(6), 995–1004.

Brooks, S. (1997). Of hope and hospice. *Contemporary Longterm Care, 20*(7), 56–61.

Brown, D. (1998). Home care nursing as a philosophy of care. *Home Healthcare Nurse, 16*(3), 164–165.

Bull, M. J. (1990). Factors influencing family caregiver burden and health. *Western Journal of Nursing Research, 12*, 758–776.

Children's Defense Fund. (1998) *The state of America's children yearbook 1998*. Washington, DC: Author.

Clarke, P., & Cody, W. (1994). Nursing theory-based practice in the home and community: The crux of professional nursing education. *Advances in Nursing Science, 17*, 41–53.

Dougherty, G. (1998). When should a child be in the hospital?: A. Frederick North, Jr, M.D. Revisited. *Pediatrics, 101*(1), 19–25.

Franz, A. (1997). Prognosis: Home care nursing. *Home Healthcare Nurse, 15*(12), 876–877.

Hafkenschiel, J. H. (1990). Home care past and future. *HMQ*, Third Quarter.

Hickey, M. (1998, July). Disease management improves patient care, cuts costs. *Physicians Management*, p. 214.

Hospice Foundation of America. (1999). "*What is Hospice?*": http://hospicefoundation.htm.

Jerant, A. (1999). Home telemedicine: Merging the old and new ways. *American Family Physician*, 60(4), 1096–1098.

Jerant, A. F., Schlachta, L., Epperly, T. D., Barnes-Camp, J. (1998). Back to the future: The telemedicine house call. *Family Practice Management, 5*, 18–22, 25–26, 28.

Keeling, B. (1978, March). Making the most of the first home visit. *Nursing, 78*, 24–28.

Kenyon, V., Smith, E., Hefty, L. V., Bell, M. L., McNeil, J., & Maraus, T. (1990). Clinical competencies for public health nursing. *Public Health Nursing, 7*, 33–39.

Kiecolt-Glaser, J. K., Glaser, R., Shuttleworth, E. C., Dyer C. S., Ogrocki, B. S., & Speicher, C. E. (1987). Chronic stress and immunity in family care givers of Alzheimer's disease victims. *Psychosomatic Medicine, 49*, 523–535.

Kincade, K. (1997). Growing home-care business benefits from telemedicine TLC. *Telemedicine*, p. 4.

Kubler-Ross, E. (1975). *Death: The final stage of growth*. New York: Simon and Schuster.

Kubler-Ross, E. (1969). *On death and dying: What the dying have to teach doctors, nurses, clergy and their own families*. New York: Macmillan.

Levine, C. (1999). Home sweet hospital: The nature and limits of private responsibilities for home health care. *Journal of Aging and Health Care, 11*(2), 341–360.

Lovejoy, D. (1997). *Making the transition to home health nursing*. New York: Springer.

MacLaren, E. (1994). Basics of managed care. *NurseWeek*, pp. 10–11.

Maraldo, P. (1989). Home care should be the heart of a nursing sponsored national health plan. *Nursing and Health Care, 10*(6), 301–306.

Martinson, I. M. (1993). Hospice care for children: Past, present and future. *Journal of Pediatric Oncology Nursing, 10*, 93–98.

Milone-Nuzzo, P. (1998). Beyond venipuncture as the qualifying service for Medicare: Seeing the forest for the trees. *Home Healthcare Nurse, 16*(3), 177–183.

National Association of Home Care (NAHC). (2000 and 2001). *Basic statistics about home care*. Washington, DC: Author.

National Institute on Disability and Rehabilitation Research and Training Center. (1996, November), *U.S. Department of Education Disability Statistics Abstract* (Number 17). University of California, San Francisco.

Neal, L. (1977). Current clinical practice of home care nursing. *Home Healthcare Nurse, 15*(12), 881–882.

Nugent, D. (1999). Providing solutions for the growing trend toward home health care. *Health Management Technology, 20*(8), 28–31.

Oleske, J., & Czarniecki, L. (1999). Continuum of palliative care: Lessons from caring for children infected with HIV-1. *Lancet, 354*(9186), 1287–1891.

Peters, D., & Eigsti, D. (1991). Utilizing outcomes in home care. *Caring, 10,* 44–51.

The President's Advisory Commission on Consumer Protection and Quality in the Health Care Industry. (1998). *Quality First: Better Health Care For All Americans.* Washington, DC: U.S. Government Printing Office.

Pruchno, R. A., & Potashnik, S. L. (1989). Caregiving spouses: Physical and mental health in perspective. *Journal of the American Geriatric Society, 37,* 697–705.

Remington, L. (1997). Disease management programs. *The Remington Report, 5*(4), 1.

Rice, R. (1999). A little art in home care: Poetry and storytelling for the soul. *Geriatric Nursing, 20*(3), 165–166.

Rice, R. (1996). *Home health nursing: Concepts and application* (2nd ed.). St. Louis: Mosby.

Schaffer, C., & Behrendt, D. (1997). Disease state management across the continuum: Bettering lives, providing value. *The Remington Report, 5*(4), 20–23.

Schoen, M. A., & Koenig, R. J. (1997). Home health care nursing: Past and present–Part I. *Medical-Surgical Nursing 6*(4), 230–232.

Schwartz, R. (1977). News from Washington. *The Remington Report, 5* (4), 12-13.

Shamansky, S. (1988, June). Providing home care services in a for-profit environment, *Nursing Clinics of North America, 23*(2), 387–398.

Shaughnessy P. W. (1996, June 14). *Using outcomes to build a continuous quality improvement program for home care.* 11th National Nursing Symposium on Home Health Care, University of Michigan School of Nursing, Ann Arbor, MI.

Sheldon, P., & Bender, M. (1994, September). High-technology in home care, *Nursing Clinics of North America 29*(3), 508–519.

South Mississippi Home Health Orientation Manual for Registered Nurses. (1996). Hattiesburg, MS: Author.

Twohy, K. M., & Reif, L. (1997). What do public health nurses really do during prenatal home appointments? *Public Health Nursing, 14*(6), 324–331.

Warhola, C. (1980). *Planning for home health services: A resource handbook.* DHSS Pub. No. (NRA) 80-14017. Washington, DC: Public Health Service. Department of Health and Human Services.

Waters, K. (1996). Hospice: Comforting the dying patient. In R. Stone (Ed.), *Gerontology Manual.* Tacoma, WA: University of Puget Sound.

Wilson, S. (1993). Hospice and Medicare benefits: Overview, issues, and implications. *Journal of Holistic Nursing, 11*(4), 356–368.

Zelwesky, M. G., & Deitrick, E. P. (1987). Rx for care givers: Respite care. *Journal of Community Health Nursing, 4,* 77–84.

Chapter 15
Disasters in the Community

Karen Saucier Lundy and Janie B. Butts

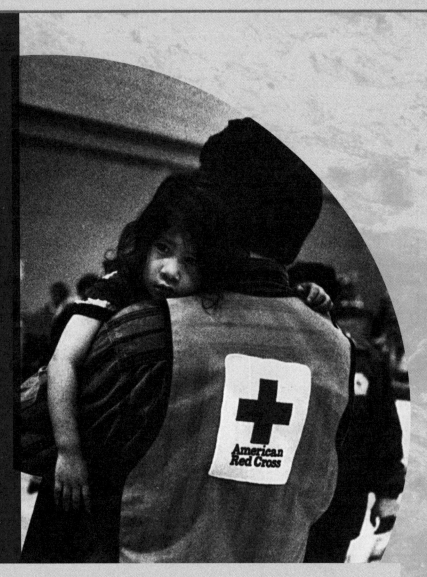

Disaster! The very word can evoke fear, panic, and a pounding heart. A major disaster occurs almost daily somewhere in the world: plane crashes, floods, hurricanes, tornadoes, fires, earthquakes, acts of terrorism, droughts, famines, and wars. The community health nurse can assist communities in preparing for disasters and limiting the damage from disasters. Communities can become stronger and healthier as a result.

QUESTIONS TO CONSIDER

After reading this chapter, answer the following questions:

1. What are the categories and types of disasters community health nurses might deal with?
2. What are the variables by which disasters can be understood?
3. What is a global disaster?
4. Who are the populations most at risk in a disaster? Why?
5. What are the stages of disaster and how does each stage impact the disaster workers and the affected population?
6. What are the steps in the disaster process?
7. What are the characteristics of a disaster plan?
8. What are the common elements of a disaster plan?
9. What is disaster response? What are the different levels of response?
10. What is disaster triage? Why and how should it be implemented?
11. What is the role of the community health nurse in the disaster relief process?
12. What specific approaches should a community health nurse use to mitigate human and material losses in a disaster?
13. What happens to the survivors in a disaster? How can a community health nurse promote recovery after a disaster?
14. What are the factors that can place individuals in a vulnerable position?
15. Why are children and elderly more at risk during a disaster? What can be done to intervene?
16. What are the sources of stress for the disaster workers and how can this be managed?

KEY TERMS

Disaster
Disaster planning
Disaster triage
Emergency
Emergency stage
Federal Emergency Management Agency (FEMA)

Human-generated (man-made) disasters
Impact stage
Interdisaster stage
Level I response
Level II response
Level III response

Level IV response
Major disaster
National Disaster Medical System (NDMS)
Natural disasters
Posttraumatic stress disorder (PTSD)

Predisaster stage
Recovery
Reconstruction, or rehabilitation, stage
Response

"Today our fellow citizens, our way of life, our very freedom came under attack in a series of deliberate and deadly terrorist acts."

President George W. Bush
after 9/11/01 terrorist attacks

The United States has experienced unprecedented disasters since the late 1980s, which include major earthquakes, hurricanes, tropical storms, floods, landslides, volcanic eruptions, severe winter storms, and wildfires (FEMA, 1997a). As a result of these catastrophic events, more than 500 people have lost their lives; another 4,500 people die each year in fires. Since 9/11 with the terrorist attacks on the World Trade Center and the Pentagon, the U.S. public has become much more aware of the devastating national and global effects of bioterrorism as a current disaster threat.

In the last two decades, natural disasters, such as earthquakes, hurricanes, floods, and volcanic eruptions, have cost approximately 32 million lives worldwide, have adversely affected the lives of at least 800 million more people, and have cost more than $50 billion in property and personal loss (Advisory Committee, 1987; Office of U.S. Foreign Disaster Assistance, 1995).

During 1998 alone, violent weather cost the world a record $89 billion, more money than was lost from weather-related disasters during the entire decade of the 1980s (Worldwatch Institute, 1998). Most of the increase in natural disaster damage was due to a combination of deforestation and climate change, including El Niño.

Imagine that you were somehow above to watch, from a distance, a major disaster unfold. You would see suffering and devastation—but that would be only part of the story. You also would see lots of people move into action—people from government agencies, private organizations, businesses and volunteer groups. You would see them working as a team to keep essential services operating, provide first aid, food and water, clear debris, rebuild homes and businesses, and prevent the disaster from happening again.

Federal Emergency Management Agency, 1997a

Community health nurses sometimes feel unprepared to react competently in a community disaster situation. For most practicing nurses, formal disaster education or training is not comprehensive. Therefore, the training that is received by nurses does not include the whole picture on levels of preparedness, which range from the basic emergency department response to the highest level of response from the community infrastructure. The disaster training that pertains to nurses' agency positions is usually the only training received, which often limits their understanding of the community's perspective on preparedness and response.

Although training may not be comprehensive in many institutions, an important goal for community health nurses is for them to feel a greater sense of disaster preparedness. When community health nurses are prepared for disaster, research has indicated that communities benefit. Study after study has revealed that improved organization in nursing care, planning the disaster response, and understanding the effects of disaster on families, communities, health professionals, and ultimately society, can prevent or reduce the detrimental short- and long-term effects of disasters.

Levels of prevention are integral in planning and responding to disasters for community health nurses, as well as other key personnel in the community infrastructure. The levels of prevention are integrated at certain points in this chapter. The levels include primary, secondary, and tertiary. Primary prevention is aimed at reducing the probability of disease, death, and disability resulting from a disaster. Secondary prevention includes the immediate identification of disaster problems and the implementation of measures to treat and prevent their recurrence or complications. Tertiary prevention involves rehabilitation of disaster victims and the community to an optimal function level, with permanency of change from the disaster assumed. The goal during rehabilitation is to minimize further damage resulting from the disaster.

By increasing community health nurses' understanding, confidence, and skill in disaster planning and care, the damage to our communities during disasters can be lessened (Garcia, 1985). Not only are lives saved and human and property damage reduced, but also the overall health of the community can be strengthened.

What are the real threats of disaster? How can community health nurses be better prepared? This chapter will help you answer these questions as you develop a better understanding of the nature of disasters and learn about the various levels of disaster preparedness in which community health nurses are involved. The role of preparedness is essential to mediate the harmful effects of catastrophes, such as the Titanic disaster of 1912, described in Box 15-1.

The Nature of Disasters
Definitions and Types of Disasters

Some of the many definitions of disaster include the definitions of an emergency and a major disaster. An **emergency** is any hurricane, tornado, storm, flood, high water, wind-driven water, tidal wave, earthquake, volcanic eruption, landslide, mudslide, snowstorm, drought, fire, explosion, or other catastrophe in any part of the United States that requires federal emergency assistance to supplement state and local efforts to save lives and protect property, public health, and safety or to avert or lessen the threat of a disaster (U.S. Congress, Section 102, Disaster Relief Act Amendments, 1974).

A **major disaster** may be any of the events listed as an emergency in any part of the United States that, in the determination of the president, causes damage of sufficient severity above and beyond emergency services by the federal government, to supplement the efforts and available resources of states, local governments, and disaster relief organizations in alleviating the damage, loss, hardship, or suffering caused thereby (U.S. Congress, Section 102, Disaster Relief Act Amendments, 1974). Erickson (1976) gave a pictorial description of disaster:

- *A sharp and furious eruption of some kind that splinters the silence for one terrible moment and then goes away*
- *An "event" with a distinct beginning and a distinct ending that is by definition extraordinary—a freak of nature, a perversion of the natural processes of life*
- *Doing a great deal of harm*
- *Sudden, unexpected, and acute*

For the purposes of this chapter, **disaster** is an event that causes human suffering and creates unmet needs and demands exceeding the abilities of the community to cope without outside assistance. Most importantly, from a public health perspective, disasters are defined by what they do to people and are therefore relative to the context in which they occur. What results in a disaster in one community might not necessarily be considered a disaster in a different community (Noji, 1997). Disasters fall into two broad categories or types: **natural disasters** are those that arise from the forces of nature, such as hurricanes, tornadoes, earthquakes, and volcanic eruptions; **human-generated (manmade) disasters** are those in which the principal direct causes are identifiable human actions, deliberate or otherwise, such as the recent 9/11 events. These two categories can be further subdivided into different types of disasters (Box 15-2).

Floods have been the most common type of natural disaster, accounting for more than one-third of all disasters between 1980 and 1990 (Office of U.S. Foreign Disaster Assistance, 1995). One example of a horrendous flood, although not necessarily a typical disaster, was the Mississippi River Flood of 1927, which has been cited as the worst natural disaster in U.S. history. In 1927, the Mississippi River swept across a geographic area larger than Massachusetts, Connecticut, New Hampshire, and Vermont combined and resulted in water as deep as 30 feet on the land, stretching from Illinois and Missouri south to the Gulf of Mexico and New Orleans. This flood forced almost 1 million people from their homes and resulted in thousands of deaths.

Many of the dead were being pulled out of the Mississippi River at New Orleans for months after the flood. When more than 40,000 homes were destroyed close to where the dam broke in Mississippi, camps were set up in the Confederate National Park in Vicksburg. American Red Cross nurses (Box 15-3) and nurses from the Mississippi State Department of Health, as well as nurses from other states, were assigned to relief efforts for several months in the spring of 1927. A total of 383 nurses worked in the Mississippi flood disaster. Nurses worked in these refugee camps, battling typhoid and nutritional deficiencies such as pellagra. The waters from the Mississippi did not recede for 3 months (Barry, 1997; Sabin, 1998).

Although disasters can be grouped according to the stated definitions, in reality the distinction between natural and human-generated disasters is often blurred, for a natural disaster can trigger secondary disasters, such as explosions, fires, and toxins released into the air after an earthquake. Such combination-type synergistic disasters are referred to as *NA-TECH disasters*. An example of a NA-TECH disaster occurred in the former Soviet Union when windstorms spread radioactive materials across the country, increasing by up to 50% the land area contaminated in an earlier nuclear disaster at Chernobyl (see Box 15-9).

....

There can be no winners in a world of man-made epidemics.
King Hussein, 1996

....

BOX 15-1 THE MAKING OF A DISASTER: THE SINKING OF THE "UNSINKABLE" TITANIC

NONDISASTER OR INTERDISASTER PHASE

The Titanic was on its maiden voyage when it sank on April 14, 1912. This ship was the crown jewel of the White Star Line, a mammoth 46-ton British liner of incomparable luxury, three football fields long and eleven stories high, which was the world's largest and purportedly safest vessel on the water. On this maiden voyage, the Titanic had as its passengers both British and American aristocracy, along with immigrants coming to the "New World" with promises of a new life. The boat deck and bridge were 70 feet above water. According to White Star Line documentation, a "trial test" of 6 to 7

BOX 15-1 THE MAKING OF A DISASTER: THE SINKING OF THE "UNSINKABLE" TITANIC—cont'd

hours total was conducted 1 month before leaving Great Britain. This trial consisted of turning circles and compass adjustment; also, the ship sailed "a short time" at full steam, but never at full speed before passengers boarded. The crew and officers of the Titanic (numbering 899) joined the ship a few hours before the passengers and went through only one drill: They lowered two lifeboats on starboard side into water. No evidence of crew duties being delineated as to task or role in event of disaster were noted by Congress. Congressional hearings found that the crew did not know their "proper stations" or assignment until after passengers had already boarded in Queenstown, Ireland. There were 1,324 passengers on board the ship, and together with 899 crew members, a total of 2,223 persons were on the maiden voyage of the Titanic. Congress found no evidence of passengers having any orientation in disaster procedures. There were 1,176 lifeboats and life jackets for all persons on board. The Titanic was considered "unsinkable," having been constructed with special watertight bulkhead compartments that could be sealed off if the ship took on water. There was no evidence of a disaster plan or safety instructions posted or provided to passengers, nor were crew members prepared for their roles in the event of a disaster. The crew staffed the Titanic round the clock and had lookouts posted in the crow's nest for any water-related hazards.

PREDISASTER OR WARNING PHASE

The Titanic had received several ice warnings on the third day of the voyage, and the captain noted them. On the day of the disaster, a warning message cited icebergs within 5 miles of the track that the Titanic was following, very near the place where the accident occurred. Congressional hearings revealed that despite repeated warnings, no general discussion took place among the officers, no conference was called to consider these warnings, and no heed was given to them. The speed was not reduced, the lookout was not increased, and the only extra vigilance noted was from the officer of the watch, who gave instructions to the lookouts to "keep a sharp lookout for ice." The speed of the ship had been gradually increased, and just before

the collision, the ship was making her maximum speed of the voyage. Passengers had no advance knowledge of any possible risks of the ship related to the icebergs.

IMPACT PHASE

At 10:13 PM on Sunday, April 14, the lookout signaled the bridge and telephoned the officer of the watch with this message: "Iceberg right ahead." The officer of the watch immediately ordered the quartermaster at the wheel to put the helm "hard astarboard" and reverse the engines. The Titanic immediately struck the ice, and the impact caused the vessel to roll slightly. The impact, which ripped a hole in the steel plating of the ship, was not violent enough to disturb the crew or passengers. During this time, the damage was reported by crew members from the boiler room related to water coming in; the captain began inspecting the ship for damage. Passengers were still not aware of the accident.

EMERGENCY PHASE

The reports by the captain after various inspections of the ship revealed that the compartments were rapidly filling with water and that the bow of the ship was sinking deeper and deeper. Through the open hatches, water promptly began overflowing into the other bulkheads and decks. No emergency alarm was sounded, no whistles were blown, and no systematic warning was given the passengers. Within approximately 15 minutes after his inspection, the captain issued a distress call to ships in the area. The call was heard by several ships in the vicinity. The Carpathia, which was 58 miles away, responded to the distress signal by turning immediately toward the sinking ship. Other ships also attempted to sail toward the sinking ship but were too far away to be of any reasonable assistance. The closest ship, the Californian, was only 19 miles north of the Titanic but did not attempt to rescue the ailing ship. Proceedings indicate that the crew of the Titanic began firing distress rockets at frequent intervals and that the crew of the Californian saw them. The captain of the Californian failed to heed the warning signals and was chastised by Congress for "indifference or carelessness" and for not responding to the Titanic's distress calls in accordance with the dictates of international usage and law. The

Continued

BOX 15-1 THE MAKING
OF A DISASTER: THE SINKING
OF THE "UNSINKABLE" TITANIC—cont'd

captain immediately gave the signal to retrieve the lifeboats, with the order to put women and children in the boats first. The proceedings report that the lack of preparation at this time was most noticeable. There was general chaos as passengers learned of the accident from each other, from some crew members who knocked on cabin doors, and from being awakened by the movement of people running on the ship. "There was no system adopted for loading the boats; there was great indecision as to the deck from which boats were to be loaded; there was wide diversity of opinion as to the number of crew necessary to man each boat; there was no direction whatever to the number of passengers to be carried by each boat, and no uniformity in loading them" (p. 548). In some boats, there would be only women and children; in others there would be an equal proportion of men and women. Only a few of the lifeboats were loaded to capacity; most were only partially loaded, which resulted in needless losses. If all of the lifeboats had been fully loaded at capacity for 1,176 persons, more than the 706 persons could have reasonably survived. Furthermore, the proceedings noted that if the sea had been rough (which it wasn't), it is questionable whether any of the lifeboats would have reached the water without being damaged or destroyed. The lifeboats were suspended 70 feet above the water, and in the event of the ship's rolling (with a rough sea), the boats would have swung out from the side of the ship and then crashed back into the ship as it was being lowered. Also, had the survivors been concentrated in fewer boats once on the water, the staff could have returned and rescued more passengers. Once the ship sank at 12:47 AM, it broke in half and people died from drowning, exposure, and trauma; 1,517 persons died, 706 survived. Survivors of the Titanic reported rowing toward the lights of a ship in the distance, which has now been established as those of the Californian. There were questions about the way passengers were evacuated relative to whether they were in first, second, or third class accommodation. Sixty percent of first class passengers survived, 42% of second class survived, and only 25% of the third class passengers survived. These statistics suggest that there may have been a distinction in the warning and evacuation based on class accommodation. Twenty-five percent of the crew were saved. The rescue of survivors came from the Carpathia crew and eventually from the crew of the Californian. After a thorough search, ships returned to New York and Nova Scotia with the survivors. A brief burial prayer service for the dead was held at 8:30 AM by the captain of the Carpathia. Public media notification occurred the evening of April 15, 1912.

RECONSTRUCTION OR REHABILITATION PHASE

The wreck of the Titanic represents in myth and reality a disaster beyond human comprehension at a time when technological advances were seen as our defense against the disasters of nature. Because of lack of preparedness and lack of planning for ship disasters, technology could not have saved the passengers on the Titanic. The recommendations that evolved from the Titanic hearings held by Congress in May of 1912 were no less than revolutionary in terms of safety preparedness. One was that inspection certificates would be contingent on sufficient lifeboats to accommodate every passenger and every member of the crew. Inspection certificates that mandate these requirements would apply to all boats who carry passengers from ports of the United States. Lifeboats should be positioned in such a way that they would not be subject to damage from height related to water level. There would be no fewer than four members of the crew, trained in handling boats, on each lifeboat. All crew members assigned to this duty would be drilled in lowering and rowing the lifeboats not less than twice per month and the "fact of such drill or practice should be noted in the log." Recommendations also included assigning passengers to lifeboats before sailing and posting the shortest route to the lifeboats in each room. Two electric searchlights were to be present on boats carrying more than 100 passengers. A radio operator must be on duty at all times, 24 hours a day. And finally, all ships from that point on would be required to meet construction standards related to watertight compartments and hulls.

Source: Kuntz, T. (Ed.). The Titanic disaster hearings: The official transcripts of the 1912 Senate investigation. New York: Pocket Books.

BOX 15-2 CATEGORIES AND TYPES OF DISASTERS

NATURAL DISASTERS

- Meteorological: hurricanes, tornados, hailstorms, snowstorms, and droughts
- Topological: landslides, avalanches, mudslides, and floods
- Disasters that originate underground: earthquakes, volcanic eruptions, and tidal waves
- Bacteriological: communicable disease epidemics (e.g., *Ebola* virus) and insect swarms (e.g., locusts)

HUMAN-GENERATED DISASTERS

- Warfare: conventional warfare (bombardment, blockage, and siege) and nonconventional warfare (nuclear, chemical, and biological; acts of terrorism)
- Civil disasters: riots and demonstrations
- Accidents: transportation (planes, trucks, automobiles, trains, and ships); structural collapse (buildings, dams, bridges, mines, and other structures); explosion; fire; chemical (toxic waste and pollution); and biological (sanitation)

Source: Modified from Garcia, 1985; Noji, 1997.

BOX 15-3 AN EARLY FIELD TEST OF THE AMERICAN RED CROSS'S NURSE ENROLLMENT CAMPAIGN: THE PURVIS, MISSISSIPPI, TORNADO OF 1908

A devastating tornado hit the small town of Purvis, Mississippi, in April of 1908, injuring 200 persons. The American Red Cross had just undertaken its first major campaign to recruit and enroll nurses nationally for such disasters, and the Purvis tornado provided a "field test" of the newly developed communication system. In the end, a head nurse and 17 staff nurses were employed from the District of Columbia, Philadelphia, and New York. These nurses managed tent hospitals and coordinated disaster relief for 3 weeks. Although the nursing was well done, recruitment and securement of nurses with the new system had been less than successful. The ARC staff had met with considerable difficulty locating the enrolled nurses and in the end had to recruit unenrolled, volunteer nurses outside the system. The disaster served to draw attention to the need for a more collaborative effort between nursing organizations together with the American Red Cross to develop a network of disaster preparedness through local volunteer nurses.

Source: Kernodle, P. (1949). The Red Cross nurse in action 1882–1948. New York: Harper and Brothers.

Disaster Characteristics

Disasters have different characteristics. Knowledge of these variables is necessary in disaster management and planning. Dynes, Quarentelli, and Kreps (1972) identified six variables by which disasters can be understood. The variables include predictability, controllability, speed of onset, length of forewarning, duration of impact, and scope and intensity of impact.

1. *Predictability is influenced by the type of disaster. A hurricane has a high degree of predictability in industrialized countries, and earthquakes are considerably less foreseeable than floods. Although we often assume that disasters are fairly rare occurrences, there are certain areas of the globe that are more prone to disasters, such as flood plains of the Ohio Valley or low-lying areas in the Louisiana swamp. The Gulf Coast of Mississippi, Texas, Louisiana, Florida, and Alabama are all vulnerable to the threat of hurricanes born from the warm waters of the Caribbean. Tornadoes are more common in Kansas, Texas, and Mississippi and less common in North Dakota and Idaho.*

2. *Controllability refers to the degree to which interventions can be used to control the disaster, such as using dams for flood control; earthquakes have very little controllability.*

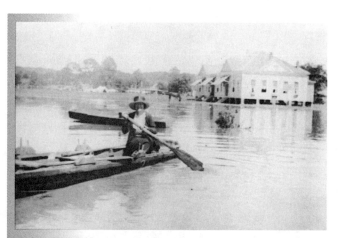

Public health nurse in disaster recovery during the worst natural disaster in the United States—the Mississippi River Flood of 1927.

3. *Speed of onset is quick with floods and tornadoes, whereas hurricanes generally are slow to develop.*

4. *Length of forewarning is the period between warning and impact. Communities in the path of a hurricane may have the luxury of a 24-hour warning, whereas a tornado warning may provide only a few minutes of preparation.*

5. *Duration of impact also varies. A tornado may be on the ground for only a few minutes, whereas a flood's impact usually lasts for days. The worst combination of variables from the viewpoint of damage is the disaster that is rapid in onset, gives no warning, and lasts a long time. An earthquake with strong aftershocks is such a disaster.*

6. *Scope and intensity of impact refers to geographic and social space dimension. A disaster such as a tornado may be limited to a mile or two, but a flood may involve hundreds of miles. The population density of an area influences this variable and can lead to widespread consequences. An example of density is the Oklahoma City bombing, which was limited to a few city blocks but affected a large, dense population. A densely affected area can result in disruption of community functions, depending on the number of persons involved and the geographic impact. The World Trade Center and Pentagon attacks of 2001 have had global consequences, including U.S. military action.*

• •

"These terrorists kill not merely to end lives, but to disrupt and end a way of life. . . . From this day forward, any nation that continues to harbor or support terrorism will be regarded by the United States as a hostile regime. Our Nation has been put on notice: We are not immune from attack. We will take defensive measures against terrorism to protect Americans. . . . Great harm has come to us. We have suffered great loss. And in our grief and anger we have found our mission and our moment. Freedom and fear are at war . . . We will rally the world to this cause, by our efforts and by our course. We will not tire, we will not falter, and we will not fail."

September 20, 2002
George Bush in Address to Congress on Terrorism

• •

Global Disaster Issues

As humans continue to migrate throughout the globe and population densities continue to increase in flood plains, along vulnerable coastal areas, and near faults in the earth's crust, we can expect these natural disasters to worsen and affect more people. The global community continues to witness complex emergencies resulting from the breakdown of traditional state structures, armed conflict, and the upsurge of ethnicity and micronationalism (Noji, 1997). One has to look no further than today's news-

paper headlines or watch CNN to find these political and cultural conflicts as they play out on a daily business, such as in Bosnia, Somalia, Rwanda, and Chechnya, to name but a few of the disaster areas. As a result of these political and cultural upheavals, refugees have become a large and vulnerable population with complex health problems.

Between 1965 and 1992, 90% of all natural disaster victims lived in Asia and Africa (IDNDR, 1994). The number of people affected (killed, injured, or displaced) by disasters worldwide rose from 100 million in 1980 to 311 million in 1991. By the mid-1990s, the number of refugees affected by a combination of natural and human-made disasters increased to an estimated 17 million throughout the world.

Earthquakes are global incidents that have been cited as causing the greatest number of deaths and the largest monetary loss of any type of natural disaster (Berz, 1984). The tragic earthquake that occurred in Istanbul, Turkey, in August 1999 is an example of high cost of human lives—thousands of deaths were reported.

Not only are these displaced vulnerable populations at risk for serious health consequences, the economic costs for their care are devastating (Noji, 1997). As United Nations Secretary General Boutros Boutros Ghali stated:

> There is no hard-and-fast division—in terms of their [disasters] effects on civilian populations—between conflicts and wars, and natural disasters. Droughts, floods, earthquakes, and cyclones are just as destructive for communities and settlements as wars and civil confrontation. Just as preventive diplomacy can foresee and prevent the outbreak of war, so the effects of natural disasters can be foreseen and contained (cited in Noji, 1997, p. xv).

Much of the destruction caused by natural disasters can be avoided. For almost every natural disaster in the world in the 1990s, "an ounce of prevention" or preparedness would have made a significant difference in terms of damage to persons and property (Noji, 1997, p. 7). Natural hazards, such as weather, earthquakes, and floods, are in fact only natural agents that "transform a vulnerable condition into a disaster" (Noji, 1997, p. 11).

People often do not know their limitations until they reach them. As technology has advanced and provided humans with opportunities to live in and explore the world without the territorial constraints of our ancestors, the probabilities that the future will be marked by periodic disasters are certainly increased. In many cases in recent disasters, building codes were ignored, communities were located in dangerous areas, warnings were not issued or followed, or plans were unknown to all community residents or were ignored (Noji, 1997).

We know much about the cause and nature of disasters, populations at risk, and the inevitable outcome when communities are not prepared for disasters. Such knowledge assists us in anticipating some of the effects a disaster may have on the health of communities. Knowing how people are injured and killed in disasters is critical prerequisite knowledge for preventing or reducing injuries and deaths during future disasters (Noji, 1997). For example, although none of the advances in science and technology have done much to arrest the force of natural disasters, we see them coming a few hours earlier and can measure their destructiveness with greater precision afterward. Yet those very advances have made us in many ways even more vulnerable to potential catastrophes, because persons often feel a "false sense of security" regarding the likelihood of serious threat from a disaster (Erickson, 1976).

International Decade for Natural Disaster Reduction

The United Nations General Assembly declared the 1990s the "International Decade for Natural Disaster Reduction" (ID-NDR) and led the way in calling for a global, scientific, technical, and political effort to reduce the impact of catastrophic acts of nature (Advisory Committee, 1987). This declaration came about because both disasters and the number of their victims have increased in recent decades (Pickens, 1992). Such massive adverse impacts on the health of global populations have now been recognized as a significant public health problem. Sudden impact disasters, such as earthquakes and tornadoes, may result in large numbers of people killed, injured, or disabled for life; health facilities damaged or destroyed; and national health care development efforts in underdeveloped countries set back for years.

As human societies have become more dense with urban migration and population growth, more people are exposed and vulnerable to the hazards of disaster than ever before. Our increasingly sophisticated and technical physical infrastructure makes more developed countries, such as the United States, even more vulnerable to destruction than in past generations. For instance, a major disaster could disrupt the computer networks of the federal government or some other large organization. Damage from natural and technological disasters tends to be more and more extensive when proper planning and precautions are not taken. In the past 50 years, much has been learned about disasters and their aftereffects. Disaster preparedness involving careful and methodical planning does make a difference in mediating the destructive nature of disasters (Noji, 1997).

Disaster as a Global Public Health Problem

The Centers for Disease Control and Prevention (CDC) has led the way and has major responsibilities to prepare for and respond to public emergencies such as disasters. The CDC is also responsible for conducting investigations into the health effects and health consequences of disaster. The first major comprehensive research study of disasters was published in 1962 by Baker and Chapman in their book *Man and Society in Disaster*. Since then, many research centers have been established to study the health effects of disaster; among them are collaborative centers under the guidance and sponsorship of the World Health Organization (WHO) and the Pan American Health Organization. The major aim of these research efforts is to assess risk for death and injury and to develop strategies for preventing or mitigating the impact of future disasters.

•••••••••••••••••••••••••••••

Will you be a hero in your daily work? . . . We may give you an institution to learn in, but it is you who must furnish the heroic feelings of doing your duty, doing your best, without which no institution is safe.

Florence Nightingale

•••••••••••••••••••••••••••••

Disasters affect communities in myriad ways. Most effects of a disaster affect health, directly or indirectly (Noji, 1997). Communication lines, such as telephones, television, and computer links, may be disrupted, as well as transportation links, such as roads and methods of transportation. Public utilities (electricity, water, gas, water, and sewer) are often disrupted early in a massive disaster. A substantial number of persons may be without homes. Casualties may require medical and nursing care. Damage to food, damage to food preparation and sources, and lack of sanitation resources may create serious public health threats. A long-term effect is the community's possible destruction of its industrial or economic base. A detailed summary of disasters and public health can be found in Box 15-4 and the health effects of disasters in Box 15-5.

Populations at Risk in Disasters

Not all persons in the world are equal regarding the probability of disaster occurrence or severity of consequences. The more vulnerable a population to a disaster, the more serious the outcomes of injury and damage to persons and property (Mizutani & Nakano, 1989). As far as individual health characteristics, persons with conditions that put them at risk, such as those with chronic diseases, elder persons, pregnant women, the disabled, homebound persons, or children, are among the most vulnerable in any society in regard to impact of disaster. Industrialized countries are buffered from disasters by characteristics and abilities that are summarized in Box 15-6.

The low death rate associated with recent disasters in the United States, such as hurricanes Hugo (1989), Andrew (1992), and Georges (1998), and earthquakes in San Francisco (1989) and Los Angeles (1994), are evidence of the success of the United States' resources in disaster warning and recovery (Noji, 1997).

BOX 15-4 PUBLIC HEALTH PROBLEMS THAT MAY RESULT FROM DISASTERS

- Excessive deaths and injuries can tax the local health services and therapeutic capabilities, which may require external assistance.
- Destruction or disruption of acute care health facilities, such as clinics and hospitals, may leave services and resources unable to provide care to the injured from the disaster and pre-disaster client population needs.
- Disruption of routine health services and preventive activities can lead to long-term consequences in terms of morbidity and mortality.
- Environmental hazards can lead to increased risks for communicable disease and injury from a damaged ecosystem.
- Psychological and social behavioral stressors, including panic, anxiety, neuroses, and depression, can be exacerbated.
- A shortage of safe, nutritional food sources may lead to severe nutritional deficiencies and sequelae in the very young and the very old.
- Displacing populations to overcrowded hospitals and shelter facilities may increase the dangers of communicable disease.

Sources: Adapted from Logue, Melick, & Hansen, 1981; Noji, 1997.

BOX 15-5 HEALTH EFFECTS OF DISASTERS

PHYSICAL

Sleep disturbance

Poor concentration

Back pain

Tachycardia

Poor diet

PSYCHOLOGICAL

Loss of self and relationships

Emotional pain

Brooding

Aggressive thoughts

Depression

SOCIOCULTURAL

Loss of intimacy

Loss of sense of belonging to once-claimed culture

Source: Procter & Cheek, 1995.

The following major factors contribute to the degree of vulnerability of populations:

- *Human vulnerability resulting from poverty and social inequality*
- *Environmental degradation resulting from poor land use*
- *Rapid population growth, especially among the poor*

Anderson (1991) estimated that 95% of the deaths that result from natural disasters occur among 66% of the world's poorest population. According to Guha-Sapir and Lechat (1986), the poor are most at risk for greatest damage for the following reasons:

- *They are likely to live in substandard housing with little structural protection.*
- *They often live in coastal locations that are at high risk for disasters.*

BOX 15-6 RESOURCES FOR INDUSTRIALIZED COUNTRIES

- Sophisticated technology to forecast storms
- Development and strict enforcement of codes for earthquake-resistant and fireproof buildings
- Widespread mandatory use of communications networks to broadcast disaster warnings, alerts, and information about disaster preparedness
- Resources to provide timely and high-quality emergency health services and accommodation
- Contingency planning to prepare the population and public agencies for possible disasters
- Shelters for evacuation widely available and used by population

Source: Adapted from Garcia, 1985.

- *They are likely to live in flood plains and other less desirable land.*
- *They are likely to live in substandard housing built on unstable geographic slopes.*
- *They are likely to live near hazardous industrial sites.*
- *They are not usually well educated about safe and appropriate lifesaving behaviors.*
- *They are more dependent on others for transportation.*

Stages of Disaster

Disasters can be divided into five chronological stages that require specific levels of prevention and levels of response at various points during each stage. Knowing the disaster stages will assist in the development of the disaster plan, role responsibilities, and the setting of priorities in each phase of the disaster plan. Refer to Box 15-1 as an illustration of the stages of disaster. The stages of a disaster are presented in the following list:

- *Nondisaster, or interdisaster, stage*
- *Predisaster, or warning, stage*
- *Impact stage*
- *Emergency stage*
- *Reconstruction, or rehabilitation, stage*

Disaster planning should begin before the disaster event. During the nondisaster, or **interdisaster**, **stage**, planning and preparation for a disaster include the two critical elements of disaster preparedness: (1) disaster training and education programs for the community and (2) the development of a disaster plan for all involved in the mitigation of a potential disaster (Noji, 1997). Mitigation is preventive in nature and defined as action taken to prevent or reduce the harmful effects of a disaster on human health and property (Malilay, 1997). Included in this critical phase of primary prevention are assessment of hazards and risks, vulnerability analysis, inventory of existing resources for coping with a disaster (human, communication, and material), and the establishment of a disaster plan. Disaster planning is discussed in more detail in a later section.

A disaster is imminent during the warning, or **predisaster**, **stage**. The disaster plan, when available, is implemented, which includes early warnings based on predictions of impending disaster and mobilization as well as implementation of protective measures for the affected communities and populations (Garcia, 1985). Because primary prevention is the focus during this stage, disaster team members, officials, and emergency personnel prepare the population for disaster by providing information via multiple communication routes. Advisories and warnings are issued, and evacuation measures are taken where indicated. Mobilization can occur in the form of evacuation to shelters, preparation such as using sandbags around riverbanks to divert flood waters, boarding up windows and tying down boats when a hurricane is forecast, and moving to the basements or inner halls of homes and schools in the event of a tornado. Health care workers may be placed "on alert call" for health facility staffing and disaster shelter management. The effectiveness of these protective measures will depend largely on the community's preparedness and contingency plans developed in the nondisaster phase (Noji, 1997).

Problems associated with the warning include the following: first, communication systems may be inadequate in transmission and/or reception, or there may not be enough time to send warnings; second, the community must recognize the warning threat as serious and legitimate. However, some people in the targeted community may deny the need for taking action based on previous experience with the specific disaster (e.g., persons who live on a fault line or on a coastline), and the presence of false alarms in the past can desensitize persons to appropriate reaction (Garcia, 1985; Janis & Mann, 1977).

The **impact stage** involves "holding on" and enduring the impact of the disaster. This stage may last from minutes (as in earthquakes, plane crashes, tornadoes, and bomb blasts) to days or weeks (hurricanes, floods, fire, and drought). People who are directly experiencing the disaster may be unable to comprehend the scope of the disaster (Garcia, 1985). If possible, a preliminary assessment and inventory of injuries and property damage should be conducted by disaster team members during the impact phase or immediately afterward so that the implementation of secondary prevention strategies of setting priorities can be set in motion. How much the impact affects community members depends on several factors: population density, the extent of the damage, the preparedness of the community, the extent of community resiliency, and response to the consequences of the damage.

During the **emergency stage**, the community faces the consequences of the disaster's impact. This stage begins during the actual impact and continues until the immediate threat of additional hazards have passed (Garcia, 1985). Secondary prevention strategies are used to minimize damage and prevent further complications. This stage is divided into three parts—isolation, rescue, and remedy—which are presented in the following list:

1. *Isolation of the affected population can occur as a result of limited access (as a result of disaster damage, such as closed roads, downed trees, or building obstruction). The community members themselves must assume responsibility for their own needs relative to the disaster until outside help arrives.*

2. *Rescue begins when outside resources arrive and provide search-and-rescue operations. Community members are often hurried, stressed, and nonproductive in this early stage. First aid, emergency medical assistance, and a command post for disaster management are established. Restoration of means of communication begins, and regional, state, fed-*

eral, and voluntary organizations and agencies converge to meet the needs of the community.

3. *Remedy begins with the establishment of organized, professional, and voluntary relief operations and organization. The panic and confusion of the earlier phases tend to subside. Community members, disaster workers, and volunteers "get on with the task" of providing appropriate medical aid, clothing, food, and shelter to the affected population. The injured and ill are triaged, transportation becomes more organized, morgue facilities are established, reunions of family members become organized, and communication networks are established to provide early data of the disaster damage (Garcia, 1985). Later in the emergency stage, surveillance of public health effects (e.g., infectious disease, sanitation issues, safety concerns) is put in place and interventions are developed. When communities are well prepared and disaster plans are in place to help people know the "what, when, and how" of disasters for their population, both self-reliance and the effectiveness of early assistance saves lives and reduces injury during this critical period (Noji, 1997).*

The **reconstruction**, or **rehabilitation**, **stage** begins when communities start the process of healing. Reconstruction or rehabilitation optimally restores the community to predisaster conditions (Noji, 1997). Health services are restored to normal. Damaged homes, facilities, and buildings are repaired and reconstructed. This period is also the time for evaluation and reflection by the community and disaster team members, community officials, and voluntary agencies as lessons learned from the disaster are shared and documented (Noji, 1997). This period, which may combine secondary and tertiary prevention, may take days, months, or years, depending on the nature of the disaster, the response of the community, and the extent of the damages. For persons in the impact area, the recovery can be a long course and, in some cases, can be a lifelong readjustment to life and community living after the disaster (Garcia, 1985).

After the 9/11 disasters, people in New York City have reconstructed their lives in varied ways. Memorials have been held, art work created, and a new community ethic of connectedness seems to have emerged. After one year, there appeared to be a need to invest in the future, to define and reach for goals and to invest energy in plans on rebuilding the city and in individual lives that had been personally touched by the trauma and loss of the 9/11 disasters. Klagsbrun (2002) suggests that by moving on in our personal lives, as well as in our communal lives, we are attempting to regain control over our destiny. Each person often reviews his or her own history and recognizes how they have overcomes losses, difficulties of all kinds, pain and failure and have succeeded in being able to go on. The crises managed in the past then become healthy patterns of coping with the present unthinkable disaster.

It is during the rehabilitative phase that victims often suffer from posttraumatic stress disorder. **Posttraumatic stress disor-**

der (PTSD) is recognized by the American Psychiatric Association (APA) with the following symptoms and circumstances: The sufferer is a victim of an extremely distressing event persistently reexperiencing the event after it is over (compulsive and obsessive thoughts and details about the event), persistently avoiding stimuli that remind the victim of the event, and experiencing numbing of responsiveness and persistent symptoms of arousal not present before the trauma (APA, 1987). In conjunction with disaster, other symptoms include flashbacks, depression, inability to form close personal relationships, and sleep disturbances (Barker, 1989). Florence Nightingale is thought to have suffered from PTSD after the Crimean War. This condition, once diagnosed, requires professional mental health intervention and follow-up (Waters, Selander, & Stuart, 1992).

Disaster Planning

A planned response to disasters must occur to lessen the terror of a disaster, to cushion the impact by providing care for the greatest number of potential survivors, and to increase society's ability to survive disasters and grow more self-sufficient and self-reliant in the process (Waeckerle, 1991). Clearly, the benefits of disaster planning for society today are more significant than ever as widespread disasters become more common and more costly, in both human and property terms.

Anticipating a disaster and planning for the possibility of multiple outcomes from disasters strengthen a community's adaptability. Consequently, the disaster team develops the ability to respond more quickly and more effectively in the face of disaster (Muench, 1996). Another benefit to planning is the delineation of roles and responsibilities of the players in disaster preparedness. The result is less confusion over who does what and the roles of the multitude of organizations and volunteers once resources become available.

Once a disaster is imminent it is too late to plan a response. A clear community disaster plan for all contingencies should be coordinated by knowledgeable and experienced leaders and officials in the community. Such a plan must be as inclusive as possible, including input from health professionals; voluntary agencies; policy makers; officials from local, state, and federal levels, such as the civil defense and the Federal Emergency Management Agency (FEMA); emergency response system personnel; and all other components of the health care delivery system from acute care to home health to residential care, including medical and nursing schools (Waeckerle, 1991).

Steps in the Disaster Process

When a major disaster has occurred, such as hurricane Andrew in 1992, the president of the United States intervenes after the governor of the affected state requests the president to declare the area a major disaster. However, all major disaster declarations must follow certain steps (FEMA, 1998c).

First, local government agencies, such as the mayor and civil defense, which includes neighboring communities and volunteer agencies, must respond. Second, if the local agencies become overwhelmed, the state responds at the governor's request through state agencies and the National Guard. Third, the local, state, federal, and volunteer organizations make a damage assessment.

Fourth, when state resources have been exhausted, the governor of the state will make a request to the president for a declaration of a major disaster. The governor bases this request on the already-completed damage assessment collected by the civil defense team and commits a certain amount of state funds and resources to the long-term recovery from the disaster.

Fifth, FEMA evaluates the request and recommends action to the White House. Sixth, the president either gives the executive order for the declaration or FEMA informs the governor the request has been denied. The whole process may only take a few days. If the executive order is given, federal and financial resources are mobilized through FEMA for search and rescue and for the provision of basic human needs. Long-term federal programs are mobilized during this time.

The Disaster Plan

The purpose of **disaster planning** is to reduce a community's vulnerability to the tremendous consequences of disasters and to prevent or minimize problems resulting from system damage associated with the disaster (Drabek, 1986). Community health nurses are involved in disaster planning, as are other health care professionals in the community. Specific ways that a nurse can be more prepared for a disaster in his or her community are described in the next section.

In a disaster, the usual strategies and process for providing care may not work. Deviating from a routine plan of care may present a few problems for nurses and other health care professionals when disaster occurs. Disaster health care is very different from daily nursing practice; it is not routine (even compared with emergency department services), and the philosophy of care is based on "providing the greatest good for the greatest number." Abiding by this standard of care is often difficult for health care professionals, especially for those in routine practice settings, who practice holistic care and provide optimal care to all who need services. The disaster plan is fundamental in the preparation of health care professionals (Waeckerle, 1991). Drabek (1986) identified general principles that can guide community health nurses who take part in disaster planning. These principles are listed in Box 15-7.

Waeckerle (1991) stated, "Disaster planning is an enormous undertaking" (p. 815). As in other areas of health care, enormous amounts of money are spent in the United States on disaster relief during the recovery period, with little funds available for communities to use in disaster preparedness and disaster planning. This poses very real challenges in the development of a disaster plan. Although the disaster plan is usually developed from

---

BOX 15-7 PRINCIPLES TO GUIDE DISASTER PREPAREDNESS FOR ALL PERSONS INVOLVED IN PLANNING

Measures used for everyday emergencies generally do not work in major disasters.
- Disasters are more uncertain, less predictable, with more unknowns, and citizens have little consensus on what needs to be done in a disaster.
- Laypersons are most likely to jump in and provide aid without direction and knowledge of prioritization and triage.

Plan for specific population needs and consider "disaster planning" as a verb, which is ongoing, rather than a noun, such as the limits of a written plan.

Provide information regularly to the community to correct misconceptions.
- Widespread looting and theft are actually quite uncommon.
- People should be given information and details about the extent of the disaster to enable them to take appropriate action, in contrast to the long-held belief of health workers that people will panic if they "know too much."

Involve the entire community in the planning process, not just officials and emergency personnel.
- Such inclusion limits confusion about who does what and where the lines of authority are.

Use routine working methods and procedures in the disaster plan, which will eliminate the need to learn new procedures and prevents confusion at the disaster site.

Disaster plans should be flexible.

Roles and responsibilities of team members should be identified by position or title, not by names of individuals, to avoid having to revise the plan when people change positions.

---

guidelines set forth by local, state, and federal officials, communities are often on their own and must rely on local officials and volunteers to do much of the work when organizing a disaster plan and evaluating its validity through mock disaster drills (Waeckerle, 1991).

Since the anthrax attacks on the U.S. and the threat of small-pox bioterrorism, disaster plans must include much more detail on protocols for managing communicable diseases and chemical agents, most of which current health care professionals have never seen. Bioterrorism, germ warfare, and disaster/bioterrorism preparation have become common terms on news shows and in the vocabulary of the American public since 9/11 (Porche, 2002). With the most recent terrorist attacks of anthrax spores distributed through the United States Postal Service as a means to produce fear and the possibility of infecting unsuspecting individuals, most citizens are unclear as to how to protect themselves. In addition to being prepared and educated about bioterrorist agents such as anthrax and small pox, disaster planners also need to prepare for even rarer organisms such as Brucellosis, plague, Tulareima, Q Fever and Botulism. Additionally, chemical agents are substances that can injure and kill through a variety of mechanisms. Such agents as choking, blood, blister or neural agents are the ones most likely to be used in an attack and will cause the highest rates of morbidity and mortality (Porche, 2002; Smith, 2000). Garrett (2000) warns that the collapse of the public health infrastructure in the United States leaves us particularly vulnerable to such epidemics. Public health is the only viable protection against epidemics, whether natural or man made and public health is responsible in most states for disaster planning. Through the last two decades, health departments have been chronically underfunded, according to Garrett (2000), because of their successes in the past century at keeping children immunized, the air breathable, factories safer, and citizens better educated about self-care. Disaster plans then must change as threats to the public's health evolve.

Characteristics of Disaster Plans

Through research of past disasters and presence or absence of disaster plans, disaster specialists have determined common characteristics of effective disaster plans (Drabek, 1986; Noji, 1997; Waeckerle, 1991). They are as follows:

- *The disaster plan is based on a realistic assessment of potential problems that can happen, such as destruction to property, material, and utilities; impairment of communication; and geographic isolation.*

- *Estimates of types of injuries that result from disasters most likely to occur in the area and the possible destruction of health facilities and alternative agency use are included in the plan.*

- *The plan is brief, concise, and inclusive of all who can provide disaster aid.*

- *The plan is organized by a timeline; it details the stages of a disaster, who must be involved, what must occur, and how each stage unfolds throughout the disaster process.*

- *The plan is approved by all agencies that provide authority endorsement, as well as sanctioned by those who have the*

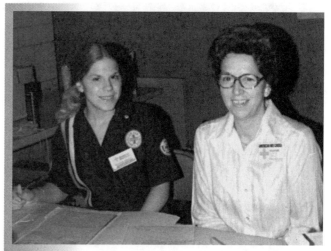

Chapter author, Dr. Karen Saucier Lundy (left), at an American Red Cross shelter after hurricane Allen in Galveston, Texas.

most power to see that the plan is updated periodically and carried out when disaster strikes.

- *The plan is regularly tested through mock drills and revised based on drill results.*

- *The plan is always considered a work in progress because needs and resources in a community relative to disaster preparedness change constantly.*

Common Elements of Disaster Plans

Although disaster plans should be targeted for the specific community, certain components should be included in all disaster plans. Each component may have more or less elaboration, detail, and specifics according to the needs of the community to which it applies. These components consist of authority; communication; supplies; equipment; human resources (health professionals, both acute and public health); emergency and disaster specialists; officials of government and voluntary agencies; engineers; weather specialists; community leaders, both lay and official; team coordination; transportation; documentation; record keeping; evacuation; rescue; acute care; supportive care; recovery; and evaluation. Details of these components are summarized in Box 15-8.

Disaster Management

The goal of disaster management is to prevent or minimize death, injury, suffering, and destruction (Taggert, 1982). Disaster management by nature is an interdisciplinary, collaborative team effort (Sullivan, 1998); however, community health nurses are integral in planning disasters and responding. Disaster management is usually coordinated by specific community officials, such as the civil defense.

Once the civil defense efforts are begun, coordination of the many networks in the community disaster infrastructure are car-

BOX 15-8 COMMON ELEMENTS OF A DISASTER PLAN

Authority: Issues warnings and official responses and is the central authority for disaster declarations and delegation

Communication: Warnings to public and how communicated, whether by weather sirens, television, radio, police loudspeakers; includes chain of notification, rumor control, and restriction and access to the press in the disaster area

Equipment and supplies: Sources and where located, usual and special needs, staging areas, and controlled access to supplies; dissemination of donated food, clothing, and storage

Human resources: Health professionals, both acute and public health; emergency and disaster specialists, utility officials, officials of government and voluntary agencies, engineers, weather specialists, community leaders, both lay and official

Team coordination: Central operations, staging area, chain of command

Transportation: Traffic control, access and escape routes, control of risk to victims, and rescuers related to transportation

Documentation: Details of disaster plan, how and where disseminated; procedures for managing records of injuries, deaths, supplies, and agency reporting responsibilities; development of brief forms with minimal duplication

Evacuation: Logistics and procedures, destination of evacuees, and routes of escape

Rescue: Search and rescue operations; details the removal of victims and immediate first aid, who is responsible, and what equipment is needed

Acute care: Casualty collection points, triage, and detailed role descriptions of health care workers for immediate emergency care

Supportive care: Shelter management

Recovery: Postdisaster team meeting, debriefing, critical incident stress debriefing, press conferences, and reports to media

Evaluation: Mock disaster drills and revision of disaster plan based on results

ried out by individuals overseeing these agencies. Some examples include the mayor, chief executive officer(s) of the local hospital(s), executive officer of the local American Red Cross chapter, the emergency medical system manager, and the emergency/triage physicians and nurses.

Other agencies or resources and staff persons who make up the disaster team include local, state, and federal disaster management agencies; private relief organizations, such as churches and the Salvation Army; fire and police departments; political leaders who function under the mayor's administration; engineers, geologists, and meteorologists; sociologists, epidemiologists, and other researchers; community volunteers; and the media, including television news reporters, cable weather broadcasters, and radio communication persons (e.g., short-wave radio, HAM radio).

Disaster Response

Disaster response is a complex plan that is sometimes difficult to coordinate and carry out. All health care and other personnel should become knowledgeable about the disaster plan and their anticipated roles. As pointed out previously, regularly evaluating the performance of all involved personnel through mock disaster drills is an important function of community health nurses and other personnel involved in coordinating disaster response (Dixon, 1986; Neff & Kidd, 1993).

Response and Recovery

The disaster team's **response** is initiated during and after the impact stage of the disaster. Local, state, regional, national, federal, and volunteer agencies assist communities in need (FEMA, 1998c). **Recovery** is a long-term process that occurs during the rehabilitation stage of the disaster. Sometimes, severe financial strain is placed on the local or state government during this time.

Levels of Disaster Response

Disasters are usually defined in terms of severity and levels of response required. Neff and Kidd (1993) identified four levels of disaster response, which are explained in the following paragraphs.

A **level I response** is limited to emergencies that require medical resources from the local hospital and community, such as minor injuries incurred in a local disaster, but also may include severe injuries incurred in multicar accidents or a plane crash. Occasionally, level I responses may include state and federal agency involvement (Neff & Kidd, 1993). In general, hospital and community resources are adequate to provide field and hospital triage, medical treatment, and stabilization for multiple casualties. All hospitals maintain a written disaster plan that corresponds with the local civil defense and community disaster plan.

Fundamental to all written level I hospital disaster plans is the assurance that a command post and chain of command will be established. Usually, the chief executive officer or a senior administrator of the hospital will be in command. Communication via telephones, cellular systems, and portable radios is limited to the commander, security, and other authorized personnel. Water conservation and backup generators are important considerations just in case they are needed. A smooth flow of clients depends on an efficient triage system in the field and within the hospital.

A **level II response** involves multiple casualties that require the use of multijurisdiction health care personnel and medical facilities across a specified region (Auf der Heide, 1989; Neff & Kidd, 1993). When more than one geographic jurisdiction is involved or required, the chain of command structure becomes unified for the sake of clarity, information flow, and minimization of duplications. Coordination and communication efforts among the agencies are emphasized at this response level.

When a mass casualty disaster occurs, a **level III response** is required (Auf der Heide, 1989; Neff & Kidd, 1993). This level of disaster, such as hurricane Andrew in South Florida in 1992 and the World Trade Center and Pentagon, is so overwhelming that medical resources at the local and regional levels are exhausted. State and federal agencies intervene.

The **National Disaster Medical System (NDMS)** is a voluntary system that was formed through the collaborative efforts of several governmental agencies in the United States (Pretto & Safar, 1991). The primary objective of the NDMS is to increase the mobilization of national resources in an effort to save as many lives as possible. Accomplishing this objective involves providing rapid medical responses, evacuating families and communities, and coordinating medical care. The NDMS efforts, such as recommendations and guidelines for disaster planning and response, filter down to state and local governments and officials, such as the civil defense office and the emergency medical services in the community.

Nurses are involved on every level of the NDMS. Some of the functions of community health and other nurses include serving on the NDMS's national-level task force and board; decision making regarding guidelines and policies; disaster planning on the state and local levels; collaborating with other disaster team members on plans, procedures, and tasks; coordinating the disaster team at various locations within the community; triaging victims at community and hospital locations; and managing the care of victims.

Level IV response occurs when the **Federal Emergency Management Agency (FEMA)** intervenes by providing financial and oversight assistance. FEMA is an independent agency that reports to the president of the United States. Level IV response efforts sometimes require an executive order from the president to declare the disaster a major disaster. (Discussion of the presidential response to FEMA was discussed in the section "Disaster Planning.") From 1964 to early 1998, there were 1,198 disasters, such as the earthquakes in San Francisco in 1989, declared by the president of the United States as level IV disasters (FEMA, 1998a).

Since its development in 1979, FEMA's mission essentially has remained the same, which is "to reduce loss of life and property and protect our nation's critical infrastructure from all types of hazards, through a comprehensive, risk-based emergency manage-

ment program of mitigation, preparedness, response, and recovery" (FEMA, 1996, p. 2). FEMA may respond during the impact stage or the rehabilitation stage of the disaster, or both. FEMA may respond early, during impact, to increase mobilization of personnel and supplies. During recovery or rehabilitation, FEMA responds as the result of an executive order (FEMA, 1998c). In the recovery process, FEMA assists in rebuilding communities so that communities and agencies can return to a functional status.

Project Impact was established by FEMA in an effort to build disaster-resistant communities (FEMA, 1998b). In the past 10 years, $20 billion has been spent by FEMA to assist families in repairing and rebuilding their communities after natural disasters. FEMA has responded to 43 major disasters, involving 27 states, declared by President Clinton.

Other Disaster Agencies
American and International Red Cross Disaster Services

The American Red Cross (ARC) is a humanitarian organization "led by volunteers and guided by the Congressional Charter and the Fundamental Principles of the International Red Cross Movement" (ARC, 1997, p. 1). The ARC provides relief to victims of disasters and helps people prevent, prepare for, and respond to emergencies.

On May 21, 1881, Clara Barton and a group of her friends founded the ARC as a result of her commitment to and hard work with the mass casualties of yellow fever, dysentery, and many other infections during the Spanish-American War (ARC, 1990; Frantz, 1998). Because of the efforts of the Red Cross nurses during the Spanish-American War, Cuba communicated the committed efforts of Clara Barton to important officials. Although Barton was not actually a nurse, her organizational skills were exceptional. She was a former schoolteacher and government worker from Massachusetts.

More than 100 years have passed, but the memory of Clara Barton lives. The Red Cross nurses of the Spanish-American War were responsible for the congressional decision of 1901 to establish the Army Nurse Corps.

The unique contribution that Barton made to the worldwide Red Cross movement was her organization of volunteers to help disaster victims (ARC, 1990). America became the 32nd nation to support the Red Cross international treaty at the Geneva Convention in 1882. In 1900, the U.S. Congress granted the ARC its charter.

Today the ARC is composed of more than 1.2 million adult and youth volunteers. Many nurses are considered disaster volunteers. Community health nurses should take a voluntary leader's role in the ARC's disaster preparedness, response, and shelter management. In 1995 and 1996, the ARC spent $216.5 million while assisting 125,120 families during disasters (ARC, 1998). The ARC constantly adapts to current needs (ARC,

1990). Increasingly, Red Cross volunteers are being trained for technological disasters, such as those involving toxic chemicals, explosive materials, radiation, and chemicals.

Salvation Army

The Salvation Army was founded in London in 1865 by William Booth (Salvation Army, 1997a). The Salvation Army was founded on Christian principles. The Salvation Army Act of 1980 described its mission, which is "the advancement of Christian religion . . . of education, the relief of poverty, and other charitable objects beneficial to society of the community of mankind as a whole" (Salvation Army, 1997a).

During a disaster, the Salvation Army provides food, water, shelter, and clothing and helps trace families. With the goal of carrying out God's mission, Salvationists reach out to suffering and needy people by providing the Word of God and basic human physical needs (Salvation Army, 1997b).

Evacuation

Community health nurses, among many other health care personnel, need to realize that wild panic reactions are different from fleeing from a threat (Auf der Heide, 1989). Mileti, Drabek, and Haas (1975) stated that panic may occur but usually only when at least one of three conditions is present: (1) a perception of immediate danger, (2) encountering blocked escape routes, and/or (3) a feeling of being isolated. When panic occurs, it is usually of short duration and not contagious, depending on the response from the media (Auf der Heide, 1989).

Evacuation traditionally has been a difficult task to carry out because of people's reluctance to evacuate (Quarantelli & Dynes, 1972; Wenger, James, & Faupel, 1985). There are several reasons for this reluctance (Auf der Heide, 1989). The primary reason for hesitancy is that some people do not believe that they are in danger. Another reason is that some people want to remain at the site to protect their property. Not wanting to evacuate until the family can be removed as a unit is another reason for hesitancy. The head of the household or another member may refuse to leave until the other family members, which may also include dogs or other pets, are safe.

Besides the concern for human lives, FEMA is concerned for the lives of animals and, more specifically, the human-animal bond (Lockwood, 1997). Many owners of pets have developed a close relationship with their pets. Lockwood explored why animal owners will risk danger to themselves and not evacuate disaster areas without assurance of their animals' well-being. The most common responses are that people love their animals and treat them as part of the family.

The key to motivating people to evacuate is to improve warning effectiveness, which consists of several strategies (Auf der Heide, 1989). The credibility of the present warning and the validity of past evacuation warnings influence a person's decision of whether to evacuate. Consistency and repetition of the warning by different sources of the evacuation command always in-

crease the chance that a person will heed the warning. Commands to evacuate by agency and community officials are taken more seriously, which promotes the belief of the message. A clear, specific message to evacuate that is understood will yield better results. Finally, an effective strategy is to ensure a course of protective actions, such as ample law enforcement officers on duty, for those people evacuating.

Role of the Media

Mass media can be a friend or foe (Auf der Heide, 1989). To enhance disaster response, the media can provide accurate information, convey instructions to the public, and stimulate donations from parts of the country not affected by the disaster.

On the other hand, the media may complicate the operations by taking a "feeding frenzy" spin on the facts. Reporters may make unreasonable demands on resources, facilities, and officials (Auf der Heide, 1989). Distortion of the facts, overreaction, and perpetuation of disaster myths are other factors that may interfere with the disaster response operations.

Good communication is vital during the evacuation operations. The Weather Bureau, radio stations, television announcements, local sirens and announcements, and computers should be used to alert the public of the impending threat. Another medium is the Emergency Broadcast System, where officials provide local, state, or national information and warnings. When the evacuation is in process, a large volume of requests place overwhelming demands on the media, as well as public officials of the city and county.

Rescue

The search-and-rescue mission is the most challenging part of the disaster operations (Silverstein, 1984; Waeckerle, 1983, 1991). Searching for and rescuing disaster victims tax the physical capabilities and emotions of rescuers. Emotional demands can be extremely traumatic to the rescuers and require psychosocial debriefing.

Teams of health care personnel, fire and security officials, and volunteers comb the designated area many times in search of casualties. Once the casualties are located, quick triage actions are necessary. After the victims are categorized by way of triage, rescue workers need to continue to search the area for undiscovered injured people or dead bodies.

Triage

The triage system normally practiced in emergency departments across the country is not the same triage system used during a disaster (Kitt, Selfridge-Thomas, Proehl, & Kaiser, 1995). Field (disaster) triage is used when mass casualties result from disaster. The initial triage that takes place in the field is called the *primary triage*. *Secondary triage* occurs at the point of entry into the medical facility, and *tertiary triage* occurs in the specified area where the client is located, such as the emergency department, pediatrics, and so on.

Disaster triage allows health care personnel to identify the most salvageable clients so that treatment can be initiated immediately. Colored tags with symbols are attached to disaster victims so that level of triage can be readily seen by health care personnel (Kitt, Selfridge-Thomas, Proehl, & Kaiser, 1995).

Several factors may affect the triage system (Dixon, 1986). The client's general state of health is one factor. For example, an elderly person may have a poor cardiovascular status, which may decrease the person's survival expectation. Another factor that may affect the outcome of triage is the health care worker's inexperience in triage and assessment. Lack of supplies or equipment is another factor. Not having proper supplies and equipment in sufficient quantities can adversely influence the disaster victim's triage status (Neff & Kidd, 1993)

Disaster Shelters

Shelters are managed by trained volunteers and/or Red Cross nurses. When help is needed, the executive director of the affected local chapter of the Red Cross calls upon nurses and other volunteers. Shelters are opened by volunteers in the community through coordination efforts of the ARC, the mayor, civil defense, and other officials of the community. Churches, schools, civic centers, and community centers are used as shelters.

It is sometimes difficult to determine or anticipate shelter needs during disasters. The local Red Cross depends on other ARC chapters, the mayor, and civil defense teams to report anticipated numbers of persons that are evacuating their premises and reporting to a shelter. In widespread disasters, shelters are opened in a number of areas that house the local residents as well as victims who have traveled a long distance to escape more immediate danger. An example of a widespread disaster was hurricane Camille in 1969, which traveled from the Mississippi Gulf Coast to North Mississippi and beyond (see box below). Persons in the most danger were on the Mississippi Gulf Coast, so they evacuated to cities and towns north of the coast, while the local residents of those areas also were evacuating their premises and relocating to the same shelters. In instances such as this, anticipating the correct number of shelter residents is difficult. However, good communication between city officials and remote areas regarding evacuation numbers should be a priority.

For each shelter, there is one team manager, at least one nurse volunteer, multiple people to keep records, and numerous volunteers trained to assist victims. Activities include keeping thorough records; coordinating meals; providing snacks, cots, blankets, and other essentials; providing health care, such as first aid treatment and over-the-counter medications that have been authorized by a physician; acting as a liaison between victims and resource agencies and their families; and protecting the victims from harm by keeping alert to possible fire outbreaks, accidents, and other mishaps.

The ARC's motto is "Help Can't Wait" (ARC, 1995). When help is needed, mass recruitment of supplies, equipment, food, and shelter is coordinated by the ARC. For example, in 1993 after the summer Midwest floods, Wal-Mart Stores, Inc., loaned the ARC a large warehouse, forklifts, and staff to expedite distribution of urgently needed supplies to the shelters (ARC, 1995). Other retail stores and pharmaceutical companies offered many supplies and a large amount of monetary assistance.

Role of the Community Health Nurse in Disasters

Why should community health nurses be involved in disaster? Aren't trauma and hospital nurses better qualified to work in disasters than nurses in the community?

FYI

Hurricane Camille

Hurricane Camille was a category 5 hurricane that hit the coasts of Mississippi, Alabama, and Louisiana with winds in excess of 200 mph. Hurricane Camille resulted in the deaths of 141 persons, 9,472 injuries, property loss and damage for 74,000 families, and more than $1 billion total damage. At the 30-year anniversary of the storm, the scars and influence of Camille still exist on the Mississippi Gulf Coast, where the most severe damage occurred. The storm produced 24-foot tidal waves in August of 1969 and remains one of the deadliest storms of the 20th century.

Comments from Survivors

"Afterwards, it looked like we had been bombed. My house was 'caddywhompas' on its foundation. All you could hear were helicopters and people crying. It was the most horrible experience I have ever had."

"The thing that I remember were the dead cows on the beach."

"The beach looked like a holocaust. A woman slipping and sliding through mud and muck clutching a lifeless child to her chest."

Source: Hattiesburg American, August 14, 1994, p. 7A.

Good questions—ones that many student nurses and practicing nurses alike may ask. Our ideas about disasters, what happens, and who is involved—both victims and rescuers—are often shaped by the media. The disaster movie formula developed as a major box office draw in the 1970s with such movies as *The Poseidon Adventure* (1972), about a sinking cruise ship; the *Airport* movie series about jet liner crashes; *The Towering Inferno* (1974), about a burning skyscraper; *The Hindenburg* (1975), about the real-life zeppelin airship disaster of 1937; and *The China Syndrome* (1979), about a fictitious nuclear power plant accident, which became an eerie prelude to the actual Three Mile Island nuclear accident that same year. During the past 30 years, U.S. and international moviegoers have been fascinated by disasters and continue to line up for top movies, such as *Armageddon* (1998), *Deep Impact* (1998), and *Titanic* (1997), the biggest movie money-maker of all time.

These movies, as well as television programs such as *ER*, portray disasters as a backdrop for story lines and romances, heroes and villains, and greatly influence the way we visualize disasters. As a result, disaster planning and disaster preparedness are given very little attention. Ironically, the most recent terrorist attacks on the World Trade Center and the Pentagon provided more specific details about actual recovery and effects of aftermath for the public through extensive media coverage. At least temporarily, the American public appear to be more aware about the need for preparedness for disaster.

Community health nurses are much better prepared than most other health care professionals to manage disasters in the community, because emergency treatment and triage are but two of many activities that help people cope with disaster.

Successful strategies often pair a community health nurse with a trauma nurse in the disaster setting. One of the major determinants of how well a disaster is managed is not only how well we carry out our individual roles in a disaster but also how well we allow others to carry out their roles (Suserud & Haljamae, 1997).

General Functions of the Community Health Nurse

Community health nurses, as well as other nurses, are involved in emergency treatment and triage during the impact stage of the disaster. Good physical assessment skills are vital for success. Only health care personnel highly skilled in assessment should triage. Most health care personnel are not trained in advanced assessment skills and cannot make acuity judgments proficiently. However, baccalaureate-prepared personnel and emergency paramedics are trained to triage and then give emergency treatment.

Because nursing is specialized, as are most health professions, community health nurses often are more knowledgeable about teamwork and interdisciplinary effort than nurses in other specialties because they rely on group efforts daily in community health nursing practice. Community health nurses are experts in program planning, community assessment, and group dynamics, skills that are critical to the effective management of a disaster crisis. Because community health nurses are population focused, assessing and intervening with vulnerable populations are second nature.

Other functions that enable community health nurses to work effectively in disasters include working with the media to inform and educate, the use of public health interventions to minimize risks from communicable diseases, and the securing of community resources for victims. These functions are accomplished while coordinating multiagency efforts in the mediation of health risks at the disaster site (Garcia, 1985). The background work of disaster management, for which community health nurses are perfectly suited, may not make it to the big screen, but such activities are what ultimately influence how well a community survives and heals from disaster.

Specific Nursing Approaches

A major goal of community health nurses is to be an asset to the community, not a burden. Specific approaches that community health nurses should accomplish to mitigate human and material losses in a community disaster include the following strategies:

1. *Personal preparedness:*
   - *Be disaster-prepared and disaster-aware.*
   - *Maintain your own emergency equipment, supplies, and skills.*
   - *Be certain that your family knows what to do during a disaster, when to do it, who to call, and where to go.*
   - *Use caution and prudence when selecting the location of your home.*

2. *Community involvement:*
   - *Become familiar with local disaster plans and emergency evacuation procedures.*
   - *Get involved in the political issues in your community that relate to disaster preparedness and recovery.*
   - *Support leaders who choose long-term, focused solutions in loss reduction and emergency preparedness rather than those who choose short-sighted, politically expedient solutions.*
   - *Help modify land use and develop ordinances that reflect the best knowledge of geography and water hazards.*
   - *Support local emergency assistance organizations by serving on advisory boards.*
   - *Assist in the education of the public in personal disaster preparedness.*
   - *Visit schools to help prepare children for assuming the lifetime responsibility of being prepared for disasters in the community.*

3. *Professional preparedness:*
   - *Become trained and certified in professional disaster nursing by the local ARC chapter.*
   - *Get involved in the development of agency and community disaster plans.*

- *Attend continuing education classes and disaster skills updates to keep current in disaster management skills.*
- *Be supportive of administrative efforts to increase disaster preparedness.*
- *Write new stories, volunteer to speak at community meetings, write letters to the editor of local newspapers, and publish articles in nursing journals about the nursing role in disaster preparedness (Garcia, 1985).*

Shelter Management and Care

Pickens (1992) emphasized the importance in roles of health care workers in disasters. Community health nurses play a vital role in disaster preparedness and response. In fact, the leadership administered by community health nurses may greatly impact the public's reception and comprehension of disaster education and warnings. See the Case Study on p. 358 for examples of successful shelter management.

The general public, as well as many nurses, do not realize the impact that nurses have before, during, and after a disaster (Demi & Miles, 1984). The leadership role that community health nurses can take may prevent deaths and property damage.

Red Cross disaster nurses and other volunteers are often trained to coordinate and manage shelters, conduct tertiary triage within the shelter, and administer first aid to sick or wounded people. Currently, the Red Cross has a pool of more than 15,000 trained disaster volunteers, many of whom are nurses (ARC, 1995). Volunteers are ready for immediate assign-

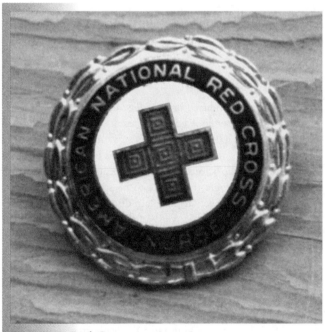

American Red Cross nursing pin.

A CONVERSATION WITH...

Because of the tremendous response from caring volunteers at the Oklahoma City bombing disaster, the first critical step was to establish a centralized system to manage the number of individuals calling to report to the emergency site. Once established, we were able to schedule, validate licenses, and orient volunteers from the Oklahoma State Medical Association, Oklahoma Nurses Association, American Red Cross, hospitals, and other entities to the expectations and limitations of the bomb site.

There was tremendous generosity from everyone. Medical supplies, equipment, and medication were immediately available and continued to be delivered at the site for many days. Public health was responsible for centralizing and assuring that these supplies were used appropriately and responsibly by licensed providers. It was important to assure that the appropriate practice guidelines were in place.

Providing disaster services as a public health function doesn't end with just providing emergency services. Public health is also responsible for ensuring that volunteers that provide ongoing emergency health services are competent and properly licensed. It is important to be familiar with your state's nurse practice act and knowledgeable regarding any actions that might be needed to invoke licensure reciprocity in the event that the disaster is such magnitude that volunteers arrive from other states or countries to assist.

Planning and ongoing networking with all players in the emergency response team is very important. While personnel may change, the fundamental needs in an emergency generally do not. Having a public health work force that is prepared in disaster response is very beneficial.

Any coordination and networking that can be in place with state and local American Red Cross chapters prior to a disaster benefits both the public health agency and the American Red Cross.

—Toni D. Frioux,
MS, CNS, ARNP, Chief, Nursing Service,
Oklahoma State Department of Health

ment for damage assessment, case management, and shelter management at a moment's notice.

The ARC shelter manager, often a community health nurse, organizes and manages the shelter operations by fulfilling the roles of administrator, leader, and supervisor (Garcia, 1985). The way the manager conducts operations impacts the flow of operations and activities within the shelter. Functions of the manager include allocating space, obtaining supplies and equipment, scheduling staff, completing reports and records, and attending to problems.

If the community health nurse volunteer happens to be the manager and the nurse on duty, the dual roles and functions can become overwhelming. Care should be coordinated by application of the nursing process (Garcia, 1985). Good assessment and planning skills are among the most important functions of the community health nurse volunteer. Interventions in this setting include preventing disease and illness, providing emotional support, protecting health, and providing intermittent, temporary care to this vulnerable population.

Anticipation of certain problems will facilitate the operations and care of the community health nurse volunteer. For instance, in the shelter population, the nurse should expect some everyday, normal occurrences, which will include chronically ill people who are dependent on medications and equipment, normal episodes of illness and infection, communicable disease, and emotional stress reactions. Evaluation of the shelter population should be ongoing, including one-on-one conferences with shelter families and staff members.

Disaster Recovery

Toffler, in his classic study *Future Shock* (1970), described future shock as "the response to overstimulation" (p. 344). He described numerous examples of stress in situations requiring constant change; among them are persons in disasters. Toffler described persons who experienced a disaster as being trapped in environments that are rapidly changing, unfamiliar, and unpredictable. Results of such situations can be devastating, even for the most stable and well-prepared person. Victims of disasters may be hurled into antiadaptive states and be incapable of the most elementary decision making (Toffler, 1970). Evidence of this reaction can be seen in pictures of a woman, after a destructive earthquake, strolling down a dangerous, debris-filled road with a dead or wounded baby in her arms, her face blank and numb, appearing impervious to the danger around her. Persons can be overwhelmed and become paralyzed as familiar objects and relationships are transformed. Where a person's house once stood, a tornado can within minutes change the environment into an unrecognizable pile of rubble and gushing water pipes. The Oklahoma City bombing destroyed life and property within minutes, replacing familiar landmarks with images of unimaginable horror and destruction.

Simple acts taken for granted hours before, such as making a telephone call or pouring a cup of coffee, are no longer appropriate or possible. Signs, sounds, and other psychological and cultural cues surround disaster victims without meaning, without recognition during and immediately after the impact. Every word, every action, every movement is characterized by uncertainty. Even in a crowd, victims often experience a sense of isolation and loneliness, abandonment, and an overwhelming sense of loss—loss of the world as they know it. Confusion, disorientation, and distortion of reality occur spontaneously; fatigue, anxiety, tenseness, and extreme irritability follow. Apathy, emotional withdrawal, and pessimism result when victims develop a sense of little hope for the future or when they see themselves as never being safe or stable again (Toffler, 1970).

In the classic study *Everything in its Path,* sociologist Kai Erickson described the 1972 Buffalo Creek flood and its aftermath in terms of disaster impact and the destruction of community (Erickson, 1976). This study provided a detailed and analyzed view of a disaster and the resulting conflict between individualism and dependency, self-assertion and resignation, and self-centeredness and community orientation. The results of this devastating disaster included loss of community connection, declining morality, rise in crime, and the rise in out-migration from the sudden loss of neighborhood and community. Organized disaster activity was largely provided by outsiders.

Collective deaths, like those in a disaster, do not permit persons to set up the usual barriers between the living and the dead, as is customary in the deaths of the hospital, where "death is screened from view, sanitized, muffled, tidied up" (Erickson, 1976, p. 169). In disaster, "death lies out there at its inescapable worst. There are no wreckers to rush the crushed vehicle away, no physicians to shroud death in a crisp white sheet or to give it a clean medical name, no undertakers to wash away the evidence of death and to knead out the creases of pain or fear . . . and the sight does not go away easily" (Erickson, 1976, p. 169).

Effects on Survivors

When death is experienced on a wide scale, such as in a disaster, survivors often experience guilt as a result of their own survival (Erickson, 1976). They may even come to regret their own survival, when others around them were killed in what seems like a meaningless and capricious way, in part because "they cannot understand by what logic they came to be spared" (p. 170). Survivor guilt has often been described in disaster research literature. Lifton (1967), in his classic study of the psychological effects of the atomic bomb in Hiroshima, found that survivors described the open eyes of corpses as evoking guilt: It was as if the eyes were saying, "Why me, why not you?"

Lifton and Olson (1976) identified five major elements that may be found in some type of combination in all disasters. Psychological difficulty or maladaptive response is more likely to occur if all five elements are found in a single disaster, as in the Buffalo Creek flood. The five elements are suddenness of the event, human callousness in causation (human-made rather than natural causation), continuing relationship of survivors to the disaster, isolation of the community, and totality of destruction.

The experience of the disaster can have both short- and long-term effects on mental health and functioning, such as dissociation, depression, and PTSD (Gerrity & Flynn, 1997). Refer to Box 15-5 for other health effects associated with disasters. Meichenbaum (1994) has compiled from disaster research a list of factors that can place individuals in a vulnerable position for developing psychological problems when all five of Lifton and Olson's (1976) elements are present in a disaster. They include the following:

- *Objective and subjective characteristics of the disaster, such as proximity of the victim to the disaster site, the duration, the degree of physical injury, and the witnessing of grotesque, graphic scenes*
- *The characteristics in the community of postdisaster response and recovery environment, such as cohesiveness of community and disruption of social support systems*
- *The characteristics of the individual or group; for example, elders, unemployed persons, single parents, children, those with previous history of mental disorders, and those with marital conflict before the disaster*

Most studies on the aftermath of disasters have reported that the first reaction of survivors is a state of dazed shock and numbness. The "disaster syndrome" consists of classic symptoms of mourning and bereavement on a communitywide scale: grief for lost community members and homes and grief for lost culture and familiar surroundings (which will never be the same again, no matter what form the recovery takes). To make this reaction worse, government and rescue workers often control access to the disaster area, keeping residents from their own homes and cleaning up wreckage without consulting the community members. Often, such work by disaster workers, although necessary, further distances the survivors from their need to be a part of the recovery process and exacerbates feelings of loss of control caused by the disaster itself.

Among the symptoms of extreme trauma that can affect an entire society, such as the Oklahoma City bombing, is a sense of vulnerability, a feeling that one has lost a certain natural immunity to misfortune, a growing conviction that the world is no longer a safe place to be (see Box 15-10 on p. 361 and Case Study on p. 358). A lingering thought grows into a prediction of sorts: If this can happen, something even more terrible is bound to happen—the line has been crossed (Erickson, 1976). Box 15-9 describes an example of the far-reaching effects of the Chernobyl disaster, which continues to threaten the well-being of affected communities.

Special Survivor Populations: Elders and Children

Children are at special risk during a disaster because of their immaturity—they have not yet developed adult coping strategies and do

---

BOX 15-9 THE CHERNOBYL NUCLEAR DISASTER: WILL IT EVER BE OVER?

On April 26, 1986, a reactor blew up in Chernobyl in the former Soviet Union, resulting in an explosion that threw out 100 million curies of dangerous radionuclides to surrounding areas of the Ukraine, Belarus, and Russia. The World Health Organization estimates that 4.9 million persons were affected, making it the largest nuclear disaster in history. The results: Livestock, vegetables, grains, the soil, and the environment continue to be hazardous for human existence, although a large population still inhabit these areas. Cancer, rare pediatric cancers, leukemia, chromosomal damage, and stress-related disorders plague the region and result in premature death and disability among all age groups. Scientists even now do not know how long the nuclear danger will remain or if it ever again the region will be safe to live in.

Source: Edwards, 1994.

---

not yet have the life experiences to help them understand what has happened to them. Also, we know that children rely on routine and consistency in their environment, relationships, and home life for a sense of security and identity. These areas are often disrupted in a disaster. Problems can emerge at school and last for much longer periods when compared with adults (Gerrity & Flynn, 1997). Children may suffer from fears, phobias, sleep disorders, nightmares, excessive dependence, fear of being alone, hypersensitivity to noise and weather conditions, and regression, such as thumbsucking, bedwetting, and "baby talk" or stuttering (Laube & Murphy, 1985).

Elders often experience significant depression and despair from losing homes and being uprooted from familiar surroundings. Many of the elderly had already lost primary family members and friends before the disaster. Among their valuables are family photos and mementos, Bibles, and keepsakes. Loss of this sort has a considerably greater effect on elders than others. There are also the compounded problems of more chronic diseases and health problems, making them more vulnerable to disaster stress (Gerrity & Flynn, 1997). Disorientation and memory disturbances have also been noted in this population (Laube & Murphy, 1985). Again, refer to Box 15-5 to review health effects in disasters.

Simple intervention methods, such as group work for children and elders and short-term counseling immediately after the disaster, have proven quite effective in helping the recovery process. Community health nurses are in an excellent position to intervene with these vulnerable populations. Community health

The Oklahoma City Bombing, April 19, 1995

On the morning of April 19, 1995, the Alfred P. Murrah Federal Building in Oklahoma City was the site of a devastating terrorist bomb. In addition to federal employees and other government workers, the building was the site of a day-care center. Because of the effectiveness of the city's disaster plan, rescue and recovery began within minutes after the explosion. Oklahoma experiences frequent, deadly tornadoes throughout the state and consequently maintains a highly organized disaster planning response.

Initial priorities the morning of the bombing included getting people out of the building, triaging injuries, and transporting the injured to six nearby hospitals. Nurses in hospitals, home health agencies, and public health and other facilities in the community quickly responded to the needs of the victims. By midafternoon of that day, the four trauma departments had seen 40 to 80 persons each. Victims were transported by ambulances, private vehicles, cabs, and vans. A family communication center was quickly set up at a local church, 5 miles from the bomb site, by the American Red Cross and FEMA. This center, which "wrapped its arms around the families of the victims of the blast," provided mental health professionals, hospice nurses, psychiatric nurses, and counselors 24 hours a day for 2 weeks after the bombing. The medical examiner's office communicated with the families of the victims there, and rescue workers from the bomb site frequently reported back to the families concerning the progress of the search teams.

A play area for children was set up, and the Salvation Army provided comfort services, including food and clothing. Pets were brought by local groups to provide solace for the victims. A Native American healer was present for tribal members. Toll-free numbers were provided by the state mental health department for direct and indirect victims' use to prevent and treat posttraumatic stress disorder. Support groups were set up, television talk shows featured survivors and disaster workers, and articles were printed in the local newspapers, all directed toward giving the people of Oklahoma a chance to talk through the horror of their collective experiences. The city's convention center became a huge hostel that fed, clothed, and housed thousands of rescue workers during this period. Roses and chocolates appeared on the pillows of disaster workers, stress management was available, massages were provided for sore muscles, and there was "always a listening ear for sore souls."

Nurses were involved at all levels of the disaster, including triage at the command center, accompanying surgeons as they removed the legs of a child in the bombed building, providing grief counseling for the families of victims and for the disaster workers themselves, providing direct care at hospitals to the injured, and visiting the families of victims in their homes for forensic identification and later on as follow-up.

According to Wilson (1996), an "important reason why the people here worked so well was because of disaster planning. When people live in an area that is nicknamed 'tornado alley,' they plan for disaster" (p. 24). "Though we will never rectify the loss of life incurred in a disaster by planning ahead, we can be ready to mobilize the resources to make all of us a little less vulnerable" (p. 25).

Source: Wilson, 1996.

nurses must be able to locate children and elders so that immediate action can be taken. The most likely place to find these populations are in community shelters.

Traditional healers and informal community resource persons have also been used effectively by recovery teams to assist the community in looking within for healing energy. Women's associations, community development schemes, family welfare workers, and church volunteers have all had significant success in mobilizing community resources to promote community healing and recovery. Such strategies reduce the need for outside resources, as well as helping the community regain its stability using its own assets of solidarity (Richman, 1993).

Collective Trauma: The Loss of Community

Erickson (1976) detailed the loss of not only the sense of community, which occurs in a mass disaster, but also the loss of communality, which consists of a network of relationships that make up their general human surround. Erickson (1976) described communality as a "state of mind shared among a particular gathering of people" (p. 189). In a sense, this community is one that cushions the pain, provides a context for intimacy, represents morality, and serves as the repository of old traditions and culture.

When a disaster demolishes a community, people find that they no longer have the collective reservoir of pooled resources, both physical and emotional, from which to draw. Communities act as a "cluster of people acting in concert and moving to the same collective rhythms who allocate their personal resources in such a way that the whole comes to have more humanity than its constituent parts. In effect, people put their own individual resources at the disposal of the group—placing them in the communal store and then drawing on that reserve supply for the demands of everyday life" (p. 194).

When a community is destroyed, people find themselves without the reservoir on which they have relied in the past. They find that they are almost empty of feeling, empty of affection, and empty of confidence and assurance. Residents feel abandoned, often expressing feelings of fear, apathy, and demoralization. Comments

from survivors often reflect despair: "I thought this was the end of the world" or "It looked like Dooms Day" (Erickson, 1976, p. 199).

. . . .

Whoever fights monsters should see to it that in the process he does not become the monster. And when you look into the abyss, the abyss looks into you.

Nietzsche

. . . .

Nurses' Reactions to Disasters

Nurses also should attend to the needs of the disaster workers themselves during and after a disaster to reduce the possibility of producing secondary victims. Rescue personnel are often reluctant to take breaks to replenish food, water, and rest when time is of essence in the search and recovery phase when they are needed. Nevertheless, nurses should be firm in reminding

A CONVERSATION WITH...

How did you become interested in disaster research?

In 1970 I was fresh out of my master's program at the University of Colorado and was asked by the local American Red Cross Chapter in Dallas to give a talk to their nurses on the psychological effects of disaster. I thought they wanted me to talk about the psychological effects of disaster on nurses (later learned that they just wanted the effects in general). I had no experience so I went to the library to research the subject and found only one reference specific to the effect on nurses— Jeannette Rayner's article written in 1958. By generalizing from publications about army nursing, plus Rayner's article, I managed to meet my assignment but felt a great need for an in depth study of the psychological effects of disaster on nurses. I later wrote a small grant to the American Red Cross for funding to survey nurses' reactions in a recent tornado close to home. While waiting on that response, Hurricane Celia hit the coast of Texas. I immediately called and requested that I be sent to that area. This was granted and I was on site within 24 hours of the disaster. That study was published in Nursing Research. *I later broadened my area of study to cover all health care providers in disaster. Not long after my first study I was invited to be a part of a task force to revise the Disaster Act to include assistance for psychological aspects of disaster. That was completed and has been carried forth ever since.*

Should BSN nurses be prepared in disaster response and recovery?

Students in baccalaureate programs should have classes and simulated experience in reducing the impact of disaster. If available, collaboration with the local Red Cross chapter is ideal. Nursing students that take their courses can earn hours toward Red Cross certification, thus shortening the time after graduation to become a Red Cross nurse.

Why do you believe BSN nurses should be prepared in disaster nursing?

Nurses are uniquely qualified by the nature or their education and experience. Nurses are prepared to work with the whole patient—physically and psychologically. They work both in crisis and chronic conditions which is necessary because a disaster victim, definitely in crisis, may also have a chronic illness. Thus, they have the basic qualifications. Updating their knowledge and skills should continue through workshops and disaster drills sponsored by/through their place of work.

—Jerri Laube, RN, PhD, FAAN

Dr. Jerri Laube is co-author, with Dr. Shirley A. Murphy, of *Perspectives on Disaster Recovery* (1985, Appleton-Century-Crofts).

workers that in order to remain useful, they must not exhaust themselves in the process. Seeing that workers are rotated and providing rest, nourishment, and relaxation for the rescuers should be considered essential responsibilities of the community health nurse.

Nurses often experience the same disturbing, and sometimes dramatic, emotional problems as those found in their clients who were victims. Nurses may experience difficulty concentrating, fatigue, irritability, insomnia, and other unique symptoms of stress. The unique symptoms include depersonalization of the victim, a macabre sense of dark humor, hypervigilance, and excessive unwillingness to disengage or leave the disaster scene or the helping role (e.g., refusal to leave after the arrival of a relief shift) (Gerrity & Flynn, 1997). Reactions of nurses are magnified when the nurse is a member of the affected community and when the nurse may have endured property and community damage, as well as stress related to family well-being. According to Laube-Morgan (1992), nurses should be considered "normal persons reacting in a very normal manner to an abnormal condition" (p. 19).

Sources of stress for the disaster nurse can be generally classified into three categories: (1) event stressors, the trauma and fatigue associated with the extreme intensity of the disaster event, of the highest intensity if the nurse lives in the affected community and has family who are potential victims; (2) occupational stress—stress related to role conflict, role overload, and role confusion; and (3) organizational stressors—factors that emerge from the organizational response itself, multiagency demands, and the complex tangle of bureaucracy that emerges in a major disaster (Hartsough & Myers, 1985). With every disaster victim treated, nurses often experience an unconscious fear that the victim could just as easily have been one of their loved ones.

Nurses are educated to maintain professional composure in any type of stressful situation, even in the face of grief, suffering, and death. This composure has been termed *detached concern* by Coombs and Goldman (1973). Detached concern is the adaptive ability to care for critically ill and injured clients while maintaining an acceptable emotional detachment. Research has revealed that nurses function effectively in disasters, and very few have long-term emotional difficulties after the disaster.

In Laube's (1973) study of the hurricane Celia disaster, the majority of nurses functioned in their role without impairment from anxiety. Major stressors that nurses may experience during disasters have been identified by researchers as excessive physical demands, concerns for personal safety, inadequate supplies, seeing people suffer and not being able to meet basic needs of all, hurt children, disorganization, and concern for their own family's welfare (Waters, Selander, & Stuart, 1992).

Family roles seem to play a critical part in the nurse's response to disaster. Health care workers who are from the disaster area have exceptional stress, because not only must they work through their own reactions to and losses of the community from the disaster, but they also must resolve the family/community role conflict (Waters,

Selander, & Stuart, 1992). In other words, when the nurse's family well-being is jeopardized, professional effectiveness decreases and stress more likely will impact the nurse's role. This finding means that outside disaster workers are indicated early in the course of disasters and should continue until the local health care providers can be assured of their own family's safety (Laube, 1985).

•••••••••••••••••••••••••••••••

It's when Mother Nature gets so angry at man and his arrogance that she whips up a little humble pie.
                    Jimmy Buffett, 1998, on a tornado
                          in Brookings, South Dakota

•••••••••••••••••••••••••••••••

Stuhlmiller (1996) contended that because nurses are typically involved with suffering and disruption of lives of their clients, they in fact may be in a better position than other disaster workers to mediate the effects of the disaster. By participating in debriefings, nurses are healing themselves as they help others begin their own process of healing. Stuhlmiller contended that we often assume that workers are at risk for post-traumatic stress and proceed with negative assumptions about how they should react. By doing so, we unwittingly hamper their "natural restorative capacities" (p. 19). In other words, looking for the negative effects may overshadow the positive outcomes on which nurses tend to focus—the positive outcomes that come from helping people in extreme need.

"Disasters challenge self-understanding and meanings just as illness does . . . what the rescuers need most then is what nurses are particularly good at providing. Nurses can foster emotional recovery and growth by attending to what approaches work best and by acknowledging the validity of the person's expressed pain, fear and grief" (p. 19). Such a view is consistent with Laube's (1973) conclusion that with all of the possible stressors nurses face with disasters, studies consistently reveal the nurses' responses to disaster do not interfere with their effectiveness as professionals (Laube, 1973).

As a result of these findings, it can be concluded that nurses are extremely vulnerable to PTSD in the aftermath of a disaster. The following Research Brief describes the nurses' reactions and feelings during and after hurricane Hugo. Box 15-10 consists of actual quotes from nurses who expressed their feelings about their work in a disaster.

Prevention Strategies for Nurses

By being prepared for a disaster through specialized training and anticipatory stress counseling, nurses can reduce the damage of a disaster to self. Simple measures such as appreciating the intensity of emotions and dealing with them; taking breaks; eating nutritious foods with smaller, more frequent meals; avoiding drink-

RESEARCH BRIEF

Chubon, S. J. (1992). Home care during the aftermath of hurricane Hugo. Public Health Nursing, 9(2), 97–102.

Chubon was in the midst of an ethnographic study of home care nurses' job stress when hurricane Hugo struck the South Carolina coast in 1989. The home health agency was heavily damaged by wind and water and was uninhabitable for more than a week. Because the nurse researcher had observed the nurses for 10 weeks before the hurricane, she was able to collect data about their response to the disaster in the context of their usual role of home health nurse. The nurses in the agency were simultaneously victims and caregivers for their home health clients. They experienced grief, anger, and frustration about their losses, as well as conflict between family responsibilities and work responsibilities. Chubon's work supported the findings of previous studies in which nurses continued to function effectively in their work roles despite their emotional responses. Because baseline data were available before the hurricane struck, this study indicated that the nurses' functioning was generally consistent with their predisaster work patterns. Sources of stress consistently related to the safety of their own loved ones and family. Suggested interventions were (1) to bring outside nurses from other home health agencies to care for assigned clients until the local nurses stabilize their own family situations and (2) to make mental health resources available in the immediate postrecovery period for the nurses in the agency.

ing large amounts of caffeine and alcohol; exercising; and sleeping as much as possible have given nurses the added strength to not only survive but flourish in a disaster. Seldom can as much attention be given to the victims as the nurse believes is necessary.

Although nurses seem to be fairly effective in mediating stressors in the disaster setting, they are certainly not immune to possible ill effects. Laube-Morgan (1992) suggested from her research of the 1989 Loma Prieta earthquake in California that prevention programs for disaster workers should be included in disaster preparedness. For primary level prevention, a crisis team should work with the disaster staff before a disaster strikes. The crisis team should include a social worker, minister, psychiatric nurse, and other mental health professionals as available. This team should have input into the disaster plan and be included in disaster drill critiques and debriefing. At a secondary level of prevention, the same team should be highly visible during the impact of the disaster. They could provide emotional support and monitor the emotional stability of the workers, intervening as necessary. At the tertiary level of prevention, after the disaster, the team should take an active role in organizing and conducting mandatory disaster debriefing sessions. Counseling referrals should be made at this time and should, again, have input into the critique of the disaster plan's effectiveness related to worker response and recovery (Laube-Morgan, 1992). Such strategic interventions can prevent burnout and emotional casualties of the health care provider.

CONCLUSION

As disasters are increasing in number and, many times, severity each year, community health nurses need to be adequately prepared more now than ever before. Lillian Wald, a famous nursing theorist and community activist, responded to her societal needs by developing the Henry Street Settlement House in 1893. Wald stated, "Nurses not only serve the individual but promote the interest of a collective society" (as cited in Kippenbrock, 1991, p. 209). This statement also applies today, especially in the face of disasters.

Being prepared for future disasters means that community health nurses must plan disaster care for multicultural populations. The hallmark of American society is multiculturalism (Sobier, 1995). The major disaster goal for nurses now and in the future is to retain maximum wellness of individuals and populations in communities (Procter & Cheek, 1995). Learning to work with appropriate resources and placing emphasis on specific approaches to enhance individuals, families, and communities are integral to protection and healing from a disaster.

Melanie Dreher, past President of Sigma Theta Tau International (1996), pointed out that nurses are very resilient and can be called *everyday heroes*. There have been numerous nurses who were outstanding in heroic acts, such as Nightingale, Alcott, and Cavell. Dreher contended that nurses with "heroine" status are recognizable by traits and actions. She stated: "They define their life's work not in terms of paychecks, working conditions and employment benefits, but in terms of the number of lives saved, families in crisis who were counseled, and patients comforted" (p. 5).

CRITICAL THINKING ACTIVITIES

1. Based on the Case Study on p. 358, answer the following questions:
   - What are the primary, secondary, and tertiary prevention disaster interventions carried out by nurses during the Oklahoma City bombing?
   - Identify activities in each of the stages of disaster recovery.
   - Give examples of the three categories of stressors that disaster nurses faced in Oklahoma.
   - Identify the components of the Oklahoma City disaster plan. What would be your recommendations for the disaster team, based on the information above?
2. How can community health nurses better prepare individuals for the present and future threat of bioterrorism and terrorism?

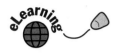 Explore Community Health Nursing on the web! To learn more about the topics in this chapter, access your exclusive web site: http://communitynursing.jbpub.com

REFERENCES

Advisory Committee on the International Decade for Natural Hazard Reduction. (1987). *Confronting natural disasters: An international decade for natural hazard reduction.* Washington, DC: National Academy Press.

American Psychiatric Association (APA). (1987). *Diagnostic and statistical manual of mental disorders* (3rd ed. rev.). Washington, DC: Author.

American Red Cross (ARC). (1990). *A history of helping others* (ARC Publication No. 4627). Washington, DC: ARC National Headquarters.

American Red Cross (ARC). (1991). *Coping with disaster: Emotional health issues for disaster workers on assignment* (ARC Publication No. 4472). Washington, DC: ARC National Headquarters.

American Red Cross (ARC). (1995). *Disaster is everybody's business* (ARC Publication No. 5061). Washington, DC: ARC National Headquarters.

American Red Cross (ARC). (1996). *Disaster services: We're there when you need us* (ARC Publication No. 4450). Washington, DC: ARC National Headquarters.

American Red Cross (ARC). (1997). *Our mission statement*: www.redcross.org/mission.html.

American Red Cross (ARC). (1998). *Disaster facts*: www.fema.gov/library/df_5.htm.

Anderson, M. B. (1991). Which costs more: Prevention or recovery? In A. Kreimer & M. Munasinghe (Eds.), *Managing natural disasters and the environment.* Washington, DC: World Bank.

Auf der Heide, E. (1989). *Disaster response: Principles of preparation and coordination.* St. Louis: Mosby.

Baker, G, & Chapman, R. (1962). *Man and society in disaster.* New York: Basic Books.

Barker, E. (1989). Care givers as casualties. *Western Journal of Nursing Research, 11,* 5.

Barry J. M. (1997). *Rising tide: The great Mississippi flood of 1927 and how it changed America.* Simon & Schuster: New York.

Berz, G. (1984). Research and statistics on natural disasters in insurance and reinsurance companies. *The Geneva Papers on Risk and Insurance, 9,* 135–157.

Buffett, J. (1998). *A pirate looks at fifty.* New York: Random House.

Chubon, S. J. (1992). Home care during the aftermath of Hurricane Hugo. *Public Health Nursing 9*(2), 97–102.

Coombs, R. H., & Goldman, L. J. (1973). Maintenance and discontinuity of coping mechanisms in an intensive care unit. *Social Problems, 20,* 342–355.

Demi, A. S., & Miles, M. S. (1984). An examination of nursing leadership following a disaster. *Topics in Clinical Nursing.* Rockville, MD: Aspen Publishing.

Dixon, M. (1986). Disaster planning—Medical response: Organization and preparation. *American Association of Occupational Health Nurses, 34*(12), 580–584.

Drabek, T. E. (1986). *Human system response to disaster: An inventory of sociological findings.* New York: Springer-Verlag.

Dreher, M. C. (1996, First Quarter). Heroism. *Reflections,* 4–5.

Dynes, R. R., Quarantelli, E. L., & Kreps, G. A. (1972, December). *A perspective on disaster planning, TR-77* (pp. 6–8). Washington, DC: Defense Civil Preparedness Agency.

Edwards, M. (1994, August). Living with the monster—Chernobyl. *National Geographic, 186,* 2.

Epstein, P. R. (1998). Watching El Nino, *Public Health Reports, 113,* 330–333.

Erickson, K. (1976). *Everything in its path: Destruction of community in the Buffalo Creek flood.* Simon & Schuster: New York.

Federal Emergency Management Agency (FEMA). (1996). *This is FEMA.* Washington, DC: FEMA Headquarters.

Federal Emergency Management Agency (FEMA). (1997a). *FEMA highlights and statistics for 1997*: www.fema.gov/library/fact97.htm.

Federal Emergency Management Agency (FEMA). (1997b). *The strategic plan: Partnership for a safer future.* Washington, DC: FEMA Headquarters.

Federal Emergency Management Agency (FEMA). (1998a). *Historical presidential disaster declarations*: www.fema.gov/library/dd-1964.gif.

Federal Emergency Management Agency (FEMA). (1998b). *Project impact*: www.fema.gov/impact/.

Federal Emergency Management Agency (FEMA). (1998c). *The federal disaster declaration process and disaster aid programs: Response and recovery*: www.fema.gov/declara/.

Frantz, A. K. (1998). Nursing pride: Clara Barton in the Spanish-American War. *American Journal of Nursing, 98*(10), 39–41.

Garcia, L. M. (1985). *Disaster nursing: Planning, assessment, and intervention*. Rockville, MD: Aspen Publishing.

Garrett, L. (2000). *Betrayal of trust: The collapse of global public health*. New York: Hyperion.

Gerrity, E. T., & Flynn, B. W. (1997). Mental health consequences of disasters. In E. K. Noji (Ed.), *The public health consequences of disasters* (pp. 101–121). New York: Oxford University Press.

Guha-Sapir, D., & Lechat, M. F. (1986). Reducing the impact of natural disasters: Why aren't we better prepared? *Health Policy and Planning, 1,* 118–126.

Hartsough, D. M., & Myers, D. G. (1985). *Disaster work and mental health: Prevention and control of stress among workers*. Rockville, MD: National Institute of Mental Health.

International Decade for Natural Disaster Reduction Promotion Office (IDNDR) (1994). *Natural disasters in the world: Statistical trends on natural disasters*. Tokyo: National Land Agency.

Janis, I. L., & Mann, L. (1977, June). Emergency decision making: A theoretical analysis of responses to disaster warnings. *Journal of Human Stress*, 35–48.

Kippenbrock, T. A. (1991). Wishing I'd been there. *Nursing and Health Care, 12*(4), 209.

Kitt, S., Selfridge-Thomas, J., Proehl, J. A., & Kaiser, J. (1995). *Emergency nursing: A physiologic and clinical perspective* (2nd ed.). Philadelphia: W. B. Saunders.

Klagsbrun, S. C. (2002). A mental health perspective on 9/11. *Journal of the Association of Nurses in AIDS Care*, Vol. 3, No. 5, September/December (p. 67).

Laube, J. (1973). Psychological reactions to nurses in disaster. *Nursing Research, 22,* 343–347.

Laube-Morgan, J. (1992). The professional's psychological response in disaster: Implications for practice. *Journal of Psychosocial Nursing, 30*(2), 17–22.

Laube, J., & Murphy, S. A. (1985). *Perspectives on disaster recovery*. Norwalk, CT: Appleton-Century-Crofts.

Lifton, R. J. (1967). *Death in life: Survivors in Hiroshima*. New York: Random House.

Lifton, R. J., & Olson, E. (1976). The human meaning of disaster. *Psychiatry, 39,* 1–7.

Lockwood, R. (1997). *FEMA: Through hell and high water: Disasters and the human-animal bond*. Washington, DC: FEMA and the Humane Society of the United States.

Logue, J. N., Melick, M. E., & Hansen, H. (1981). Research issues and directions in the epidemiology of health effects of disasters. *Epidemiological Review, 3,* 140–162.

Malilay, J. (1997). Floods. In E. K. Noji (Ed.), *The public health consequences of disasters* (pp. 287–301). New York: Oxford University Press.

Meichenbaum, D. (1994, June 14–18). *Disasters, stress, and cognition*. Paper presented for the NATO Workshop on Stress and Communities, Chateau da Bonas, France.

Mileti, D. S., Drabek, T. E., & Haas, J. E. (1975). *Human systems in extreme environments: A sociological perspective* (Monograph No. 21). Boulder, CO: Program on Technology, Environment, and Man, Institute of Behavioral Science, University of Colorado.

Mizutani, T., & Nakano, T. (1989). The impact of natural disasters on the population of Japan. In J. I. Clarke, P. Curson, S. L. Kayastha, & P. Nag (Eds.), *Population and disaster*. Cambridge, MA: Basil Blackwell.

Muench, J. (1996). Disaster training pays off for Juneau nurses. *Alaska Nurse, 46*(5), 1.

Neff, J. A., & Kidd, P. S. (1993). *Trauma nursing: The art and science.* St. Louis: Mosby.

Noji, E. K. (1997). *The public health consequences of disasters.* New York: Oxford University Press.

Office of U.S. Foreign Disaster Assistance. (1995). *Disaster history: Significant data on major disasters worldwide, 1900-present.* Washington, DC: Agency for International Development.

Pickens, S. (1992). The decade for natural disaster reduction. *Nursing & Health Care, 13,* 192–195.

Porche, D. J. (2002). Biological and Chemical Bioterrorism Agents. *Journal of the Association of Nurses in AIDS Care,* Vol. 13, No. 5, September/October, 57–64.

Pretto, E. A., & Safar, P. (1991). National medical response to mass disaster in the United States: Are we prepared? *Journal of the American Medical Association, 266,* 1259–1262.

Procter, N. G., & Cheek, J. (1995). Nurses' role in world catastrophic events: War dislocation effects on Serbian Australians. In B. Neuman (Ed.), *The Neuman systems model* (3rd ed.). Norwalk, CT: Appleton & Lange.

Quarantelli, E. L., & Dynes, R. R. (1972, February). When disaster strikes (it isn't much like what you've heard about or read about). *Psychology Today,* p. 72.

Richman, N. (1993). After the flood. *American Journal of Public Health, 83*(11), 1522–1524.

Sabin, L. (1998) *Struggles and triumphs: The story of Mississippi nurses.* Jackson, MS: Mississippi Hospital Association Foundation.

Salvation Army. (1997a). *The Salvation Army international headquarters: About us:* http://salvationarmy.org/aboutus.htm.

Salvation Army. (1997b). *The Salvation Army international headquarters: International spiritual life commission:* www.salvationarmy.org/slc.htm.

Silverstein, M. E. (1984). *Triage decision trees and triage protocols.* Washington, DC: FEMA Headquarters.

Sklar, D. P. (1987). Casualty patterns and disasters. *Journal of the World Association of Emergency Disaster Medicine, 3,* 49–51.

Smith, P. (2000). Terrorism awareness: Weapons of mass destruction: Part I, Chemical agents, *The Internet Journal of Rescue and Disaster Medicine, 2*(1), retrieved October 10, 2002, from http://www.icaap.org/iuicode?86.2.1.6.

Sobier, R. (1995). Nursing care for the people of a small planet: Culture and the Neuman systems model. In B. Neuman (Ed.), *The Neuman systems model* (3rd ed.). Norwalk, CT: Appleton & Lange.

Stuhlmiller, C. M. (1996, First Quarter). Studying the rescuers. *Reflections,* 18–19.

Sullivan, T. J. (1998). *Collaboration: A health care imperative.* New York: McGraw-Hill.

Suserud, B., & Haljamae, H. (1997). Acting at a disaster site: Experiences expressed by Swedish nurses. *Journal of Advanced Nursing, 25*(1), 155–162.

Taggert, S. D. (1982). *Emergency preparedness manual.* Salt Lake City: University of Utah.

The anniversary of hurricane Camille. (1994, August 14). *Hattiesburg American,* p. 7a.

The many graces of Oklahoma City nurses. (1996). *Reflections, 22*(1), 10–12.

Toffler, A. (1970). *Future shock.* New York: Random House.

Waeckerle, J. F. (1983). The skywalk collapse: A personal response. *Annals of Emergency Medicine, 12,* 651.

Waeckerle, J. F. (1991). Disaster planning and response. *New England Journal of Medicine, 324,* 815–821.

Waters, K. A., Selander, J., & Stuart, G. W. (1992). Psychological adaptation of nurses post-disaster. *Issues in Mental Health Nursing, 13,* 177–190.

Wenger, D. E., James, T. F., & Faupel, C. E. (1985). *Disaster beliefs and emergency planning.* New York: Irving Publishers.

Wilson, J. S. (1996). Healing Oklahoma's wounds. *Home Healthcare Nurse, 14*(1), 23–25.

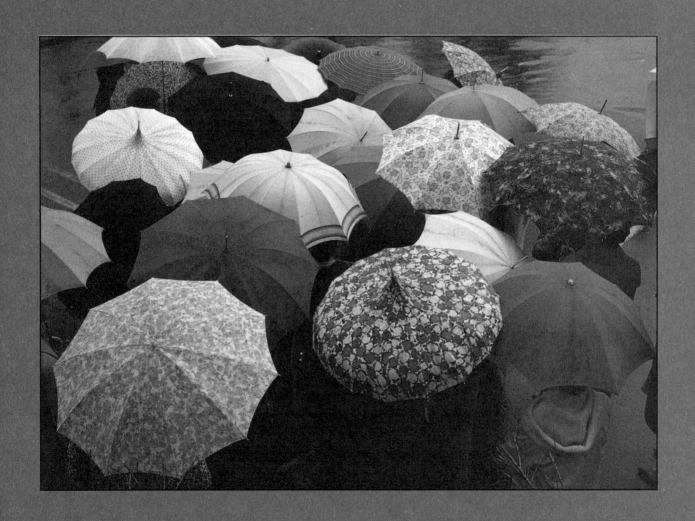

PART THREE

Community-Based Nursing Care

Recent changes in society have had a profound impact on the health care delivery system in the United States. There has been an explosion of technology accompanied by an increase in health care costs to the consumer, with resulting changes in the *setting* and *focus* of health care delivery. Managed care and controlling health care costs are primary foci of the health care industry. The family, as the oldest and most basic of all social institutions, has undergone dramatic change in structure and function. Through the family, health care needs are identified and addressed, from birth to death. The portion of the U.S. population that is older than 65 is the fastest growing segment, as well as the group that requires the most health care dollars. Individuals with higher acuity levels, that in the past were treated in acute care institutions, are now being discharged to the community and treated in the home. The nurse of the 21st century will require a firm foundation in both acute and community-based/community-focused nursing health care to assist individuals in making the transition not only from acute care to home care but to and from other community settings, such as school and work.

Through the family, children are socialized to norms, values, and behavior. As such, the family is a powerful influence on the health beliefs and behavior of its members. The assessment of family functioning and its ability to meet the health needs of its members is a critical aspect of the community health nurse role.

Research indicates that gender influences the seeking, acquisition, and use of health services and health behavior. Women are less likely to be diagnosed with heart disease because it has long been associated as a male health problem. Men, in turn, often seek health care later than their female counterparts, which often results in less successful outcomes.

When children receive appropriate health-promotion and disease-prevention services, they are less likely to develop health problems. Nursing has a role in providing anticipatory guidance to parents and children regarding health-promotion and disease-prevention activities.

Community-based settings for mental health care have dominated for several decades. With the mental health clients, this is more cost-effective than institutionalization, and outcomes for the family are positive. Local community mental health centers provide care for all levels of mental health care needs. Lack of reimbursement and appropriate identification mechanisms for locating the mentally ill require creativity on the part of the community health nurse to meet community mental health needs.

Because Americans are living longer, myriad age-appropriate additional health care services for the aging population will be necessary. The health and care of the elder client is but one of the challenges associated with this age group. Ample research has documented that the caregiver is also at high risk from impaired health. Poor health of the caregiver is often a deciding factor in making the decision to place an elderly family member into institutionalized care. Community health nurses must develop and implement strategies that promote physical and mental health for both the elder and the caregiver.

Unit V
Care of Families in Community-Based Nursing

Chapter 16
Foundations of Family Care
Ruth A. O'Brien

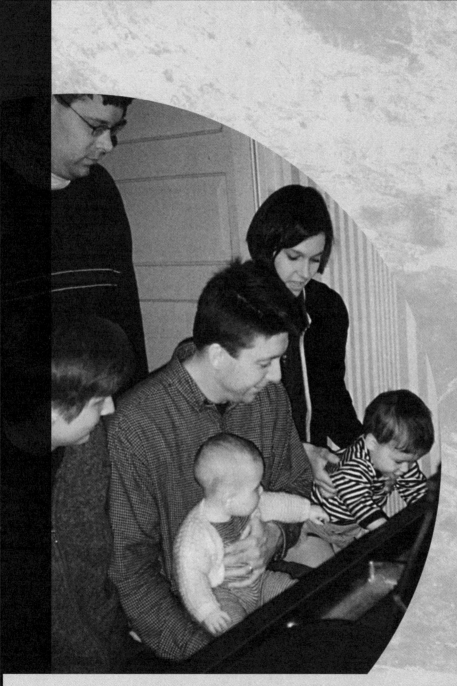

The family is two or more individuals who manifest some degree of interdependence in their interactions with each other and their environment in meeting basic human needs for affection and meaning. Moreover, our family is who we think it is.

QUESTIONS TO CONSIDER

After reading this chapter, answer the following questions:
  1. How is *family* defined?
  2. What are the health responsibilities of the family?
  3. What is the difference between family-oriented and family-focused nursing care?
  4. What is an example of a conceptual framework for family assessment?
  5. How is the self-efficacy model of family interventions used in promoting the health of families?

KEY TERMS

Affect	Family	Interdependence	Positive feedback
Beliefs	Family developmental	Meaning	Power
Communication	tasks	Negative feedback	Self-regulation
Contracting	Function	Nonsummativity	Structure
Environment			

Joyce Williams, a school nurse at Sagebrush Elementary, reflected on her recent meeting with Mrs. Carson, the first grade teacher for Kevin Johnson. Mrs. Carson had contacted her to discuss Kevin's increasing episodes of toileting accidents and inattention in class over the past 2 months. Mrs. Carson questioned whether Kevin's behavior was indicative of problems coping with his parents' divorce; she told Joyce that the third grade teacher who had Kevin's sister in class related that the children's father recently remarried and moved to another city about 50 miles away. According to Kevin's school file, Mrs. Johnson was a legal secretary for a large law firm downtown. Recognizing the strains that a single, working parent raising two children, 6 and 8 years old, might be experiencing, Joyce decided that she would call Mrs. Johnson to schedule a home visit to talk with her about the problems Kevin's teacher had reported. A home visit, rather than a conference at the school, would provide an opportunity for her to observe parent-child interaction and also to gain a better appreciation of how Mrs. Johnson is handling being a single parent and what other supports are available.

FYI

Two-thirds of women work for pay during the same years that they are bearing and raising children.

Source: International Law Office. (1999). Maternity Protection at Work. *Geneva, Switzerland: International Labor Office.*

Definition of Family

Dramatic changes in family structure over the past few decades are highlighted in contrasting media images portrayed in popular television sitcoms, such as *Ozzie and Harriet* and *Father Knows Best* in the 1950s and 1960s and *Murphy Brown* in the 1990s. The popular image of the family as a nuclear two-parent unit raising their own children, with father as the breadwinner and mother as the homemaker, as portrayed in *Ozzie and Harriet* and *Father Knows Best,* is no longer the dominant pattern in American society. In fact, only 1 in 5 families of the 1990s fits this popular stereotype (Ahlburg & De Vita, 1992).

Single-parent, stepfamilies or blended families, dual-career families in which both parents work, married couples without children, cohabitating couples, and gay and lesbian families were typical of the diverse family patterns of the 1990s (Bianchi & Spain, 1996). *Murphy Brown,* the popular sitcom featuring a successful career woman who chooses to have a baby without a husband, illustrates one of the changes in the demography of the family over the past 40 years. And the Johnson family described in the case vignette at the beginning of the chapter represents yet another form of family diversity resulting from divorce and remarriage.

Social, demographic, and economic factors have all contributed to the changing composition of the family. U.S. Census Bureau statistics indicate that 1 in 3 births in 1995 were to unmarried women. Contrary to common perceptions that teens are responsible for most of the out-of-wedlock births, rates of out-of-wedlock births are highest among single women in their 20s (Snyder & Moore, 1996). Based on the trend toward a higher proportion of births to single women, coupled with the higher incidence of divorce, about half of all children today are expected to spend some part of their time in a single-parent home (Bianchi & Spain, 1996). And given that more than 75% of people who divorce remarry, demographers estimate that stepfamilies or blended families (approximately 19% in 1990) will become the norm in the 2000s (Ahlburg & De Vita, 1992). The number of dual-career families also has markedly increased, with almost three-fourths of married mothers with children in 1996 reporting some paid employment. Furthermore, the continued growth of the older population will increase both the number of elderly couples and the number of frail elderly persons living alone who will require supportive services in an era when adult daughters hold jobs and are not as readily available as earlier generations to be family caregivers (Bianchi & Spain, 1996).

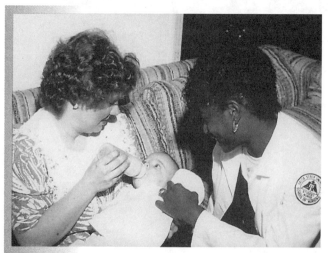

The single-mother family has increased in number during the past decade. These families are at special risks for poverty and a lack of health insurance.

Heightened attention to demographic changes in the composition of the family over the past 40 years has generated considerable debate among social scientists on whether the family is declining in importance in our society. In reflecting on the passion that often surrounds the debate, Cowan, Field, Hansen, Skolnick, and Swanson (1992) asserted, "Families mattered in the past; they continue to matter in the present; and they will matter still, in the uncertain years of our future" (p. 481). Valuing the family, however, should not be confused with valuing a particular family form. They urged that rather than viewing demographic changes in the composition of the family unit as indicative of family decline, we need to reconsider traditional definitions of family that emphasize legal and biological ties between members and conceptualize how diverse types of families fulfill different functions to address the complexity of their health needs.

How should we define the family for community health nursing assessment and intervention? Although community health nursing's primary target of service is the community (Williams, 1996), work with the family as a population is one strategy that nurses may use to improve the health of communities. Thus, community health nurses need a broad conceptual perspective of the family that recognizes diverse compositions. **Family** in this chapter refers to two or more individuals who identify themselves as family and manifest some degree of interdependence in interactions with each other and their **environment** in meeting basic human needs for affection and meaning. Themes central to this definition are members' **interdependence** in meeting basic needs and members' **beliefs** that they are a family. This purposefully broad view of family encompasses the traditional two-parent nuclear family, single-parent families, stepfamilies or blended families, and childless couples, as well as relationships that are not built on legal or biological ties, such as gay or lesbian families.

Health Responsibilities of the Family

How well the family functions has a great impact on individual family members' well-being and health behaviors. Health professionals' encounters with the family are episodic, with the family assuming responsibility for a least 75% of the health care of its members (Duffy, 1988). An assessment of family functioning in promoting and protecting its members' health requires a clear understanding of its responsibilities in this arena. Five major responsibilities of the family for members' health are presented.

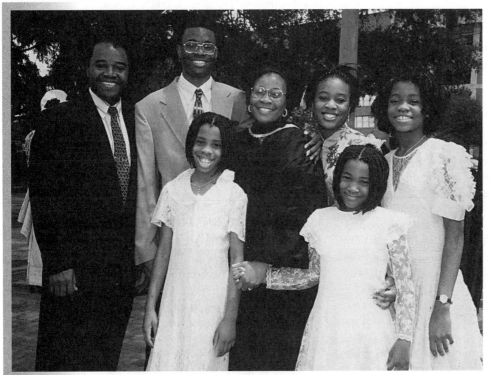

The family provides security where children can get a sense of who they are and what they can accomplish.

Development of Members' Sense of Personal Identity and Self-Worth

The family plays a significant role in the development of one's mental health (Hanson & Boyd, 1996; Loveland-Cherry, 1996). Family interactions may facilitate or impede members' access to (1) **affect,** the sense of loving and being loved; (2) **power,** the freedom to decide what one wants and the ability to obtain it; and (3) **meaning,** a sense of who and what one is. The functionally healthy family is one that maintains a balance between all members' access to affect, power, and meaning so that no member consistently and systematically is denied actualization of these basic human needs. Community health nurses often receive referrals to conduct a family assessment in situations in which parents have experienced difficulties in meeting the socioemotional needs of infants and young children, resulting in impaired attachment and inadequate weight gain associated with the syndrome referred to as *failure to thrive.* Early parent-infant attachment is critical to the development of trust and ability to form intimate relationships with others later in life. Parents who have difficulty forming appropriate attachments with their infants may have lacked appropriate role models as young children themselves. Such individuals often are suspicious of professionals, and much interpersonal skill and patience is needed to establish working relationships with them. By conveying warmth and caring, coupled with a nonjudgmental attitude, nurses can assist parents in learning how to meet the socioemotional needs of their children.

Emotional Support and Guidance During Life Cycle Transitions

As individuals grow and mature, they are expected to meet new performance expectations consistent with their current life stage. For example, a child is expected to learn to read when he or she goes to school. Should the child find reading difficult, school progress is slowed and the child's sense of personal worth is threatened. Support and guidance from the family is essential in helping individuals achieve their developmental tasks across the life cycle (Duvall & Miller, 1985). In fact, the family as a whole is described as having responsibilities, goals, and developmental tasks that parallel the developmental tasks of individual family members. Thus, while children are expected to learn to read and develop other cognitive skills when they go to school, the family has the corresponding developmental task of encouraging children's educational achievement and learning to relate to the educational system in an effective manner.

Community health nurses have many opportunities to provide guidance to families undergoing life cycle transitions. Prenatal and postpartum visits for new parents can offer health teaching to ease the transition to parenthood. Changes in family structure as a result of divorce and/or remarriage also present new developmental tasks for family members, such as single par-

enthood and the addition of a stepparent into children's lives. As noted in the introductory paragraph, Kevin's teacher, in making a referral to the school nurse, questioned whether his toileting accidents in school might be symptomatic of difficulty in coping with his parents' divorce and the subsequent move and remarriage of his father.

....

For good or ill, our families and the environment in which we live are the backdrop against which we play out our entire lives. Families shape our futures; our early family experiences heavily influence and to a degree determine how we forever after think and behave.
    Hillary Rodham Clinton, *It takes a village and other lessons children teach us,* 1996

....

Socialization of Family Members to Value and Maintain Health

Family members acquire values about health and learn personal health practices relative to nutrition, exercise, smoking, alcohol consumption, and hygiene through their family of origin and later transmit these values and beliefs to their children as they become parents. Recognition that lifestyle factors are the single most important determinant of most of our chronic diseases has focused attention on the importance of the family's responsibility to teach its members how to maintain and preserve health (Antonovsky, 1987; DHHS, 1990).

Healthy People 2010 (DHHS, 2000) offers a vision for preventing unnecessary death and disability, enhancing the quality of life for all Americans through the establishment of specific health promotion and disease prevention objectives. Many of the objectives focus on lifestyle risks that have their origin in health practices learned within the family context. In their interactions with families, nurses may assist members to assess health risks and to incorporate health promotion into their lifestyle (Duffy, 1988). Schools and the workplace also offer natural loci for helping children and adults to improve their health knowledge and develop attitudes that facilitate healthier behaviors.

Education About When and How to Use the Health Care System

The family also serves as the basic referent for defining illness and what should be done about it (Doherty & Campbell, 1988). The process by which the ill person seeks information and advice from family, friends, neighbors, and other nonprofessionals has been labeled the "lay referral network." Whether a family member's symptoms should be treated with home remedies and over-the-counter medications or professional help should be sought is negotiated within the family based on interpretations of the seriousness of the symptoms, the possible cause, and the impact that illness may have on the member's fulfillment of role responsibilities (Doherty, 1992). While *Healthy People 2010* has shifted national attention toward primary prevention by emphasizing health promotion and health protection activities, secondary prevention, which involves early detection and treatment of illness, is also recognized as another important approach for fostering healthy communities. In some families, one is defined as ill only when symptoms are severe enough to impact role performance. Teaching women the importance of breast self-examinations and having yearly Pap smears and a mammogram after age 50, or teaching males the importance of regular testicular and digital rectal examinations are examples of ways nurses can encourage family members to value the early detection of disease and to use the health care system in a more proactive way.

Care Provision and Management for Chronically Ill, Disabled, and Aging Family Members

Families assume a major share of the responsibility for intergenerational support and assistance. Among older disabled persons who live in the community, more than 90% relied in part on family for care (Ahlburg & De Vita, 1992). Two distinct caregiving roles that may be assumed by the family are direct care provider and indirect care manager. The direct care provider actively assists family members with those activities and tasks that they are no longer able to perform independently. Stevenson (1990) reported that 80% of family caregivers provided care for the impaired relative 7 days a week for an average of 4 hours per day. In contrast, the indirect care manager identifies the needed services an impaired relative requires and manages their provision by others. Problems in meeting societal expectations of families for caring for disabled and aging members are emerging because the caregiving role previously filled by women has dramatically changed as a result of the increase in dual-career families. Recognition of the latter has led to the rapid expansion of home health services and hospice programs to facilitate care of family members within their home environment.

Theoretical Approaches to the Family

Theory provides the practitioner with a systematic way of viewing a particular phenomenon. There are varied theoretical frameworks that have been used to describe family interaction and behavior. No single theory is sufficiently broad to deal with the complex dynamics that undergird the family's competence to fulfill its health responsibilities. Thus, an integrated approach that blends family systems theory with family development and human ecology theory will be used. This ecological systems perspective is particularly relevant to the discipline of nursing because it considers interrelationships between individuals within the family as well as between the family unit and the community over time.

Human Ecology Theory

Human ecology theory emphasizes the importance of social contexts as influences on human development. Bronfenbrenner (1986) notes that the parent-child relationship is enhanced as a context for development to the extent that the family's interrelationships with social networks, neighborhoods, communities, institutions, and cultures are supportive of its efforts to care for children. A similar perspective is presented by Hillary Rodham Clinton in her book, *It Takes A Village: And Other Lessons Children Teach Us.* Thus, the extent to which work settings provide quality day care or flexible working hours can strongly influence the success of dual-career couples in fulfilling their child-rearing functions. Similarly, adolescent parents are more likely to be able to continue to meet their own developmental needs for education when school policies support pregnant teens remaining in school throughout the pregnancy and/or provide child care for teens returning to school after the baby's birth.

••••••••••••••••••••••••••••

Nothing is more important to our shared future than the well-being of children. For children are at our core—not only as vulnerable beings in need of love and care but as a moral touchstone amidst the complexity and contentiousness of modern life. Just as it takes a village to raise a child, it takes children to raise up a village to become all it should be. The village we build with them in mind will be a better place for us all.
Hillary Rodham Clinton,
It takes a village and other lessons children teach us, 1996

••••••••••••••••••••••••••••

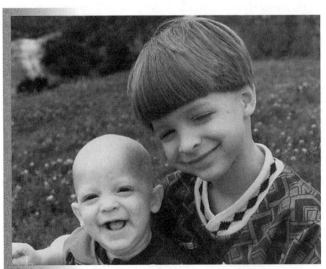

The socialization of children is one of the most important functions of the family.

Another distinctive feature of human ecology theory is its recognition that the family is both influenced by and actively influences the larger social systems with which it interacts. This perspective of human ecology theory encourages us to look at interactions between the family and its multilevel environment as reciprocal rather than unidirectional processes. For example, although governmental policies often strongly impact the health care services available to a family, families can impact and shape policy. Parents concerned about pressures from health maintenance organizations (HMOs) and insurance companies, which often forced mothers and their newborns to be discharged within 24 hours of birth, joined professional and citizen lobby groups to help pass a 1996 law titled "The Newborns' and Mothers' Health Protection Act." This bill requires insurers to cover a minimum stay of 48 hours for mothers and their newborns.

Family Systems Theory

Although human ecology theory provides us with a conception of how interrelationships between the family and its social context influence the family's capacity to foster health, it does not address how internal processes within the family may facilitate or impede health. Family systems theory, however, does provides us with several key concepts to understand the role of internal family processes on health. First is the concept of **nonsummativity,** which states that the family as a whole is greater than the sum of its parts; a change in one family member affects all family members (Wright & Leahey, 1994). Because the whole is more than and different from the sum of its parts, the family's ability to fulfill its health responsibilities cannot be predicted from knowledge about an individual's behavior and health practices. Rather, the nurse must assess how family relationships and their social environments either impede or foster health (see the Research Brief above).

For example, one cannot judge that an infant is developing adequate attachment without assessing the relationships between the parent and infant. Are bids of the infant to mother for attention when distressed responded to with soothing behaviors on the part of the mother? Healthfulness is reflected in the dyad's capacity to achieve patterns of interaction that are mutually rewarding (Robinson, Emde, & Korfmacher, 1997). Another example of the principle of nonsummativity is illustrated in the brief vignette presented at the beginning of this chapter. Rather than simply viewing Kevin's toileting accidents and inattention as indicators only of a potential underlying physical health problem, the school nurse and teacher recognize the importance of considering that Kevin's symptoms may reflect problems he is having in coping with changes in family relationships. Moreover, the school nurse chooses to follow up on the problem by scheduling a home visit to gather more data on how the mother is handling the transition to being a single parent.

Two other concepts important in understanding how the family operates as a system are structure and function. **Structure** refers to the organization of relationships among family mem-

RESEARCH BRIEF

Deatrick, J. A., Brennan, D., & Cameron, M. E. (1998). Mothers with multiple sclerosis and their children: Effects of fatigue and exacerbations on maternal support. Nursing Research, 47(4), 205–210.

A study of 35 mothers with multiple sclerosis and their children found that both mothers and children perceived that mothers were less physically affectionate when mothers' symptoms of illness were exacerbated. Mothers, however, significantly underestimated the changes in their physical affection compared with children's perceptions. Qualitative data further revealed that affective issues were linked with tremendous fears of the children, particularly the younger children, as reflected in the following comments: "I cry when she's sick. Sometimes I think that she is going to die."

bers (i.e., roles), whereas **function** defines the purposes or goals of the family, such as activities necessary to ensure health and growth of its members (Walsh, 1982). Structure and function are interrelated in that the structure of a family influences how well it is able to fulfill its purposes or goals. Roles within a family must be integrated much as the meshing of gears in a finely-tuned engine to facilitate attainment of common goals. Nurses working in the community often encounter families who are struggling with children's behavioral problems because the parents cannot agree on what are reasonable bedtimes for young children or how to consistently set limits, and consequently each defines different expectations for the child. Although adults may learn to balance multiple role expectations (e.g., spouse, parent, worker, volunteer), young children need clarity in role expectations to begin to develop a sense of identity and self-worth (one of the family's five health responsibilities).

Finally, understanding the role that self-regulation processes play in how the family functions in meeting its health responsibilities is important for nurses working in the community. A balance between stability and change is needed for a family to effectively address the differing needs of its members over time (Klein & White, 1996). Self-regulation involves processing the internal as well as external feedback that a family receives regarding its behavior. Feedback can be positive or negative. **Positive feedback** moves the family toward change, whereas **negative feedback** tends to promote stability. In assessing a family, the nurse seeks to identify those behaviors that are detrimental to health and provides feedback in the form of health teaching. In the previous example in which parents are having difficulty in agreeing on limits for their children, teaching by the nurse about realistic expectations for the child's developmental age and the importance of consistency in parental discipline would be directed toward behavioral change. On the other hand, in working with a mother who the nurse observes reads to her toddler, teaching about how parents can facilitate language development of toddlers would reinforce and expand on the mother's existing behaviors.

Family Development Theory

Family development theory highlights that change is an inherent aspect of family life. The family life cycle is described in terms of developmental stages characterized by major family events—in particular, the addition and exiting of members (Carter & McGoldrick, 1989). The concept of **family developmental tasks** refers to growth responsibilities that must be achieved by a family during each stage of its life cycle to successively meet the health and developmental needs of its members. For example, the birth of a child necessitates that other family members learn new role behaviors for protecting and fostering the health and development of the infant. Variations in the family life cycle and its developmental tasks are changing with the increasing diversity of family types. Although the single-parent family experiences the same life cycle changes as the traditional two-parent nuclear family, the absence of the second parent to carry a share of the family tasks with respect to support, child rearing, companionship, and gender role modeling for children may result in increased stressors for single parents. Divorce and possibly remarriage, with their losses and shifts in family membership, create new developmental tasks. For example, after divorce, spouses need to work through resolution of the attachment to one another while promoting ongoing parental contact between the ex-spouse and children (Carter & McGoldrick, 1989). With stepparent or blended families, crucial developmental tasks involve the restructuring of family boundaries and roles to allow for inclusion of new family members (stepparent and possibly stepchildren). Bain (1978) has advanced a theory to predict the capacity of families to cope with life cycle transitions that helps integrate human ecology and family systems with family development theory. According to his theory, families who are likely to have the least capacity to cope with life cycle transitions, or who are at most risk, are (1) those who are experiencing a greater number of concurrent life cycle changes involving (2) role transitions of great magnitude (e.g., blended families) and who (3) have a social support network that is small and nonsupportive, and (4) live in a community that has few available services to assist them with the transitions confronting them.

Family-Oriented Versus Family-Focused Nursing Role

Nurses working in the community generally advocate a family approach in the delivery of services. In reality, a family approach has varied meanings in practice. Many times, nursing interventions are directed toward the health concerns of referred individuals, with other family members being considered only as a support system for helping the individual cope with his or her health concerns. This family-oriented approach is most typical of nurses working in ambulatory care centers and home health agencies. For example, in working with a newly diagnosed diabetic, the nurse may assess the extent to which other family members understand and support the diabetic individual's need to modify dietary patterns to manage the disease effectively and prevent further complications. The complexity of health issues confronting families may, at times, necessitate a more sophisticated holistic approach. With a family-focused approach, as contrasted with a family-oriented approach, the family as a whole is viewed as having specific health responsibilities, and the extent to which family processes support these functions is the nursing focus. Assessments of the family as a group are made and interventions are directed toward helping the family grow in its abilities to meet its health responsibilities. A typical example often encountered by nurses working in public health departments is the family with a 13-year-old pregnant adolescent. From an ecological systems perspective, the adolescent's pregnancy necessitates role changes for all family members as the new baby is incorporated into the family. Hence a family-focused approach is needed to help family members deal effectively with the life cycle transitions triggered by the adolescent's pregnancy.

As nurses move into community settings, they need to be aware of the differences between a family-oriented and family-focused approach and select the one that is best suited to the needs of the health care situations they encounter. The mission of the health care delivery system in which the nurse works also may influence the choice of approach. For example, where the mission of the organization is disease control or rehabilitation, the family-oriented approach may be a better fit. Nurses working in organizations such as health departments, which have a population-focused perspective and emphasize health promotion and disease reduction, are likely to find more support for a family-focused approach.

A Conceptual Framework for Family Assessment

A conceptual framework provides direction to the collection, organization, and interpretation of data about the family's health situation. The conceptual framework for family assessment presented in this chapter builds on the perspective of the family as an ecological system and is designed to assist nurses in evaluating the extent to which a family is able to fulfill its health responsibilities (Box 16-1). The conclusion reached by conducting the assessment is an evaluation that the family is functioning more or less optimally in meeting its health responsibilities, as opposed to an evaluation regarding the health status of a particular family member.

To meet its health responsibilities, a family needs to be conscious of the health needs of its members at varying stages in the

BOX 16-1 FAMILY HEALTH RESPONSIBILITIES

Promote mental health of family members by providing opportunities for each to achieve a satisfactory sense of personal identity and self-worth.

Provide support and cognitive guidance for family members to achieve developmental tasks associated with life cycle transitions.

Socialize family members to adopt health practices that foster health and reduce risks for disease.

Educate family members about when and how to use health care services when disruptions in health occur.

Assist ill, disabled, and aging family members to meet their basic needs either through direct care provision or through helping them access community services.

EXPANDING FAMILY HEALTH POTENTIAL.

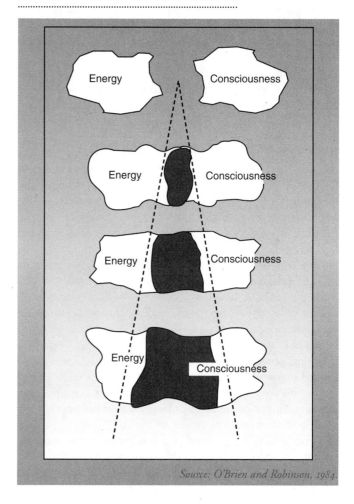

Source: O'Brien and Robinson, 1984.

life cycle and have sufficient energy to undertake the desired healthful behaviors (O'Brien, 1979; O'Brien & Robinson, 1984). At times, a family may have sufficient energy but lack the necessary awareness of members' needs to use its energy constructively to attain desired goals. The reverse also may be true. Thus, it is only when energy and consciousness interface and overlap that the family has the potential to effectively fulfill its health responsibilities (see the figure on the right).

A more detailed discussion of these two core concepts as well as those family attributes and processes that may influence the level of energy and consciousness within a family system is presented below.

Energy

To teach family members good health practices, to use the professional care system to foster health maintenance, to provide members with supportive and effective relationships necessary for positive mental health, and to actively cope with life cycle transitions all require the investment of energy (Newman, 1994; Rogers, 1983). A critical issue in family functioning is the regulation of energy flow to attain balance as opposed to imbalance—too much or too little energy (O'Brien & Robinson, 1984). When the energy flow within families is too much, behavior is likely to be chaotic and ineffectual, resulting in crisis-oriented problem solving when members' needs or concerns become too great to ignore. The latter is often the case in families that lack clear boundaries and where extended kin, neighbors, and friends move in and out of the household at will. In contrast, when energy is low or depleted, family members' needs are likely to be unmet, as illustrated in the following experience related by a mother suffering from postpartum depression.

My husband and son got back from the store. I think my 3-year-old son wanted to tell me about something that happened. It was physically so hard to listen that I really remember just trying to pull up some kind of wall so that I wouldn't be battered to death. At this point I was really sitting on the couch trying to figure out whether I could ever move again, and I started to cry. My son started hitting me with his fists, and he said, "Where are you, Mom?" It was really painful because I didn't have a clue as to where I was either. He was really trying to wake something up, but it was just too far gone. There was no way that I could retrieve the mom that he remembered and hoped he would find, let alone the mother I wanted to be for my new baby.
                                                                    Beck, 1996

In addition to assessing the energy that the family has available to invest in meeting members' health needs, it is important to identify how it replenishes its energy. The potential sources of energy vary from family to family, from individual to individual. For some, the source may be religious beliefs, cultural traditions, shared time together, school or work activities, or social relationships with friends. The nature of the sources is unimportant, provided that the family acquires sufficient energy to meet the demands placed on it. With a family that manifests a low energy level, nursing intervention may take the form of helping the family identify new ways of acquiring energy.

Pertinent questions to consider in assessing a family's energy level include the following:

- *How does the family acquire energy?*
- *What are its sources?*
- *Is there sufficient energy to meet the varying needs of its members? If not, where is the family's energy directed?*
- *Does the expenditure of energy in meeting family demands occur repeatedly at the expense of one particular family member?*

Consciousness

Consciousness is being aware of one's own feelings, needs, and actions as well as what is happening with others; in essence, it is the information that a system has available to effectively fulfill its functions (Newman, 1994). Growth and change within a family are directly linked to the family's level of consciousness, because it enables knowledge to be translated into goal-directed behavior. That is, the greater the consciousness, the more aware the family will be of its health responsibilities at any given stage of the life cycle, and the repertoire of choices generated for meeting those responsibilities will be more refined (Newman, 1994; O'Brien & Robinson, 1984). A thoughtful assessment of the family's level of consciousness provides the foundation for planning health promotion activities.

Another important aspect of the family's consciousness is the myths it creates about how it operates as a family (O'Brien & Robinson, 1984). For example, a family may describe relationships among members as close and intimate because all members spend a lot of time watching television together. Yet an observer might note that family members hardly ever communicate with one another during the time spent in the same room. Quite obviously, family myths may at times impede addressing family members' needs because the family is unable to recognize the need for behavioral change as a result of the belief that it is already behaving in the desired way. A useful assessment technique to begin to help family members become more aware of their own behavior is to engage them in reflective exercises. For example, in responding to a mother who complains that her son is "always misbehaving and won't listen" to her, the nurse might ask the mother to describe in detail a typical incident, including what her son was doing at the time and how she responded to his behavior. A common error that parents make in setting limits is to tell the child what not to do but offer no explanation for why the behavior is unacceptable.

Pertinent questions to consider in assessing a family's level of consciousness include the following:

- *How aware and knowledgeable is the family of specific health and developmental needs of its members?*
- *Does it hold incorrect beliefs that are likely to lead to unsound health practices?*
- *Is its perception of how it functions congruent with reality?*
- *What are the sources that the family utilizes in acquiring knowledge?*
- *How do past family experiences influence its consciousness of health issues?*
- *Does it actively seek to expand its level of consciousness or does it respond only to crisis demands?*

Role Structure

Roles define the goals and actions that are expected to characterize the occupant of a specific position such as mother or father (Hardy & Conway, 1988). Identification of the varying roles of family members provides the nurse with important information about the organization of relationships among family members, such as who is expected to do what and for whom. Flexibility of role definitions enables the family to deal more effectively with developmental transitions and situational crises resulting from illness or disability of one of its members (Boss, 1988).

Difficulty in the performance of one's role is defined as role insufficiency. A basic concept in role theory is that roles are reciprocal in that they are patterned to complement that of a role partner. Thus, the mothering role cannot be understood without looking at the corresponding role of the child at a particular developmental stage. Role behaviors expected of mothers of infants will differ from those expected of mothers whose children are in their adolescent years. When role insufficiency occurs, one or more family members' health and developmental needs are likely to be unmet.

In assessing family members' role performance, nurses need to be aware that role behaviors are learned according to the cultural values of the family. Collecting information about the family's customs and traditions is important for interpreting whether family members' roles are appropriate within their social context. For example, the maternal grandmother often assumes the mothering role for young children in African American single-parent families (Burton & deVries, 1995). Furthermore, it often is helpful to gather information about their early role models and how these experiences have affected present role behaviors (Friedman, 1998). It is not uncommon for parents' expectations and behaviors toward children to be similar to those they experienced in their families of origin (see the Research Brief on p. 380).

Role overload leading to increased stress and reduced levels of wellness has been cited as an issue for single-parent families (Burden, 1986; Popenoe, 1995). The single parent must fulfill

RESEARCH BRIEF

Hall, L. A., Sachs, B., & Rayens, M. K. (1998). Mothers' potential for child abuse: The roles of childhood abuse and social resources. Nursing Research, 47, 87–95.

A study of 206 low-income single mothers of young children found that the mothers' child abuse potential was positively associated with the levels of physical and sexual abuse experienced in their own childhood; sexual abuse displayed the strongest association. Compared with mothers who were not sexually abused in childhood, those reporting violent sexual abuse as children were almost six times more likely to have high potential for physically abusing their children.

both mother and father roles, often in addition to the work role, whereas role ambiguity and conflict are often major sources of stress in stepparent and blended families as members attempt to define whether the stepparent should assume the role of parent or nonparent and how children of the respective parents should relate as siblings. A typical example of resulting role conflict is the stepfather who disciplines his wife's child for misbehavior and is confronted by his wife for "overstepping" the boundaries of his role as a stepfather. In addition, ongoing relationships with the biological parent and the addition of relationships with the kin of the stepparent further compound the clear definition of family roles (Carter & McGoldrick, 1989). It is important for the nurse to carefully assess role strain and conflict occurring within the family because tension and conflict may negatively impact members' emotional well-being. Clarity of role expectations is crucial to helping family members develop a sense of personal identity and self-worth. Moreover, role strain and conflict, if left unresolved, may deplete the usable energy available for meeting the family's other health responsibilities, such as teaching members basic practices to maintain health and how to use health care services appropriately (Pratt, 1976, 1982).

Pertinent questions to consider in assessing a family's role structure include the following:

- *What roles do each of the family members fulfill? How competently do members perform their roles?*
- *How do past family experiences influence members' role performance?*
- *If role strain or conflict exists, what are the contributing factors?*
- *Is there flexibility in roles when needed?*

Decision-Making Processes

Decision making is central to the fulfillment of family responsibilities in meeting members' health and developmental needs. It is a process that involves (1) recognizing the need for a decision,

(2) identifying and weighing alternatives, and (3) selecting an alternative and facilitating its implementation. Central to effective decision making is the processing of information; the decision maker must be able to discriminate between what is important and what is not, between what is relevant and what is irrelevant, between actions that will achieve goals and those that will not. The family's use of health care services often provides insight into their decision-making processes. As noted, families often seek the advice of extended kin and friends about how to interpret untoward symptoms and whether they are sufficiently serious to warrant professional care. In some families, illness may be equated with inability to perform one's expected roles, resulting in a delay in seeking health care until symptoms are advanced. Studies have shown that poor health-related decision-making skills often reflect difficulty in decision making in other areas of family life. On the other hand, parents who make general lifestyle decisions that are growth-oriented and motivated toward change are more likely to practice and encourage health promotion behaviors for themselves and their children (Duffy, 1988). Nursing assessment of the family's decision-making processes focuses on identifying strengths or limitations in the information-processing function as well as the generation of alternative solutions. Immediate closure through the selection of a single option without explicit ranking or elimination of alternatives is characteristic of dysfunctional families, whereas healthy, functioning families explore numerous options, and if one alternative does not work, the family backs off and tries another, instead of trying to just make one option work (O'Brien & Robinson, 1984; Walsh, 1982). Of equal importance to note are those situations in which families arrive at no decision. Discussions finish inconclusively and are then decided by events, as with a couple who argues about what form of birth control to use until the wife discovers she is pregnant. Such an event is called *de facto decision making* in that things are allowed to happen without planning. De facto decision making is characteristic of multiproblem fam-

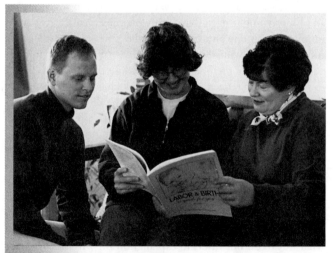

Chapter author, Dr. Ruth O'Brien (right), counsels a prenatal family about birth options.

ilies, many of whose members feel powerless and/or lack the energy to actively manage their lives. It also may occur in healthy families dealing with highly stressful situations when members' abilities to process information is reduced (Friedman, 1998).

Observations about family decision-making processes also help clarify its power structure. Families tend to reach decisions either by consensus or accommodation (Friedman, 1998). With consensus, a particular course of action is mutually agreed on by all concerned. With accommodation, some members assent to allow a decision to be reached. Accommodation occurs by use of compromising, bargaining, and coercion. Thus, by recognizing situations involving accommodation and who was identified with the decision reached, the nurse can identify the "power" brokers in the family. Identification of who has the power in family decision making is crucial for nurses working with families because interventions must be designed to include these family members (see the following Research Brief).

Pertinent questions to consider in assessing family decision making include the following:

- *Who makes what decisions?*
- *Are there particular health needs/issues that are not recognized or addressed?*
- *Is the family able to discriminate between information that is relevant and that which is irrelevant to the decision?*
- *Are alternative solutions generated and weighed? Is the selected alternative implemented?*
- *Who holds the power in family decision making? To what extent do family decisions involve consensus or coercion?*

RESEARCH BRIEF

Cole, R., Kitzman, H., Olds, D., & Sidora, K. (1998). Family context as a moderator of program effects in prenatal and early childhood home visitation. Journal of Community Psychology, 26(1), 37–48.

The ability of a nurse home visitation program for first-time mothers and their infants to affect changes in the quality of the caregiving environment was found to vary with household structure. Mothers who lived alone and those who lived with their husbands or boyfriends were able to create safer and more stimulating child-rearing environments than mothers who lived with grandmothers or with other adults. The investigators interpreted these findings as suggesting that where the mother is able to plan and take a course of action on her own, or in concert with someone over whom she is likely to exert some decision-making influence such as a husband or boyfriend, she is more able to implement changes in the home suggested by nurse home visitors.

Communication Patterns

Observation of a family's communication patterns yields valuable information about the meaning accorded to various family members as well as the clarity of interpersonal boundaries (Sieburg, 1985). **Communication** is a transactional process between two or more individuals in which feelings, needs, information, and opinions are shared. One of the most basic assessments regarding the family's communication patterns is the identification of who communicates what with whom. Individuals within the family may selectively disclose feelings, needs, and information to other members. Thus, communication patterns are linked to the family's level of consciousness. When individuals share their ideas and feelings freely and completely, they have a broad base of cues and provisional solutions on which to base their final actions. Problem solving is more effective in such families because members contribute to the solution of concern and are more likely to be committed to the decisions reached.

Still another important assessment is the identification of covert rules governing communication among family members. Satir (1983) defines rules as the "shoulds" and "should nots" of family life. For example, a family rule may be that only positive feelings should be expressed or that sex is not an appropriate topic of discussion. An illustration of the importance that family rules play in understanding communication exchanges among family members may be found in a spousal argument over the wife's allowing the couple's 10-year-old son to attend a movie with a group of friends. After much heated discussion, the husband acknowledges that he did not object to his son's having gone to the movies with his friends, but he felt his wife should have consulted him before giving the son permission. In reality, the argument between husband and wife stems from the husband's perception that his wife violated a family rule, namely that decisions about the son's peer activities are joint parental decisions. One fundamental principle of communication theory is that every exchange not only conveys information or content, but a definitional meaning of how one views self and others (Sieburg, 1985). In fact, the recognition accorded to the other is more crucial than the content. By attending to the recognition accorded to others, the nurse can gain an understanding of how communication shapes member's feelings of self-worth and self-efficacy. Confirming messages validate the intrinsic worth of the person and endorses the other's self-experience as unique and valuable. Confirmation is conveyed by direct verbal acknowledgment of the other's message, expanding or elaborating on its content, requesting clarification of what another has said—all behaviors reflective of active listening.

Child: "Mom, look I tied my own sneakers."

Mother: "Let me see. Yes, you did do a fine job of tying your laces. You have worked very hard at learning to do that. I'm proud of you."

In contrast, disconfirming messages question the other's perception or validity of self-experience through such behaviors as looking away from the other when speaking, interrupting the other, turning to speak to a third person while the other is still talking, interjecting comments that are irrelevant, engaging in other activities while talking, exiting while another is talking, or remaining silent when a response is required or expected (Sieburg, 1985). Obviously, such behaviors leave the recipient with a feeling of powerlessness and, over time, result in lowered self-esteem.

> *Child: "Mom, look I tied my own sneakers."*
>
> *Mother: "Don't bother me now. Can't you see that I'm reading the newspaper?"*

Another important principle of communication relates to the congruence between the verbal and nonverbal aspects of the exchange. Verbal language conveys the substance of the message, whereas nonverbal language transmits the more subtle nature of the intent of the message. The degree of congruence and balance between the verbal and nonverbal portions of an exchange define the degree of clarity of the message for the recipient. Given that much verbal conflict among family members often stems from faulty interpretation of nonverbal aspects of communication, it is particularly important to assess the extent to which family members are able to elicit feedback and validate messages to minimize misinterpretation of cues and faulty mind reading (Sieburg, 1985).

Communication patterns also are the most observable indicators of the clarity of interpersonal boundaries among family members. The use of "I" statements as opposed to "we" statements and the extent of mind reading and censorship (e.g., "You shouldn't say that," "You have no reason to feel angry") present in members' communications with one another provide important clues to the clarity of interpersonal boundaries and members' sense of separateness and personal autonomy (Sieburg, 1985). Clear and functional communication among family members is considered a cornerstone of the healthy family (Goldenberg & Goldenberg, 1996; Janosik & Green, 1992; Satir, 1983). It is foundational in enabling the family to fulfill its health responsibility in assisting members to develop a sense of personal identity and self-worth. Moreover, clarity and openness of communication among family members facilitates effective decision making when disruptions to health arise. Families whose members lack good communications skills also often have difficulty accessing community services to help with their needs.

Pertinent questions to consider in assessing a family's communication patterns include the following:

- *Who talks to whom?*
- *What feelings or issues are closed to discussion?*
- *Are members able to clearly state their needs and feelings?*
- *Is there congruence between verbal and nonverbal aspects of communication?*
- *How well do members listen when others are communicating?*
- *Do members elicit feedback and validation in communicating with one another?*
- *What are the predominant patterns of acknowledgment accorded various members?*
- *Is communication among members age appropriate?*

Values

Knowledge of the value orientations of the family provides direction to understanding the why of family dynamics. A family's configuration of values ascribes meaning to certain health events and suggests ways to respond to them (Friedman, 1998). The identification of family values, however, is often compounded by the family's own lack of awareness of how it ascribes worth to people, events, and things. It is important to distinguish both the overt and covert values operative in family behavior.

A particularly important value orientation to assess is how the family views itself in relation to the environment. The family that feels it has little control over what happens does not take the initiative to seek out new ideas, information, or resources and apply them to the solution of family problems or to minimize health risks (Boss, 1988). Similarly, the time orientation of the family impacts the extent to which it actively addresses life cycle transitions and change. Families that emphasize past traditions may experience life cycle transitions as more stressful (Carter & McGoldrick, 1989). Likewise, a predominant focus on the present is likely to minimize anticipatory planning and emphasize de facto decision making (Duffy, 1988). As noted in the discussion of family decision making, families that rely on de facto decision making are less likely to engage in health promotion activities or use preventive health services.

Furthermore, there is a hierarchical nature to family values that influences the family's perceptions of risks and benefits of taking certain actions. The relative ranking of health in the family's hierarchy of values is important in determining the extent to which forces within the family tend to sustain or undermine health care behaviors. For example, the family who places a high value on home ownership may choose to forego preventive health care if economic resources are limited. An accurate assessment of a family's value system should help tailor interventions to goals that are important to the family.

A family's values are a reflection of its subculture, as well as of the community in which it resides. Obviously, the greater the degree of congruence between a family's subcultural values and the community's values, the more the community supports the family's identity. Incompatibility in values between the family and community generates conflict that increases stress within the family as a whole or between varying members of the family who have assimilated the community's values in differing degrees. Such stress may deplete the energy available to meet health responsibilities as well as negatively affect members' self-esteem (Friedman, 1998; Pratt, 1982).

It is equally important to recognize that nurses often have their own personal as well as professional values that define how the "ideal family" should behave. Unless nurses are aware of their own values, interactions with families may become conflictual as they pursue interventions directed toward expectations they hold for the family that are incongruent with its own values and beliefs. Generally, nursing's code of ethics encourages respect for the family's autonomy to make its own choices involving health matters unless such choices are likely to result in serious harm for others, such as spread of communicable disease and physical or sexual abuse of children.

Given that values cannot be seen directly, Friedman (1998) advocates the use of a "compare and contrast" method to assist the nurse in identifying specific family values. The compare and contrast method involves using a list of central values of the dominant culture or the family's subcultural reference group to engage the family in a discussion of their own values. Through discussion with the family, the nurse seeks not only to identify values held by the family and their overall relative importance to one another, but also to identify value differences and clashes between family members.

Pertinent questions to consider in assessing a family's values include the following:

- *What are the important values held by the family?*
- *To what extent do family values foster active coping and mastery of concerns?*
- *What is the family's orientation to the past, present, and future?*
- *What is the relative ranking of health in the family's hierarchy of values?*
- *Are there value conflicts evident within the family, between the family and subculture/community, or between the family and nurse?*

Family Boundaries

Family boundaries serve to distinguish the family from the social contexts or environments with which it interacts. In essence, family boundaries serve as a conceptual filter controlling the degree of exchange that family members have with their environ-

ment (Klein & White, 1996). Having selectively permeable boundaries allows for family growth and change, because the use of resources outside the family is enhanced (see the Research Brief below). The latter can contribute to family functioning by developing awareness of alternative courses of action (e.g., greater consciousness) and by increasing understanding of personal health practices and the value of self-directed action for promoting health (Pratt, 1982). Conversely, the amount of information a family can handle adequately is limited, and loose boundaries that result in an excess of information or conflicting information from the environment may amplify and create family disorganization (Walsh, 1982).

Markedly restricted interchange with the environment creates a greater reliance on inner family resources. Relatively closed families may exhibit more energy, in the form of tension, than they can discharge in constructive ways. Studies repeatedly have noted that child abuse clusters in families that are isolated from other families, neighbors, and society. In healthier isolated families, the members tend to believe that all or most of the needs of the members can be met within the family or the family's reference group (Sedgwick, 1981). Yet such exclusive reliance on internal resources may occur to the detriment of one or more family members in situations involving long-term chronic illness or disability, as evidenced by caregiver burden (Kramer & Kipnis, 1995; Smith, Tobin, & Fullmer, 1995).

Pertinent questions to consider in assessing family boundaries include the following:

- *Are family boundaries overly rigid or overly loose?*
- *What ongoing relationships does the family maintain with extended kin, friends, or other social groups?*
- *Do interactions with its support network foster or impede the family's ability to cope with its health responsibilities?*
- *Is the family satisfied with its support network?*
- *Is the family willing and able to access community services?*

Although the framework for family assessment presented in this chapter emphasizes critical areas of family functioning that have been found to contribute to the family's effectiveness in meeting its health responsibilities, one usually begins by obtaining basic identifying data about the family and its immediate environment: names and ages of family members, health history of each family member, racial/ethnic background, education, employment, income, health insurance, housing, characteristics of the immediate neighborhood, and availability of health and other basic services in the neighborhood (e.g., grocery stores, schools, churches, transportation). The purpose or reason for the nurse's contact with the family guides the initial information collected about pertinent areas of family functioning. For example, in making a home visit to the Johnson family to follow up on Kevin's toileting accidents and inattention in school, the nurse might begin by asking Mrs. Johnson what she thinks may be contributing to the changes in Kevin's behavior. Initial

RESEARCH BRIEF

Jepson, C., McCorkle, R., Adler, D., Nuamah, I., & Lusk, E. (1999). Effects of home care on caregivers' psychosocial status. Image: The Journal of Nursing Scholarship, 31(2), 115–120.

A sample of 161 caregivers of cancer patients were randomly assigned to a home care nursing intervention or to a control group that received no home care. At 3 and 6 months, caregivers in the home care intervention group showed improved psychosocial functioning (fewer depressive symptoms) compared with caregivers in the control group.

Family Life Cycle Transition: Teenage Pregnancy

Nancy, a 16-year-old unmarried Caucasian teen, lives in a housing project with her mother, her mother's current boyfriend, and two brothers—Jerome, 17 years old, and Derrick, 3 years old. She is 25 weeks pregnant. The pregnancy was unplanned; she was not using any form of contraception. Ronald, her 26-year-old boyfriend, is the father of the expectant child. Ronald has two previous children (ages 2 and 4 years) by another woman whom he rarely sees.

Nancy did not seek prenatal care until the beginning of her second trimester of pregnancy. To date, she has gained 13 pounds. Her health practices include the use of home remedies and self-comfort measures that she learned from her grandmother. She began smoking at age 13 and now smokes 1 to 2 packs of cigarettes a day. A frequent problem is urinary tract infections. Nancy told the clinic nurse who made the referral, "I can hardly get up in the morning to face the day now that I am pregnant. Sometimes life just doesn't seem worth it."

The two-bedroom apartment is too small for the five-person family; Nancy sleeps on a pull-out couch in the living room. She complains that she never has any privacy. The home is cluttered and in need of cleaning. Much cigarette smoke permeates the environment. Nancy says she feels unsafe in her neighborhood, where groups of males congregate outside the project complex; thus, she stays indoors most of the day.

Nancy dropped out of school in the ninth grade to stay home and care for Derrick while her mother works. She states that she knows that she will not be able to get a very good job in the future without finishing high school and wishes she could find a way to continue her education. Her mother works long hours as a certified care assistant in a nursing home trying to support herself and her children. The mother's current boyfriend is looking for employment because he had to quit his job in construction as a result of a back injury from an automobile accident.

Nancy is ambivalent about her pregnancy. She reports that Ronald has become more distant as her pregnancy has progressed; she is concerned that he may not assume financial responsibility for the baby and that this will be a further strain on her mother. She expresses confidence about being able to take care of a baby because she has had significant responsibility for her younger brother. The nurse observes that Nancy displays much warmth and patience in interactions with Derrick during the visit.

Nancy receives Medicaid and help from the Women, Infants and Children (WIC) Program. Although she could not be specific as to how Ronald makes a living, she states, "He always seems to have plenty of money." He has given her some money to buy baby equipment and clothes.

1. What initial family diagnosis would you make?
2. What other information would you need to know to assist Nancy in promoting a healthy pregnancy?
3. What community resources could you use to promote family health in this family?

---

information shared by the family will help guide the nurse in determining what other data to collect. The data are synthesized to identify family strengths in meeting its health responsibilities and areas where the family could use help to cope more effectively. The latter serves as a guide for negotiating the nurse's continuing role and activities with the family.

A Self-Efficacy Model for Nurse-Family Intervention

Because the family's ability to effectively fulfill its health responsibilities requires self-direction and self-governance, the nurse-family intervention should facilitate the family's active participation in dealing with the health concerns or issues that it is experiencing. Indeed, the family's active participation in nurse-family interactions may be a significant variable in determining the effectiveness of nursing intervention (O'Brien & Robinson, 1984). The **contracting** process provides a means for enhancing family participation in its own health maintenance. Contracting is based on the belief that families have the potential for self-growth and the right to self-determination. It calls for an active participative as well as a collaborative role for both family and nurse because the goal is to build family self-efficacy in addressing its needs. The contracting process may be subdivided into five interlinking, sequenced phases (Sloan & Schommer, 1982). As with any relationship, the phases denote an ebb and flow of movement rather than discrete points at which something begins or ends. In the description that follows, each phase is discussed separately, although in reality they may overlap.

Identification of Family Health Concerns and Needs

This phase begins with the initial contact between the family and the nurse. Data, both subjective and objective, are gained about each other through observation and exchange of information. The use of a conceptual framework for assessing family functioning facilitates a clear identification of how the family is meeting its health responsibilities and any accompanying concerns (see Appendix A). The preferable outcome of this first phase is an agreement between the nurse and family on the definition of the problems, needs, and concerns to be addressed in subsequent interactions. Two other outcomes are also possible: (1) referral to a more appropriate service or (2) termination because congruence between nurse and family does not exist and effective problem solving is not feasible (Williamson, 1981).

Mutual Setting of Goals

What does the family hope to accomplish? This is a crucial question, and one that is not asked often enough by nurses. By asking what the family hopes to gain from the intervention, the nurse assists the family to focus on its own goals and priorities. The nurse also can gain a sense of congruency between individual member and family goals, often a source of potential conflict (Lynch & Tiedje, 1991). In essence, this phase involves collaborative negotiations and democratic compromise rather than the nurse deciding goals. The nurse, however, expands the family's consciousness by sharing observations and knowledge that can facilitate the family's identification of goals.

The communication style used by the nurse can foster or hinder the family's acceptance of a suggested goal. For instance, "Perhaps we need to work on ways to reduce the distress your son's behavior is causing" is likely to be met with a more favorable response than, "You need to work on improving your relationships with one another." The second approach will invariably raise the family's defenses, whereas the first fosters its willingness to allow the nurse to help them work toward a solution to their concern. Helping the family to set realistic, attainable goals is one of the nurse's key functions. Goals should be stated in a precise manner capable of being monitored and a time frame for accomplishment specified. For example, "Mother will spend half an hour each evening in some planned activity with children" is a more measurable goal than, "Mother will improve attention given to children." Even when specific goals are set, there may be lack of progress. The family's prioritizing of goals may conflict with the nurse's. The nurse may need to support the family's priorities to free its energy for other goal attainment. If the nurse cannot offer such support because of possible injury to a particular family member, the family needs to be informed of what action will be taken.

Delineation of Alternatives

Once the goals are established, the nurse and family need to discuss how they can be attained. This process involves (1) the exploration and determination of the family's strengths and available resources, (2) the steps or actions needed to attain the goals, (3) the negotiation and division of responsibilities of the family and nurse for goal attainment, and (4) the establishment of a reasonable time limit for implementing the plan.

Emphasizing the already existing family strengths reinforces the family's belief in its own ability to solve problems and meet goals. In working with a mother having difficulty with limit setting and discipline with a toddler, the nurse might begin by acknowledging the attempts the mother has made to solve the problem and emphasize how well she is managing other areas of child care. Such an approach fosters esteem and confidence in the mother and facilitates her acceptance of the nurse as a helping person. A temptation to be avoided is the offering of numerous suggestions about how to do something better or differently before recognizing and drawing out the family's estimation of its own resources and potential solutions. The nurse can then supplement the family's developing knowledge base by introducing family and/or community resources not identified for its consideration.

Equally important in the planning process are decisions on the sequence of activities and the time frame needed to achieve the goal. The nurse generally plays a supportive role in this process, encouraging the family to make specific and detailed plans that are likely to maximize goal attainment. Agreement on the nurse's role and ways to monitor progress are crucial outcomes of this phase.

Implementation of the Plan

The plan and division of responsibilities mutually agreed on are tried. The nurse plays particularly vital roles during this phase. First is the anticipation of problems or setbacks that may arise, followed by helping the family recognize and deal with them in as positive a way as possible. A series of minor setbacks can discourage and demoralize family members to the extent that the carefully negotiated plan may be prematurely abandoned. Frequent contacts for guidance and support during the implementation phase can help individual family members accomplish their tasks. Second, the nurse has an important role-modeling function in that nursing responsibilities are carried out as agreed, within the given time limit. If problems are encountered in fulfilling the agreed-on nursing activities, the nurse should communicate them openly to the family and seek help in making alternative plans.

Evaluation

Evaluation is an ongoing process throughout all phases of the nurse-family transaction as well as an end phase. Results may range from successful goal attainment to discovering that the selected solution is not acceptable to the family. The latter may happen when the family and nurse fail to identify the "real" problem,

CASE STUDY

Application of Nurse-Family Intervention Model: Johnson Family

Mrs. Williams, the school nurse at Sagebrush Elementary, called Mrs. Johnson and scheduled a home visit for 5:30 PM. She began the visit by clarifying for Mrs. Johnson the changes in Kevin's behavior that his teacher had noted in recent months and asked her if she had observed similar problems at home. Mrs. Johnson reported that Kevin had begun to have episodes of nighttime bedwetting and she felt he was more moody and at times, quite argumentative with her when she would not let him "have his way." She stated that she had spoken with Kevin's pediatrician about the bedwetting, and he felt that Kevin was probably having trouble with the changes with his father. Kevin had no history of bedwetting or toileting accidents since about 3 years of age. The pediatrician encouraged her not to scold Kevin for his accidents and to try to give him a little more attention to help him deal with his separation from his father.

When asked what she thought of the pediatrician's advice, Mrs. Johnson acknowledged that she knew the divorce had been hard for the children. Their father's former job had made it possible for him to be home with them after school, and he had spent a lot of time with Kevin, helping him with schoolwork, games, and other activities. Since her ex-husband's remarriage, he has spent less time visiting with the children. She knew that Kevin missed his father's attention, but planning time to do all the things his dad had done was difficult for her along with working and managing the home. Moreover, she knew Kevin resented going to the "after-school program" because of her work hours. In fact, she sometimes had to ask her mother-in-law to pick up the children from the child-care center because she had to work late. Mrs. Johnson indicated that she didn't want to refuse her boss's request to work late because she was hoping to qualify for a promotion. One of the women she worked with was retiring in another 6 months, and her position as office manager would need to be filled. Although her mother-in-law was always willing to be helpful with caring for the children, she didn't like to ask too often. She felt that her in-laws might have

some feelings that she contributed to the divorce because of her interest in "getting ahead in her career." Her own parents did not live close.

During the visit, Mrs. Williams observed that Mrs. Johnson often seemed impatient with Kevin, responding rather sharply to him when he came into the room where they were meeting to ask questions. She often redirected him to go to his sister for help. At one point, Mrs. Johnson even remarked to the nurse that she had difficulty coping with Kevin's many requests of her and that it hurt her when he made comments to her about how things were different "when Daddy lived here." When she set limits with him, he often remarked, "I want to go live with my Daddy."

Using Mrs. Johnson's descriptions of the problems she was facing in dealing with Kevin at the time of the divorce (Kevin's bedwetting and increased demands for her attention, his remark that "things were different when Daddy lived here") and her own observations about parent-child interactions, and Mrs. Johnson's hesitation to turn down requests for overtime work and to ask for too much help from in-laws, the nurse felt it appeared that the family was experiencing difficulty with new family developmental tasks resulting from the divorce and remarriage of the father, such as learning to be a single parent and promoting ongoing parental contact between the ex-spouse and children. In discussing with Mrs. Johnson ways that she thought the nurse might be helpful, they identified the goal as helping Mrs. Johnson to assist her children with the divorce and developed the following immediate plan:

- The nurse would set up a conference with the school psychologist for Mrs. Johnson to have some counseling about how to deal with Kevin's reaction to the divorce and his behavior.

- Mrs. Johnson would take children to the neighborhood library on the weekend and borrow some children's books that deal with parental divorce. Together she and children would read the books.

- Mrs. Johnson would try to spend half an hour each evening with children in some planned activity that the children helped choose.

- The nurse would revisit in 2 weeks to follow up on Mrs. Johnson's meeting with the school psychologist and to assess how children had responded to books on parental divorce and the mother's efforts to plan some activity with them each evening.

they select unrealistic solutions, or unforeseen outcomes occur. As in other phases, the family should be encouraged to participate equally by sharing feelings and concerns about its course as well as about the nurse's role in accomplishing outlined responsibilities. Emphasis on positive strides, although they may be small, can bolster the family's sense of self-efficacy.

Crucial questions to consider in end-phase evaluation include the following:

- *Was the goal(s) achieved?*
- *Was the selected solution(s) appropriate?*
- *What factors facilitated or impeded goal attainment?*
- *Should the nurse-family relationship be terminated or should other goals and plans be developed?*

The manner in which the nurse-family relationship is concluded is as vital as the way in which it is begun. The establishment of a plan for continuity of care, if needed, is crucial. Often, after a period of intensive nursing supervision, a plan for periodic reassessment of the situation is warranted. This is particularly applicable to families dealing with long-term chronic illness or disability. The family should know how to contact the nurse should unanticipated changes occur before the scheduled interval for reappraisal.

CONCLUSION

Understanding the family as a focal unit for nursing care will become more important in the future as health care delivery increasingly takes place in community settings. A family is two or more individuals who manifest some degree of interdependence in their interaction with each other and their environment in meeting basic needs for affection and meaning. The family life cycle is described in terms of developmental stages corresponding to major family events—in particular, the addition and exiting of members.

Families who are likely to have the most difficulty coping with life cycle transitions are those who experience a large number of concurrent life cycle changes involving transitions of great magnitude; who have a small, nonsupportive social network; and who live in a community with few resources to assist them.

Health responsibilities of the family include (1) the provision of opportunities for members to achieve a sense of personal identity and work, (2) emotional support and cognitive guidance for members experiencing life cycle transitions, (3) education of members about how to maintain health and when and how to use professional services, (4) the socialization of members to value health and to accept personal responsibility for its maintenance, and (5) care provision for chronically ill, disabled, or aging family members. To fulfill its health responsibilities, the family needs sufficient energy and knowledge to invest in goal-directed behavior.

Nurses' work with families is facilitated through the use of a conceptual framework for collecting, organizing, and interpreting data about how the family is fulfilling its health responsibilities and issues and concerns they are experiencing. The self-efficacy model for nurse-family intervention involves a contracting process in which the nurse and family pursue mutually established goals.

CRITICAL THINKING ACTIVITIES

1. Reflect on your own experience in growing up in a family. Identify how your family met each of the five health responsibilities. How are your beliefs about health and ways to maintain your health similar to or different from those practiced in your family?

2. Using the case study on *Family Life Cycle Transitions: Teenage Pregnancy*, address the following questions.

   - What are some factors that may have led Nancy to become pregnant? As you answer this question, think about her life history.

   - What are the potential health threats to Nancy and her unborn baby, given her current health habits and living situation?

   - Using the framework for assessment presented in this chapter, how would you assess the family's current capacity to deal with this life cycle transition given the information provided?

   - What additional information would you want to gather?

   - What ethical principles should guide your interactions with Nancy and her family?

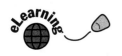 **Explore Community Health Nursing on the web!** To learn more about the topics in this chapter, access your exclusive web site: http://communitynursing.jbpub.com

REFERENCES

Ahlburg, D. A., and De Vita, C. J. (1992). New realities of the American family. *Population Bulletin, 47*(2), 1–44.

Antonovsky, A. (1987). *Unraveling the mystery of health: How people manage stress and stay well.* San Francisco: Jossey-Bass.

Bain, A. (1978). The capacity of families to cope with transition: A theoretical essay. *Human Relations, 8,* 675.

Beck, C. T. (1996). Postpartum depressed mothers' experiences interacting with their children. *Nursing Research, 45*(2), 98.

Bianchi, S. M., & Spain, D. (1996). Women, work, and family in America. *Population Bulletin, 51*(3), 1–48.

Boss, P. (1988). *Family stress management.* Newbury Park, CA: Sage Publications.

Bronfenbrenner, U. (1986). Ecology of the family as a context for human development. Research perspectives. *Developmental Psychology, 22*(6), 723–742.

Burden, D. S. (1986). Single parents and the work setting: The impact of multiple job and homelife responsibilities. *Family Relations, 35*(1), 37–43.

Burton, L., & deVries, C. (1995). Challenges and rewards: African-American grandparents as surrogate parents. In L. M. Burton (Ed.), *Families and aging.* Amityville, NY: Baywood.

Carter, E. A., & McGoldrick, M. (Eds.). (1989). *The changing family life cycle: A framework for family therapists* (2nd ed.) New York: Gardner Press.

Clinton, H. R. (1996). *It takes a village: And other lessons children teach us.* New York: Simon & Schuster.

Cole, R., Kitzman, H., Olds, D., & Korfmacher, J. (1998). Family context as a moderator of program effects in prenatal and early childhood home visitation. *Journal of Community Psychology, 26*(1), 37–48.

Cowan, P. A., Field, D., Hansen, D. A., Skolnick, A., & Swanson, G. E. (Eds.). (1992). *Family, self, and society: Toward a new agenda for family research.* Hillsdale, N.J.: Lawrence Erlbaum.

Deatrick, J. A., Brennan, D., & Cameron, M. E. (1998). Mothers with multiple sclerosis and their children: Effects of fatigue and exacerbations on maternal support. *Nursing Research, 47*(4), 205–210.

Department of Health and Human Services (DHHS). (2000). *Healthy People 2010: Conference edition.* Washington, DC: U.S. Government Printing Office.

Doherty, W. J. (1992). Linkages between family theories and primary health care. In R. Sawa (Ed.), *Family health care* (pp. 30–39). Newbury Park, CA: Sage Publications.

Doherty, W. J., & Campbell, T. L. (1988). *Families and health.* Newbury Park, CA: Sage Publications.

Duffy, M. E. (1988). Health promotion in the family: Current findings and directives for nursing research. *Journal of Advanced Nursing, 13.*

Duvall, E. M., & Miller, B. L. (1985). *Marriage and family development* (6th ed.). New York: Harper & Row.

Friedman, M. M. (1998). *Family nursing: Research, theory and practice* (4th ed.). Stamford, CT: Appleton & Lange.

Goldenberg, I., & Goldenberg, H. (1996). *Family therapy: An overview* (4th ed.). Monterey, CA: Brooks/Cole.

Hall, L. A., Sachs, B., & Rayens, M. K. (1998). Mothers' potential for child abuse: The roles of childhood abuse and social resources. *Nursing Research, 47,* 87–95.

Hanson, S. M. H., & Boyd, S. T. (Eds.). (1996). *Family health nursing: Theory, practice and research.* Philadelphia: Davis.

Hardy, M. E., & Conway, M. (1988). *Role theory: Perspectives for health professionals.* New York: Appleton-Century-Crofts.

Janosik, E. H., & Green, E. (1992). *Family life.* Boston: Jones & Bartlett.

Jepson, C., McCorkle, R., Adler, D., Nuamah, I., & Lusk, E. (1999). Effects of home care on caregivers' psychosocial status. *Image: The Journal of Nursing Scholarship, 31*(2), 115–120.

Klein, D. M., & White, J. M. (1996). *Family theories: An introduction.* Thousand Oaks, CA: Sage Publications.

Kramer, B. J., & Kipnis, S. (1995). Eldercare and work-role conflict: Toward an understanding of gender differences in caregiving burden. *The Gerontologist, 35*(3), 273–278.

Loveland-Cherry, C. (1996). Family health promotion and health protection. In P. J. Bomar (Ed.), *Nurses and family health promotion* (2nd ed., pp. 22–35). Philadelphia: W. B. Saunders.

Lynch, I., & Tiedje, L. B. (1991). Working with multiproblem families: An intervention model for community health nurses. *Public Health Nursing, 8*(3), 147–153.

Newman, M. A. (1994). *Health as expanding consciousness* (2nd ed.). New York: National League for Nursing Press.

O'Brien, R. A. (1979). *A conceptualization of family health. Clinical and scientific sessions.* Kansas City: ANA.

O'Brien, R. A., & Robinson, A. G. (1984). Family as client. In J. A. Sullivan (Ed.), *Directions in community health nursing.* Boston: Blackwell Scientific.

Popenoe, D. (1995). The American family crisis. *National Forum, 75*(3), 15–19.

Pratt, L. (1976). *Family structure and effective health behavior: The energized family.* Boston: Houghton Mifflin.

Pratt, L. (1982). Family structure and health work: Coping in the context of social change. In H. I. McCubbin, A. E. Cauble, & J. M. Patterson (Eds.), *Family stress, coping, and social support* (pp. 73–89). Springfield, IL: Charles C. Thomas.

Robinson, J. L., Emde, R. N., & Korfmacher, J. (1997). Integrating an emotional regulation perspective in a program of prenatal and early childhood home visitation. *Journal of Community Psychology, 25*(1), 59–75.

Rogers, M. E. (1983). Analysis and application of Rogers' theory of nursing. In J. W. Clements & F. B. Roberts (Eds.), *Family health: A theoretical approach to nursing care* (pp. 219–228). New York: Wiley.

Satir, V. (1983). *Conjoint family therapy* (3rd ed.). Palo Alto, CA: Science and Behavior Books.

Sedgwick, R. (1981). *Family mental health: Theory and practice.* St. Louis: Mosby.

Sieburg, E. (1985). *Family communication: An integrated systems approach.* New York: Gardner Press.

Sloan, M. R., & Schommer, B. T. (1982). The process of contracting in community health nursing. In B. W. Spradley (Ed.), *Readings in community health nursing* (2nd ed., pp. 197–204). New York: Little, Brown.

Smith, G. C., Tobin, S. S., & Fullmer, E. M. (1995). Elderly mothers caring at home for offspring with mental retardation: A model of permanency planning. *American Journal on Mental Retardation, 99*(5), 487–499.

Snyder, N. O., & Moore, K. A. (1996). *Facts at a glance.* Washington, DC: Child Trends.

Stevenson, J. P. (1990). Family stress related to home care of Alzheimer's disease patients and implications for support. *Journal of Neuroscience Nursing, 22*(3), 179–188.

Walsh, F. (Ed.). (1982). *Normal family processes.* New York: The Guilford Press.

Williams, C. A. (1996). Community-based, population focused practice: The foundation of specialization in public health nursing. In M. Stanhope & J. Lancaster (Eds.), *Community health nursing: Promoting health of aggregates, families and individuals* (4th ed., pp.21–34). St. Louis: Mosby.

Williamson, J. A. (1981). Mutual interaction: A model of nursing practice. *Nursing Outlook, 29,* 104.

Wright, L. M., & Leahey, M. (1994). *Nurses and families: A guide to family assessment and intervention* (2nd ed.). Philadelphia: Davis.

APPENDIX A

FAMILY ASSESSMENT GUIDE

1. Family Composition and Identifying Data
   - *Names, ages of family members*
   - *Address*
   - *Racial/ethnic background*
   - *Education/school attendance*
   - *Employment*
   - *Income*
   - *Health insurance*

2. Environmental Data
   - *Is housing adequate to meet family's needs?*
   - *What are the characteristics of the immediate neighborhood and community?*
   - *What health and other basic services are available in the neighborhood? in the community?*
   - *What is the availability of public transportation?*

3. Energy
   - *What are the sources of energy for the family?*
   - *Is there sufficient energy to meet the varying health needs of its members? If not, where is the family's energy directed?*
   - *Does the expenditure of energy in meeting family demands occur repeatedly at the expense of one particular family member?*

4. Consciousness
   - *How aware and knowledgeable is the family of specific health and developmental needs of its members?*
   - *Does it hold incorrect beliefs that are likely to lead to unsound health care practices?*
   - *Is its perception of how it functions congruent with reality?*
   - *What are the sources that the family utilizes in acquiring knowledge?*
   - *Does it actively seek to expand its level of consciousness or does it respond only to crisis demands?*
   - *How do past family experiences influence its consciousness about health issues?*

5. Role Structure
   - *What roles do each of the family members fulfill?*
   - *How competently do members perform their roles?*
   - *How do past family experiences influence members' role performance?*
   - *If role strain or conflict exists, what are the contributing factors?*
   - *How are role conflicts resolved?*
   - *Is there flexibility in roles when needed?*

6. Decision-Making Processes
   - *Who makes what decisions?*
   - *Are there particular needs/issues that are not recognized or addressed?*
   - *Is the family able to discriminate between information that is relevant and that which is irrelevant to the decision?*
   - *Are alternative solutions generated and weighed?*
   - *Is the selected alternative implemented?*
   - *To what extent does family decision making involve consensus or coercion?*

- *Does the mode of decision making affect its implementation?*
- *Is the family satisfied with the results of their choices?*

7. Communication Patterns
   - *Who talks to whom?*
   - *What feelings or issues are closed to discussion?*
   - *Are members able to clearly state their needs and feelings?*
   - *Is there congruence between verbal and nonverbal aspects of communication?*
   - *How well do members listen when others are communicating?*
   - *Do members elicit feedback and validation in communicating with one another?*
   - *What are the predominant patterns of acknowledgment accorded varying members?*
   - *Is communication among members age appropriate?*

8. Values
   - *What are the important values held by the family?*
   - *To what extent do family values foster active coping and mastery of concerns?*
   - *What is the family's orientation to the past, present, and future?*
   - *What is the relative ranking of health in the family's hierarchy of values?*
   - *Are there value conflicts evident within the family, between the family and subculture/community, or between the family and nurse?*

9. System Boundaries
   - *Are family boundaries overly rigid or overly loose?*
   - *What ongoing relationships does the family maintain with extended kin, friends, or other social groups?*
   - *To what degree do interactions with its support network foster or impede the family's abilities to cope with its health responsibilities?*
   - *Is the family satisfied with its support network?*
   - *To what extent is the family willing and able to access community services?*

Chapter 17

Caring for the Family in Health and Illness

Linda Beth Tiedje

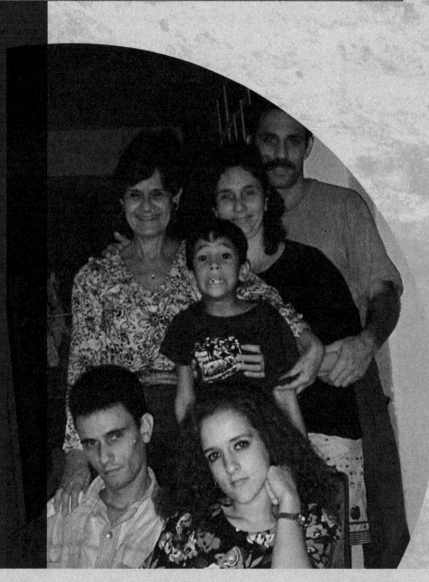

Caring for families in health and illness is not new to nurses. Lillian Wald, Margaret Sanger, and Mary Breckinridge are a few of the nurses who helped establish a tradition of family care. Indeed, some count public health nurses as one of the unique contributions America has made to the cause of public health. Much has changed in the social and economic system since the days of Wald, Sanger, and Breckinridge. Each generation of nurses must reclaim this tradition of family care: keeping relevant wisdom from the past and learning new ways to help families in the ever-changing world in which we live.

CHAPTER FOCUS

Thinking Differently About Family Health
Thinking Upstream
Thinking of a Bottom-Down Health System
The Human Ecology Model: Thinking in Layers

Community-Based Services for Promoting Family Health
Preventive Support Services for All Families
Targeted Programs for More Vulnerable Families
Families in Crisis

Characteristics of Successful Interventions: Creating Healthy Families and Communities
Relationship-Focused Care
Intensity and Timing of Interventions
Nursing Skills and Strategies

Issues in Family Nursing Today

Values: A Challenge for the Future

Healthy People 2010: Objectives Related to Families

QUESTIONS TO CONSIDER

After reading this chapter, answer the following questions:
1. What is thinking upstream and its relevance to caring for families?
2. What are community-based services in the promotion of health for families?
3. What are characteristics of successful family interventions?
4. What is the nurse role in relationship-focused care?
5. What are necessary nursing skills and strategies in promoting positive family interventions?
6. What are current issues in family nursing?
7. What are current nursing values?

KEY TERMS

Ad Hoc Committee to Defend Health Care
Bottom-down health system
Caring
Comprehensive community initiatives (CCIs)
Courage
Human ecology model
Inclusion
Intensity
Intensive services
Least possible contribution theory
Nursing skills and strategies
Preventive support services
Social responsibility
Strength-based approach
Reflective thinking
Relationship-focused care
Targeted programs
Think upstream
Timing

What is family health, and what does it mean to care for the family in health and illness? Family health is a whole series of activities that are designed to promote health, to prevent disease and injury, to prevent premature death, and to create conditions in which we can all be safe and healthy (Levy, 1998). There are many examples of activities nurses do every day to promote family health:

- *Supporting a family with a chronically ill child to find community resources and respite care*
- *Working with a family with a schizophrenic young adult to establish consistent drug therapy and vocational training*
- *Discussing eating patterns learned in families of origin when providing support and information for weight reduction*
- *Reflecting on family learned values as we attempt to understand others for whom health is not a priority*
- *Assessing whether other women in the family have breast-fed in the process of helping a new mother initiate breast-feeding*
- *Working for the enforcement of laws that prohibit sales of tobacco to minors and eliminating cigarette vending machines*
- *Being part of school curriculum committees to ensure a focus on social skills so that students learn skills such as sharing, listening to others, and working cooperatively in groups*
- *Teaching parenting competency skills in parent education classes*
- *Participating in community-based sex education committees*

A more specific example of family nursing to prevent disease, injury, and premature death occurred in Hawaii. A group of emergency department (ED) nurses there noted the numbers of individual children who were coming to the ED as a result of drownings and near drownings. Some of the children were resuscitated; others died. Over time the nurses collected data from families and found that none of the pools in which the children drowned had fences. Working with families, the fire department, and other community groups, they raised funds to help families fence their private pools, and the accidental drownings among children decreased. This is an example of a family-focused, community-targeted intervention that served to prevent disease and injury and premature death. Nurses in EDs each day save children in tertiary care settings; they can also move beyond this "downstream" approach to thinking about how to work with families in *preventing* such accidents from occurring in the first place.

Thinking Differently About Family Health

As novice health care providers, we may view provision of health care to families as an "extra," a nonessential part of individually focused, technically oriented care. As we become more confident of our physical assessment, communication, and psychomotor skills, we learn that health care is more than the provision of individual-level physical care. Indeed, we begin to appreciate that factors at the level of the family, group, and society affect the health of individuals within them. Overall family health challenges us to think in new ways about influences on the family. Specifically, this new way of thinking challenges us to (1) **think upstream**, always asking, "What would have prevented this in the first place?" (Butterfield, 1991; McKinlay, 1979); (2) think of working with families in a **bottom-down health system** (Hancock, 1993) where homes and neighborhood meeting places are the basis of health care delivery, not hospitals; and (3) to use the **human ecology model** (Bronfenbrenner, 1986) in thinking beyond what happens within individual families to factors outside families that influence family health.

Thinking Upstream

If we think of illness as people drowning in swiftly flowing water, thinking upstream means we have to think beyond rescuing people from the water and look upstream to see what is "pushing" the people into the dangerous water in the first place (McKinlay, 1979). Rescuing people is a "downstream endeavor." In health care, downstream endeavors are short-term, individually focused interventions such as lung transplants for two-pack-a-day smokers or treating myocardial infarctions instead of the sedentary, stressful lifestyles that lead to them. Upstream interventions focus on the social and physical environments in which families live. Upstream interventions focus on changing the behavioral, social, political, and environmental factors that lead to poor health, not waiting "downstream" for poor health to occur (Butterfield, 1991).

In the late 1990s, school violence erupted throughout the United States: Springfield, Oregon; Littleton, Colorado; Pearl, Mississippi; Paducah, Kentucky; Fayetteville, Tennessee; Jonesboro, Arkansas; and Edinboro, Pennsylvania. School violence was a rare and unpredictable phenomenon that fueled a search for "answers." The answers and the causes, of course, were multifaceted. A steady diet of violent media, the availability of guns, increasing feelings of alienation and unchecked rage, racism, and a lack of communication within families all were implicated as causes. School violence is a complicated phenomenon with no easy answers. In the real world, downstream thinking (dealing with consequences of school violence) and upstream thinking (dealing with its prevention) are both required. To focus only on downstream thinking is a mistake. The other mistake often made is to focus blame on singular causes. President Bill Clinton, in a radio address to the nation (May 1, 1999), urged all citizens to focus on responsibility instead of blame. What responsibility could be taken by each citizen to help prevent such violence in the future? Thinking responsibly means thinking upstream about what would prevent such school violence in the first place. Consider these comments taken from a *USA Today* story the week of the Littleton, Colorado, shootings. Recall that in Littleton the student gunmen targeted people of color and athletes:

> "I think one of our jobs as students is to include everybody; I would want to do that." Mario Francisco Penaiver, 18-year-old student from Puyallup, Washington.

HEALTHY PEOPLE 2010

OBJECTIVES RELATED TO FAMILIES	**Maternal, Infant, and Child Health**
Educational and Community-Based Programs	*Breast-Feeding, Newborn Screening, and Service Systems*
Health Care Setting	16.19 Increase the proportion of mothers who breast-feed their babies.
7.7 Increase the proportion of health care organizations that provide patient and family education.	**Nutrition and Overweight**
	Food Security
	19.18 Increase food security among U.S. households and in doing so reduce hunger.
	Source: DHHS, 2000.

"These kids were not genetically programmed to be racist. They have been taught by the people around them." Stanley Wilson, 39, Montgomery, Alabama.

"We, as a society, have to ask, 'What is the impact of a steady diet of violent media content on a growing child?'" Kathryn Montgomery, the Center for Media Education.

Urging parents to take any guns in their homes to the police, Rosie O'Donnell, talk show host, said, "If you have a gun in the house, you are 43 times more likely to be a victim of gun violence."

The National Association of Attorneys General and the National School Boards Association have also published a manual with tips on preventing violence in schools, focusing on parents as a key in prevention. Some of the upstream thinking includes encouraging parents to participate and volunteer at school and encouraging students and teachers to talk about problems. The National School Safety Center also encourages parents to talk with their children about fears and feelings and to be part of their children's lives. Community health nurses, in the spirit of such upstream thinking, could start school-based parent groups. If parental involvement is one of the keys to prevention, parents need to know *how* to communicate, offer support, and open the dialog. Community health nurse–led parent groups would be a preventive start. See above for selected *Healthy People 2010* objectives focusing on families.

Thinking of a Bottom-Down Health System

Hancock (1993) suggests that instead of thinking of a health care delivery system based in tertiary or hospital-/specialty-based care, we should focus on how to keep people healthy (see the figure to the right). Such a system would be a health system, as opposed to the current illness-focused system. Most resources would then be prevention-focused at the neighborhood and community level. In a bottom-down health system, the services

link people and families with others in support groups, neighborhood activities, parent training groups, early childhood education, and after-school recreation programs. Such services can be provided by primary care teams in the home and primary health centers based in schools and neighborhoods.

A bottom-down health system is based on the concept of social capital (Kawachi, Kennedy, Lochner, & Prothrow-Stith, 1997; Lomas, 1998) and the importance of increasing social cohesion in communities. Features of social capital in communities

BOTTOM-DOWN HEALTH SYSTEM.

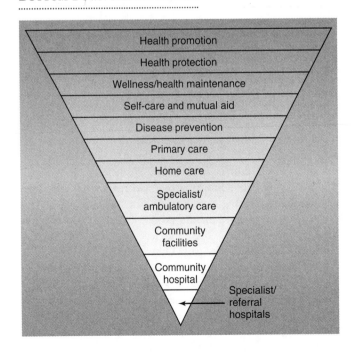

RESEARCH BRIEF

Lantz, P. M., House, J. S., Lepkowski, J. M., Williams, D. R., Mero, R. P., & Chen, J. (1998). Socioeconomic factors, health behaviors, and mortality: Results from a nationally representative prospective study of US adults. Journal of the American Medical Association, 279(21), 1703–1708.

A recent study investigated the difference in mortality rates (death) between those with higher and lower levels of education and income. Four behaviors were examined in the low- and high-income group. The four behaviors were cigarette smoking, alcohol drinking, sedentary lifestyle, and weight. It was thought that the differences in mortality between the groups would be due to a higher rate of these behaviors in those with low education and income. Results indicated that the risk of dying was higher in the lower-income group. However, the four health behaviors together only explained 12% to 13% of the effect of income on mortality, a modest amount. This means that differences in death rates between the rich and poor would persist even with improved health behaviors.

If health risk behaviors do not explain higher mortality in people of lower education and income, what does? Several factors have been suggested: more exposure to occupational and environmental health hazards in poor neighborhoods; differential access to health care; social variables such as lack of social support; a lost sense of mastery, optimism, control, and self-esteem; heightened levels of anger and hostility; and chronic stress at home and work, including racism and classism.

The Human Ecology Model: Thinking in Layers

In Chapter 16, the family was presented as an ecological system using general systems and human ecology theories. These theories focus on the external influences that affect families and their ability to function. These forces outside the family have a powerful influence on what goes on inside the family. Some of these systems outside the family are neighborhoods, institutions, the media, and government. The human ecology model (see the following figure) shows how individual and family health are nested within and influenced by these macro-level forces, like Russian dolls stacked neatly one inside the other (Bronfenbrenner, 1986).

In this human ecology model, many factors inside and outside the family influence family health. Are community factors more important than family factors? Are individual factors more important than family factors? Are community factors more important than individual factors? Each of the three broad categories of factors—community, family, and individual—contributes about the same amount to making people within families, especially children, resilient and resistant to stress.

Most traditional interventions focus mainly on individuals, occasionally on families, and less often on institutions and communities. For example, when a community health nurse makes a home visit to an adolescent mother, her baby, and her extended family, traditionally, the primary focus has been on individuals within that family, such as how much the baby weighs and health follow-up for mother and baby. Bronenfenbrenner (1986) would encourage us also to look at the family and community: Does the workplace or school have a designated place to pump breast milk? Do friends support the adolescent mother by providing child care from time to time? What encouragement is the mother

include "social organization such as networks, norms and trust that facilitate coordination and cooperation for mutual benefit" (Putnam, 1995, p. 66). This can be done by creating meeting places, sports leagues, clubs, and associations. Creating spaces in communities for people to come together allows for idea exchange and fosters trust. Building a community structure is the focus for health, not the individual (Minkler, 1998). Some experts now think that social capital is the most important determinant of our health (Lomas, 1998).

An example of building social cohesion in a community occurs in Grand Ledge, Michigan, each spring. On a spring weekend, several activities are planned to bring people of all ages together. Children gather to make May baskets to deliver to friends, and a May Pole dance is held at a city park. Other activities include a teddy bear tea, a quilt show, and a pie contest. Such community building is "for health" because it increases social contact. A vast group of studies has already linked social support networks to health outcomes (House, Landis, & Umberson, 1988). But more than that, a new body of research is emerging that supports the additional health benefits of cohesive, caring communities (Lomas, 1998).

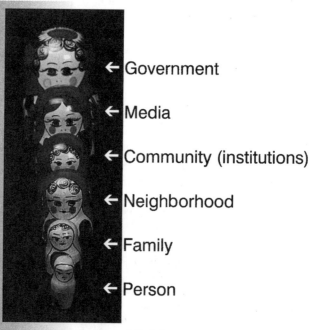

The Human Ecology Model.

FACTORS THAT CONTRIBUTE TO INVULNERABILITY OR RESISTANCE OF STRESS IN CHILDREN.

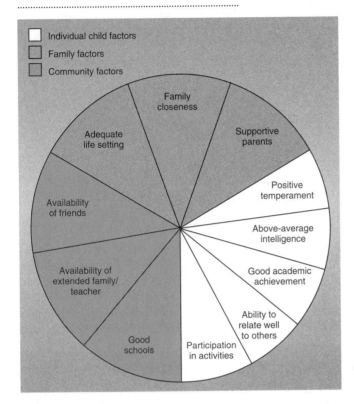

receiving to return to school? Does the mother have a list of friends she can keep by the phone to call when she needs to talk? What messages do the media (e.g., television, magazines) provide to adolescent women? Do local churches provide quality drop-in child care? What are school policies regarding child care for adolescent parents? What are government programs for employment or educational support for teen parents? Does this adolescent mother have access to contraceptive services?

The human ecology model emphasizes that "the way we organize our society, the extent to which we encourage interaction among the citizenry, and the degree to which we trust and associate with each other in caring communities is probably the most important determinant of our health" (Lomas, 1998, p. 1181).

Community-Based Services for Promoting Family Health

Recall that in the introduction to this chapter one aspect of family health was to create conditions in which we can all be safe and healthy. "Every community must have a range of family-based programs, starting with **preventive support services** for all families, continuing through **targeted programs** for more vulnerable families, and ending with highly **intensive services** for families in crisis" (Children's Defense Fund, 1994, p. 4, emphasis added).

BOX 17-1 APPLICATION EXERCISE

KEY CONCEPT: THE HUMAN ECOLOGY MODEL

Think of an individual client you have taken care of in the past. List family, neighborhood, community, media, and government factors that influence his or her health or illness. Then identify one prevention-targeted intervention that would help prevent disease and injury or promote health. For example, research has established connections between asthma and the exposure to environmental chemicals and passive smoke. In addition to treating asthma (tertiary care), a more prevention-oriented approach would examine family, neighborhood, community, media, and government factors that influence asthma and then develop interventions targeted at prevention of these factors. For instance:

- *Government:* E-mail legislators about air quality standards.
- *Media:* Use principles of marketing, public relations, and advertising to design a public service campaign working with the state health department, such as public service announcements to increase awareness of asthma and who is affected. Use experts such as William DeJong and Jay Winsten, who have written *The Media and the Message: Lessons Learned from Past Public Service Campaigns.* (This book provides guidelines and is available from the National Campaign to Prevent Teen Pregnancy, 2100 M Street NW, Suite 300, Washington DC, 20037).
- *Community:* Petition local restaurants to provide no smoking sections.
- *Neighborhood:* Plan test cigarette buys using teens to see which businesses are not enforcing bans on cigarette sales to minors.
- *Family:* Role-play with clients ways to persuade those they live with not to expose them to passive smoke.
- *Individual:* Encourage those with asthma to write about their stressful experiences. A recent study documented the positive effects of such a writing intervention for people with asthma (Smyth, Stone, Hurewitz, & Kaell, 1999).

Preventive Support Services for All Families

In contrast to the United States, where programs are most commonly developed for "at-risk" groups with problems, in other parts of the world, community-based social support for all families is part of a comprehensive program of health care. *All* families

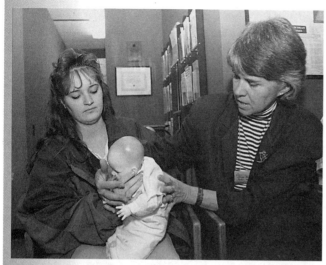

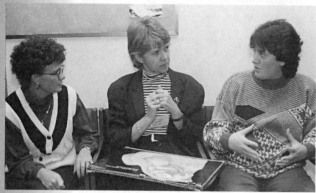

Chapter author, Dr. Linda Beth Tiedje, works to promote health with teen mothers through hands-on education and by including family members in interventions.

receive postpartum home visits after they leave the hospital, and health visitors continue to see *all* families of preschool children on a regular basis (Crockenberg, 1985).

Another example of preventive support services for all families is a preterm birth prevention program begun in France, based on a communitywide public health approach. In contrast to approaches in the United States, which have unsuccessfully attempted to identify women at risk for preterm birth, in France all families, regardless of income, were targeted by a national media campaign. The purpose of the campaign was to make everyone more aware of symptoms of preterm labor. In addition, the effects of employment, such as long-term standing, were also widely publicized as affecting preterm labor. This universal preterm birth prevention approach has become a successful national policy in France and has markedly reduced infant mortality there (Papiernik, Bouyer, Yaffe, Winisdorffer, Collin, & Dreyfus, 1986).

Another example of preventive support services for all families is a widely disseminated program created by the Search Institute in Minneapolis. The program uses a **strength-based approach** and focuses on building assets broadly in all individuals, families, and communities (Roehlkepartain, 1995). The assumptions include that all people and environments possess strengths that can be used toward improving their quality of life and that all environments, even the most bleak, contain resources.

Targeted Programs for More Vulnerable Families

What does an "at-risk" family look like? Who is vulnerable? Some define vulnerable populations as groups who experience limited resources and have a consequent high risk for morbidity and premature mortality (Flaskerud & Winslow, 1998), such as families with a chronically ill child who do not have respite care. Families who are least likely to cope with life cycle transitions are

CASE STUDY

Strength-Based Approaches

At a prenatal clinic, a nurse approached a teenage mother and her boyfriend with their new baby who seemed thin for her age of 6 weeks. The father was holding the baby and burping her, vigorously pounding on her back. Overcoming her urge to negatively comment on the father's burping technique, the nurse asked how things were going. The family related that the baby had already had surgery for pyloric stenosis and had several repeat visits at child health clinic to check on her small head circumference. Later in a discussion with other families in the clinic waiting room, the father strongly voiced his
opinion that babies needed lots of holding and "couldn't be spoiled." Reflecting back on this encounter, if the nurse had acted on her initial impulse to judge this teen couple and their child-care techniques, she would have missed the opportunity to see their real strengths: attentiveness at keeping health care appointments, shared care of the child, and knowing that the child needed holding and touch. This strength-based approach is in keeping with Search Institute programs.

1. How could the nurse be most effective in working with this young family?

2. What might be a priority intervention for these parents?

those defined to be most at risk, such as families with a history of abuse who are moving to a new city with a new baby. Vulnerable families might also have a small and nonsupportive social network or live in communities with few available services. All of these factors may make families at risk from time to time.

Economic factors also help define risk in families, poverty being an especially potent factor. One-third of all children in the United States will live in poverty at some time before reaching adulthood. Surprisingly, fewer than 20% of poor families live in inner-city urban areas (Federman, Garner, Short, Cutter, Kiely, Levine, McGough, & McMillen, 1996). Individuals in these poor families are indeed vulnerable, facing multiple problems such as joblessness, substance use, crime, violence, and poor schools. These multiproblem families vary in size, composition, location, and the nature of problems they present (Lynch & Tiedje, 1991).

Although not all poor families are multiproblem families, certain family qualities help define families as multiproblem. Women in multiproblem families often feel exploited and powerless in relationships with males. Men in these families, if present, often do not see themselves as responsible for taking care of children either physically or emotionally. Children in multiproblem families depend on proximal control and lack home orientation to school norms (Lynch & Tiedje, 1991). These defining qualities are not intended as value judgments or descriptors for *each* family in this category. Multiproblem families have problems both within the family and between the family

FYI

Refugee Families

In 1999 in Kosovo, thousands of families were displaced, causing crisis and chaos. Once refugee camps were established to provide for basic needs, schools were set up to provide education and a unifying social support for the families. Finally, the United Nations trained preventive mental health workers to work with groups of children. Health care workers assisted the children in playing games, telling stories, and expressing their grief, because many of them were separated from parents. The components of these interventions are common to interventions for all families in crisis.

RESEARCH BRIEF

Byrd, M. E. (1999). Questioning the quality of maternal caregiving during home visiting. Image: The Journal of Nursing Scholarship, 31(1), 27–32.

Field research examined 53 maternal-child home visits made by one nurse over a period of 8 months during 1995 and 1996. The nurse provided information about infant feeding, sleeping, elimination, and development. Although the visits were not exclusively with multiproblem families, two issues emerged that have implications for services to these families. With the most vulnerable of the families, the nurse's visits were primarily "child-focused," and the mother-nurse interactions centered on assessing, then doubting, the ability of the mother's caregiving. Both factors may limit positive outcomes, particularly when maternal caregiving behaviors are doubted. A more successful strategy is to form a supportive interpersonal relationship with the mother. The approach advocated is one of caring and supporting the mother so that she can care for the child.

and the wider community. They often feel insecure and fearful in the wider community. Multiproblem families span both vulnerable and crisis family categories and are known for both the chronic problems that make them vulnerable and the crises they frequently experience. Comprehensive, community-based services targeting family economics, social support, and education are more successful with multiproblem families than services that focus narrowly on one type of problem at a time.

Families in Crisis

A family may be in crisis for several reasons. Families may run out of food. Home fires may leave a family without shelter. Families in which physical and emotional abuse occur are certainly families in crisis. Families displaced by war are also families in crisis. Regardless of the cause, interventions to help families in crisis share common components. First, their basic needs of food, clothing, and shelter must be provided for and their safety ensured. Next, both social and community support networks must be initiated or maintained. Finally, longer term mental health prevention programs must be referred to or established.

Characteristics of Successful Interventions: Creating Healthy Families and Communities

Launching and sustaining work with families is difficult. Successful nursing interventions with families contain several similar components: (1) **relationship-focused care**, (2) attention to **intensity** and **timing** of the interventions, and (3) particular **nursing skills and strategies**.

Relationship-Focused Care

The ability of sensitive nurses to develop ongoing, meaningful relationships with families makes a difference in the ultimate

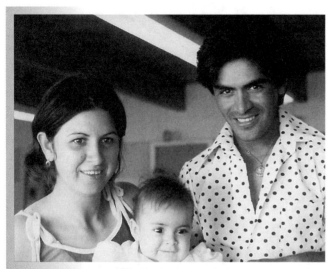

The family provides the framework for learning about health risks and health behavior.

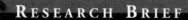

RESEARCH BRIEF

Heinicke, C. M. (1993). Factors affecting the efficacy of early family intervention. In N. J. Anastasiow & S. Harel (Eds.), At-risk infants: Interventions, families and research (pp. 91–100), Baltimore: Paul H. Brookes.

Using intervention studies available addressing the family formation period, Heinicke and his colleagues concluded that the most effective programs provided 11 or more contacts with parents over at least a 3-month period. The intensity of the intervention allowed for an ongoing, nurturing, and supportive relationship with staff delivering the intervention.

effectiveness of an intervention. Nursing is more than a series of tasks to be performed "on" families or information delivered to educate them. Through interactions with families, nurses weave a "tapestry of care" (Gordon, 1997). Interpersonal connections become the foundation for effectively influencing health behaviors and helping people take charge of their health and healing (Remen, 1996; Tanner, 1995; Zerwekh, 1997).

Intensity and Timing of Interventions

Programs with successful results offer opportunities for multiple contacts with families over a short time. Programs during the childbearing years are particularly useful because they furnish potential continuity over time and multiple contacts. Multiple contacts in and of themselves do not ensure success, however. Other factors, such as provider credibility, are also important for successful results.

School-based clubs and groups offer opportunities for multiple contacts over time. One such group, begun by a school nurse, targeted preadolescent girls, who during the second decade of life appear to be substantially more vulnerable than boys to environmental and psychological stressors (Pipher, 1994). A school nurse started a girls club with girls from the fourth grade. The girls met weekly over the noon hour at school, at first to talk. A softball team, field trips to sporting and cultural events, and a presentation on grooming and hygiene were soon club activities. Such a club, building assets such as self-esteem

CASE STUDY

Establishing Trust for Relationship-Focused Care

At the request of a children's clinic, a nurse made a home visit because clinic personnel were concerned that a 6-month-old child had not been brought in for cast changes. The cast was the result of treatment for congenital foot deformities. At the first home visit, the mother was guarded and uncommunicative and admitted the nurse to her home with obvious reluctance. The dominant feature in the dark, cluttered room was a slate pool table. The nurse, sensing that so costly an item in all probability was highly prized, shared that observation with the mother. The nurse then admired the pool table,

noting its many features. The mother responded immediately. She explained at length about how much it meant to the family to have it, how friends and neighbors gathered to use it, and its contribution to her life. She then angrily described the previous nurse who had scolded her for spending money foolishly instead of using her resources to better meet the needs of her children. She was grateful to the current nurse for being a more understanding person and immediately switched the conversation to questions she had about her children. She then proceeded to plan with the nurse how she could arrange for necessary clinic follow-up for the 6-month-old, thanked the nurse for all her help, and asked when she would return.

Source: Lynch & Tiedje, 1991.

and communication skills, is health promoting and helps prevent adolescent pregnancy. Positive, asset-building activities with preadolescent girls are prime examples of intensive interventions.

In addition to intensity, most family interventions require time and living through difficulties. Unlike quiz shows, family interventions do not provide immediate answers. It takes time for families to experiment with new ideas and strategies. It takes time for families to come to their own solutions.

For example, there is a growing number of community-based programs for couples who present for domestic violence counseling and want to be treated jointly (Johannson & Tutty, 1998). Although controversial, in cases of domestic abuse, the conjoint treatment of couples is increasing because unless both men and women are treated, the cycle of abuse repeats even when a relationship with a particular abusive partner ends. Conjoint treatment requires patience and time. Most conjoint groups last 12 weeks and are preceded by gender-specific (all-men or all-women groups) 24-week treatment groups. The conjoint groups are often held in community centers, schools, or YWCAs and emphasize alternatives to domestic violence. Cessation of physical violence between the partners is a condition for group membership.

•••••••••••••••••••••••••••••

Most people learn how to avoid emotional hijackings from the time they are infants. If they have supportive and caring adults around them, they pick up the social cues that enable them to develop self-discipline and empathy.

Hillary Rodham Clinton, 1996

•••••••••••••••••••••••••••••

Nursing Skills and Strategies

Nurses delivering interventions to families must have skills specific to the intervention delivered. Five skills are particularly important: communicating, problem solving, listening, connecting, and evaluating.

Communicating

In addition to the skills nurses need to communicate, communication is also a core issue in families and communities. Community health nurses can facilitate communication and also teach particular communication skills to people in families and groups. The following program example is one way nurses may provide parents with practical advice about ways of communicating with their children. The content area is human sexuality.

In New York, Jo Leonard and Marcia Siegel (1998) implemented a workshop for mothers and daughters called "Mother-Daughter Workshop: Getting Your Period." Offering the class to girls ages 9 to 13, no class is bigger than eight mother-daughter pairs. The class is based on the premise that parents are the first and most important sexuality educators and that family support and guidance have a significant effect on sexual activity. The class provides opportunities for parents and children to practice communicating about sexuality. It also provides opportunities to ask questions about sexuality in a neutral atmosphere. The class is a prime example of a strategy nurses may use to enhance family communication.

•••••••••••••••••••••••••••••

At work, you think of the children you've left at home.
At home, you think of the work you've left unfinished.
Such a struggle is unleashed within yourself; your heart is rent.

Golda Meir, Former Prime Minister of Israel

•••••••••••••••••••••••••••••

Problem Solving

Problem solving is a skill that must be done with and not for families and communities. Nurses may have "rescue fantasies" as helpers, wanting to take on the problem and tell others what to do. Coming to terms with who owns the problem leads to mutual goal setting and gives clients the power of solving their own problems.

For example, a nurse in a prenatal clinic was discussing the importance of finishing high school with a pregnant mother who had dropped out of school. The pregnant woman was accompanied by her mother, who also was a high school dropout. As the nurse talked with both women, it was obvious that the grandmother was proud of her longstanding job as a hotel maid. She also believes high school had been unnecessary for her achievement. For the nurse to assume an authoritarian, directive role in this situation and insist on high school completion would have been unproductive. Instead, talking with the mother and daughter about education, jobs, and life success over the course of the pregnancy helped the nurse better understand the mother-daughter perspective. The mutual problem solving that evolved enabled the daughter to "own the problem" of high school completion and take the necessary steps for it to happen.

Listening

Nurses have vast amounts of health information to share with families and communities in an effort to improve health outcomes. Often, our first impulse is to give advice and information. Sometimes, especially in response to particular client questions, advice is appropriate. However, we have entered an era in which health information is no longer a commodity exclusively owned by health systems. Many individuals, families, and communities can access health information from many sources. Self-care and wellness reflect a growing awareness that maintaining and enhancing health is a shared enterprise between providers and consumers. In such a shared enterprise, listening becomes a more vital skill. What does the client already know? What experiences has the client already had? Listening through storytelling has recently been reclaimed as a powerful educational and therapeutic tool (Banks-Wallace, 1998). When a nurse truly listens to clients' or families' stories, he or she can more fully understand where they are coming from. Storytelling can reveal the way clients and families think about health issues, as well as gaps in their understanding. The use of storytelling as an educational tool also has been expanded to include groups of clients within prenatal and other clinic settings (Banks-Wallace, 1999).

Connecting

Caring for families in health and illness requires the ability to connect with other agencies and programs, to coordinate and reinforce interventions. Being assertive, phoning other providers, planning family meetings—all this requires skill and a definite lack of shyness! Nurses often know the many other agencies involved with a family and initiate care conferences to coordinate services. Long before case managers were popular, community health nurses were coordinating services for individuals and families. It is nurses who often are the best client advocates, articulating family needs for and with families.

During the late 1980s and the early 1990s, an approach emerged to facilitate connecting: **comprehensive community initiatives (CCIs)**. Instead of focusing on one type of problem at a time, CCIs focus on creating systems of comprehensive services (e.g., health care, social services, education, housing) through a variety of programs and community building to better the lives of urban poor families (Stagner & Duran, 1997). The overall purpose is to provide neighborhood conditions in which families can succeed. CCIs share certain attributes such as emphasizing participation and providing a variety of services with their predecessors: settlement houses (early 1900s), neighborhood programs (1930s), war on poverty programs (1960s), and community action agencies (1970s).

Evaluating

Outcomes of what community health nurses do are important. To measure those outcomes, evaluation knowledge and skills are especially critical. In addition to evaluating interventions with individuals and families, nurses are often asked to serve on evaluation teams to review the impact of community planning or intervention efforts. Traditional evaluation methods include pretesting and post-testing, interviews, surveys, record review, and focus groups (Minkler, 1998). A new approach that expands on some of these traditional methods is called *empowerment evaluation*. It is used as a tool for both evaluation and community building (Fetterman, Kaftarian, & Wandersman, 1996).

Empowerment evaluation was used in the evaluation of a human immunodeficiency virus (HIV) prevention community planning effort funded by the Centers for Disease Control and Prevention in 1994, and consists of four steps. The first step in the empowerment evaluation process is taking stock. This involves a review of documents (e.g., budgets, reports, organizational charts) and interviews and focus groups with community participants to uncover background experiences. The purpose of this step is to reveal a common history and broad shared experience. In the second step, setting goals, the evaluator helps community group members identify where they want to go and the

kind of evaluation they want to create. Note that the evaluation process is not a preconceived idea of the evaluator.

The third step, that of developing strategies, is often difficult. Uneasy group dynamics and underfunding often create hassles and obstacles as communities struggle to decide on particular strategies to meet high expectations. In the example of the HIV prevention planning, one team encountered many difficulties when generating strategies. In an effort to overcome these difficulties, participants were asked to name the biggest hassle of community planning and to identify what they particularly appreciated in each of the other participants. The written responses were then organized into hassles, uplifts, and ways of changing course. These responses were circulated and then discussed at a community meeting. This helped the participants move beyond the difficulties to the work they needed to do: developing strategies.

The fourth and final step of empowering evaluation is documenting the process, that is, keeping a written record of what occurred and why, in a way accessible to all participants. The usefulness of this step was apparent in the HIV prevention planning process when the planning group, after nearly a year, faced some difficult decisions. Planning group members were on a 3-day retreat and faced a vote about how to proceed. Behind-the-scenes maneuvering, miscommunication, and longstanding alliances left the planners angry and divided. The empowering evaluation team found some data collected after an ice breaker exercise early in the planning process when participants had been asked to share their personal mottoes and messages for the world. One of the messages was from a group member who had died of acquired immunodeficiency syndrome (AIDS) just a few months before. Stunned, the group was reminded of their collective vision, and they were then able to vote in a more unified spirit. This use of data is a prime example of how documenting the process can be used to empower communities in evaluation efforts (Roe, Berenstein, Goette, & Roe, 1996).

The five nursing skills and strategies of communicating, problem solving, listening, connecting, and evaluating are a necessary foundation for community health nurses as they seek to provide services to individuals, families, and communities. These skills are necessary but not sufficient in a health care system where changes are massive, swift, and without precedent. Therefore, in the next section, issues in family nursing resulting from large-scale integrated health care enterprises, managed care plans, intense market competition, and a pervasive concern for operational efficiency and cost reduction are discussed.

Issues in Family Nursing Today

The health care climate in which we practice may constrain what we want to do with families and communities. For example, many states have community programs in which nursing visits are reimbursed in a fragmented way for childbearing families: maternal support services for mothers, infant support services for children, Women, Infants and Children (WIC) for nutrition, and family planning services for contraception. The "family" sees many health care providers, with little concern for coordination of services. As nurses in that situation, we may find ourselves in situations we have not created and without much power. It is difficult to provide family-centered care in an environment that reimburses for individual services and that is not designed for time with families. Difficult, but not impossible. The nation's estimated 2.5 million nurses make up the clinical backbone of the care delivery system. Nurses are uniquely suited in this emerging health care system. We have the exact skills the health care delivery system needs: communicating, problem solving, listening, connecting, and evaluating.

Nursing reinvented itself in the past when social changes demanded it. Before the Depression, most nurses worked in private duty. As the Depression grew worse, nurses moved into hospitals and were employed at a salary. We can reinvent ourselves again, as we have done before (Sharts-Hopko, 1998). How do we accomplish this reinvention?

One strategy is based on the **least possible contribution theory** (Weisman, 1981). A little can go a long way, and the least possible contribution is the one with the best chance of making a difference, however small. Making one small, insignificant contribution furnishes a foundation on which one can continue to add other contributions until something surprising but substantial results. Of course, least possible contribution does not mean doing as little as possible. Least possible contribution means doing something that the nurse is really good at and something that is only a little bit beyond the ordinary (Weisman, 1981).

An example of the least possible contribution theory in action occurred in 1997 when a group of Massachusetts health care providers created the **Ad Hoc Committee to Defend Health Care.** Together these physicians and nurses worked to reestablish caregiving from those who were trying to make health care a business driven by the bottom line. This committee has become a national movement against "a corporate-driven health care system" (Shindul-Rothschild, 1998). The committee's agenda is based on the following legislative initiatives: (1) Give the public information so that they can make informed choices; (2) assure patients that they will be cared for by registered nurses; and (3) extend whistle-blower protection to all health care workers so that they are not put in the position of choosing between a job and advocacy for clients. Only through such group efforts can the health care delivery scale be tilted back toward care instead of profits. Human and capital resources can then be put back into direct client care instead of where the true inefficiencies lie in the delivery system—in the huge administrative overhead.

Values: A Challenge for the Future

The value of inclusion rather than exclusion and the embracing of diversity as a means of enriching the social fabric remain two of our greatest challenges in community health. To deliver relationship-focused care to families, nurses must get emotionally free to focus on the family without judgment or bias. As nurses we may perceive people's situations differently because of our own value systems, which are created by our own experiences. We live in a heterogeneous society, a society with many different kinds of people and families. There are recent immigrant families from all over the world, as well as families whose ancestors came from Northern Europe, England, Eastern and Southern Europe, and Scandinavia. We must not only assess minorities for cultural norms, customs, and rituals; the majority culture also has cultural norms, customs, and rituals that must be owned. To ignore cultural assessment of everyone is to imply that the majority culture is the "norm" and is beyond assessing.

The structure of families is also increasingly diverse: single parent, two parent, gay or lesbian parent, and so on. Therefore, health care providers often find themselves relating to families that are different from the ones they grew up in either in culture or structure. It is common when confronting such differences to feel strange or uncomfortable. Sometimes, health care providers react by thinking of ways all people and families are

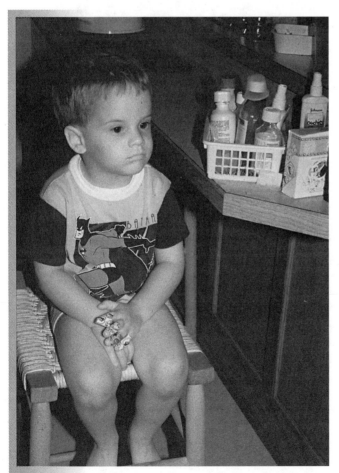

Children learn how to care for themselves in the family.

alike, such as that we all have similar needs (e.g., food, clothing, shelter) and we all need love and affection. As health care providers, we also need to preserve the differences in people and families. That is more difficult. At times, we may just want everyone to be like us.

To better meet the values challenges of a diverse culture, three activities are outlined in this section. The first is a self-assessment quiz in Box 17-2 to increase value and community awareness. The second is a critical thinking exercise in Box 17-3 about providing support for families when there are scarce resources. Decisions about such family support ultimately involve values. The third activity is to recall how core nursing values may help us meet the challenges of a diverse society.

In the area of values, looking where we have come from may help us in where we are going. Nursing may provide guidance to meeting the values challenges in providing care to families and communities in a diverse culture. Salmon (1999) reminds us that there are five core values in nursing: **caring, courage, inclusion, reflective thinking,** and **social responsibility.** The value of caring is what has allowed us to move from the "doing for" approach to the current focus on enabling and empowering. The second value of courage needs to be shared and taught with exemplars and living models. We need to share and call attention to the daily courageous acts of nurses, particularly as they care for diverse groups. The third nursing value of inclusion seems most appropriate for the values challenge of working with diverse

---

BOX 17-2 SELF-ASSESSMENT QUIZ FOR PROVIDERS WORKING WITH FAMILIES AND COMMUNITIES

In the spirit of thinking of similarities and differences in people, this self-assessment is intended as a means for you as a provider to become more aware of your values. In addition, questions 4 to 9 are intended to assess your awareness of your community, because community cohesion and the degree to which you associate with others in creating caring communities will be important to your success as a community health nurse.

1. Do you respect others' beliefs?
2. Do you believe that life is good and positive?
3. What is your ethnic/cultural heritage? List some norms/customs/rituals.
4. When was the last time you took public transportation?
5. Have you given blood recently?
6. Have you ever served on a jury?
7. How many of your neighbors do you know by name?
8. When was the last time you went to a free public event or amusement like a museum or the zoo?
9. When was the last time you checked a book out of the local library?
10. Do you do volunteer work in your community?

Source: Questions 1 to 3 are based on Benson, 1996; questions 4 to 10 are based on a community quotient quiz adapted by the Utne Reader (Cordes & Walljasper, 1997).

BOX 17-3 VALUE CHECKPOINT: CRITICAL THINKING

The issue of who is responsible for children affects not only how we as health care providers care for families, but also how resources get allocated in our society. People from widely different points of view can agree that valuing families is important in our society. What is harder is agreeing on how much the family needs to be supported by social institutions, including churches, schools, community agencies, and government (Schorr, 1989).

The conservative view is that families should be self-reliant and self-sufficient, not relying on community and government support. The liberal view is that "parents are and should be the most important people in their children's lives. But that doesn't mean they can or should raise their children without any help" (Children's Defense Fund, 1994). Liberals maintain that many forms of assistance are needed to maintain strong families, including sufficient family income and access to health care, child care, and adequate housing.

Think for a moment about your attitudes and beliefs regarding family support. How much family support is needed? What kind of support is needed? Should government ensure basic health care for all families, including children and parents? How does increasing the supply of affordable housing promote health in families? What is the best environment for families if we want to create families who are self-reliant, self-sufficient, and responsible? At what point does the conservative model threaten the overall health of the community? At what point does the liberal model threaten self-reliance in families?

CONTINUUM OF SERVICES.

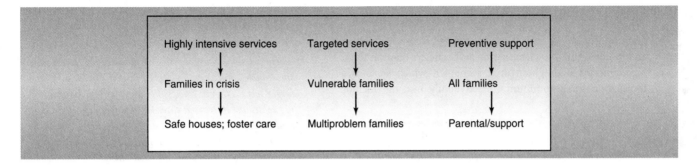

Highly intensive services   Targeted services   Preventive support

Families in crisis   Vulnerable families   All families

Safe houses; foster care   Multiproblem families   Parental/support

groups. But have we as nurses, so long marginalized and excluded, learned our lessons so well that we in turn oppress others? Listen to Salmon on this point: "I wonder what we teach our students about inclusion. Do they understand that our health care system serves only some people, and that more than 40 million others have no real access to care? . . . Does our science teach students to care only for those who are part of the system? . . . Or do we convey the value that nursing's job is not complete until all receive the care they need?" (p. 23).

The fourth nursing core value is that of reflective thinking, not easy to come by in our fast-paced lives. However, as community health nurses, we must become more than just technicians. "We must also educate people who are equipped intellectually to deal with the meaning of what they do and who they are in the context of humanity" (Salmon, 1999, p. 24). It is reflection that is needed as we deal with the issues of value conflicts in a complex and diverse society.

Finally, the last core value, the linchpin for all the others, is social responsibility. Nightingale's vision of nursing's responsibility to the common good was based on social responsibility. She saw a society like ours in which certain groups were marginalized and in poor health because of unjust systems. "Her response was to engage nursing in addressing these injustices" (Salmon, 1999, p. 25). Nursing is only as good as what it does for all the people. Do we, like Lillian Wald, have a firm grasp of the way in which society functions to impact the health of individuals? Our sense of social responsibility will help us meet the challenges of values conflicts in a diverse culture.

CONCLUSION

Community health nurses must not only care for individuals and families, but also create caring and cohesive communities. Key concepts highlighted in this chapter, which serve as a foundation for a community-based family nursing, include the following:

- *Family health is a series of activities designed to promote health, to prevent disease and injury, to prevent premature death, and to create conditions in which we all can be safe and healthy.*

- *Family health challenges us to think in new, broader ways. Thinking differently about family health means (1) thinking upstream about prevention, (2) thinking of a bottom-down health system focused on increasing cohesion in communities and providing services at the neighborhood level, and (3) thinking in layers in terms of the human ecology model about the many external influences on family health.*

- *There are three general strategies for promoting family health: preventive services for all families, targeted pro-*

grams for more vulnerable families, and intensive services for families in crisis.

- *There are three characteristics of all successful interventions with families embedded in neighborhoods and larger social systems. Successful interventions involve (1) relationship-focused care, (2) attention to intensity and timing of interventions, and (3) the use of the nursing skills and strategies of communicating, problem solving, listening, connecting, and evaluating.*

- *The issues in family nursing today are varied and complex. Most important are the constraints of the health care delivery system.*

- *There are many challenges facing community health nurses as they build and organize communities for health. A special challenge is the value conflicts that result when we work with diverse families and communities.*

- *Salmon's five core values of nursing are proposed as ways to meet the value conflicts of diversity. The five core values are caring, courage, inclusion, reflective thinking, and social responsibility.*

CRITICAL THINKING ACTIVITIES

1. As a community health nurse, you have been assigned to a community action committee to design a parent support group for parents of teens in your local high school. The purpose of the group is to teach communication, conflict resolution, and problem-solving skills and to provide a forum for social support for parents. A major emphasis will be on practicing skills. Explore the following questions and give rationales for your decisions:

   - Would you have a group for parents only, for parents and teens, or separate groups for parents and teens?

   - What resources would you use to teach communication, conflict resolution, and problem-solving skills? Remember that a major emphasis of the groups is to practice these skills.

   - The teaching of social skills to children is important, especially children who feel alienated and left out. In a recent book, *Why Doesn't Anybody Like Me?*,

Hara Estroff Marano gives several suggestions to parents. How would you incorporate some of these suggestions into your parent group? What activities would you use to make the suggestions come alive?

- How many weeks will the groups meet, when (e.g., evening, weekend), and how long (e.g., 1 hour, 2 hours)?

- Who would you have lead the groups? What experts in your community would you utilize to help you if you were chosen to lead the groups?

2. Using the research of Lantz, House, Lepkowski, Williams, Mero, and Chen (see the Research Brief on p. 396), explore the factors contributing to the gap in mortality between the rich and the poor. Especially look at factors other than health behaviors. Explain how some of the other factors suggested by the research might contribute to increased mortality in the poor. How might these factors affect physical health? What are interventions that would address these other factors?

Other factors: *Intervention:*

- Lack of social relationships and social supports

- Personality factors such as a lost sense of mastery, optimism, sense of control, and self-esteem

- Factors such as a heightened level of anger and hostility

- Chronic and acute stress in jobs and at home as a result of lack of resources

- The stress of racism and classism and other stresses related to the unequal distribution of power and resources

- Differences in exposure to occupational and environmental health hazards (poor people tend to have more exposure to these hazards, e.g., lead)

- Differences in access to health care

3. Think of a family you are currently working with. Name one skill that each family member possesses that is a strength. Does the documentation system used in your nursing agency, hospital, or community clinic have a place for listing strengths of individuals and families?

4. Most conjoint domestic abuse after-treatment groups are co-led by a man and a woman. Leaders should have experience in counseling, group work, and family violence. Assume you are co-leading a conjoint after-treatment group.

- What safety considerations would you have for the formerly abused women in the group?

- What skills would be particularly important for couples to practice in the groups?

- What built-in strategies would you use to monitor current physical abuse in these relationships?

- What system would you have in place for crisis intervention if abuse developed between sessions?

Continued

CRITICAL THINKING ACTIVITIES—CONT'D

5. Explain why someone in a family or community would respond differently to a problem than you do. Discuss the following questions with the family/community to enhance their problem solving (adapted from Schorr, 1997).

- What do you think is the problem?
- What do you think you should do?
- What would help?
- What have you done in the past when this happened? Did it work?
- What are your options?
- Who might help you?

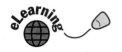

Explore Community Health Nursing on the web! To learn more about the topics in this chapter, access your exclusive web site:
http://communitynursing.jbpub.com

REFERENCES

Banks-Wallace, J. (1998). Emancipatory potential of storytelling in a group. *Image: The Journal of Nursing Scholarship, 30*(1), 17–21.

Banks-Wallace, J. (1999). Storytelling as a tool for providing holistic care to women. *American Journal of Maternal Child Nursing, 24*(1), 20–24.

Benson, H. (1996). *Timeless healing. The power and biology of belief.* New York: Simon & Schuster.

Bronfenbrenner, U. (1986). Ecology of the family as a context for human development. Research perspectives. *Developmental Psychology, 22*(6), 723–742.

Butterfield, P. G. (1991). Thinking upstream: Nurturing a conceptual understanding of the societal context of health behavior. In K. A. Saucier (Ed.), *Perspectives in family and community health* (pp. 66–71). St. Louis: Mosby.

Byrd, M. E. (1999). Questioning the quality of maternal caregiving during home visiting. *Image: The Journal of Nursing Scholarship, 31*(1), 27–32.

Children's Defense Fund. (1994). *Helping children by strengthening families: A look at family support programs.* Washington, DC: Author.

Clinton, H. R. (1996). *It takes a village: And other lessons children teach us.* Carmichael, CA: Touchstone Books.

Cordes, H., & Walljasper, J. (Eds.). (1997). *Goodlife: Mastering the art of everyday living.* Minneapolis: Utne Reader.

Crockenberg, S. B. (1985). Professional support and care of infants by adolescent mothers in England and the United States. *Journal of Pediatric Psychology, 10,* 413–428.

Federman, M., Garner, T. I., Short, K., Cutter, W. M. IV, Kiely, J., Levine, D., McGough, D., & McMillen, M. (1996). What does it mean to be poor in America? *Monthly Labor Review, 119*(5), 3–17.

Fetterman, D. M., Kaftarian, S. J., & Wandersman, A. (Eds.). (1996). *Empowerment evaluation: Knowledge and tools for self-assessment and accountability.* Thousand Oaks, CA: Sage Publications.

Flaskerud, J. H., & Winslow, B. J. (1998). Conceptualizing vulnerable populations: Health-related research. *Nursing Research, 47*(2), 69–78.

Gordon, S. (1997). *Life support: Three nurses on the front lines.* Boston: Little, Brown.

Hancock, T. (1993). Re-designing healthcare from the bottom down. In *Healthier communities action kit* (vol. 2). San Francisco: The Healthcare Forum.

Heinicke, C. M. (1993). Factors affecting the efficacy of early family intervention. In N. J. Anastasiow & S. Harel (Eds.), *At-risk infants: Interventions, families and research* (pp. 91–100), Baltimore, MD: Paul H. Brookes.

House, J. S., Landis, K. R., & Umberson, D. (1988). Social relationships and health. *Science, 241*(4865), 540–545.

Johannson, M. A., & Tutty, L. M. (1998). An evaluation of after-treatment couples' groups for wife abuse. *Family Relations, 47*(1), 27–35.

Kawachi, I., Kennedy, B. P., Lochner, K., & Prothrow-Stith, D. (1997). Social capital, income inequality, and mortality. *American Journal of Public Health, 87*(9), 1491–1498.

Lantz, P. M., House, J. S., Lepkowski, J. M., Williams, D. R., Mero, R. P., & Chen, J. (1998). Socioeconomic factors, health behaviors, and mortality: Results from a nationally representative prospective study of US adults. *Journal of the American Medical Association, 279*(21), 1703–1708.

Leonard, J., & Siegel, M. (1998). Mother and daughter workshops. *Childbirth Instructor Magazine,* March/April, 34–35.

Levy, B. S. (1998). Creating the future of public health: Values, vision, and leadership. *American Journal of Public Health, 88*(2), 188–192.

Lomas, J. (1998). Social capital and health: Implications for public health and epidemiology. *Social Science and Medicine, 47*(9), 1181–1188.

Lynch, I., & Tiedje, L. B. (1991). Working with multiproblem families: An intervention model for community health nurses. *Public Health Nursing, 8*(3), 147–153.

McKinlay, J. B. (1979). A case for refocusing upstream: The political economy of illness. In E. G. Jaco (Ed.), *Patients, physicians, and illness* (3rd ed., pp. 9–25). New York: The Free Press.

Minkler, M. (Ed.). (1998). *Community organizing & community building for health.* New Brunswick, NJ: Rutgers University Press.

Papiernik, E., Bouyer, J., Yaffe, K., Winisdorffer, G., Collin, D., & Dreyfus, J. (1986). Women's acceptance of a preterm birth prevention program. *American Journal of Obstetrics and Gynecology, 155,* 939–946.

Pipher, M. (1994). *Reviving Ophelia: Saving the selves of adolescent girls.* New York: Ballantine.

Putnam, R. D. (1995). Bowling alone. American's declining social capital. *Journal of Democracy, 6,* 65–78.

Remen, R. N. (1996). *Kitchen table wisdom.* New York: Riverhead Books.

Roe, K. M., Berenstein, C., Goette, C., & Roe, K. (1996). Community building through empowering evaluation. In Meredith Winkler (Ed.), *Community organizing & community building for health* (pp. 308–322). New Brunswick, NJ: Rutgers University Press.

Roehlkepartain, J. L. (1995). *Building assets together.* Minneapolis: The Search Institute.

Salmon, M. E. (1999). Thoughts on nursing: Where it has been and where it is going. *Nursing and Health Care Perspectives, 20*(1), 20–25.

Schorr, L. B. (1997). *Common purpose: Strengthening families and neighborhoods to rebuild America.* New York: Anchor Books.

Schorr, L. B. (1989). *Within our reach: Breaking the cycle of disadvantage.* New York: Anchor Books.

Sharts-Hopko, N. C. (1998). On chaos, wholeness, and long-standing values: Direction for nursing's future. *American Journal of Maternal Child Nursing, 23,* 11–14.

Shindul-Rothschild, J. (1998). Nurses week tribute: A nursing call to action. *American Journal of Nursing, 98*(5), 36.

Smyth, J., Stone, A. A., Hurewitz, A., & Kaell, A. (1999). Effects of writing about stressful experiences on symptom reduction in patients with asthma or rheumatoid arthritis. *Journal of the American Medical Association, 281(*14), 1304–1309.

Stagner, M. W., & Duran, M. A. (1997). Comprehensive community initiatives: Principles, practice, and lessons learned. In R. E. Behrman (Ed.), *The future of children: Children and poverty* (vol. 7[2]). Los Altos, CA: The Center for the Future of Children.

Tanner, C. A. (1995). Living in the midst of a paradigm shift. *Journal of Nursing Education, 34*(2), 51–52.

University of Massachusetts, Cooperative Extension. (1990). *Building communities of support for families in poverty.* Amherst, MA: Author.

U.S. Public Health Service (USPHS). (1991). *Healthy People 2000: National health promotion and disease prevention objectives.* (Publication No. PHS 91-50213). Washington, DC: Dept. of Health and Human Services.

Weisman, A. D. (1981). Understanding the cancer patient: The syndrome of caregiver's plight. *Psychiatry, 44,* 161–168.

Zerwekh, J. V. (1997). Making the connection during home visits: Narratives of expert nurses. *International Journal for Human Caring, 1(*1), 25–29.

Unit VI

Care of the Individual in Community-Based Nursing

Chapter 18
Men's Health

A. Serdar Atav, Sharyn Janes,
and Joseph E. Farmer

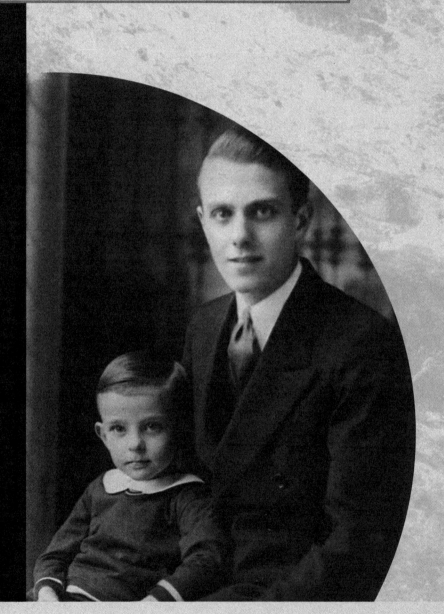

*Historically, most research studies have been based on male subjects. In many Western cultures,
years of a predominantly male workforce have resulted in health care systems and policies being established by men. Despite this dominance of men in health care systems, women still
have longer life expectancies than men.*

CHAPTER FOCUS

Men's Health
Genetic Factors
Sociocultural Factors
Environmental Factors
Behavioral Factors
Healthy People 2010

Health Care System Utilization
Ambulatory Care
Hospital Care
Preventive Care

Specific Male Health Issues
Prostate Cancer
Testicular Cancer

Erectile Dysfunction (Impotence)
Cardiovascular Disease

Selected At-Risk Populations
Men with HIV/AIDS
Homosexual Men and Families

Community Health Nursing Roles
Client Advocate
Educator
Facilitator

Men's Health Research Issues

Healthy People 2010: Objectives Related to Men's Health

QUESTIONS TO CONSIDER

After reading this chapter, answer the following questions:

1. What are some of the major factors affecting men's health?
2. How are risk factors for illness or injury different for men compared with women?
3. How does the threat of testicular and prostate cancer affect the lives of young and middle-aged men?
4. What is the nurse's role in the treatment of erectile dysfunction?
5. What are some roles for the community health nurse in the promotion of men's health?

KEY TERMS

Erectile dysfunction	Health status	Socialization process	Viagra
Fertility	Homosexuality	Stress	Violence
Gender differences			

Most nursing students have at least been introduced to, if not completed a course on, women's health or women's issues, but health issues specifically concerning men are a neglected topic in nursing. The role of the community health nurse in improving the health of men is explored in this chapter.

Men's Health

The data on mortality rates by gender are clear—women live longer than men. Men are many times more likely to die of lung cancer, motor vehicle accidents, cirrhosis of the liver, heart disease, and acquired immunodeficiency syndrome (AIDS) than women. Suicide rates are three times higher for men. Possible factors involved in such **gender differences** in health are (1) genetic factors, (2) sociocultural factors, (3) environmental factors, and (4) behavioral factors.

Genetic Factors

Genetic factors related to gender influence a man's physiological and psychological well-being. According to the genetic approach, some gender differences are natural in origin. They are driven from instinctual, hormonal, structural, or neurological characteristics of the male gender (Sabo & Gordon, 1995). For example, gender differences in ischemic heart disease mortality may be a result of the protective effects of female sex hormones and men's tendency to accumulate fat in the upper abdomen (Fackelmann, 1998; Waldron, 1995). Similarly, women with cancer generally have a more optimistic prognosis, probably because of the role of female sex hormones (Adami, Bergstrom, Holmberg, Klareskog, Perrson, & Ponten, 1990). For as yet unknown reasons, girls with medulloblastoma, a common brain tumor in children, have a much better prognosis than boys (Weil, Lamborn, Edwards, & Wara, 1998). It is also argued that higher levels of testosterone contribute to men's predisposition to **violence** (Stillion, 1995). Some of the other physiological differences between men and women include the following (Tanne, 1997):

- *Men's brain cells die faster than women's as they age.*
- *There are structural differences between men and women in the mitral valve, which separates the left atrium of the heart from the left ventricle.*
- *Women's hearts beat more rapidly than men's hearts.*
- *Men have weaker immune systems than women.*

Sociocultural Factors

In many cultures, particularly Western cultures, the male **socialization process** has emphasized traits such as the following (Torres, 1998):

- *Assertiveness*
- *Preoccupation with achievement and success (individualism, status, aggression, toughness, and winning)*
- *Restricted emotionality and affectionate behavior*

- *Concerns about power and control*
- *Fear and bias related to **homosexuality***

As a result, most males tend to conform to these stereotyped gender expectations and behaviors, leading to definite health consequences. Some men may experience more frequent trauma because of their belief that taking physical risks is a sign of masculinity. Boys are socialized into competitive games at an early age and learn to endure physical punishment as part of having fun or as a prerequisite to becoming a man (Stillion, 1995). From Little League on, a boy is told to "act like a man." Hence, to admit to having pain or some other health problem may be seen as a confession of weakness. This male denial factor is pervasive and not related to occupation, age, race, or socioeconomic status (Male Health Center, 1998a). High death rates from coronary heart disease for men in the United States may be due in part to these stereotyped gender expectations, which increase the risk of the disease (Helman, 1994).

The lack of healthy emotional channels for men contributes to higher risks among men for suicide, heart disease, accidents, and violence. The traditional male socialization process has historically emphasized restricted emotionality and affectionate behavior. This traditional male gender role is inconsistent with the provision and receipt of social support, particularly emotional support that includes expressiveness and disclosure. Such characteristics may have adverse health consequences. The lack of expressiveness becomes especially significant in the way men deal with **stress** and depression. Most men tend not to cry and try to keep emotions hidden. They are far less likely to seek psychological counseling than are women. Along with other cultural messages that men need to be strong, powerful, and independent, men are taught not to react to physical, psychological, or spiritual pain. Some men are unwilling to seek health care simply because they fear the risk of appearing "unmanly" (Men's Health Network, 1998).

••••••••••••••••••••••••••••••

I think we have a national crisis of boys in America. For some boys who are not allowed tears, they will cry with their fists or they will cry with bullets.

Dr. William Pollack,
Psychologist, Harvard Medical School, August 20, 1999

••••••••••••••••••••••••••••••

The sociocultural differences between men and women must be considered when planning and developing intervention and prevention programs. Strategies that target the general population may not consider the diversity of expectations and behaviors of men. Although some publicly funded programs may attempt to target as many people as possible, programs with more specifically focused segments or populations may be more effective with men. The nurse must consider the vast number of socialization possibilities that exist within male societies. Health interventions directed toward men may be more effective when men are separated from women, divided into age-specific groups, or grouped into a larger audience. For example, instead of a smoking cessation program for all people, with an emphasis on the long-term effects of smoking, a program targeting men ages 15 to 25, with an emphasis on the sex appeal of nonsmokers, may be more effective.

Environmental Factors

Physical and occupational environments affect the **health status** of men. More men are employed than women, and male-dominated occupations such as mining, construction, and farming are often more hazardous. Accidents on the job are a major contributor to higher death rates among men. In addition, men in these types of occupations are more likely to be exposed to carcinogens and other toxins that are associated with higher rates of pneumoconiosis (black lung), asbestosis, leukemia, and cancer of the bladder. Men's greater exposure to occupational hazards account for about 5% to 10% of the gender difference in mortality (Waldron, 1995).

The high number of men in high-risk employment settings may be advantageous to community health nurses, who can use these environments to introduce men to health care. Prevention and screening programs in the workplace can be effective interventions for men who would not seek health care in other settings.

Behavioral Factors

Unlike genetic factors, behaviors such as diet, tobacco use, alcohol consumption, illicit drug use, lack of physical exercise, physical and sexual risk taking, and suicide and violence are controllable and subject to human influence and intervention. Individuals can make wiser choices such as always wearing their seatbelts; exercising and eating right; not using tobacco, drugs, or alcohol, or at least not driving while under the influence of alcohol or drugs; not bungee jumping; or not committing acts of violence against themselves or others. Partly as a result of the cul-tural expectations of society and the gender socialization process, men's behavior is consistently less healthy than that of women. As a result, behavior is the cause of the largest differences in mortality between men and women (Stillion, 1995).

Data in the United States indicate that men's diets have had higher ratios of saturated to polyunsaturated fat, which contribute to higher ischemic heart disease mortality among men. More males than females smoke cigarettes and drink heavily. Men's smoking habits account for as much as 90% of gender differences in cancer mortality and roughly one-third of gender differences in ischemic heart disease mortality. Similarly, men's drinking contributes to higher mortality in liver disease, accidents, suicide, and homicide (Waldron, 1995).

Diet

Obesity and consumption of fatty foods increase the risk of cardiovascular disease, which is a major killer for men. Men consume a large amount of fatty foods and are less likely than women to change their eating habits, even though more than 33% of men meet the definition of obesity (a body mass index [BMI] of 27.8 kg/m^2). Researchers suggest that low-fat diet programs for men should target work site and peer-group organizations and place emphasis on adapting usual recipes (Coakley, Rimm, Colditz, Kawachi, & Willett, 1998; Nguyen, Otis, & Potvin, 1996).

Tobacco

Gender differences in smoking prevalence have been decreasing for decades, but still more males than females smoke cigarettes. In 1994, 27.8% of males were smokers, compared with 23.3%

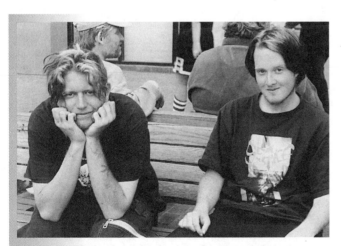

Attitudes about health change during adolescence, and teen males may have needs that go unmet.

CIGARETTE SMOKING IN ADULTS BY EDUCATION AND GENDER, 1994

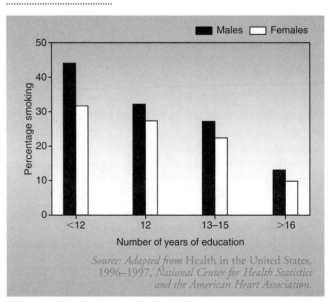

Source: Adapted from Health in the United States, 1996–1997, *National Center for Health Statistics and the American Heart Association.*

of females (American Heart Association, 1998). Smoking is positively correlated with men's higher mortality from bronchitis, emphysema, and asthma.

Men, especially rural men, are more likely to use smokeless (chewing) tobacco. Despite the general declining trends in the use of cigarettes, there has not been a decline in the use of smokeless tobacco. Smokeless tobacco use is associated with higher risks of cardiovascular disease and cancers of the oral cavity, as well as gum recession and nicotine addiction. Heavy marketing efforts by tobacco companies toward rural men might explain the slight increase in the use of smokeless tobacco (Nelson, Tomar, Mowery, & Siegel, 1996).

Alcohol

Alcohol abuse is well known for its devastating effects on physical and emotional health. Not including alcohol-related motor vehicle accidents, there were 20,000 alcohol-related deaths in 1995, and most of the victims were men. More men (68%) drink than women (55%), and men are five times more likely to drink heavily. Higher numbers of male drinkers contribute to males' higher mortality, related to chronic liver disease, cirrhosis of the liver, accidents, and homicide. In addition, male drivers have substantially higher risk of fatal motor vehicle accidents because they are more likely to have high blood alcohol levels (Waldron, 1995).

Alcohol use must be taken into consideration in developing strategies to prevent the transmission of sexually transmitted diseases (STDs), including human immunodeficiency virus (HIV), because alcohol consumption is related to risky sexual behavior. A number of studies have suggested that people who drink more heavily are more likely to have multiple partners, and among young men, consistent use of condoms decreases at higher levels of alcohol use (Graves, 1995). It is estimated that two-thirds of all alcoholics are men; more than 80% of those who have serious drug addictions are men; more than 80% of those who die of drug abuse are men; and 90% of those arrested for alcohol or drug abuse are men.

Suicide and Violence

Deaths by suicide and violence are a predominantly male phenomenon. Approximately four of five deaths by suicide are men. Between the ages of 20 and 24 men are six times more likely to commit suicide than women; and over the age of 85, men are more than 11 times more likely to kill themselves than women (Men's Health Network, 1998). Suicide rates for specific groups of men, such as veterans, divorced men, and homosexual teenagers, are even higher. Researchers argue that men's higher suicide rates are due to men's greater frequency of substance abuse, subjection to more stress, lack of emotional channels, and use of more violent, immediately lethal means of taking their lives in comparison with women.

The world of men is much more violent than that of women. White men are three times more likely to die in a homicide than

white women, and African American men are five times more likely to die in a homicide than black women (Stillion, 1995). The persons at greatest risk for violence victimization, as well as becoming the perpetrators of violence, are young males who are members of underrepresented ethnic groups and live in poor urban communities. In 1991, nearly half of all homicide victims were males 15 to 34 years of age. These young men risk injury to themselves, disrupted personal lives, damaging criminal records, extended imprisonment, and in some cases, capital punishment (DHHS, 1995a).

Much of the violent actions of men are directed at women. In the United States female murder victims are most often killed by their husbands, boyfriends, other male family members, or close male friends (Gerlock, 1997). Violence against women will not cease until greater emphasis is put on prevention and treatment programs for the men who perform the violent acts. The nursing literature that addresses the issue of working with men who batter women and children is almost nonexistent, yet nurses who work in hospitals and community settings deal with the results of domestic violence every day. Because nurses are on the front line, they are in the best position to intervene in ways that are sensitive to both the perpetrators and the victims of family violence. Nurses working in settings such as schools, churches, and work sites can conduct education programs to promote awareness of the potential for family violence (Rynerson & Fishel, 1998).

Healthy People 2010

The purpose of *Healthy People 2010* is to improve the health of Americans with specific objectives in many health-related areas. Selected objectives are listed in the following *Healthy People 2010* box.

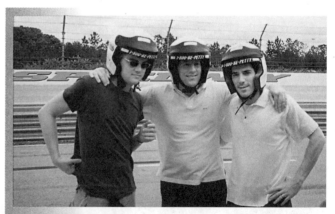

Young males are likely to be involved in risk-taking behavior. However, as role model Leonardo DiCaprio and friends demonstrate, risk can be decreased through the use of protective gear.

HEALTHY PEOPLE 2010

OBJECTIVES RELATED TO MEN'S HEALTH

Cancer

3.2 Reduce the lung cancer death rate.

3.7 Reduce the prostate cancer death rate.

3.10 Increase the proportion of physicians and dentists who counsel their at-risk patients about tobacco use cessation, physical activity, and cancer screening.

Family Planning

9.6 Increase male involvement in pregnancy prevention and family planning efforts.

Heart Disease and Stroke

Heart Disease

12.1 Reduce coronary heart disease deaths.

Stroke

12.7 Reduce stroke deaths.

Blood Pressure

12.8 Reduce the proportion of adults with high blood pressure.

HIV/AIDS

13.2 Reduce the number of new AIDS cases among adolescents and adult men who have sex with men.

13.3 Reduce the number of new AIDS cases among females and males who inject drugs.

13.4 Reduce the number of new AIDS cases among adolescent and adult men who have sex with men and inject drugs.

Injury and Violence Prevention

Unintentional Injury Prevention

15.15 Reduce deaths caused by motor vehicle crashes.

15.21 Increase the proportion of motorcyclists using helmets.

15.22 Increase use of helmets by bicyclists.

Violence and Abuse Prevention

15.32 Reduce homicides.

15.33 Reduce physical fighting among adolescents.

15.34 Reduce weapon carrying by adolescents on school property.

Mental Health and Mental Disorders

Mental Health Status Improvement

18.1 Reduce the suicide rate.

Occupational Safety and Health

20.1 Reduce deaths from work-related injuries.

Substance Abuse

Adverse Consequences of Substance Use and Abuse

26.1 Reduce deaths and injuries caused by alcohol- and drug-related motor vehicle crashes.

26.2 Reduce drug-induced deaths.

Substance Use and Abuse

26.12 Reduce average annual alcohol consumption.

26.13 Reduce steroid use among adolescents.

Tobacco Use

Tobacco Use in Population Groups

27.1 Reduce tobacco use by adults.

27.2 Reduce tobacco use by adolescents.

Source: DHHS, 2000.

Health Care System Utilization

Patterns of health care utilization by men are cited as an important contributor to the inferior health status of men. One-third of American men do not have a checkup every year. Nine million men have not seen a doctor in 5 years (Male Health Center, 1998a). Men visit doctors 25% less often than women. At the same time, men account for 66% of the clients admitted to emergency rooms (Men's Health Network, 1998). Men tend to have fewer contacts with the health care system, perhaps as a result of psychological and sociological factors such as a reluctance to admit that they need assistance. This situation is exacerbated by the fact that the American health care system tends to focus on health from an illness perspective, with relatively little attention paid to prevention. As a result, unlike women who have annual gynecological examinations that include screening for other conditions, men are less likely to enter the health care system for a physical examination on a routine basis. Moreover, although men come in contact with many health care professionals in a wide variety of settings, they have no specialist to whom they can go for their specific care needs. Men have to be to attended by generalists, such as family practitioners, or by other specialists such as urologists who also see women.

Strategies to improve men's utilization of preventive health care must target all ages. Men must establish a committed relationship with preventive health care as early as possible. For men to use preventive health care, programs that present health prevention as masculine and strengthening must be developed and implemented. The required school physical before participation in extracurricular activities may be used in the resocialization of men for the active and lifelong usage of preventive health care.

Ambulatory Care

Of the 860.9 million ambulatory care visits made to physician offices, hospital outpatient departments, and hospital emergency department in 1995, 353.8 million (41.1%) were made by men. This means that men made 153.3 million fewer trips to ambulatory care settings than women. Men have significantly lower rates of visits to physician offices and hospital outpatient departments than women, but the visit rates to hospital emergency departments do not differ by sex. Overall, men made 2.8 visits to ambulatory care settings per person and women made 3.8 visits (Schappert, 1997). This difference is even greater for ages 15 to 24 and 25 to 44.

By age 75, men have had approximately 395 contacts with physicians, whereas women have had about 517 contacts. This discrepancy persists even when the contribution of pregnancy and birth control–related issues is not counted in women's contacts. The patterns in physician contacts indicate that, for all ages, the difference between men and women has been increasing. In 1989, physician contacts were 4.8 per person for men and 5.9 per person for women. By 1992, physician contacts were 5.1 for men and 6.6 for women. In 3 years, the difference in contacts went up by 0.5 visits. Men do not go to the doctor, partly because of fear, denial, embarrassment, and threatened masculinity (Male Health Center, 1998a). Although the total number of physician contacts is lower for men, men are seen more frequently than women for chronic diseases, such as heart and lung disease, which are more prevalent among men.

Hospital Care

Hospitalization rates and length of stays in hospitals vary by sex. Hospital discharge rates, the numbers used to determine usage, from short-stay hospitals are higher for women (138 per 1,000 women) than for men (96 per 1,000). However, in 1995, men had more days of hospital care (5.8 days on the average per person) than women (5 days) (Graves & Owings, 1997). When gynecological disorders in women and reproductive disorders in men are excluded, rates of hospitalization for men are about the same as for women. The lower rate of discharge and longer hospital stays may be due to the fact that when men are hospitalized, their conditions are more severe.

Preventive Care

Men and women differ in their ability to seek preventive care for the early diagnosis of health care problems. Unlike women, who seek routine reproductive health screening, most men do not have routine checkups that would detect health problems at an early stage. Men are more likely to have examinations at the insistence of their employers, and they do not perceive that they need a regular source of care. More often than women, men perceive their health as very good or excellent and therefore may not think that they need to be involved in health promotion activities (Clark, 1999). Women are more likely than men to exhibit stronger health promotion behaviors in terms of blood pressure checks, dental flossing, diet, smoking, drinking, physical activity, weight, and hours of sleep. Men tend to view exercise as sufficient to compensate for unhealthy behaviors such as fatty diets. As a result, men are at greater risk for

ANNUAL RATE OF AMBULATORY CARE VISITS BY CLIENT'S AGE AND GENDER

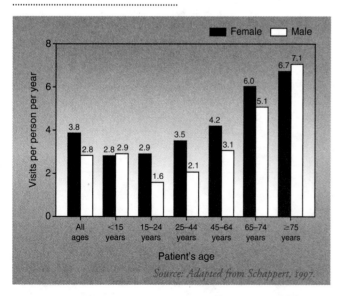

Source: Adapted from Schappert, 1997.

several of the top killers such as heart disease, cancer, suicide, accidents, and violence. Because most of these killers are preventable, changes in eating habits, workplace environments, and educational strategies are needed to improve preventive care for men.

Specific Male Health Issues

Prostate Cancer

The American Cancer Society lists prostate cancer as the second leading cause of cancer death in American men after lung cancer (Brock, 1997; Male Health Center, 1998b). Prostate cancer is most common in men older than 40, and the risk increases with each decade thereafter (Brock, 1997). Most often, prostate cancer is asymptomatic until the disease has progressed. Symptoms that may indicate prostate disease include the following (Male Health Center, 1998b):

- *Difficulty or pain with urination*
- *Painful ejaculation*
- *Blood in urine or semen*

Although prostate cancer is the second leading cause of cancer deaths in American men, how many prostate cancer prevention and awareness campaigns have you seen? Can the same be said for breast cancer? Consider the financial appropriations and expenditures for cancer in the United States detailed in Table 18-1.

Information about the necessity of digital rectal examinations beginning at age 40 for all men, with possible earlier intervention for those with signs and symptoms of problems or a positive family history, must be included and incorporated into health fairs and promotions. Information related to prostate-specific antigen (PSA) blood testing that is used in conjunction with the digital rectal examination should also be provided. In 1986, the U.S. Food and Drug Administration approved the PSA test for prostate cancer screening. Many physicians believe that the subsequent fall in prostate cancer mortality rates can be

FYI

Several high-profile men came forward in the 1990s to talk about their experiences with prostate cancer in an effort to remove the embarrassment surrounding the disease. As a result of the openness of men like former U.S. Senator and presidential candidate Bob Dole, professional golfer Arnold Palmer, and retired General H. Norman Schwarzkopf, many books and journal articles appeared and support groups surfaced all over the country.

attributed to early diagnosis with PSA testing (Feuer & Merrill, 1999). The importance of the procedure and information regarding signs, symptoms, and the screening process should be emphasized in promotions. Nurses should also include written information for distribution because some men are ill at ease discussing the procedure and testing in public.

The community health nurse can also organize targeted prostate-specific screenings, during which the men actually have the digital rectal examination and PSA blood tests. In a study that explored the relationship between attitudes toward digital rectal examinations and prostate screening among African American men, the results revealed that fear of the procedure did not prevent men from participating in the screening (Gelfand, Parzuchowski, Cort, & Powell, 1995).

Testicular Cancer

Testicular cancer accounts for only 1% of all cancers in men (National Cancer Institute, 1998; Walbrecker, 1995). However, testicular cancer is the most common form of cancer in men between the ages of 20 and 34 (Brock, Fox, Gosling, Haney, Kneebone, Nagy, & Qualitza, 1993; Clore, 1993; DHHS, 1995b; National Cancer Institute, 1998; Peate, 1997; Rosella, 1994; Walbrecker,

---

TABLE 18-1   **BREAST VERSUS PROSTATE CANCER EXPENDITURES**

	BREAST	**PROSTATE**
National Cancer Institute research	$1.8 billion	$376 million
Department of Defense research	$455 million	$20 million
U.S. government:		
Per person diagnosed	$3,000	$250
Per death	$12,000	$2,000

Jaffe, 1997.

1995). It is the second most common cancer for men between the ages of 35 and 39 and the third most common for men between the ages of 15 and 19 (National Cancer Institute, 1998). This type of cancer is 4.5 times more common among Caucasian men than African American men (DHHS, 1995b; National Cancer Institute, 1998), with rates for Hispanics/Latinos, Native Americans, and Asians falling somewhere in between (National Cancer Institute, 1998).

. . . .

I'm prouder of being a cancer survivor than I am of winning the Tour de France. If I never had cancer, I never would have won the Tour de France. I'm convinced of that. I wouldn't want to do it all over again, but I wouldn't change a thing.

Lance Armstrong,
winner of the Tour de France (21-day, 2287-mile bicycle race) and testicular cancer survivor (Montville, 1999)

. . . .

Epidemiological data show an increase in the incidence of testicular cancer over the past 20 years (Clore, 1993; Koshti-Richman, 1996). As recent as the early 1980s, testicular cancer was fatal (Brock et al., 1993) for 8 of 10 clients (Walbrecker, 1995). But today, because of advances in chemotherapy and improved surgical techniques (Brakey, 1994; Brock et al., 1993), testicular cancer is one of the most curable forms of cancer (Rosella, 1994). Testicular cancer has a nearly 100% cure rate with early detection and treatment (Brakey, 1994; Clore, 1993; Peate, 1997; Rosella, 1994; Walbrecker, 1995). This optimistic prognosis with early intervention makes testicular self-examination (TSE) a critical component of health teaching for young men (American Family Physician, 1999; Rosella, 1994; Walbrecker, 1995), especially because most cases of testicular cancer are found by the clients themselves (National Cancer Institute, 1998). Boys should begin TSE around age 13 and make it a lifelong practice because, although testicular cancer is most likely to occur before the age of 40, it can occur at any age. In fact, the incidence rises again after the age of 70 (Brakey, 1994).

The characteristics that put men at higher risk for testicular cancer include Caucasian race, young age, high socioeconomic status, or family history, as well as having a mother who took estrogen during her pregnancy (Brakey, 1994; Kinkade, 1999). Males with undescended testicles or late descending testicles (after age 6) have a 3 to 17 times higher than average risk for developing testicular cancer (National Cancer Institute, 1998; Walbrecker, 1995). Despite this information, the health education literature suggests that most of the men who are most susceptible to testicular cancer are unaware of the signs and symptoms of the disease and how to detect them (Rosella, 1994). Research has indicated that although information has been readily available to young women regarding breast self-examination (BSE) and the importance of regular Pap smears, the information related to TSE has not been as widely communicated (Turner, 1995; Walker, 1993).

Nurses are in the best position to provide young men with the information to learn the self-examination techniques needed for early detection and cure (Peate, 1997; Walbrecker, 1995). TSE education and screening programs can be set up in high schools and presented simultaneously with BSE and screening programs. Models can be used for practicing self-examination with lifelike lumps and abnormalities to teach young men what they should be looking for. Testicular examination and TSE education should be part of every routine physical examination for adolescent and young adult males. Instructions for self-examination of the testicles are given in Box 18-1.

The only way a positive diagnosis of testicular cancer can be made is through surgical removal (orchiectomy) of the affected testicle for direct examination (Henkel, 1996; Walbrecker, 1995). Because testicular cancer occurs most often in men of reproductive age, **fertility** is a major concern. Although sperm count may be lowered, a unilateral orchiectomy usually does not affect sexual function or fertility (Brakey, 1994; Henkel, 1996; Walbrecker, 1995). However, abnormalities in the remaining

---

BOX 18-1 TESTICULAR SELF-EXAMINATION

- Self-examination should be done once a month after a warm bath or shower because heat relaxes the scrotum and loosens the skin, making the testes easier to examine.

- Visually inspect the scrotum for any swelling or changes in color.

- Examine each testicle with both hands by placing the index and middle fingers under the testicle with the thumbs placed on top. Roll the testicle gently between the fingers and thumbs, feeling for any changes such as lumps, swelling, or painful spots.

- The first sign of testicular cancer is usually a hard, painless lump about the size of a pea. However, if there are any kinds of changes or abnormalities, immediately notify your health care provider, because only he or she can make a positive diagnosis.

Sources: Adapted from American Family Physician, 1999; Henkel, 1996; & Walbrecker, 1995.

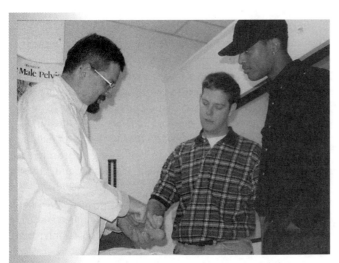

Chapter author, Joseph Farmer, uses a model to teach young men how to do a testicular self-examination.

testicle or the effects of radiation and chemotherapy may have adverse effects on sexual function and fertility (Brakey, 1994), although studies have shown that many men recover fertility within 2 to 3 years after chemotherapy (Henkel, 1996).

A Conversation With...

I love my job. I absolutely love what I do. Cancer controls your life, and I didn't want cancer to take me off the ice.

Shock and fear are the first two things that you feel. Then you feel a feeling of anxious desperation. And then when the diagnosis was complete, and I heard there was a treatment, it was non-stop humor. My goal is to find a way to laugh every day.

For people with testicular cancer that are going through their treatments and challenges, feel fortunate that there is a treatment. Understand that it will be a hard episode in your life. Understand that the treatment will try to defeat you and damage your spirit. But you can fight back and win.

—Scott Hamilton,
Olympic Figure Skating Champion
and Testicular Cancer Survivor
Source: A chat with Scott Hamilton
(excerpts from a chat on ABC News:
http://vix.com/menmag/tcschotth.htm.)

Erectile Dysfunction (Impotence)

Many sexual topics are now discussed openly, but **erectile dysfunction** is still a subject that causes fear and anxiety for many men and women (Male Health Center, 1998c). Although a significant amount of scientific data is available about erectile dysfunction (also called *impotence*), large segments of the public, including health care professionals, are still uninformed, or even worse, misinformed. A lack of accurate information, as well as reluctance on the part of many health care providers to deal openly with sexual issues, has left many clients without a source of help for their sexual concerns. Improving both public and professional knowledge and attaining a comfort level in talking about erectile dysfunction will provide both men and their sexual partners with an avenue for obtaining needed information and effective treatment (NIH, 1992).

What Is Erectile Dysfunction?

Erectile dysfunction is the inability to achieve or maintain a penile erection sufficient for sexual intercourse. About 15 million American men suffer from erectile dysfunction, and the incidence increases with age. Approximately 5% of men experience erectile dysfunction by the age of 40, increasing to between 15% and 25% by the age of 65 (National Kidney and Urologic Disease Information Clearinghouse, 1998). Erectile dysfunction is often assumed to be a normal part of the aging process, but that assumption is incorrect (Male Health Center, 1998d; National Kidney and Urologic Diseases Clearinghouse, 1998; NIH, 1992). In fact, sex researchers Masters and Johnson discovered that although sexual activity slows down with advancing age, it does not end. Several reports indicate that most men and women between the ages of 50 and 60 are still interested in remaining sexually active (Male Health Center, 1998c, 1998d).

Causes

Most cases of erectile dysfunction have a physical cause such as disease, injury, or drug side effects. Diabetes mellitus, kidney disease, multiple sclerosis, atherosclerosis, chronic alcoholism, hypertension, and vascular disease account for approximately 70% of all cases of erectile dysfunction. Of men with diabetes mellitus, 35% to 50% experience erectile dysfunction (National Kidney and Urologic Diseases Information Clearinghouse, 1998; NIH, 1992). Various kinds of surgeries are also associated with increased incidence of erectile dysfunction. The most common are surgeries that can cause injury to nerves and arteries near the penis. These include surgeries for prostate, colon, rectal, and bladder cancers. Vascular surgery can also be high risk. Many common medications list erectile dysfunction as a side effect, including drugs used to treat hypertension, antihistamines, antidepressants, sedatives, tranquilizers, appetite suppressants, and pain medications (Male Health Center, 1998c; National Kidney and Urologic Disease Information Clearinghouse, 1998; NIH, 1992). Smoking has also been shown to have an adverse effect on

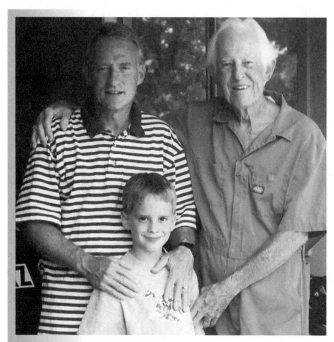

Men with at least two close relatives with prostate cancer have a very high risk of developing the disease before the age of 70. Men with a family history of prostate cancer should have PSA screenings and prostate examinations between the ages of 50 and 70.

erectile function by increasing the effects of other risk factors such as vascular disease or hypertension. Vasectomy, however, has not been associated with increased risk for erectile dysfunction (NIH, 1992).

In 10% to 20% of cases of erectile dysfunction the cause is deemed to be psychological. Factors such as stress, anxiety, guilt, depression, low self-esteem, and fear of sexual failure can cause erectile dysfunction without the presence of any physical problems or can be secondary reactions to underlying physical causes (National Kidney and Urologic Disease Information Clearinghouse, 1998; NIH, 1992). Important facts that should be emphasized when counseling a man and his sexual partner about erectile dysfunction include the following (Male Health Center, 1998c):

- *Most men experience erectile dysfunction related to stress or alcohol at some time in their lives.*

- *Past sexual practices, including masturbation, do not cause erectile dysfunction.*

- *Physical disorders can directly affect sexual functioning.*

- *An occasional problem with erectile dysfunction does not mean a chronic problem will develop.*

- *A man can sabotage his ability to have an erection by worrying about it.*

Treatment

Treatment varies according to the severity and cause of the dysfunction. Health care providers start with the least invasive treatment and progress to more invasive treatments until erectile dysfunction is corrected. Reducing the dosage or eliminating drugs that may be causing erectile dysfunction is the first step. Psychotherapy and behavior modifications are next. Vacuum devices, oral drugs, drugs injected into the urethra, and finally surgically implanted penile devices or vascular surgery are offered as treatment if the problem persists (National Kidney and Urologic Disease Information Clearinghouse, 1998; NIH, 1992).

In 1998, a new "wonder drug" called *sildenafil citrate* (commonly known as **Viagra**) was approved by the U.S. Food and Drug Administration. Viagra is taken 1 hour before sexual intercourse and works by boosting the effects of nitric oxide, a chemical produced by the body to relax smooth muscle in the penis and allow increased blood flow during sexual stimulation. This drug does not trigger automatic erection as other drugs used to treat erectile dysfunction do, but rather just allows the man to respond to sexual stimulation (National Kidney and Urologic Disease Information Clearinghouse, 1998). The drug is very successful in treating many forms of erectile dysfunction, although some fear the drug may be overused by middle-aged and older men who may not actually suffer from erectile dysfunction but just want to "boost" their sex lives.

Role of the Community Health Nurse

The most important things the community health nurse can do for men with erectile dysfunction are to provide accurate and easily understandable information and to encourage the man and his sex partner to talk openly and comfortably about the problem. Including the man's sex partner in the discussion acknowledges his or her importance in the relationship. The partner may also have questions, doubts, and insecurities that need to be addressed. Many persons whose partners are impotent blame themselves for the problem. The partner may also feel hurt and angry because the male has withdrawn physically and emotionally. Understanding that he or she is not to blame can go a long way in enabling the partner to support the diagnosis and treatment (Male Health Center, 1998c). It is important for the nurse to be sensitive to the needs of clients whose values or sexual orientation may be different from the nurse. Not all partners of male clients will be their wives. In fact, some of the sex partners of male clients may also be male. Whatever the relationship of the partners, all couples should be treated with dignity and respect.

Cardiovascular Disease

Cardiovascular disease is the single greatest cause of death in men. Approximately 1 in 3 male deaths is related to cardiovascular disease. Similarly, more than one-third of men dying between the ages of 45 and 65 die of a heart attack. Cardiovascular disease is caused by the accumulation of fatty deposits within the artery wall that causes stiffness and reduced blood flow. When the brain interprets reduced blood flow as low blood pressure, it sends a signal to the heart to compensate. The heart works faster with less rest and increases the pressure on each contraction. Normal blood pressures for men range from 120/70 to 150/80 depending on age. With severe hardening of the arteries, blood pressure may increase to 200/100 mm Hg (Men's Health Network, 1998). Although there are many explanations for higher cardiovascular disease rates among men than women, research points to two major factors:

1. *Men's diets have higher ratios of saturated to polyunsaturated fat, which contributes to cardiovascular disease.*

2. *Men's sociocultural environments lead to higher levels of stress, which contributes to cardiovascular disease.*

Cardiovascular disease and hypertension can often be prevented by changes in behavior, including stopping smoking, increasing activity, and improving diet. Community health nurses can design educational programs that target men to promote behavior changes that reduce the risk of cardiovascular disease. These recommendations may include the following:

- *Losing weight*
- *Reducing salt intake*
- *Quitting smoking*
- *Eating foods rich in natural sources of fiber and antioxidant vitamins*
- *Exercising*
- *Relaxing*

RESEARCH BRIEF

Johnson, J. V., Stewart, W., Hall, E. H., Fredlund, P., & Theorell, T. (1996). Long-term psychosocial work environment and cardiovascular mortality among Swedish men. American Journal of Public Health, 86, 324–331.

A sample of 12,517 Swedish men were studied over 14 years to examine the effect of cumulative exposure to work organization (in terms of psychological demands, work control, and social support) on cardiovascular disease mortality. The study identified 521 deaths from cardiovascular disease. Using a nested case-control design, work environment scores were assigned to cases and controls by linking lifetime job histories with a job exposure matrix. Cardiovascular mortality risk in relation to work exposure after adjustment for age, year last employed, smoking, exercise, education, social class, nationality, and physical job demands was analyzed. The results of the study indicated that workers who had combined work exposure to low control and low support had higher risks for cardiovascular disease mortality.

In addition, consumption of moderate amounts of alcohol and sexual activity are associated with reduced risks of cardiovascular disease (Men's Health Network, 1998).

Selected At-Risk Populations
Men with HIV/AIDS

According to the Centers for Disease Control and Prevention (CDC, 1998a), by 1994 AIDS had become a leading cause of death in the United States for men between the ages of 25 and 44. With the introduction of new medications in recent years, AIDS-related death rates have steadily declined, but the incidence of new HIV cases continues to rise (CDC, 1998b). AIDS has historically been viewed in the United States as a disease targeting a specific population—homosexual men. Although the initial cases in the United States, Canada, Australia, and Western Europe were found among this population, this was not the case for the rest of the world. After two decades of the pandemic, many still view HIV/AIDS as something that will not affect them. As a result of this apathy, the safer sexual practices adopted in the homosexual communities have not been applied as readily in heterosexual communities. High-risk behaviors, such as alcohol and drug use and unprotected sex with numerous partners, continue to put heterosexual men at risk. Heterosexual transmission rates continue to escalate, especially in the African American and Hispanic communities, where 41% of all new reported cases are found (CDC, 1997).

The introduction of new medications has reduced the number of AIDS-related deaths, which can be interpreted to mean persons with HIV are living longer. What does this mean to younger men? An entire generation of sexually active men has never known of a world without HIV or AIDS. To some, this may be interpreted as, "Why bother to protect myself, because I can always take the medications." Some are applying safer sexual practices haphazardly, thus allowing the introduction of drug-resistant strains of HIV into their bodies. To others, especially an alarming number of young homosexual men, the principle of "I'd rather die young and beautiful" applies. Intervention and prevention programs must address these issues and concerns. The community health nurse's best option would include the education of young men who would act as role models for their peers.

What does the increase in HIV cases within the African American and Hispanic communities mean to the community health nurse? Intervention and prevention programs need to specifically target these communities. The church is an institution generally accepted as having a powerful influence within both of these communities. By securing the commitment from religious leaders and their congregations, the community health nurse can create positive change from within the system. Developing role models and implementing prevention programs that utilize members of the community results in much more effective outcomes.

For example, the community health nurse working within a community often develops a relationship with community

CASE STUDY

You are a nurse working in a community clinic. One of your clients is Rick Fernandez, a 34-year-old married man who complains about fever and swollen glands. Fearing the possibility of HIV, you ask Rick the typical textbook questions to assess his HIV risk behaviors: You ask if he uses intravenous drugs, if he has had any blood transfusions, if he has sex with men, and if he is homosexual. He responds with a no to all questions. Based on his replies, you do not pursue HIV testing. When he comes back a few months later with complaints of recurrent skin lesions, you again ask about his HIV risk behaviors and receive the same answers as before. Rick insists that he is a happily married man in a monogamous relationship and does not use any sort of drugs. Rick seems offended by your questions. You approach the physician and ask if he has considered testing Rick for HIV. The physician has assessed the risk behaviors and concluded that Rick does not have any of the risk factors associated with HIV. When Rick returns to the clinic for a third visit, you are more assertive and convince Rick to have an HIV test. The test comes back positive. Rick reveals to the HIV counselor that he had been imprisoned a while back and that his only potential exposure to HIV might have been through another inmate who raped him.

1. What is your reaction to Rick's situation?
2. Do you feel that your personal beliefs and values influenced your reaction?
3. Why do you think Rick did not disclose the key information earlier?
4. What could you have done to obtain the accurate information?
5. What specific questions could you have asked Rick to obtain this information?

members. Once a trusting relationship has been established, the nurse can approach some of the unofficial leaders within the community to enlist their support and discuss strategies and objectives to decrease the epidemic of infection affecting the population. This needs to be done in a nonjudgmental manner, in which the nurse details the problems and possible solutions without passing blame or creating fear. By enlisting the members' support in the initial stages, the nurse can formulate plans and develop goals that are perceived as important to the community, thus securing support for the intervention.

Homosexual Men and Families

The special needs of homosexual men include more than just HIV/AIDS education. Homosexual men and their families exist in virtually every community, regardless of how restrictive or liberal the community proclaims to be. However, societal stigmatization of **homosexuality** forces many to remain "in the closet" (Giger & Davidhizar, 1995). Homosexual myths and stereotypes abound, particularly in cultures that value male dominance or masculinity. Homosexual men and their sexual practices run the entire spectrum, just as in the heterosexual community. Also, homosexual men may be married or have children, live alone or with a partner. Individuals define who makes up their family group, not nurses or institutions.

The community health nurse's role in interactions with any group of men is inclusion instead of exclusion. Nurses should ask questions in such a manner that the man does not feel obligated to give an answer he believes the nurse expects. When using such

items as risk assessments, questions should be phrased in a general manner. For example, the nurse should ask about "the number of sexual partners" instead of "the number of women." Nurses should maintain a nonjudgmental tone and manner throughout all interactions. Just as in any interaction, including the entire family whenever possible is recommended. By developing a trusting and honest relationship, the nurse can be instrumental in generating assistance and implementing change of unsafe or risky behaviors.

Community Health Nursing Roles

The community health nurse assumes a wide range of duties and responsibilities while providing health care to men. A typical week could include hundreds of miles traveled, diverse teaching methods and strategies, and numerous new encounters. Community health nursing roles may include client advocate, educator, and facilitator.

Client Advocate

As a client advocate, the role of the community health nurse includes interfacing with health care providers and health care agencies to support the best care for the client. For instance, a nurse realizes that a recently diagnosed HIV-positive man has been prescribed AZT alone, rather than the more effective cocktail combination medications. A proper assessment must be made to determine whether alternative medications could have been prescribed. With the permission of the client, the nurse can contact the appropriate health care provider and discuss the client's options with a nonthreatening and nonjudgmental stance to allow for future interactions. Any new information must be shared with the client.

Educator

The role of a health educator for men can often be challenging. Education can occur in any setting from the stockyards to the corporate boardroom. Safety issues, violence, diet, and physical exercise are examples of topics that may be addressed. The community health nurse must customize education efforts to the specific needs of the clients. The first step involves a correct assessment of the educational needs of the individuals. The nurse determines the level of the learners to ensure that the level of the educational program is neither too low nor too high for the specific group. Providing educational programs for men in their own environments requires versatility and flexibility.

Facilitator

The community health nurse as facilitator brings various people and groups together to talk about issues and needs. The most significant facilitator role involves helping people and groups of different views to reach a compromise so that they can find a common ground to solve problems and bring about positive changes to alleviate a specific community health problem. For instance, a community health nurse, as the facilitator, may initiate positive change through programs with specific targeted groups such as adolescent boys. This can be accomplished by teaching safer sexual practices to prevent STDs and teenage pregnancies by bringing together parents, school administrators, politicians, health care providers, and teens.

Men's Health Research Issues

Despite the advances in medical technology and research, men still continue to live an average of 7 years less than women. Although most medical research was historically based on men, men's health issues no longer dominate the research agenda because of recent federal mandates. Research on men's health must focus on the areas where prevention, early detection, and treatment efforts will significantly improve the quality of life of men across the life span. Table 18-2 includes some priority areas of research on men's health issues.

In addition, research studies must be more inclusive and utilize subjects that represent the diversity within the male population. Studies need to report findings based not only on middle-aged, middle class, Caucasian males, but also on other males representing various ethnic and socioeconomic groups.

TABLE 18-2   MEN'S HEALTH RESEARCH PRIORITIES

RESEARCH AREA	JUSTIFICATION FOR RESEARCH PRIORITY
Prostate cancer	The likelihood that a man will develop prostate cancer is 1 in 11; one-third of the cases are expected to die from the disease; the death rate for prostate cancer has grown at almost twice the death rate of breast cancer in the last decade.
Testicular cancer	It is one of the most common cancers in men aged 15–34, and, when detected early, has an 87% survival rate.
Lung disease	85% of the cases are expected to die from the disease.
Colon cancer	Nearly one-third of the cases are expected to die from the disease.
African American men	Highest incidence of prostate cancer in the United States.
Drunk driving and other alcohol-related problems	Men are seven times as likely as women to be arrested for drunk driving and three times as likely to be alcoholics.
Health promotion	Significant numbers of male related health problems such as prostate cancer, testicular cancer, infertility, and colon cancer, could be detected and treated if men's awareness of these problems was more pervasive. Women visit the doctor more often than men, enabling them to detect health problems in their early stages.

Adapted from 103d Congress H. B. Res. 209 As introduced in the house.

CONCLUSION

Men's health care is not easily defined as a single issue with a limited focus or target population. Although men constitute half the population, their needs and health system utilization vary greatly from those of women. Issues faced by men must be addressed to improve their overall health and decrease the variance in life expectancy between men and women.

The community health nurse can be instrumental in securing access to and promoting the utilization of health care by men. Health promotion and screening programs can be implemented with specifically targeted groups of men. The community health nurse also assumes the roles of client advocate, educator, and facilitator to secure the most advantageous outcomes for the improvement of men's health.

CRITICAL THINKING ACTIVITIES

1. *Smoking is a behavior issue that plays an important role in the reduction of the length and quality of life of men. As a community health nurse, what programs would you develop to improve this situation? What groups would you specifically target? How would you most effectively implement your plans?*

2. *Based on the information provided regarding men's utilization of preventive health care, what would be the most effective intervention(s) to ensure participation? Where should the intervention(s) be implemented? How would the intervention(s) be modified to address differences in age, religion, education, or socioeconomic status?*

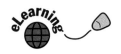 Explore Community Health Nursing on the web! To learn more about the topics in this chapter, access your exclusive web site: http://communitynursing.jbpub.com

REFERENCES

Adami, H., Bergstrom, R., Holmberg, L., Klareskog, L., Perrson, I., & Ponten, J. (1990). The effect of female sex hormones on cancer survival: A register-based study in patients younger than 20 years at diagnosis. *The Journal of the American Medical Association, 263*(16), 2189–2193.

American Family Physician. (1999, May 1). Testicular cancer—What to look for. *American Family Physician, 59*(9), 2549–2550.

American Heart Association (AHA). (1998). *Risk Factors*: www.amhrt.org/Scientific/Hsstats98/08rskfct.html.

Brakey, M. R. (1994, September). Myths and facts . . . About testicular cancer. *Nursing, 24.*

Brock, D. L. (1997). Male genital cancers. In C. Varricchio (Ed.), *A cancer source book for nurses* (7th ed., pp. 327–334). Atlanta: American Cancer Society.

Brock, D., Fox, S., Gosling, G., Haney, L., Kneebone, P., Nagy, C., & Qualitza, B. (1993). Testicular cancer. *Seminars in Oncology Nursing, 9*(4), 224–236.

Centers for Disease Control and Prevention (CDC). (1998a). *Trends in the HIV/AIDS epidemic.* Washington, DC: Department of Health and Human Services.

Centers for Disease Control and Prevention (CDC). (1998b, April 24). Diagnosis and reporting of HIV and AIDS in states with integrated HIV and AIDS surveillance—United States, January 1994–June 1997. *Morbidity and Mortality Weekly Report*, pp. 309–315.

Centers for Disease Control and Prevention (CDC). (1997, February 28). Update: Trends in AIDS incidence, deaths, and prevalence—United States, 1996. *Morbidity and Mortality Weekly Report*, pp. 165–173.

Clark, M. J. (1999). *Nursing in the community* (3rd ed.). Stamford, CT: Appleton & Lange.

Clore, E. R. (1993). A guide for the testicular self-examination. *Journal of Pediatric Health Care, 7*(6), 264–268.

Coakley, E.H., Rimm, E. B., Colditz, G., Kawachi, I., & Willet, W. (1998). Predictors of weight change in men: Results from the Health Professionals Follow Up Study. *International Journal of Obesity, 22,* 89–96.

Department of Health and Human Services (DHHS). (1995a). Counseling to prevent youth violence. In *Guide to clinical preventive services: Report of the U. S. Preventive Services Task Force* (pp. 687–698). Washington, DC: U.S. Government Printing Office.

Department of Health and Human Services (DHHS). (1995b). Screening for testicular cancer. In *Guide to clinical preventive services: Report of the U. S. Preventive Services Task Force* (pp. 153–157). Washington, DC: U.S. Government Printing Office.

Department of Health and Human Services (DHHS). (1991). *Healthy people 2000: National health promotion and disease prevention objectives.* Washington, DC: U.S. Government Printing Office.

Fackelmann, K. (1998). An enzymatic sex difference. *Science News, 153*(13), 204.

Fareed, A. (1994). Equal rights for men. *Nursing Times, 90*(5), 26–29.

Feuer, E. J., & Merrill, R. M. (1999). Cancer surveillance series: Interpreting trends in prostate cancer—Part II: Cause of death misclassification and the recent rise and fall in prostate cancer mortality. *Journal of the National Cancer Institute, 91*(12), 1025–1032.

Gelfand, D. E., Parzuchowski, J., Cort, M., & Powell, I. (1995). Digital rectal examinations and prostate cancer screening: Attitudes of African American men. *Oncology Nursing Forum, 22,* 1253–1255.

Gerlock, A. A. (1997). New directions in the treatment of men who batter women. *Health Care for Women International, 18,* 481–493.

Giger, J., & Davidhizar, R. (1995). *Transcultural nursing: Assessment and intervention.* St Louis: Mosby.

Graves, E. J., & Owings, M. F. (1997). 1995 summary: National hospital discharge survey. *Advance Data Form Vital and Health Statistics,* p. 291.

Graves, K. L. (1995). Risky sexual behavior and alcohol use among young adults: Results from a national survey. *American Journal of Health Promotion, 10*(1), 27–36.

Helman, C. G. (1994). *Culture, health, and illness* (3rd ed.). London: Butterworth-Heinemann.

Henkel, J. (1996, January/February). Testicular cancer: Survival high with early treatment. *FDA Consumer:* www.vix.com.

Jaffe, H. (1997, September). Dying for dollars. *Men's Health*, p. 134.

Johnson, J. V., Stewart, W., Hall, E.H., Fredlund, P., & Theorell, T. (1996). Long-term psychological work environment and cardiovascular mortality among Swedish men. *American Journal of Public Health, 86*(3), 324–331.

Kinkade, S. (1999, May 1). Testicular cancer. *American Family Physician, 59*(9), 2539–2544.

Koshti-Richman, A. (1996). The role of nurses in promoting testicular self-examination. *Nursing Times, 92*(33), 40–41.

Male Health Center. (1998a). *Why men don't go to the doctor?* www.malehealthcenter.com.

Male Health Center. (1998b). *What do various symptoms mean?* www.malehealthcenter.com.

Male Health Center. (1998c). *How erections really happen*: www.malehealthcenter.com.

Male Health Center. (1998d). *Getting older and having sex*: www.malehealthcenter.com.

Men's Health Network. (1998). *National campaign to significantly improve male health and longevity*: www.menshealthnetwork.org.

Montville, L. (1999, August 9). Tour de Amerique. *Sports Illustrated, 91*(5), 68–72.

National Cancer Institute. (1998). *Screening for testicular cancer*: www.cancernet.nci.nih.gov.

National Institutes of Health (NIH). (1992, December 7–9). Impotence. *NIH Consensus Statement, 10*(4), 1–31: www.text.nlm.nih.gov.

National Kidney and Urologic Disease Information Clearinghouse. (1998). *Impotence*: www.niddk.nih.gov.

Nelson, D. E., Tomar, S. L., Mowery, P., & Siegel, P. Z. (1996). Trends in smokeless tobacco use among men in four states, 1988 through 1993. *American Journal of Public Health, 86*(9), 1300–1303.

Nguyen, M. N., Otis, J., & Potvin, L. (1996). Determinants of intention to adopt a low-fat diet in men 30 to 60 years old: Implications for heart health promotion. *American Journal of Health Promotion, 10*(3), 201–207.

Peate, I. (1997). Clinical. Testicular cancer. The importance of effective health education. *British Journal of Nursing, 6*(6), 311–316.

Rosella, J. D. (1994). Testicular cancer health education: An integrative review. *Journal of Advanced Nursing, 20*(4), 666–671.

Rynerson, B. C., & Fishel, A. H. (1998). Expressions of men who batter: Implications for nursing. *Journal of the American Psychiatric Nurses Association, 4*(2), 41–47.

Sabo, D., & Gordon, D. F. (1995). Rethinking men's health and illness. In D. Sabo & D. F. Gordon (Eds.), *Men's health and illness: Gender, power, and the body* (p. 21). London: Sage Publications.

Schappert, S. M. (1997). Ambulatory care visits to physician offices, hospital outpatient departments, and emergency departments: United States 1995. *Vital Health Statistics, 13*(129).

Stillion, J. (1995). Premature death among males. In D. Sabo & D. F. Gordon (Eds.), *Men's health and illness: Gender, power, and the body* (pp. 47–67). London: Sage Publications.

Tanne, J. H. (1997). Medicine's new motto: One sex does not fit all. *American Health For Women, 16*(5), 54–58.

Torres, J. B. (1998). Masculinity and gender roles among Puerto Rican men: Machismo on the US mainland. *American Journal of Orthopsychiatry, 68*(1), 16–26.

Turner, D. (1995). Testicular cancer and the value of self-examination. *Nursing Times, 91*(1), 30–31.

Walbrecker, J. (1995, January). Start talking about testicular cancer. *RN*, pp. 34–35.

Waldron, I. (1995). Contributions of changing gender differences in behavior and social roles to changing gender differences in mortality. In D. Sabo & D. F. Gordon (Eds.), *Men's health and illness: Gender, power, and the body* (pp. 22–35). London: Sage Publications.

Walker, R. (1993). Modeling and guided practice as components within a comprehensive testicular self-examination educational program for high school males. *Journal of Health Education, 24*(3), 162–168.

Weil, M. D., Lamborn, K., Edwards, M. S. B., & Wara, W. M. (1998). Influence of a child's sex on medulloblastoma outcome. *The Journal of the American Medical Association, 279*(18), 1474–1476.

Chapter 19

Women's Health

Norma G. Cuellar, Karen Saucier Lundy, and Venus Callahan

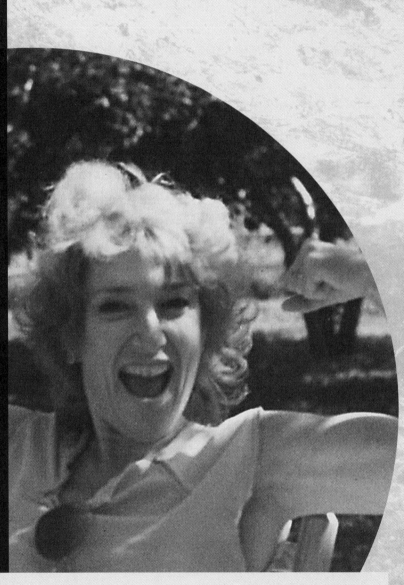

Women now live an average of 30 years longer than they did 100 years ago. A woman born in 1900 was expected to live 49 years; today's baby girl can expect a life span of 79 years. Significant changes and increased opportunities in the lives of American women have broadened the focus of women's health to include physiological, emotional, social, cultural, and economic well-being.

QUESTIONS TO CONSIDER

After reading this chapter, answer the following questions:
1. How are demographic variables related to women's health status?
2. As women age, what specific health concerns and issues are most prevalent?
3. What are special health concerns of lesbians, women of color, and elder women?
4. What are the special ethical issues related to health that concern women?
5. What populations of women are more vulnerable to health risks?
6. How can nurses provide preventive-based care to the diverse population of women in the promotion of health?
7. What are sources of empowerment for women related to improved health?
8. What future issues will likely influence the health of women?

KEY TERMS

Caregivers
Commission on the Status of Women
Constructed knowledge
Empowerment

Feminism
Feminization of poverty
Heterosexism
Homophobia

Hormone replacement therapy
Mammography
Perimenopausal period
Procedural knowledge

United Nations Platforms for Action for Women
Urinary incontinence
World Conference on Women

For much of the 20th century, women's health focused almost exclusively on reproductive functions such as menstruation, childbearing, and menopause. In 1990, a landmark report by the General Accounting Office (GAO) revealed shocking gaps in research on women's health issues. During the 20th century, women had been left out of most research on cancer, heart disease, and interventions, such as the development of new technology and medications. Such inequities resulted in women's health being considerably behind in advances known to benefit men (Allen & Phillip, 1997).

In the 1990s, the federal government mobilized the greatest effort ever to improve women's health through research and services. We now have better and safer **mammography** and breast cancer treatment, more effective ways to prevent and treat osteoporosis, and we know more about alternatives for women during the **perimenopausal period**. As the lives of women have been extended, chronic diseases and disabilities have taken the place of acute illness and childbirth as leading causes of death. Women are living longer lives, challenging community health nurses to help women improve the quality of these added years.

Women, as the primary **caregivers** of families, are key to achieving the goal of healthy communities. However, women face significant barriers in gaining access to health care. Often, inadequate education and low socioeconomic status prevent women from assuming the responsibilities of their own health and well-being. As consumers of health services, women must be involved in the development of health policy to achieve parity in availability and access to health care resources for women. Community health nurses play key roles in collaborating with women to achieve the national goal of health care for all. This chapter provides information about the context of women's health and how community health nurses can assist women of all ages to meet health needs.

Demographic Profile of Women's Health

Population Characteristics

Currently, 84% of women in the United States are Caucasian (Phillips, Sexton, & Blackman, 1996). In subsequent generations, however, the racial and ethnic diversity of women is expected to increase markedly. The mean age for women in the

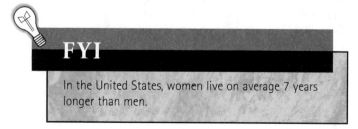

FYI

In the United States, women live on average 7 years longer than men.

United States is currently 34 years. As baby boomers begin to age, the care of the elderly population, who will be predominantly women, will have a significant impact on health care.

Proportion of Women

The U.S. Census Bureau (1999) reports a ratio at birth of 105 males to 100 females. However, in most countries, women typically have longer life spans than men and consequently make up 52% of the world's population. In the United States, the average life span for a woman is 78.6, compared with 72.3 for men. Because males are more likely to die at any given age, the proportion of females to males increases over the life span (U.S. Census Bureau, 1997). This fact should alert the community health nurse that special needs for the elderly may predominately center around women's gerontological issues.

* * *

We grow neither better nor worse as we get old, but more like ourselves.

Mary Lamberton Becker

* * *

Education

Education is positively correlated with health status (National Center for Health Statistics, 1993). According to the U. S. Census Bureau (1999), more women are completing educational degrees, although a higher percentage of women than men are only graduating from high school and community colleges. Above this educational level, the numbers reverse, with more men than women completing baccalaureate programs (16.8% and 15.4%, respectively), master's programs (5.9% and 4.9%, respectively), and doctoral programs (1.5% and 0.6%, respectively). In the

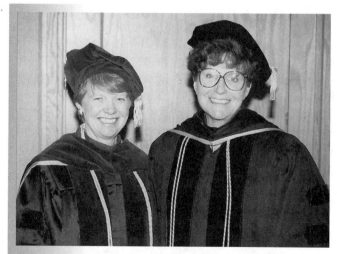

As women become better educated, health indicators improve also.

past, the predominant roles women chose were in education, nursing, library science, and social work. However, in the last two decades, more women have entered professions traditionally held by men such as engineering, theology, medicine, law, and dentistry, making up 50% of student enrollment. A continuing concern is that ethnic minority women have been slow to enter these major areas of study (Pollard & Tordella, 1993). An emerging trend, according to the U.S. Census Bureau, reflects an overall increase in college enrollment among African Americans and Hispanics since 1970 (Allen & Phillips, 1997). Such a trend holds promise for increasing the number of women pursing advanced specialty degrees as these cohorts move through the educational ranks.

Employment

More women are in the workforce than ever before and are entering the workforce at an earlier age. However, increased opportunities in the workforce are creating more challenges and risks for their families, such as child and elder caregiving issues. The job market remains male dominated, with average annual salaries differing by gender. Recent data indicate that women earn $0.71 to every $1.00 earned by men (U.S. Census Bureau, 1997).

....

Since every woman's problem occurs in part because of the nature of being female in this culture, which programs us to put the needs of others ahead of our own, we need to make radical changes in our minds and in our lives to get and stay healthy.
Christine Northrup

....

Traditional female occupations generally pay less than comparable men's jobs and have fewer benefits. Sixty-five percent of women are in the workforce as librarians, teachers, social workers, and nurses with low salaries. Working women continue to assume responsibility for child care, housework, and elder care (Wuest, 1993). More than 50% of women with an infant are in the workforce, up 35.3% since 1978. The percentage of new mothers who work tends to increase both with age and education (Taeuber, 1991). Men are more likely to be employed in higher-level management positions, with jobs that offer health benefits, medical leave, and insurance. Women with limited health benefits may not seek out health care when needed and are less likely to practice preventive health care.

Poverty

Women earn less than men and, as a result, make up two-thirds of all poor adults. In 1996, 24% of women lived in poverty, a number increasing every year (U.S. Census Bureau, 1997). This statistic is greatly influenced by culture and race, with the largest increases among African American and Hispanic women.

Women in poverty are usually 18 to 24 years old, live in the south (50% of the U.S. women in poverty live in this region), and reside outside central cities. Many factors contribute to poverty, including the gender wage gap, single mothers as heads of households, teenage birth rates, lack of adequate child care, and lack of enforcement of child support payments. Of all the countries in the industrialized world, the United States is the only country without a system that provides subsidized child care for working parents.

Dual-earner families are least likely to live in poverty, with a median salary reported at $36,389, compared with families headed by a man at $26,827 and by a woman at $15,346 (U.S. Census Bureau, 1999). These factors have been called the **feminization of poverty**. In the community setting, women should be aware of social services, child-care programs, nutritional resources, and other resources for family needs.

Marital Status/Family Configuration

Women's roles in marriage and the family are in a state of transition and have been since the 1960s. The traditional role of the unemployed mother working in the home has become a small minority. Only 6% of households have a male working full-time supporting a full-time homemaker with children in the home. The necessary goal of any family, however defined, is to maintain the integrity of self and members, including safety, well-being, and health of the family. In today's society, 28% of married couples do not have children; 32% of families are headed by single women, with an increase seen in female heads of households in all racial groups; and 25% of families live in single-dwelling homes (U.S. Census Bureau, 1999).

Racial differences in lifestyles can affect attitudes and beliefs about health. African Americans, as compared with Caucasians, are more often single or married with no spouse present or living with extended families. More Caucasians are divorced or widowed and tend to have fewer children than African Americans and Hispanics. Families maintained by women with no husband present are more likely to be poor. Among those men who are present in their families, African American and Hispanic men tend to spend more time with their family tasks than Caucasian men (Lawton, Rajagopal, Brody, & Kleban, 1992).

Childbearing

Trends in U.S. birth rates have major implications for the growth of the population and future trends in health care. Fertility rates dropped in 1997, with an overall decline in birth rates (U.S. Census Bureau, 1999). The numbers of births are expected to decline further as the baby boomers age and pass their childbearing years. More women are delaying childbearing or choosing to remain childless. Birth rates vary by age and ethnicity, with the number of births for unmarried women declining in all age groups. Table 19-1 illustrates the birth rate by age and race in 1996.

TABLE 19-1	1996 Percentage of Birth Rates of Women by Age and Race				
Age Group	Total Births	Caucasian	African American	American Indian	Asian or Pacific Islander
10–14	11,242	50%	46%	2%	2%
15–19	494,272	70%	26%	2%	2%
20–24	951,247	77%	19%	>1%	3%
25–34	1,982,740	83%	11%	>1%	5%
35–44	472,473	82%	11%	>1%	6%
45–49	2,980	80%	9%	>1%	10%

Source: CDC, 1997.

There are 6 million pregnancies in the United States each year. Three million of these pregnancies are unplanned, with 1.5 million ending in abortion (Pasquale, 1994). The leading method of contraception remains female sterilization, followed by the oral contraceptive pill (U.S. Census Bureau, 1997).

In 1995, 81.3% of mothers began prenatal care within the first trimester, the highest ever recorded. Twice as many African American women deliver low-birth-weight babies compared with Caucasian women. Of women of childbearing age, 25% are not covered by insurance and 25% are insured but without maternity insurance coverage. Medicaid is used to help pay for 34% of all deliveries, and approximately 15% of childbearing mothers receive food stamps (U.S. Census Bureau, 1997). Parenting classes, health care for children, quality day-care facilities, and flexible employment opportunities for working mothers are not consistently available to women in the United States; the health and well-being of working families has not been a national funding priority. Many countries throughout the world have established policies that ensure protection and support of mothers, infants, and families and can serve as role models for such positive family investments.

Health Status

Life expectancy steadily increased for both men and women in the 20th century. The life expectancy of women has increased to nearly 80 years, with women older than 50 making up the fastest growing segment of the U.S. population (U.S. Census Bureau, 1999). With a decline in mortality in certain diseases for men (e.g., cardiovascular disease) and an increase in the numbers of women who assume many lifestyle behaviors and health habits previously characteristic of men (e.g., cigarette smoking, alcohol use, full-time work in the labor force, head of household responsibilities), the differences in life spans for women and men (currently 78.6 and 72.3 years, respectively) may not be so great in the future.

Morbidity

Women experience higher morbidity than men and use acute care health services at a higher rate than men. Women are hospitalized more than men and experience more chronic conditions, including arthritis, depression, orthopedic problems, diabetes, chronic obstructive pulmonary disease (COPD), hemorrhoids, hypertension, chronic bronchitis, asthma, and chronic sinusitis. Although research has shed some light, these gender differences are still not fully understood. Twice as many women as men are

Most women have contact with the health care system during their reproductive years. Venus Callahan, chapter author, examines an expectant mother.

FYI

For all persons who live to be 100 years of age, there will be five women for every two men.

limited in physical activity, reporting more missed days from work or school, and in research studies they report their health conditions as worse than those of men.

The three major chronic conditions women experience are heart conditions, arthritis, and hypertension, which all increase with age (U.S. Census Bureau, 1999). Differences in morbidity exist by age. The leading chronic condition in younger women is chronic sinusitis and hay fever, followed by orthopedic problems. For middle-aged women, arthritis, hypertension, and COPD are the most common. For women older than 65, arthritis and hypertension remain the leading chronic illnesses. However, older women also have all the consequences of aging, including sensory impairments, heart disease, and mobility impairments.

Mortality

The leading causes of death in women are heart disease, cancer, and stroke, with differences by age and across racial groups. The leading causes of death for young women younger than 24 are accidents, homicide, suicide, human immunodeficiency virus/acquired immunodeficiency syndrome (HIV/AIDS), and complications of pregnancy. For women ages 25 to 64, the leading causes of death are cancer, HIV/AIDS, heart disease, and COPD. The leading causes of death in women older than 65 are heart disease, cancer, cerebrovascular accident (CVA), pneumonia, and influenza. These diseases can be caused by lifestyle and environmental and social factors and are often preventable. Alcohol and drug use and abuse, unprotected sex, cigarette smoking, lack of exercise, obesity, and environmental threats are all implications in the mortality rate (Allen & Phillips, 1997).

Some investigators claim that the mortality of women may be influenced by their own perceptions of health. Some women may delay seeking care when sick because of family and work obligations, may not take symptoms of pain seriously, and may not pursue health care. Also, physicians have been accused of minimizing women's complaints and not treating women as aggressively as their male cohorts (Mark, Shaw, & DeLong, 1994). All of this may contribute to women entering the health care system at a high acuity level.

• •

Aging is very much a woman's issue. That's because women are most valued for their childbearing capacities. Once we've used up those capacities and our supposed sexual attractiveness, our social worth is gone.

Gloria Steinem, 1999

• •

Reproductive Risks

Women are uniquely at risk during pregnancy and childbirth, including the risks of induced and spontaneous abortions. Even now in the 21st century, women die during childbirth, with pulmonary embolism the leading cause of death in pregnant women. However, through partnerships between community health nurses and the health care system, maternal mortality has been dramatically reduced through prenatal care, education related to maternal risk factors, blood transfusions, anesthesia, and antibiotics. Racial discrepancies persist in number of deaths, with women of color having a threefold greater incidence of death during pregnancy than Caucasian women (Williams & Thomas, 1997). This is attributed to lack of prenatal care, poor nutrition, and substandard living conditions. Concurrent infant death rates are also disproportionate among races, with twice the number of infants of color dying than Caucasian infants.

Health Promotion and Prevention Across the Life Span

Community health nurses, because of their unique relationship to clients and their awareness of community problems and resources, occupy a pivotal role in influencing women's beliefs and practices for health promotion and illness prevention. Community health nurses, as educators of women about health issues, incorporate the health promotion and disease prevention of *Healthy People 2010* (see the *Healthy People 2010* box on p. 438 for selected objectives) to accomplish the primary goal of identifying and implementing behavioral and social interventions that are effective in motivating women to use preventive health services across the life span.

Adolescence (12 to 18 Years Old)

Community health nurses can play an important role in promoting the health of adolescent females through teaching, counseling, and role modeling. Community health nurses need to establish trusting relationships with adolescents, thereby gaining their confidence. Nurses need to be able to ask questions that might reveal alcohol and other drug abuse, high-risk sexual activity, or emotional distress. Community health nurses working with adolescents face challenges in communication, peer influences, and the stigma of being seen in local health clinics or settings. Effective programs that have a positive impact on the health of adolescents are often specifically targeted to teens in schools, night clinics, and malls, as well as through celebrity and teen role model spokespersons.

Young women in adolescence have many issues to deal with, including puberty; menarche; body image; eating disorders; and sexual issues, including sexual identity, contraception decisions, and sexually transmitted diseases (STDs). Attitudes about these issues are influenced by peers, society, and family relationships. *Healthy People 2010* objectives should guide direction for efforts in this age group. School-based health programs for health promotion, exercise and fitness, sex education, and prevention of drug use should address social concerns for this age group. Because the greatest number of new smokers are adolescent females, primary lung cancer prevention must start at the elementary school level with aggressive counseling programs to decrease the number of new smokers among young girls. Successful programs with teen

HEALTHY PEOPLE 2010

OBJECTIVES RELATED TO WOMEN'S HEALTH

Arthritis, Osteoporosis, and Chronic Back Conditions

Osteoporosis

2.9   Reduce the overall number of cases of osteoporosis.

2.10   Reduce the proportion of adults who are hospitalized for vertebral fractures associated with osteoporosis.

Cancer

3.3   Reduce the breast cancer death rate.

3.4   Reduce the death rate from cancer of the uterine cervix.

3.11   Increase the proportion of women who receive a Pap test.

3.13   Increase the proportion of women aged 40 years and older who have received a mammogram within the preceding 2 years.

Family Planning

9.4   Reduce the proportion of females experiencing pregnancy despite use of a reversible contraceptive method.

9.11   Increase the proportion of young adults who have received formal instruction before turning age 18 years on reproductive issues, including all of the following topics: birth control methods, safer sex to prevent HIV, prevention of sexually transmitted diseases, and abstinence.

9.12   Reduce the proportion of married couples whose ability to conceive or maintain a pregnancy is impaired.

9.13   Increase the proportion of health insurance policies that cover contraceptive supplies and services.

HIV

13.3   Reduce the number of AIDS cases among females and males who inject drugs.

Injury and Violence Prevention

Violence and Abuse Prevention

15.34 Reduce the rate of physical assault by current or former intimate partners.

15.35 Reduce the annual rate of rape or attempted rape.

Maternal, Infant, and Child Health

Maternal Death and Illness

16.4   Reduce maternal deaths.

16.5   Reduce maternal illness and complications due to pregnancy.

Prenatal Care

16.6   Increase the proportion of pregnant women who receive early and adequate prenatal care.

Nutrition and Overweight

Iron Deficiency Anemia

19.12 Reduce iron deficiency among young children and females of childbearing age.

19.14 Reduce iron deficiency among pregnant females.

Sexually Transmitted Diseases

STD Complications Affecting Females

25.6   Reduce the proportion of females who have never required treatment for pelvic inflammatory disease (PID).

25.7   Reduce the proportion of childless females with fertility problems who have had a sexually transmitted disease or who have required treatment for pelvic inflammatory disease.

25.8   Reduce HIV infections in adolescent and young adult females aged 13 to 24 years that are associated with heterosexual contact.

Source: DHHS, 2000.

girls and the prevention of smoking initiation have focused on assertiveness training and decision-making models of accountability.

The Youth Risk Behavior Surveillance System under the auspices of the Centers for Disease Control and Prevention (CDC, 1993) monitors health-risk behaviors among youth and young adults. These health-risk behaviors contribute to unintentional and intentional injuries, tobacco use, alcohol and other drug use, sexual behaviors, dietary behaviors, and physical activity, and should guide the community health nurse in planning interventions directed toward the female adolescent. Schools, churches, and recreational groups all provide the community health nurse with opportunities to influence health decisions through education (U.S. Adolescent Health Summary, 1997).

Young Adulthood (19 to 35 Years Old)

Two main concerns of women in this age group include making career choices and establishing relationships that may lead to marriage and pregnancy (Allen & Phillips, 1997). Community health nurses can address health promotion interventions in the context of these two life tasks. Nurses need to be knowledgeable regarding the various resources that are available in the community to assist women in this age range with such decisions. The nurse can be an effective model/mentor for young women in this developmental stage and should be able to address such concerns as fertility counseling, parenting skills, contraception options, domestic violence, and occupational health issues. Women in young adulthood face concerns such as STDs, contraceptive choices, safety, intentional and unintentional injury, stress management, alcohol and drug abuse, unhealthy dietary behaviors, physical activity, and role stress and strain. As women marry and establish families, they face issues such as learning to balance work and children, sexual harassment in the workplace, and establishing habits of self-care. The community health nurse must be cognizant of the problems of this age group and skillful in locating and accessing the resources available to therapeutically intervene.

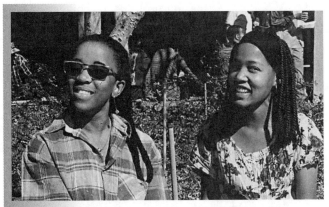

African American women have higher risks for cancer and hypertension and are less likely to use preventive health service.

Perimenopausal/Menopausal (36 to 55 Years Old)

The community health nurse must address health priorities with this age group of women, which include the following:

- *Benefits and risks of **hormone replacement therapy** (HRT)*
- *Early signs and symptoms of a cardiovascular disease*
- *Benefits of monitoring and controlling cholesterol and blood pressure levels*
- *Maintaining bone strength and density*
- *Maintaining healthy weight*
- *Exercising regularly*
- *Benefits of a regular mammogram*

It is during this time that breast cancer becomes a greater threat to a woman's longevity (Allen & Phillips, 1997). As women delay childbearing and with advanced reproductive technology, more and more women may be having their first child during this late reproductive stage. Women may also be caring for their own parents during this time while building careers, creating even greater time and energy demands. Table 19-2 is the recommended preventive health care calendar for adult women according to the American Medical Association (AMA, 1997).

The perimenopausal years are ages 36 to 50. During this period of a woman's life, the ovaries begin to slow down and eventually cease production of estrogen. Because of this decrease in estrogen, women may experience symptoms such as hot flashes, vaginal dryness, or night sweats. All perimenopausal women should be counseled about the benefits of taking hormone replacement therapy. Without estrogen, bones will begin to lose density and become thinner, weaker, brittle, and more prone to fracture. The lack of estrogen also decreases the high-density lipoprotein (HDL) cholesterol and raises the low-density lipoproteins (LDL) cholesterol, which increases the risk of cardiovascular problems such as myocardial infarction and CVA.

Women may react differently to these premenopausal physiological changes in the body. During this time, a woman may reexamine her life, which may result in a new self-identity. Women must explore what aging means to them and go through an acceptance of what their life has been and what it may still become. Sexuality of women changes during this time. Despite the fact that the public does not consider older women to be sexually active, most report positive experiences with sex during this time (Fogel & Woods, 1995). Many women view this time as the best years of their lives—children are grown, job is secure, and acceptance of self-identity has been established. For women who have devoted early years to childrearing, they may be returning to school or reentering the career market.

Mature (55 and Older)

As more women are reaching the mature stage of the life cycle, the community health nurse must realize that a shift of health emphasis from infectious and acute diseases to chronic diseases

TABLE 19-2   **RECOMMENDED HEALTH CARE CALENDAR**

TEST OR PROCEDURE	WHO NEEDS IT?	HOW OFTEN?
General physical exam (including blood pressure and lifestyle counseling)	Everyone	Every year
Pelvic examination	Everyone	Every year
Dental examination	Everyone	Every year
Eye examination	Everyone	Every year
Breast examination	Everyone	Every year
Breast self-examination (BSE)	Everyone	Every month
Skin cancer check	Everyone	Every 3 years
Rectal examination	Everyone	Every year
Pap smear	Everyone	Every year
Blood cholesterol	Everyone	Every 3 years (if first test was normal); as recommended by doctor if level is elevated
Mammogram	Everyone	Every 1 to 2 years between ages 40 and 49; once a year after age 50
Tests for sexually transmitted diseases	Anyone who is sexually active	Every 6–12 months if multiple partners, otherwise as recommended by doctor
Electrocardiogram	Anyone with two or more of the following risk factors for heart disease: family history, smoking, high cholesterol, diabetes, high blood pressure	Every 3 to 5 years
Sigmoidoscopy	Anyone over 50	Every 3 years
Fecal occult-blood test	Everyone	Every year
Tuberculin skin test	Anyone who is at increased risk	Every year or as recommended by doctor
Tetanus booster	Everyone	Every 10 years
Diphtheria booster	Everyone	Every 10 years

Source: AMA, 1998.

occurs in this age group of women. Because of the chronic nature of diseases in this age group, the historical definition of health (absence of disease) is less applicable. Rather, an emphasis should be placed on functional health, independence, and au-

tonomy. Health promotion should be aimed at preserving the mature woman's ability to function at the highest spectrum of wellness. Health-promoting activities to enhance wellness are listed in Box 19-1.

BOX 19-1 HEALTH PROMOTION ACTIVITIES FOR THE MATURE WOMAN

HEALTH SCREENINGS

Blood pressure, early cancer detection, hearing and vision screenings

HEALTH EDUCATION

Stress reduction, nutrition, general health, smoking cessation, classes about seasonal health issues such as hypothermia, heart related illness, colds/flu

IMMUNIZATIONS

Influenza shots

SAFETY

Safe driving courses, self-protection measures

EXERCISE

Walking, aerobics, water aerobics, weight lifting, weight-bearing exercise

Health Concerns Across the Life Span

Adolescence (12 to 18 Years Old)

Violent deaths, homicide, suicide, and accidents, particularly motor vehicle accidents, are responsible for the majority of deaths in this age group. Adolescents' misconception that they are "immortal" leads to risk-taking behaviors that make them more susceptible to injury and death. Female adolescents face potential threats to health such as substance abuse, pregnancy, acne, menstrual disorders, eating disorders, and STDs. Every year, nearly one-fourth of all new HIV infections, one-fourth of all new STD infections, and 1 million pregnancies occur among our nation's teenagers (U.S. Adolescent Health Summary, 1997).

The community health nurse can be a pivotal force in promoting the health of adolescents through health assessment, risk analysis, screening, anticipatory guidance, health teaching, and counseling with the adolescent as well as the parents. The most common health care request of adolescent females is related to pregnancy. Included in this visit, the community health nurse must conduct a health screening assessment, including last missed menstrual period, contraception being used, living arrangements, and financial status. If an adolescent is pregnant, anticipatory guidance is needed. This includes referral to a local prenatal health clinic or health department, encouragement of open communication regarding pregnancy with family or significant other, and referral to local department of human services for Medicaid enrollment if necessary. Health teaching must include the effects of alcohol and drugs on the fetus, the potential side effects of x-rays on the fetus, nutrition, and Women, Infant and Children (WIC) nutrition program enrollment. The counseling services of the nurse must include conducting a meeting with the adolescent and parent to inform them of the pregnancy. For sexually active adolescents who are not pregnant, the nurse should encourage enrollment in family planning clinic for contraceptives and STD education.

. . . .

I'm not the usual celebrity size. And I think that people who like to see images of themselves reflected back feel strongly connected to me.

Rosie O'Donnell, 1997

. . . .

Young Adulthood (19 to 35 Years Old)

For young adults and college students, as for adolescents, violent death or injury, alcohol and substance abuse, unwanted pregnancies, and STDs are major health threats. Most health problems in this stage are related to lifestyle behaviors. Weight concerns and eating problems are often reported as concerns for young women. Media images and social influences pressure young women desiring to be thin into abusive habits, such as purging, vomiting, laxative and diuretic abuse, and poor nutrition (Fogel & Woods, 1995). Young women should be aware of

interventions to delay onset of osteoporosis, including increasing calcium intake and weight-bearing exercises to promote bone density and decreasing cola intake, which decreases reabsorption of calcium.

The community health nurse can play a vital role in educating this group regarding behaviors that will positively affect their lifestyles. The proper use of condoms to help prevent STDs and the availability and variety of different contraceptive choices to prevent an unwanted pregnancy must be discussed with the young adult. Addressing these concerns and seeking a solution together will accomplish the ultimate goal of improved health.

Perimenopausal/Menopausal (36 to 55 Years Old)

A comprehensive assessment of women in this age group should include the changes of life that this woman goes through, including physiological, psychological, and emotional changes. The community health nurse must assess the woman's knowledge regarding the changes in her body, including her beliefs about menopause and the implications for her health. The nurse must be aware of complementary therapies women may chose for their health care and should be open-minded about what is acceptable for their client. Cardiovascular disease, cancer, and osteoporosis are the three major diseases that occur during the perimenopausal/menopausal period of a woman's life.

Cardiovascular Disease

Cardiovascular disease is the leading cause of death in American women, accounting for more than 359,000 deaths from coronary heart disease and 87,000 deaths from strokes in 1990 (Smith, 1995). Most effective for disease reduction is primary prevention through risk factor modification. The modifiable risk factors are cigarette smoking, hypertension, hypercholesterolemia, and physical inactivity, with less direct but still important risk factors of obesity, diabetes, stress, and menopause.

Community health nurses need to first be aware of the modifiable risk factors and then develop a cardiovascular health plan with an emphasis on prevention. When a woman seeks health care, either for herself or a family member, the community health nurse should seize the opportunity to emphasize heart health. The relationship between estrogen and cardiovascular disease, along with cardiac risk factors, must be discussed and assessed. The use of medications in the home should be reinforced by client teaching, including when to take prescribed nitroglycerin and when to seek medical attention for chest pains. By empowering the woman with knowledge, she will be able to seek medical care early and hopefully extend not only her longevity but her quality of life as well.

Cancer

Cancer is the second leading cause of death for women (Allen & Phillips, 1997). The most common types of cancer in women are lung, breast, colorectal, ovarian, and pancreatic. Lung cancer has surpassed breast cancer as the leading cause of cancer deaths. Tobacco is the single most toxic carcinogenic substance responsible for the occurrence of lung cancer and has been linked to cancers of the mouth, pharynx, larynx, esophagus, pancreas, uterine cervix, kidney, and bladder (McGinn & Haylock, 1993). Smoking cessation programs for women who smoke need to be readily accessible (see the following Research Brief).

. . . .

Cancer got me over unimportant fears, like growing old.
Olivia Newton John, 1998
Actress, singer, and breast cancer survivor
who had a modified radical mastectomy
to remove a cancerous tumor in July 1992

. . . .

Breast cancer is the second leading cause of cancer death in women overall and is the leading cause of cancer deaths in women aged 50 to 54. It is imperative that community health nurses educate women regarding signs and symptoms of breast cancer such as a lump, thickening or swelling, dimpling, skin irritation, distortion, retraction, scaliness, pain, and nipple tenderness, discharge, or inversion (American Cancer Society, 1995). A trained health care provider must investigate these

symptoms as soon as possible. If cancer is detected in the early stages (localized), the 5-year survival rate is 94%.

When a woman is receiving chemotherapy for cancer, the nurse should be aware of the side effects of chemotherapy and what can be done in the home to decrease or alleviate symptoms of discomfort (e.g., nausea, vomiting, pain). They must also be aware of local resources to ensure that women have prompt access to care as soon as a definite cancer diagnosis has been obtained, along with support groups and referral agencies for cancer victims. See Box 19-2 for Cancer Support Groups.

Osteoporosis

Bone mass peaks at the end of the growth period, usually around age 17. There are some small gains in bone mass up to age 30; this is then followed by a progressive loss of bone mass. Twenty-eight million Americans, 80% of whom are women, have osteo-

RESEARCH BRIEF

Marcus, B., & Albrecht, A. (1999). The efficacy of exercise as an aid for smoking cessation in women. Archives of Internal Medicine, 159(11), 1229–1235.

This descriptive research study examined the effectiveness of exercise as an aid for smoking cessation in women. The sample was composed of 281 healthy but sedentary female smokers between the ages of 18 and 65 who had smoked routinely for at least 1 year. The subjects were followed in a 12-week smoking cessation program. Of the 134 women who exercised three times a week, 19.4% gave up smoking for at least 2 months after their program ended, compared with 10.2% of the 147 nonexercisers. Three months later, 16.4% of the exercisers were still not smoking, compared with 8.2% of the nonexercisers. One year after the study, the difference was 11.9% and 5.4%, respectively. The study provides evidence that vigorous exercise leads to improved rates of continuous abstinence from smoking in women.

BOX 19-2 CANCER SUPPORT GROUPS

American Cancer Society
1599 Clifton Rd. NE
Atlanta, GA 30329
800-ACS-2345

Candlelighters Childhood Cancer Foundation
1312 18th St. NW, 2nd Floor
Washington, DC 20036-1808
800-366-2223

National Alliance of Breast Cancer Organizations
1180 Avenue of the Americas, 2nd Floor
New York, NY 10036
212-719-0154

National Coalition for Cancer Survivorship
323 8th St. SW
Albuquerque, NM 87102
505-764-9956

SHARE: Self-Help for Women With Breast Cancer
19 W. 44th St.
New York, NY 10036
212-719-0364
Hot line 212-382-2111

Y-ME National Organization for
   Breast Cancer Information and Support
18220 Harwood Ave.
Homewood, IL 60430
800-221-2141
24-hour hot line 708-799-8228

TABLE 19-3	OSTEOPOROSIS RISK FACTOR PROFILE FOR WOMEN

RISKS	MODIFIABLE FACTORS
65 years and older	Slender build
Family history of osteo-porosis	Estrogen deficiency
	Sedentary lifestyle
Caucasian or Asian	Low calcium intake
Postmenopausal, espe-cially premature	Failure to achieve peak bone mass
History of atraumatic fracture	Cigarette smoking
	High alcohol consumption
Loss of 1 inch or more in height	Weight below normal
	Steroid use

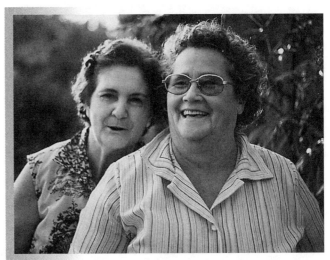

As women age, friendships become more important in promoting a sense of well-being.

porosis, representing a major public health problem in the United States. Vertebral fractures generally occur in women 55 years and older, and result in back pain, height loss and kyphosis, anterior rib pain, negatively changed body image, difficulty in fitting clothes, a protuberant abdomen, and abdominal discomfort (as a result of reduced lumbar vertebral height). Hip fractures occur twice as often in women older than 75 than in men and are associated with excess mortality of 5% to 20% as a result of preoperative and postoperative complications, such as deep vein thrombosis, pulmonary embolism, and pneumonia.

The community nurse must be aware of the lifestyle changes to prevent osteoporosis, including calcium intake, weight control, and weight-bearing exercise, as well as hormone replacement therapy used to treat osteoporosis. The osteoporosis profile (Table 19-3) can be used by nurses to identify risk factors for women.

Mature (55 and Older)

Mature women deal with many health care issues as they age. Many of the illnesses discussed in the section on menopausal women apply here also. However, as women live longer, their chronic conditions may increase in severity. Depression, dementia, and **urinary incontinence** are some of the illnesses that occur later in life. Arthritis, osteoporosis, hypertension, and cardiovascular disease continue to be health concerns for women in this age group (Fogel & Woods, 1995).

Community health nurses often must deal with depression in mature women. Many may have outlived their spouses and are dealing with the loss daily. This depression often goes untreated. Many medications may also contribute to the depression. If dementia is present, safety considerations in the surrounding environment should be made. Urinary incontinence is seen twice as often in women than in men; it is found in 30% of elderly women (Fogel & Woods, 1995). Nurses must also be aware of

medications that may cause urinary retention or urinary incontinence, possibly leading to urinary tract infections.

Diversity and Women's Health
Cultural Influences

The impact of culture on women is imperative for the community health nurse to understand. Gender roles are influenced by culture. An awareness of family dominance patterns is essential when teaching clients and communicating with family members. In some cultures, women may not speak unless they are given permission by a spouse or father. It is also important to understand how men and women interact in each culture (Lipson, Dibble, & Minarik, 1996; Purnell & Paulanka, 1998). Although most cultures are still largely patriarchal, matriarchal influences are also important. Acceptable ways of communicating and touching should be assessed by community health nurses and included in any interventions for the client. Guidelines for a cultural communication assessment appear in Box 19-3.

Sexual Orientation

As lesbianism has become more accepted, its impact on families and health care should be acknowledged by the community health nurse. Family structures are no longer made up only of the typical married couple with children. Gay and lesbian couples have openly taken residence together and may live with other persons, including communal communities where responsibilities are shared based on common beliefs. Many lesbian women choose to adopt children or conceive a child through artificial insemination or heterosexual intercourse (Zeidenstein, 1990). However, most cultures continue to stigmatize homosexuality, forcing homosexuals to remain "in the closet" (Giger & Davidhizar, 1995). Health care continues to be prejudiced toward heterosex-

BOX 19-3 QUESTIONS FOR ASSESSING CULTURAL COMMUNICATION PATTERNS

1. Is the individual willing to share thoughts, feelings, and ideas?

2. What does touching mean in the culture? Is touching certain body parts appropriate?

3. What does silence mean in the culture? a loud voice?

4. What spatial and distancing characteristics when communicating are observed for family members versus strangers?

5. What eye contact is used (avoidance, changes among family, friends, strangers, or socioeconomic groups)? Is it a sign of respect or insult?

6. What facial expressions are used? Do they smile a lot, show emotions?

7. How are people greeted?

Source: Adapted from Purnell & Paulanka, 1998.

Old Ladies

Hurrying, late again,
I rounded the corner too fast.
They were caught, frozen on one
frame of my mind's camera.
Two old ladies sitting on the porch swing
so near the narrow winding road
I could have touched them.

Both were white-haired and
comfortably padded,
both wearing red dresses,
turned to almost face each other,
both laughing, faces lined but serene.

Old ladies are sometimes poor,
sometimes stuck with raising children's
children. I know. But still
I think of those two old ladies
wearing red dresses, swinging and laughing.

A measure of wisdom and grace
and peace seem theirs.
Oh sure, they must peer into the dark tunnel
and see the train growing larger. And maybe
they lie alone in silent dark room. And maybe
wisdom and grace and peace
sometimes elude them.

But still
I hope I live to be an old lady
and wear red dresses
and sit in a porch swing
and laugh.

Jeanne Ezell, Ph.D.
July 1993

ual relationships by ignoring specific health care considerations of this population.

Lesbian women are more likely to neglect their own health care needs and avoid examinations by health care providers because of the stigma and humiliation that often goes along with the disclosure of being a lesbian. They are more likely to reveal their identity to practitioners who are open and nonjudgmental (Stevens, Tatum, & White, 1996). Lesbians are at low risk for vaginal infections, STDs, and HIV. In contrast, they are at higher risk for breast and uterine cancer than their heterosexual cohorts (Rosser, 1994). They also are more likely to experience stress and depression because of social isolation. Substance abuse is reported in 30% of lesbian women, compared with 7% in the general population (Deevey & Wall, 1992). **Heterosexism** and **homophobia** contribute to prejudice, fear, and continued discrimination against lesbians.

The community health nurse should learn to communicate without bias with women of all sexual orientations. Lesbians are often insulted when health care workers assume they are heterosexual and ask questions gender specific, such as "What form of birth control do you use?" Alternative questions should be phrased in the form of open-ended, nongender statements like "Tell me about your sexual activity." The nurse should encourage lesbian women to have regular pelvic examinations and to avoid unprotected oral sex by using latex barriers (Zeidenstin, 1990). Mental health counseling and support networks are also options for dealing with the psychosocial issues and sexual practices associated with relationships.

Women and Aging

The elderly population will more than double by the year 2050, with the oldest old—those older than 85—the most rapidly growing segment. Twenty percent of elders will be from underrepresented populations (U.S. Census Bureau, 1997). These women are much more likely to be widowed, live alone, and live in poverty. Women belonging to underrepresented racial and ethnic groups have been termed "quadruple jeopardy" because they are elderly, minority, female, and poor. Elderly women are also reported to have high levels of depression related to loneliness (Bennett, 1987).

Differences have been identified regarding why women are living longer, including differences by gender, exposure to environmental hazards, health habits, personality styles, and reactions to illness. Men have traditionally held jobs that expose them to more hazardous environmental factors, such as asbestos and carcinogens. Women have traditionally smoked less and managed stress better (Golub & Freedman, 1985). These differences are expected to narrow in the future as a result of changes in our society, equal rights for women, and greater participation of women in the workforce.

••••••••••••••••••••••••••••

Freedom is what you do with what's been done to you.

Jean-Paul Sartre

••••••••••••••••••••••••••••

Because women generally outlive men, more women live alone or live in long-term care facilities. Women currently outnumber elderly men by 6 to 5 from age 65 to 69, and by 5 to 2 over age 85 (U.S. Census Bureau, 1997). More families are opting to care for their elderly parents at home; however, women (especially Caucasian women) continue to make up a larger percentage in nursing homes, with 50% childless or having outlived their own children (Golub & Freedman, 1985). The financial consequences for elderly women are of major concern. Elderly women often have saved little, because many grew up in a male-dominated time in which women did not have to consider financial affairs. The few resources that these women have must be used for a longer period. With rising health care costs, many elderly women rely on Medicare and Medicaid resources (Benderly, 1997).

Elderly women often report they are disappointed with health care and their treatment by health care personnel. As the women age, they report that physicians often dismiss their complaints as compared with their male cohorts. An example of this is often seen in women with cardiac conditions. Until recently, women have been ignored in cardiovascular research and have not been offered the same interventions that men traditionally have—such as cardiac rehabilitation. Many elderly women report feeling disrespected and mistreated. Discrimination by race and sexual orientation is also a concern. Elderly lesbian women are often discounted in health care practices, with their significant other being eliminated from major health care decisions. Elderly women may not have been socialized to deal with finances, and this may place them at significant risk. Rural elderly women may also be disadvantaged because a large number of them have a low educational and socioeconomic status (Golub & Freedman, 1985).

Community health nurses must acknowledge the diverse needs of elderly women. Health promotion should be encouraged, including sleeping, exercising, weight control, and diet. Nurses in the community should work with elderly women, listening to their needs and problems, making life less stressful for these women. The cultural prejudices against the elderly in the United States influence the way women perceive themselves as they age, how they care for themselves, and how they relate to health care providers.

Global Issues and Women's Health

The **Commission on the Status of Women** is one of the first bodies established by the United Nations Economic and Social Council to monitor the situation of women and promote their rights in all societies around the world. The United Nations Fourth **World Conference on Women** was held in Beijing, China, in 1995. Ethical issues related to women were determined, setting universal standards regarding equality between women and men. Women's concerns should be brought to the forefront with issues related to human rights. Mutilation of female body parts, prostitution for survival, and female child slavery are all considered culturally acceptable in some countries. Women must participate in the political arena and in decision making related to legislation to fully address these ethical concerns. Women should also have a role in the contribution of development of their countries, including policy, employment, education, the economy, and the environment. Above all, women must have a voice in the fight against poverty and violence against women.

Issues Affecting Women's Health
Violence

Violence can take many forms, including physical assault, sexual assault, and homicide. Age has been identified as the most significant trait that puts women at risk for a violent attack, because younger women are more likely to be victims of sexual and domestic abuse (Allen & Phillips, 1997). The health consequences of violence against women include physical, psychological, and social effects. Violence touches 1 in 4 families and is responsible for more than 1 in 3 female murder victims. It involves 6 out of every 10 couples and kills as many women every 5 years as the total number of Americans killed in the Vietnam War. Violence is the single largest cause of injury to women in the United States—more common than automobile accidents and muggings combined, creating 100,000 days of hospitalization, 30,000 emergency department visits, and 40,000 trips to the doctor's office each year. Thirty-five percent of hospital visits by women are attributed to violence, with the women seeking treatment for symptoms related to ongoing abuse. However, only 5% of these domestic violence victims are so identified (AMA, 1998).

The cost to business is perhaps as much as $5 billion annually in lost productivity as a result of absenteeism. Community

FYI

An excellent resource, the National Resource Center on Homelessness and Mental Illness provides technical assistance and information about services and housing for the homeless and mentally ill population. It is sponsored by the Center for Mental Health Services, Substance Abuse and Mental Health Services Administration at 800-444-7415.

health nurses should be aware of "red flag" identifiers associated with domestic violence, such as women who (1) always seem to have bruises on the limbs, torso, and face; (2) come to the clinic with vague symptoms of illness such as pain in lower abdomen, chronic diarrhea, or pain of undetermined origin; (3) have trouble making eye contact; (4) have controlling partners; and (5) consistently wear sunglasses, even indoors.

Community health nurses should be aware of local resources that can be accessed to assist women who find themselves in an abusive situation. National crisis lines such as the Domestic Violence Crisis Line and the Sexual Assault Crisis Line are accessible nationwide.

Homelessness

Homelessness is a growing problem in all urban and rural regions. Single women head approximately 40% of the homeless families (Allens & Phillips, 1997). For women, many factors can lead to homelessness, such as divorce, poverty, eroding work opportunities, decline in public assistance, domestic violence, substance abuse, and mental illness. Substance abuse often accompanies homelessness and increases the risk of homeless women for prostitution and other health-related conditions such as HIV, STDs, tuberculosis, and malnutrition.

The community health nurse can assist homeless women and families through primary, secondary, and tertiary prevention interventions at the individual, community, and national levels. The community health nurse may be the referral for financial assistance and act as an advocate to assist the client through the "red tape" of the bureaucratic process. Nurses must work in the community by challenging government officials to examine the homeless problem and soliciting concerned citizens to develop shelters and programs for homeless individuals and families.

Incarceration

In the last 10 years, due to the decline in economic conditions and the crack down on drugs and crime, the number of women in prison has increased to 138,000 (Wheeler, 2000). Women account for 5.8% of the prison population and 9.3% of the jail population (Gilliard & Beck, 1994). The typical conviction is for property crimes, for example, check forgery and illegal credit card use. About 80% of women in prison report an income of $2,000 per year before being incarcerated. Ninety-two percent report incomes under $10,000. Single mothers account for 90% of the women incarcerated, with 54% being women of color (www.igc.apc.org/justice/prisons/women/women-in-prison.html).

The majority of incarcerated women have a dependency on drugs and/or alcohol and are usually from a low socioeconomic group. With these lifestyle patterns, health care has usually been neglected before they are incarcerated. Many of the women have a host of chronic medical problems such as tuberculosis, HIV, and other STDs. Historically, the prison systems have not had

the resources to provide sufficient health care for these women. Community health nurses need to be politically active and petition legislative bodies to allocate monies for health care for this vulnerable population. The community health nurse needs to assume the role of client advocate in regard to child care and visitation while incarcerated. Parenting and child-care classes should be made available to the inmates. Programs that provide occupational training and promote self-esteem and assertiveness have been linked with better outcomes for women who are released from prison.

Poverty

Poverty dramatically affects women's health. Poor women have limited access to health care and preventive health care services, which results in delay of diagnosis of disease and injury, and consequently, shorter life spans. Factors unique to women in regard to poverty include the following:

- *Women are usually responsible for children, and many are single parents with no extended support.*
- *Women are not traditionally trained to assume the bread winner role and usually accept lower-paying jobs, often leading to a choice between public assistance and inadequate child care while they work.*
- *Health care is an expendable luxury when placed alongside child care, food, and lodging.*

RESEARCH BRIEF

Trossman, S. (1999, May/June). RN Explores Agent Orange's Lasting Effects on Women Vets. American Nurse, *p. 24.*

Eighty-nine percent of female veterans who served in the Vietnam War were nurses. Agent Orange, a toxin used in Vietnam to clear out dense vegetation and crops, is well known for its serious adverse health affects and role in cancer and Hodgkin's disease in men. Virtually no research had been conducted on the women who were exposed to Agent Orange. Dr. Linda Schwartz has studied this "forgotten population" and found that they are at great risk for increased cancer rates and miscarriages. Agent Orange was used to keep down weeds around the camps, and the empty containers often used to store supplies and as barbecue grills. Nurses handled the containers and were exposed to the toxin as well. The outcome of this study has been to influence policy in the Veteran's Association to compensate women for these damages.

- *Jobs women take may not have health care benefits comparable to men's jobs.*

Community health nurses need to be knowledgeable about local resources to assist women who are poor to gain access to health care. Ways to reach women in poverty for preventive health care, such as church-based programs, should be identified. Some local resources that are available in most areas include county and state health departments, federal health clinics, The United Way, Medicaid, and Social Security Administration.

Workplace Health

Women represent almost half of the current workforce. Many factors have contributed to this increasing number of women in the workforce, including economic necessity, fewer women having children, changes in women's attitudes of work, and changes in society. Women face a variety of concerns in the workplace, including reproductive risks, job stress, role conflict, sexual harassment, discrimination, and salary inequality. Women make up the largest percentage of health care workers in this country, including nurses, technologists, physicians, therapists, dietitians, and clerical workers. Major occupational hazards for health care workers include biolog-

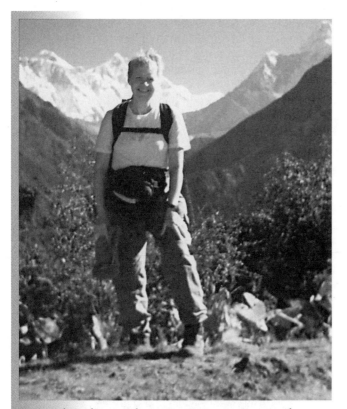

Research indicates that women can enjoy good health and an active lifestyle over a lifetime with attention to regular exercise and strength training.

ical, chemical, environmental, physical, and psychosocial hazards (Fogel & Woods, 1995).

All of these factors may influence a woman's health, both physically and mentally, in the workplace. The community health nurse in the occupational setting must address sensitive issues for women, including effects of cancer, reproductive problems (e.g., menstrual disorders, reduced fertility, genetic damage, spontaneous abortion, stillbirths), back problems, and carpal tunnel syndrome (Fogel & Woods, 1995). At-risk occupations for women must be identified. Even though many factors affect women's health in the workplace, very little research has been conducted with regard to women. Most research has been based on males as workers, resulting in biased research findings. This has led to designs and practices that compromise the working woman's health and safety. Community health nurses must be advocates for women in the workplace by conducting research based on female workers and educating women about specific gender risks associated with work.

Toward the Future
Women's Ways of Knowing

Women must play a major role in their acquisition of knowledge to make informed health decisions. Historically, most women have not been as well educated as men in basic or health sciences. The way in which women have been educated directly influences their health knowledge. Poorly educated women may participate in the health care system in silence—afraid to ask questions, feeling inadequate, with minimal knowledge of their own health care. They may accept answers without question. They may not be able to understand the complex health care system or understand why they are expected to change from old patterns. Some distrust anyone of authority and reject science and medicine, relying on tradition or family influence.

As women become better educated through college, life and work experiences they learn **procedural knowledge,** including critical thinking and logical reasoning skills. Some women will acquire **constructed knowledge** and are able to synthesize knowledge from many areas. The logic of women's ways of knowing stems from the fact that fewer women than men graduate from baccalaureate or higher degree programs (Rosser, 1994). Education can play a key role in eliminating the subservient way women react to the health care industry. Community health nurses play a critical role in the education of women throughout the life span.

....

When you don't like a thing, change it. If you can't change it, change the way you think about it and stop complaining and whining. Whining is not only graceless, it is hazardous—it can alert a brute that a victim is in the neighborhood.

Maya Angelou

....

Feminism

The politics of women's health care issues have long been in the forefront of the feminist movement. Until recently, few women have been invited to attend or participate in legislative forums related to women's health. Women have often been absent in the establishment of research priorities related to their health. Feminism and the promotion of women's rights in society today are closely associated with the promotion of a national women's health agenda.

• •

I myself have never been able to find out precisely what feminism is: I only know that people call me a feminist whenever I express sentiments that differentiate me from a door mat.

Rebecca West, 1913

• •

• •

Feminism's agenda is basic . . . . It asks that women be free to define themselves—instead of having their identity defined for them, time and again, by their culture and their men.

Susan Faludi

• •

Feminist theory deals with gender by race and class, along with individuals, groups, and communities. There are many feminist theories, including liberal feminism, Marxist feminism, socialist feminism, African American feminism, lesbian separatist feminism, conservative feminism, existential feminism, psychoanalytic feminism, and radical feminism.

FYI

The Pill That Launched a Social Revolution

Some medical historians say that the development of a foolproof contraceptive for women in 1960 influenced the role of women more than any single factor in the history of humankind. In 1950, the Planned Parenthood Federation provided funds to conduct research on the development of a safe, reliable oral contraceptive to a biologist, Gregory Pincus. Ten years later, the oral contraceptive, marketed under the name Enovid-10, was approved by the U.S. Food and Drug Administration, in 1960. Within 2 years, 1.2 million women were taking it to control the size of their families. In 1999, 10 million women used an oral contraceptive. The "pill" was indeed revolutionary in changing lives, attitudes, values, and society of women and men.

Women's issues focus on economics, health care, and violence toward women. The correlation between the feminist movement and the political arena and the impact on women's health are clearly obvious. Women must continue in their quest for a voice in health care policy and the implementation of policies that affect women (Rosser, 1995). Community health nurses can promote the feminist agenda through public policy activism and serving on boards where women's health issues are concerned.

• •

For us who nurse, our nursing is a thing, which unless we are making progress every year, every month, every week, take my word for it, we are going back.

Florence Nightingale,
1872, graduation address, St. Thomas School of Nursing

• •

Empowerment

Empowerment is based on the assumption that all people are created equal. Each person has the opportunity to recognize his or her own assets and develop from them on a professional, physical, spiritual, and emotional level. Recognizing and respecting the fact that all people have assets supports humility and dismisses the threat that others are better, eliminating any jealousy or threats of insecurity. People feel powerful in themselves when they feel secure. Community health nurses can be the "mirror" that reflects the woman's steps toward recognizing her own special assets. By affirming and reinforcing the woman's ability to recognize these assets, the woman gains confidence to move forward in the search for security and improved self-esteem.

One of the most empowering events for women has been the formation of the **United Nations Platforms for Action for Women** with the purpose to challenge governments to raise the status of women. The most recent conference was the 1995 Fourth World Conference on Women in Beijing, China, and identified commonly held beliefs about women's rights to health care. The

BOX 19-4 STRATEGIC OBJECTIVES OF THE WORLD CONFERENCE ON WOMEN

1. Increase women's access throughout the life span to appropriate, affordable, and quality health care, information, and related services.
2. Strengthen preventive programs that promote women's health.
3. Undertake gender-sensitive initiatives that address sexually transmitted diseases, HIV/AIDS, and sexual and reproductive health issues.
4. Increase resources and monitor follow-up for women's health.

A CONVERSATION WITH...

While the education of girls and women is obviously desirable for its own sake, it is especially crucial to lowering birthrates because of the different possible futures it opens up. . . . By opening the doors of education and social participation for the world's women and children, we can not only help our human family to a better life, but reduce our pressure on the planet as well.

—Carl Pope,
Executive Director of the Sierra Club.
Source: Pope, C. (1999). Solving the population problem: The key is to improve the lives of women. *Sierra Magazine, 84*(5), 14–15.

four strategic objectives for women's health are listed in Box 19-4. A specific action plan has been specified by the U.S. Congress to achieve each of the four objectives.

Health Care Policy

Policy makers in health care have historically ignored women's issues when developing health care policy. However, many policies were made in the last decade of the 20th century that influence the health promotion and well-being of women.

The Women's Health Equity Act of 1990 identified the inequality of research in women's health issues with requirements that women and underrepresented racial and ethnic groups be included in research. At the same time, the National Institutes of Health established the Office of Research in Women's Health based on the concept that women's research must expand from the traditional focus of women's reproductive systems to include all body systems and behavioral factors that influence women's health care. Recommendations for priority research for the next two decades for women include health promotion and wellness, eliminating barriers to health care services, prevention of illness, health education, and recognizing differences among women. In 1993, the Women's Health Initiative, a 14-year descriptive and intervention study of women and diseases, was launched to examine postmenopausal women of all races and socioeconomic levels, with specific considerations of the effects of interventions on heart disease, stroke, cancer, and osteoporosis. Box 19-5 identifies areas of research needed for women across the life span.

The Family Medical Leave Act was passed in 1993, allowing for 12 weeks of unpaid leave time from work for family or medical reasons. Employees are guaranteed the same job, pay, and benefits when they return to work after a leave. Because women are the primary family caregivers in the United States, this legislation is considered of major benefit for women.

BOX 19-5 RESEARCH AREAS FOR WOMEN ACROSS THE LIFE SPAN

Adolescence	Prevention of accidents, suicide prevention, HIV, sexuality, alcohol, tobacco, diet and exercise
Young adult/ college	Low-birth-weight babies, pregnancies dangerously complicated by hypertension, ectopic pregnancies resulting in death, infertility, sexuality transmitted diseases, cancer prevention (breast), safety (alcohol/drugs), health education, contraception, eating disorders, discomforts of pregnancy, obesity, HIV, family planning
Midlife	Disease prevention (cancer, hypertension, stroke, heart disease), health promotion, health education, strengths of single family head of households, multiple role adaptation, obesity, influence of diet on osteoporosis, domestic violence, early detection of cancer, arthritis, pain
Perimenopausal	Heart disease, health promotion, health education, impact of diet on osteoporosis, domestic violence, urinary incontinence, hormone replacement therapy, dietary influence on breast cancer, calcium and vitamin D supplements
Mature	Coping with chronic illnesses and disability, urinary incontinence, depression, institutionalization, respite care, social and economic contributions to health status, older women and health policy, racial/cultural influences on health care, caregivers, cost-effectiveness of health care to elder women

Women are the dominant caregivers in our society, making up 75% of caregivers in the home (Biegel, Sales, & Schulz, 1991). Caring for family members has long been an expectation of women. In addition to working outside the home, women are required to care for children, spouses, and aging parents. Women often must give up their employment to care for family members, with loss of wages, employee benefits—health and retirement—and social support. Many women who lack health insurance may not have adequate resources for health care. With the extra stresses of caregiving, women may end up divorced, with the added loss of security from the employee benefits of their spouses (e.g., health insurance) (Hogan, 1990). To address these issues, in 1991, the Family Caregiver Support Act was proposed entitling a caregiver to $2,400 a year for support services; however, this bill was not passed (Riggs, 1991). Health care policy for female caregivers must not be ignored, but rather mandated, including monetary reimbursement and respite services. Changes in health care policy that relate to the problems of female caregivers could help these women improve their quality of life.

Health behaviors of women are affected by the availability of health care resources and influenced by education and income. Women get health insurance either through employment or marriage. Well-educated women are more likely to practice positive health promotion such as healthy eating, exercising, not smoking, and drinking less alcohol (Fogel & Woods, 1995). Poverty and lack of education have a negative influence on health, with an increase in stress, depression, and poor health promotion habits. Usually, these women wait until an acute episode to seek health care. Many may rely on home remedies or alternative medicine for health care. The fact remains that inadequate health care access results in needless suffering and often death.

Despite the reality that more women are caregivers to our country, they play a small role in public decision making regarding health care issues. Women have traditionally been a small percentage of physicians, legislators, and health care administrators. This trend is changing, however, as more women are entering male-dominated professions and being elected to public office. There are more women in Congress than ever before. Women should be encouraged by community health nurses to become more involved in increasing community awareness regarding women's health issues.

RESEARCH BRIEF

Wilcox, S., & Stefanick, M. (1999). Knowledge and perceived risk of major disease in middle-aged and older women. Health Psychology, 18(4), 346–353.

This study examined the perceived health risks of middle-aged and older women related to mortality risks, personal risk, control, and preventability of risk diseases. The sample consisted of 200 women from 41 to 95 years of age. One in two women will eventually die of heart disease or stroke, and one in twenty-five will die of breast cancer. Middle-aged women and older women were more likely to know the leading cause of mortality for men in their age group than for women. Only 34% of the older women in the study knew that coronary heart disease was the leading cause of death in older women. Women in both age groups overestimated a woman's risk of death from breast cancer and underestimated the risk from lung and colon cancer. The authors speculate that heart disease is known as a "man's disease" and breast cancer has received a great deal of media attention and is more closely identified as a "woman's disease." This has implications for health providers in the education of women about the need for heart disease screening and for taking action to reduce their risks for all diseases.

CASE STUDY

Frances Benton is a 68-year-old widow who has recently been referred to your community health clinic by Rachel Jackson, a concerned neighbor. According to Ms. Jackson, Mrs. Benton's husband died about 8 months ago. Mr. Benton had been Mrs. Benton's caretaker. The couple did not have children, and there are no close relatives. Mrs. Benton had fallen and sustained a hip fracture approximately 1 year ago and recently a cracked vertebra. She has begun to have lapses of memory and has lost her way home from the grocery store. Two days ago, Mrs. Benton was out in the yard with only her slip on, which is definitely out of character according to Ms. Jackson. The landlord stopped by several times to collect the rent but could not get Mrs. Benton to understand that she had not paid it in 3 months. He had spoken with Ms. Jackson and was planning to evict Mrs. Benton.

1. What are your nursing diagnoses in this situation?

2. What secondary and tertiary preventive measures might be appropriate in working with Mrs. Benton?

3. What community resources could you collaborate with to address the health risks for Mrs. Benton?

CONCLUSION

Community health nurses are invaluable in assisting women with health care needs in the community. They should be knowledgeable regarding the various health concerns that women face, such as violence, homelessness, incarceration, poverty, osteoporosis, and cancer, and be able to define these needs. They should be aware of the local resources that are available and be skilled in linking these resources with the clients and their communities. Finally, they should be able to evaluate the process, fill in the gaps, and provide continuity of care for the individual client and the community.

CRITICAL THINKING ACTIVITIES

1. You are a rural community health nurse working on a mobile van visiting a large migrant community at a local farm. Selena King, a 16-year-old Hispanic female, comes into the van to have her blood pressure checked because she has been feeling tired and nauseated lately and is having difficulty working in the fields. She is also complaining of a coin-shaped rash on her arms, palms, and trunk. In completing your history, you find that she has not had any medical care since she was 8, when she had her appendix removed in Florida. Her blood pressure is 100/68 mm Hg. She cannot remember when her last menstrual period was, but she thinks it was 2 month ago. She is sexually active and uses condoms occasionally. She lives with her mother, four sisters, two brothers, and her father (who has forbidden her to see her boyfriend, Juan) in a travel trailer that they pull from town to town.

   • What are your nursing diagnoses in this situation?

   • How would you address the two dimensions of secondary prevention (diagnosis and treatment) of pregnancy and secondary syphilis?

   • What secondary and tertiary preventive measures might be appropriate in working with Miss King?

   • What resources could you as a community nurse tap to assist Miss King?

2. Mrs. Wise, a 67-year-old woman, is being discharged from the hospital after having surgery to repair a broken hip and bilateral wrist fractures. She will have bilateral casts for 8 weeks. She is a widow and has two sons who live within 2 miles of her. She lives alone. Her daughters-in-law will be the main caretakers. Both daughters-in-law work outside the home, neither have had any medical training, and they are afraid of assuming the health care of their mother-in-law. Mrs. Wise is reluctant to move in with her sons and would rather return to her small townhouse. The discharge diagnosis includes hip and wrist repair as a result of osteoporosis, diabetes, hypertension, and obesity.

   • What are your nursing diagnoses in this situation?

   • How would you address considerations of competence, time management, and supervision in planning the care of Mrs. Wise?

CRITICAL THINKING ACTIVITIES—CONT'D

- What resources could you as a community nurse use to assist this family in caring for Mrs. Wise and at the same time address Mrs. Wise's concerns regarding her independence?

3. Empowerment of women may well be seen in a depiction of the Greek Goddess Sarasvati (sa-RAS-vah-tee). She is the goddess of knowledge and is credited with the creation of the fruits of civilization, arts, and music. Her color and brightness represents the powerful, pure light of education, which destroys the darkness of ignorance. Sarasvati is depicted with four arms, showing that her power extends in all directions. In one of her hands, she holds a book (representing learning) and in another a strand of beads (representing spiritual knowledge). In the other hands, she holds and plays the vina, an Indian lute, representing the art of music (Waldherr, 1996).

- How does this depict our society of women in the United States today?
- Is education encouraged in women?
- What is spirituality, and how is it seen in our society? How is it seen in Sarasvati?
- What does music represent to Sarasvati or to the women of many other cultures and diversities?
- What is the darkness of ignorance?

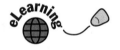

Explore Community Health Nursing on the web! To learn more about the topics in this chapter, access your exclusive web site:
http://communitynursing.jbpub.com

REFERENCES

Allen, K., & Phillips, J. (1997). *Women's health across the lifespan: A comprehensive perspective*. Philadelphia: J. B. Lippincott.

American Cancer Society. (1995). *Cancer facts and figures*. Atlanta: Author.

American Medical Association (AMA). (1998). *Women's health overview*: www.ama-assn.org/insight/h_focus/wom_hlth/40-60.htm.

Benderly, B. (1997). *In her own right: The Institute of Medicine's guide to women's health issues*. Washington, DC: National Academy Press.

Bennett, M. (1987). Afro-American women, poverty and mental health: A social essay. *Women and Health Care, 12*, 213–228.

Biegel, D., Sales, E., & Schulz, R. (1991). *Family caregiving in chronic illness*. Thousand Oaks, CA: Sage Publications.

Center for Disease Control and Prevention (CDC). (1999, September 11). *Monthly Vital Statistics Report, 46, 1*(2), 2: www.cdc.gov/nchsww/datamu46_l52.pdf.

Deevey S., & Wall. L. (1992). How do lesbian women develop serenity? *Health Care Women International, 13*, 199–208.

Department of Health and Human Services (DHHS). (1991). *Healthy people 2000: National objectives for health promotion and disease prevention*. Washington, DC: U.S. Government Printing Office.

Division for the Advancement of Women. (1995, September). *The United Nations fourth world conference on women*: www.undp.org/fwcw//daw1.htm.

Fogel, C., & Woods, N. (1995). *Women's health care: A comprehensive handbook*. Thousand Oaks, CA: Sage Publications.

Garner, C. (1991). Midlife women's health. *NAACOG Clinical Issues, 2,* 473–481.

Giger, J., & Davidhizar, R. (1995). *Transcultural nursing: Assessment and intervention*. St Louis: Mosby.

Gilliard, D. K., & Beck, A. J. (1994, June). *Prisoners in 1993: Bureau of Justice statistics*. Washington, DC: U.S. Department of Justice.

Golub, S., & Freedman, R. (1985). *Health needs of women as they age*. New York: Haworth Press.

Hogan, S. (1990). Care for the caregiver: Social policies to ease their burden. *Journal of Gerontological Nursing, 16*(5), 12–17.

IGC. www.igc.apc.org/justice/prisons/women/women-in-prison.html.

Lawton, M., Rajagopal, D., Brody, E., & Kleban, M. (1992). The dynamic of caregiving for a demented elder among black and white families. *Journal of Gerontology, 47*(4), S516–S164.

Leading causes of mortality and morbidity and contributing behaviors in the United States. (1997). In *United States adolescent health summary*: www.cdc.gov/nccdphp/dash/ahsumm/ussumm.htm.

Lipson. J., Dibble, S., & Minarik, P. (1996). *Culture & nursing care: A pocket guide*. San Francisco: UCSF Nursing Press.

Mark, D., Shaw, L., & DeLong, E. (1994). Absence of sex bias in the referral of patients for cardiac catheterization. *New England Journal of Medicine, 330,* 1101–1106.

McGinn, K. A., & Haylock, P. J. (1993). *Women's cancers*. Alameda, CA: Hunter House.

National Center for Health Statistics. (1993). *Health promotion and disease prevention: United States, 1990* (Series 10, No. 163, DHHS Publication No. 1850. Hyattsville, MD: Department of Health and Human Services.

Pasquale, S. A. (1994). Helping patient make informed contraceptive decisions. *Contemporary OB/GYN, 39*(10), 12–22.

Pollard, K, & Tordella, S. (1993). Women making gains among professionals. *Population Today, 21,* 1–2.

Phillips, J., Sexton, M., & Blackman, J. (1996). Demographic overview of women across the life span. In K. Allen & J. Phillips (Eds.), *Women's health across the lifespan*. Philadelphia, J. B, Lippincott.

Purnell, L., & Paulanka, B. (1998). *Transcultural health care: A culturally competent approach*. Philadelphia: F.A. Davis.

Riggs, J. (1991). The family caregiver support act. *Caring, 10*(12), 18–21.

Rosser, S. (1995). *Women's health—missing from U.S. medicine*. Bloomington: Indiana University Press.

Smith, P.A. (1995). Preventive Services. In D. P. Lemcke, J. Pattison, L. A. Marshall, & D. S. Cowley (Eds.), *Primary care of women* (p. 53). Norwalk, CT: Appleton & Lange.

Stevens, P., Tatum, N., & White, J. (1996). Optimal care for lesbian patients. *Patient Care, 30*(5), 121–134.

Taeuber, C. (1991). *Statistical handbook on women in America*. Phoenix: Oryx Press.

U.S. Census Bureau. (1997, June). National Center for Health Statistics: *New report document trends in childbearing, reproductive health*: www.cdc.gov/nchswww/releases/97facts/97sheets/nsfgfact.htm.

U.S. Census Bureau. (1999, April 29). National Center for Health Statistics: *National vital statistics reports*: www.cdc.gov/nchswww/data/nug47_18.pdf.

Waldherr, K. (1996). *The book of goddesses*. Hillsboro, OR: Beyond Words Publishing.

Wheeler, S. (September, 2000). Female prisoners in the United States. *Gender Policy Review*. Online: www.igc.org/igc/gateway/wnindex.html.

Williams R., & Thomas, D. (1997). Women's health. In J. Swanson & M. Nies (Eds.), *Community health nursing* (2nd ed.). Philadelphia: W. B. Saunders.

Wuest, J. (1993). Institutionalizing women's oppression: The inherent risk in health policy that fosters community participation. *Health Care Women International, 14,* 407–417.

Zeidenstein, L. (1990). Gynecological and childbearing needs of lesbians. *Journal of Nurse Midwifery, 35,* 10–18.

Chapter 20

Adolescent Pregnancy

Loretta Sweet Jemmott, Michelle Cousins Mott, and Susan Oliver Dodds

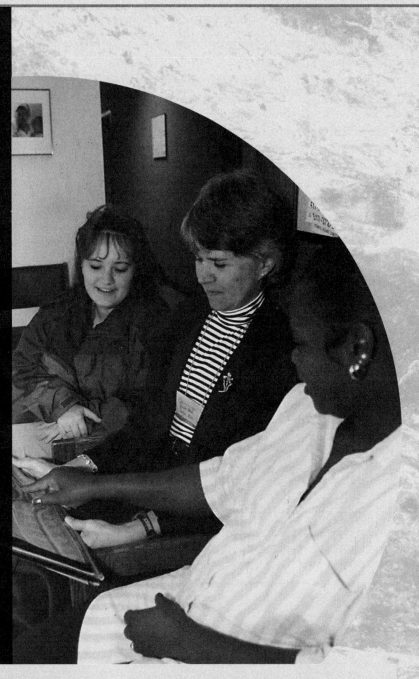

Adolescent pregnancy is a major public health problem, affecting not only the pregnant adolescent and her infant, but also families and communities nationwide.

QUESTIONS TO CONSIDER

After reading this chapter, answer the following questions:
  1. What are the factors contributing to adolescent pregnancy?
  2. What are the health outcomes for adolescent mothers?
  3. What is the effect of adolescent pregnancy on the family?
  4. How are adolescent fathers affected by their partner's pregnancy?
  5. What are the health outcomes for babies born to adolescent mothers?
  6. What kinds of community-based prevention programs are available?
  7. What is the role of the community health nurse in primary, secondary, and tertiary prevention efforts for adolescent pregnancy?

KEY TERMS

Abortion
Abstinence
Acculturation
Adolescent fathers
Adoption

Childhood victimization
Condoms
Contraception
Family dynamics
Health outcomes

Gynecological age
Peer education
Low birth weight (LBW)
Prenatal care

Repeat pregnancy
Primary prevention
Secondary prevention
Tertiary prevention

Adolescent pregnancy has often been depicted as affecting only poor, urban, minority teens, but the problem extends across all ethnic groups, socioeconomic classes, and geographic boundaries. Adolescents living in rural areas are affected at rates comparable to their urban peers (Loda, Speizer, Martin, Skatrud, & Bennett, 1997). Despite our investment of a significant amount of attention, time, research, and money on prevention efforts, the results remain discouraging, as adolescent pregnancy rates in the United States remain higher than those in most other industrialized countries (Foster, 1997).

Community health nurses can play a significant role in reducing the incidence of adolescent pregnancy and improving the quality of **health outcomes** of adolescent mothers, their children, and communities overburdened by this problem. By implementing creative interventions that address adolescents, families, and the community, community health nurses can be important weapons in the battle against adolescent pregnancy. However, it is important for the community health nurse to understand the contributing factors to adolescent pregnancy, the impact of adolescent pregnancy on adolescents and families, and the role of the community health nurse before these interventions are implemented.

Sexual Behavior and Pregnancy Rates

More than three-fourths of American adolescents have had sexual intercourse by the time they are 19 years of age, and adolescents are initiating sex at earlier ages (AGI, 1994, 1998; CDC, 1991; Hatcher, Trussell, Stewart, Stewart, Kowal, Guest, Cates, & Policar, 1994; Sonenstein, Pleck, & Leighton, 1989). Much of this sexual activity occurs without the use of safer sex measures, and consequently, adolescents are at risk for becoming pregnant and acquiring sexually transmitted diseases (STDs), including human immunodeficiency virus (HIV). Lack of protection is more likely among younger teens and adolescents, who have less sexual experience, making pregnancy particularly likely during the initial sexual intercourse encounters (AGI, 1998; Polaneczky,

FYI

One in eight adolescents in the United States ages 15 to 19 becomes pregnant each year.

Half of all initial adolescent premarital pregnancies occur within the first 6 months after initiation of coitus; 20% occur in the first month alone.

Media images of adolescent pregnancy often show minority adolescent teens, but adolescent pregnancy is not only a minority issue. Caucasian teenagers consistently account for the largest percentage of adolescent pregnancies and births.

Source: AGI, 1994, 1998; Pittman & Adams, 1988.

1998; Pratt, Mosher, Bachrach, & Horn, 1984; Spitz, Velebil, Koonin, Strauss, Goodman, Wingo, Wilson, Morris, & Marks, 1996; Taylor, Kagay, & Leichenko, 1986; Zabin, Kantner, & Zelnik, 1979; Zelnik, Kantner, & Ford, 1981).

More than 1 million adolescents become pregnant each year, with the majority of those pregnancies being unintended. Recent statistics report that, overall, adolescents account for 30% of all nonmarital births in the United States and 25% of unplanned pregnancies (AGI, 1998). Eighty-three percent of low-income adolescents become pregnant (Kirby, 1997), and many of these pregnancies are linked to negative future educational and employment outcomes (Coyle, Kirby, Parcel, Basen-Engquist, Banspach, Rugg, & Weil, 1996). The phenomenon of closely spaced (repeat) births among teens is also significant. More than 25% of adolescents who become pregnant will become pregnant again within 2 years (AGI, 1998; Campaign for Our Children, 1996). Multiple pregnancies intensify the negative consequences associated with adolescent pregnancy.

Factors Contributing to Adolescent Pregnancy

Many factors have been associated with adolescent pregnancy. Factors including earlier age of onset of puberty, earlier age of initiation of intercourse, increased sexual activity, nonuse or inconsistent use of contraceptives, lack of knowledge about sex and conception, developmental age, and social/environmental status have contributed to an increased risk for teenage pregnancy. For the community health nurse to develop appropriate interventions to prevent adolescent pregnancy, it is essential to understand the contributing factors.

Developmental Stage

Adolescence is a time of uncertainty and experimentation, as young people strive to develop their identity in preparation for adulthood. For many young people, it is a time of sexual experimentation. This experimentation is in response to the adolescents' physical, hormonal, cognitive, and psychosocial development. Unfortunately, the consequences of such experimentation far too often include increased risk of pregnancy.

Psychosocial Development

Adolescent psychosocial development progresses through three stages: early, middle, and late adolescence. Early adolescence (ages 11 to 13) is characterized by turmoil stemming from physical changes and emotional fluctuation influenced by changing hormone levels (Drake, 1996). In this stage, adolescents are often seeking control, may show defiance to authority figures, and may use sex as an outlet for the expression of their perceived control (Drake, 1996; Flavell, Miller, & Miller, 1993). Middle adolescence (ages 14 to 16) is characterized by development of self-identity and sexual identity. In search of their identity, adolescents may imitate the behaviors they see around them from media, older peers, parents, and other adults (Foster, 1997; Males, 1993). Late adolescence (ages 17 to 20) is characterized by the adaptation of self-identity and development of coping strategies that will be used in adulthood (Drake, 1996). Adolescents who do not have a strong self-identity and sexual identity may not be able to assert themselves and apply coping strategies such as the sexual negotiation skills that are used with a sexual partner (Flavell, Miller, & Miller, 1993). As a result, adolescents may give in to sexual pressure from their peers and sexual partners.

Intrapersonal Issues and Development

The development of self-concept is a major task of adolescence. For adolescents who have a poor sense of self and have a history of unsuccessful life experience, the need for love and attention may lead to sexual intercourse and pregnancy. As a mother, the adolescent may sense that she will be the center of attention in the family and have a feeling of importance and belonging (Fisher, 1984).

Adolescents may view sexual intercourse and pregnancy as a link to a sexual partner. They may believe that having sex or becoming pregnant is a way that they can ensure a continued, exclusive, caring relationship with that partner. As a result, some adolescents may feel pressured into sexual relations because they fear losing their partner if they do not comply (Davis, 1980; Toledo-Dreves, Zabin, & Emerson, 1995). This is a particularly important factor for adolescents who do not feel needed or cared for within the family unit.

In general, pregnancy as a strategy to compensate for unmet needs, to have self-esteem, or to assert independence is not particularly beneficial or successful. Parenting provides ample opportunity for failures, which are not helpful to adolescents already faced with repeated failures in their lives. An infant cannot meet all the nurturing expectations of the adolescent and has significant nurturing and attention needs of its own.

Social and Environmental Factors

Environment significantly influences adolescent ideas about sex and pregnancy and their resulting behavior. Each society has implied messages about sexuality, social behavior, and pregnancy. The clarity of the messages the community provides influences the sexual behaviors and expectations of its members (Foster, 1997). Several social and environmental factors have been identified as contributing to the high rates of adolescent pregnancy in the United States. Influences from family, culture, socioeconomic status, peers, sexual partners, drugs/alcohol use, previous sexual abuse, and STDs have all been identified (Kenney, Reinholtz, & Angelini, 1997; Plouffe & White, 1996; Robinson & Frank, 1994; Toledo-Dreves, Zabin, & Emerson, 1995; Widom & Kuhns, 1996; Zoccolillo, Meyers, & Assiter, 1997).

The Family of the Adolescent

An understanding of **family dynamics** is essential for the community nurse to work effectively with the pregnant adolescent and her family. Every family is governed by its own rules and ex-

pectations, which determine expected behavior for its members (Bowen, 1971). Problems occur when there is poor communication and conflicting messages about sex and pregnancy (DiIorio, Hockenbeery-Eaton, Maibach, Rivero, & Miller, 1996). Adolescents may hear mixed messages from the family, which often come from the family's own discomfort and embarrassment about sex and pregnancy. As a result, adolescents may perceive affirming attitudes about adolescent sexuality.

The Ethnicity/Culture of the Adolescent

Differences in culture may affect the family and peer reactions to adolescent pregnancy, which in turn influences an adolescent's perception of pregnancy. Many factors contribute to cultural identity, and it is not suggested that all members of a particular cultural group will behave in an identical fashion; however, the community nurse must be aware of and sensitive to cultural influences on adolescent pregnancy.

Mainstream American culture has a negative view toward adolescent pregnancy, yet the rates of adolescent pregnancy remain higher in the United States than in other industrialized nations (Desmond, 1994; Trad, 1999). The existence of many subcultures and various culturally based beliefs may contribute to the higher rates of adolescent pregnancy. For example, in traditional, patriarchal Latino culture, females are expected to respond to male demands, and marriage and motherhood/fatherhood are viewed as catalysts to adulthood (Orshan, 1996). As a result, Latino adolescents may have a positive attitude toward pregnancy. However, the extent to which these common culturally based beliefs impact attitudes toward pregnancy may depend on the adolescent's level of acculturation. **Acculturation** is a dynamic, multidimensional phenomenon in which the ideals and beliefs of one culture are incorporated into that of another (Orshan, 1996; Reynoso, Felice, & Shragg, 1993). Acculturated American Latino adolescents from traditional Latino families may receive contradictory sexual messages from mainstream American society and the more traditional messages of their Latino culture. To the adolescent who is developing an identity, these conflicting views may lead to inconsistent feelings about sexual activity and contraceptive use.

Similarly, African American adolescents who grow up in single-parent families may receive mixed messages about adolescent pregnancy. These adolescents may see a pattern of intergenerational out-of-wedlock teen pregnancies but hear disapproving messages about adolescent pregnancy (Desmond, 1994). Compounding the issue, there may be poor communication between the adolescent and parent about sexual issues.

Cultural influences are not limited to adolescents in minority cultures. Caucasian adolescents may also be influenced by cultural issues. In some European American cultures, discussion about sex and pregnancy is taboo. Adolescents who live in these environments may look to their peers and the media for rules of acceptable sexual conduct. Uneducated peers may provide misinformation, and the media may provide a false image of sex and pregnancy risks.

Socioeconomic Factors

There exists a vicious cycle between lower economic status and adolescent pregnancy (Males, 1993). Lower socioeconomic status has been correlated with higher rates of sexual activity and adolescent pregnancy, and adolescent pregnancy is associated with higher rates of school dropout. Adolescents who drop out of school have a decreased likelihood of attaining gainful employment. Data have shown that few adolescent parents are adequately prepared to assume the economic, social, and psychological responsibility of child care and child rearing (Stevens-Simon, Kelly, Singer, & Cox, 1996). This phenomenon has been seen across the various cultures and ethnic groups in the United States (Desmond, 1994; Farber, 1994).

Lower socioeconomic status may be linked to decreased access to care, which translates to decreased access to family planning and prevention information. Decreased access to care and contraceptive information may contribute to a higher rate of **repeat pregnancy** in the adolescent and may impact the health of the child (AGI, 1994).

The Adolescent's Peers

One of the single most influential factors in adolescent sexual activity and pregnancy is the influence of peers (Coyle et al., 1996). Formation of peer groups and an increased need for peer acceptance are normal developmental milestones of adolescence. However, this increased need for acceptance may cause adolescents to give in to the requests of their peers or imitate the actions of their peers, which may include sexual experimentation and risky sexual behavior. Moreover, sexual information is often exchanged by adolescent peers and may lead to misconceptions and result in unintended pregnancy.

The Adolescent's Sexual Partner

It is important to understand the male partner of female adolescents because female adolescent sexual activity often is submissive to male sexual desire (Jemmott & Jemmott, 1990). In addition, the typical contraceptive methods on which adolescents rely before seeking prescription contraceptives are male methods, such as condoms and withdrawal before ejaculation (Morrison, 1985).

Male attitudes toward contraceptive use, especially **condoms,** have been described as negative (Jemmott & Jemmott, 1990, 1992; Jemmott, Jemmott, & Fong, 1998; Morrison, 1985; Sorensen, 1973). For instance, many males view condom use unfavorably because they believe it reduces the pleasure or spontaneity of sexual activities. Adolescent males commonly believe that **contraception** is a female's responsibility (Jemmott & Jemmott, 1990).

Little attention has been paid to the age of sexual partners of adolescents. It has been reported that the majority of male sexual partners of adolescent females are approximately 5 years older (average age 20 to 24) (AGI, 1998), with only 30% of adolescent pregnancies resulting from **adolescent fathers.** Adolescent females may view their relationships with older partners as providing an escape from poverty, a show of defiance, a display of sexuality, and a boost to self-esteem. However, adolescent females with an in-complete perception of self may not feel able to negotiate and assert sexual boundaries, such as condom use with their older partners, and may submit to the older partner's sexual demands. Consequently, many adult-adolescent relationships result in an adolescent pregnancy (Toledo-Dreves, Zabin, & Emerson, 1995).

Adolescent males have similar risk factors for pregnancy as their female peers. Often, adolescent males struggle with development and may attempt to demonstrate independence, belong to peer groups, and demonstrate physical and sexual maturity by engaging in sexual activity. As adolescents, males may also lack future-oriented thinking and concrete thinking abilities. Together, these factors contribute to increased potential for participating in risky sexual behaviors that may lead to pregnancy (Jemmott, 1993). Adolescent males may also view pregnancy as a catalyst toward manhood and may purposely have unprotected intercourse. In the African American community, the risk for an adolescent-fathered, teenage pregnancy may be higher. The mean age for sexual initiation among African American males has been estimated to be as low as 11.1 years (Jemmott, 1993; Jemmott & Jemmott, 1990). See the Research Brief below.

Substance Use Among Adolescents

Several studies have found that the use of alcohol or drugs during sexual activity is associated with risky sexual behavior, such as intercourse with multiple partners and failure to use condoms (Jemmott & Jemmott, 1992). Alcohol and drug use may change the nature of the sexual behavior in which people engage because

RESEARCH BRIEF

Robinson, R. B., & Frank, D. L. (1994). The relation between self-esteem, sexual activity, and pregnancy. Adolescence, 29(113), 26–35.

A study by nurse researchers examined self-esteem in relation to sexual behaviors for adolescents. A sample of 141 male and 172 female adolescents of diverse ethnic backgrounds was surveyed to determine levels of self-esteem, sexual activity, pregnancy, and fatherhood status. The Coopersmith Self-Esteem Inventory was also used to obtain qualitative data related to self-esteem, demographics, and sexual activity. Analysis revealed no differences in the self-esteem of males versus females. Sexual activity or virginity had no relationship to self-esteem in males or females. Self-esteem levels were no different for pregnant teens in comparison with nonpregnant teens. However, males who had fathered a child had lower self-esteem than nonfathers. The findings support a multifocused approach to sex education for pregnancy prevention and also emphasize a need to include males in both pregnancy intervention efforts and further research on adolescent pregnancy.

logic and good judgment are clouded and inhibitions are loosened when people are "high" or because intoxication provides an excuse to engage in risky behavior (Crowe & George, 1989; Fortenberry, Orr, Katz, Brizendine, & Blythe, 1997; Jemmott & Jemmott, 1992; Kokotailo, Langhough, Cox, Davidson, & Fleming, 1994). However, there is a second, simpler explanation of the relationship between alcohol and drug use and risky sexual behavior. Adolescents who use alcohol and drugs more frequently than their peers may also engage in more sexual activity than their peers; consequently, they may engage in more risky sexual activity compared with their peers. The argument is not that alcohol and drug use causes adolescents to engage in different, more risky sexual behavior, but rather that adolescents who use alcohol and drugs engage in sexual activity more frequently (Jemmott & Jemmott, 1992).

Sexual and Physical Abuse of Adolescent Females

Childhood victimization may be linked to promiscuity and adolescent pregnancy. Adolescent females who were physically and/or sexually abused may be more likely to initiate sexual intercourse at a younger age, use drugs and alcohol, and engage in more promiscuous relationships than nonabused adolescents (Kenney, Reinholtz, & Angelini, 1997). Childhood abuse has been associated with low socioeconomic status, unemployment, family dysfunction, substance use, and psychological dysfunction. Because many of the risk factors for childhood abuse are interrelated and linked to adolescent pregnancy, it is difficult to separate the effect of each factor in a child's environment that may influence behavior (Fiscella, Kitzman, Cole, Sidora, & Olds, 1998).

Adolescents who have experienced physical or sexual abuse may use sex in an effort to attain loving nonabusive relationships or may view pregnancy as a way out of the abusive environment at home (Widom & Kuhns, 1996). However, the adolescent who has not fully developed emotionally may not be in the position to be assertive and use sexual negotiation skills, leaving them at greater risk for experiencing further sexual exploitation by present and future partners.

Knowledge Deficit Regarding Sex, Conception, and Contraception

The increased sexual activity among adolescents has not been accompanied by increased knowledge about sexual function, procreation, or birth control. Studies indicate that many adolescents remain woefully ignorant about conception and the menstrual cycle (Darabi, Jones, Varga, & Hourse, 1982; Davis & Harris, 1982; Jemmott & Jemmott, 1990; Landry, Bertrand, Cherry, & Rich, 1986). In addition to lack of information on sex and conception, adolescents lack correct information on birth control methods and the correct use of contraceptives (Davtyan, 2000; Morrison, 1985; Pollack, 1992).

Even though contraceptive information has become more available, many adolescents do not use birth control on a regular basis (Box 20-1). Adolescents generally engage in sexual intercourse for some time before obtaining reliable contraception. Reluctance to obtain and use contraception is associated with certain attitudes and psychological and social factors. Stevens-Simon,

FYI

One of five pregnant adolescents is physically and/or sexually abused (hitting, unwanted touching, sexual advances, or intercourse) by a family member or partner during their pregnancies.

BOX 20-1 WHY ADOLESCENTS DO NOT USE CONTRACEPTION IN THEIR OWN WORDS

- I didn't mind getting pregnant.
- I didn't want to appear to my partner to be prepared to have sex.
- I wanted to get pregnant.
- I wasn't planning to have sex.
- I didn't know how to get birth control.
- I thought my boyfriend was sterile.
- I didn't think that I could get pregnant.
- I didn't know how to use birth control.
- I wanted to have a baby so my boyfriend would love me.
- I thought my partner would be angry with me if I used birth control.
- I was afraid my family would find out.
- I wanted a baby to love.
- I was afraid of the side effects.
- I thought other people would find out that I was using birth control.
- It's hard to talk to my partner about birth control.
- I was embarrassed about using birth control.
- My boyfriend wanted me to get pregnant.
- I just did not get around to it.
- My partner didn't want to use birth control.
- Birth control can be expensive.
- Using a condom interferes with sexual pleasure.
- Getting birth control is inconvenient.

Source: Adapted from AGI, 1981; Howard & McCabe, 1992; Jemmott & Jemmott, 1990, 1992; Jemmott, Jemmott, & Fong, 1998; Loda et al., 1997; Zelnik & Kantner, 1979.

Kelly, Singer, and Cox (1996) reported that adolescents' attitudes include "I don't mind getting pregnant" or "I want to get pregnant." Adolescents who feel this way may neglect to use contraception or be inconsistent users of contraception.

Impact of Adolescent Pregnancy

Adolescent pregnancy has significant, far-reaching consequences. Pregnancy can affect the adolescent's health, development, education, and socioeconomic status. The family and community may also feel the effects because the majority of adolescents are unwed, live with their families, and depend on public assistance (Coley & Chase-Lansdale, 1998). In addition to psychosocial and economical outcomes, the adolescent mother experiences physical consequences that may affect her health.

Psychosocial and Health Outcomes of the Mother

Pregnancy is a time of increased demands on a woman's body. These demands can be harmful to a developing adolescent, especially if there is no focus on the increased needs of pregnancy, such as nutrition and rest. In general, adolescents experience greater health problems with pregnancy than do women older than 20 years of age. The consequences are especially severe to the youngest adolescents, those 12 to 15 years of age (Levy, Perhats, Nash-Johnson, & Welter, 1992; Trad, 1999).

Adolescents are at greater risk for developing pregnancy-induced hypertension and toxemia (AGI, 1981), anemia, nutritional deficiencies, and urinary tract infections (Bulcholz & Gol, 1986). Adolescent girls are more likely to deliver prematurely, experience rapid or prolonged labor, develop abruptio placenta, or have fetal or maternal infections (Mott, 1990).

Lack of Prenatal Care

One of the major reasons for negative health outcomes for mothers and infants is lack of **prenatal care**. More pregnant adolescents delay seeking prenatal care, access less prenatal care, or do not receive regular care as often as adult women (Cockey, 1997; Geronimus, 1986). The same teenagers at greatest risk for pregnancy—those from poor families—are also at greatest risk for poor prenatal care. This lack of care contributes to poorer health outcomes for both mother and infant. Most adolescents do not receive prenatal care in the first trimester, with nearly 20% accessing care in the last trimester only. In general, this group tends to be more illness-oriented than prevention-oriented in their health practices. The reasons for this delayed initiation of prenatal care are varied and include denial of the pregnancy, lack of knowledge, lack of access to health care, concern about concealing the pregnancy, developmental immaturity (Cockney, 1997; Zuckerman, Walker, Frank, Chase, & Hamburg, 1984), and an orientation toward concrete, present-centered reasoning (Geronimus, 1986).

Repeated Pregnancy

Several studies have shown that many young mothers have more than one child during their teen years. Obtaining exact numbers is difficult because U.S. Census data does not report repeat pregnancy rates, but estimates range from 15% to 60%, depending on the study (Brown, Saunders, & Dick, 1999; Cockey, 1997).

Adolescent mothers who have repeat pregnancies continue to be at higher risk for poor outcomes. Although it might be reasonably assumed that adolescent mothers would be more savvy in a second pregnancy, seeking and receiving more timely prenatal care, this is often not the case. One study examined the outcomes of first and second adolescent pregnancies among Caucasian and African American teenagers. The results revealed that a poor outcome in the first pregnancy was associated with a three times greater risk of repeating that outcome in the second pregnancy. The recurrence rate of preterm delivery was especially severe for African American adolescents (Blankson, Cliver, Goldenberg, Hickey, Jin, & Dubard, 1993). These results are critical because they provide a specific target for the **secondary prevention** efforts of nurses working in the community.

Psychosocial Outcomes

Although pregnancy can become a stimulus for positive growth in an adolescent, generally the results are more negative than positive. Motherhood or fatherhood in the adolescent years can cause severe disruption in the normal psychosocial development of adolescents. Pregnancy places an additional psychosocial burden on teenagers, who are already attempting to cope with the normal maturational crisis of adolescence (Bulcholz & Gol, 1986; Trad, 1999).

Adolescents typically cope with the confusion and conflict in their lives by finding safety and acceptance in their peer groups. However, adolescent parents, especially mothers, may find them-

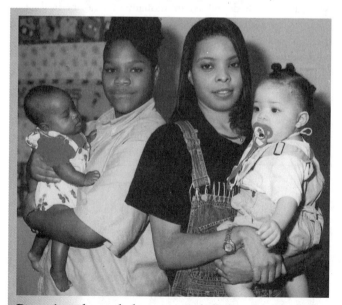

Parenting classes help teen mothers bond with their babies.

selves isolated from their peer groups at a critical time in their development. The degree of isolation may vary depending on the norms accepted by different cultural peer groups.

A primary goal of adolescence is attainment of independence. Although pregnancy may enhance independence in some ways by forcing the adolescent to take charge of a difficult situation, this forced rapid ascension into adulthood certainly is not without negative consequences. After delivery, as adolescent parents cope with the demands of a new infant, their own needs and desires are no longer first priority. The increased stress of being an adolescent parent can lead to more self-doubt, uncertainty, loneliness, and helplessness (Lieberman, 1980). The adolescent's inability to effectively cope with these feelings is reflected in the increased incidence of child abuse and neglect within this cohort (Marshall, Buckner, & Powell, 1991).

Education and Economic Disruption

Adolescents who become pregnant are less likely than their nonpregnant peers to complete their education. For example, whereas 90% of women who delay childbearing beyond adolescence complete a high school education, only 70% of adolescent mothers ultimately reach this goal (AGI, 1994). Without a complete education, many adolescent mothers find employment opportunities out of their reach and rely on low-paying jobs or public assistance programs (Grogger & Bronars, 1993).

Impact on the Family

An unplanned adolescent pregnancy can seriously jeopardize quality of life not only for the young mother and infant but also for the extended families. Families are often called on to shoulder considerable economic and emotional burdens. The strain on the family is often intensified because adolescent mothers are more likely to live in single-parent households (AGI, 1994). The long-term impact on the family is unknown, but as families compensate to deal with adolescent pregnancy, they may normalize the experience and set the stage for future adolescent pregnancy. From generation to generation, this trend may develop into a cycle. The children of adolescent parents are at increased risk of perpetuating the cycle by becoming adolescent parents themselves and dropping out of school (Campaign for Our Children, 1996).

Impact on the Adolescent Father

For every adolescent conception that occurs outside marriage, there is a father as well as a pregnant mother, yet there is limited research focusing on adolescent males who become fathers. The impact of adolescent pregnancy has been largely focused on adolescent females despite the obvious involvement of males. Even though adolescent males are the fathers in only 30% of adolescent pregnancies, it is important for the community health nurse to address the problem of teenage pregnancy with this group. Adolescent fathers may be more at risk for continued educational and social problems. Fagot, Pears, Capaldi, Crosby, and Leve (1998) found that adolescent fathers had more arrests and substance use problems than did nonfathers of the same age. The adolescent father's reaction to the pregnancy, his own psychosocial developmental issues and needs, and his behavior as a young father are critical to developing positive health outcomes for the child and impacting the behaviors of these young men before adulthood.

The adolescent father's reaction to the pregnancy is a crucial factor in determining what role he will play in the pregnancy and delivery and in the child's life. Some adolescent males react positively, but others do not. Reactions to pregnancy are influenced by many factors, including family reaction, peer group reaction, and relationship with the mother of the child. Another factor that may influence the reaction is the developmental stage of the father, because many may not be able to cope effectively with a pregnancy. Problems that impact the adolescent male revolve around the acknowledgment of the child, his financial responsibility, his school commitment, and his work situation (Males, 1993). Adolescent fathers report feeling frightened and disturbed by the responsibilities and neglected in the decision-making process, although few abandon the mother during pregnancy. Unfortunately, the young father may abandon the adolescent mother after pregnancy.

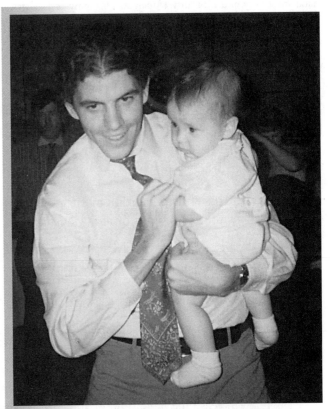

Nurses can use celebrity role models like Will Turpin, bass guitarist for Collective Soul (shown here with his son, Tristan), to demonstrate the rewards of waiting for marriage and fatherhood.

Regardless of the good intentions of most men, the fate of most adolescent fathers is similar to that of teenage mothers. Most are ill prepared to assume the role of fatherhood, and few relish the opportunity. Generally, having come from poor, relatively uneducated backgrounds, they experience serious social and economic disadvantages compared with young men who postpone fatherhood until a later age (Sonenstein, Stewart, Lindberg, Pernas, & Williams, 1997). Most of the fathers lack the necessary skills to provide a stable home environment for their families even if they want to. In short, poverty is the tie that binds most adolescent fathers and mothers. Although some manage to cope with their situation, continue educational and vocational pursuits, and mature into self-sufficient, productive members of society, the odds are stacked against them.

Psychosocial and Health Outcomes of the Newborn

Infants born to adolescents are at risk for various health problems as a result of complications with the adolescent mother's pregnancy and with the birth. These health problems include the increased incidence of preterm deliveries (before 38 weeks' gestation), increased incidence of **low-birth-weight** (**LBW**) infants (birth weight of less than 2,500 g), and increased incidence of perinatal morbidity and mortality (American Academy of Pediatrics, 1989; Blankson et al., 1993; Leppert, Namerow, & Barker, 1986).

There has been considerable debate over whether young maternal age alone is an independent risk factor for complications,

and the results are still unclear (DuPlessis, Bell, & Richards, 1997). More recent research suggests that other mediating factors (e.g., low socioeconomic status, poor prenatal care, race/ethnicity, unfavorable sociocultural circumstances) play a critical role (Plouffe & White, 1996; Yoder & Young, 1997).

Role of the Nurse

It is apparent that pregnancy during the adolescent years presents some unique risks and special needs for the adolescent, her pregnancy, and her infant. Obviously, **primary prevention** of pregnancy is a crucial component of any adolescent intervention program. However, if young girls become pregnant, it is imperative that they receive secondary and tertiary preventive care, including adequate prenatal care coupled with long-term postpartum follow-up to ensure a healthy outcome for both mother and child. Community health nurses, because of their expertise in assessment, health teaching, and program development, are well suited to this task. Their accessibility to adolescent populations places them in a pivotal position to play a significant role in the delivery of care before sexual activity, during pregnancy, and during long-term follow-up with the parents and child.

Healthy People 2010 addresses specific goals for adolescent pregnancy prevention (see the *Healthy People 2010* box below for selected objectives). The community health nurse may use these national objectives to guide the development of nursing interventions.

HEALTHY PEOPLE 2010

OBJECTIVES RELATED TO FAMILY PLANNING

9.2   Reduce the proportion of births occurring within 24 months of a previous birth.

9.6   Increase male involvement in pregnancy prevention and family planning efforts.

9.7   Reduce pregnancies among adolescent females.

9.8   Increase the proportion of adolescents who have never engaged in sexual intercourse before age 15 years.

9.9   Increase the proportion of adolescents who have never engaged in sexual intercourse.

9.10   Increase the proportion of sexually active, unmarried adolescents aged 15 to 17 years who use contraception that both effectively prevents pregnancy and provides barrier protection against disease.

9.11   Increase the proportion of young adults who receive formal instruction before turning age 18 years on reproductive health issues, including all of the following topics: birth control methods, safer sex to prevent HIV, prevention of sexually transmitted diseases, and abstinence.

Source: DHHS, 2000.

The majority of adolescents behave as if their states were that of moratorium. That is, adolescence is a time for experimenting with how one might want to be as an adult.

Rew (1998) quoted in Frisch and Frisch (1998)

Primary Prevention

Because primary prevention is a critical component of effective community health nursing, there are tremendous opportunities for nurses to address the multifaceted problem of teen pregnancy and make important contributions to developing and implementing interventions to reduce the incidence of adolescent pregnancy. Table 20-1 provides a list of issues to be considered when planning nursing interventions. An example of primary prevention is education and counseling for adolescents about sexual health issues, including, but not limited to, pregnancy prevention, family life education, family planning, and the postponement of pregnancy into adulthood. A comprehensive program in primary prevention targeting adolescent pregnancy includes three goals:

1. *Delaying or halting participation in sexual activity*
2. *Providing access to contraception and sufficient knowledge and skills to use contraception appropriately*
3. *Strengthening life goals and encouraging long-term planning*

Some prevention programs focus selectively on one goal, whereas others address all three.

One task in primary prevention is contraceptive education targeted at both males and females, encouraging adolescents to practice responsible sexual behavior. For adolescents to use contraceptives (including condoms) consistently, they need not only the correct knowledge on how to use the method, but also technical skills on how to use them correctly and on how to negotiate contraceptive use, especially condoms, with their partners. Adolescents need confidence and self-efficacy in their ability to use contraceptive methods, and the desired method must be available and accessible. Finally, adolescents need positive attitudes toward contraceptive use, especially condoms (Jemmott & Jemmott, 1992, 1998). Community health nurses should carefully explore an adolescent's knowledge base and correct any misconceptions about birth control methods. This is the important first step in providing adolescents with clear, accurate directions regarding the use of birth control. Some recent trends in contraceptive use among adolescents are encouraging. For example, two-thirds of adolescents reportedly use some form of contraception at first intercourse, with a significant increase in prevalence of use at first intercourse among 15- to 19-year-old females (AGI, 1994, 1998). Kahn, Brindis, and Glei (1999) claim that more than 1 million adolescent pregnancies were averted in 1995 because of consistent contraceptive use. These pregnancies

would have led to approximately 480,000 live births, 390,000 abortions, 120,000 miscarriages, 10,000 ectopic pregnancies, and 37 maternal deaths.

The two most popular methods of contraception used by adolescents have traditionally been the birth control pill and the condom (USPHS, 1997). Although it is beyond the scope of this chapter to fully discuss contraceptive options, it is particularly important for nurses working with adolescents to recognize the type of methods, side effects, and potential barriers that influence contraceptive choice.

Considering the variety of factors that contribute to an adolescent's increased risk for pregnancy, it is clear that there is not one reason why teens become pregnant. However, there are clear solutions and programs. These solutions and programs differ according to their target and the problem identified.

Adolescent Pregnancy Prevention Community-Based Programs

A comprehensive review of adolescent pregnancy prevention research reveals many successes and failures. Kirby (1997) concludes that programs with positive outcomes share important characteristics (Box 20-2). There is no clear agreement on what exact combination of these elements makes up the ideal prevention program. Clearly, programs must be tailored to match the needs of the particular target population. Ideally, members of the target population should be involved in the program development and implementation. There is a pressing need for prevention programs that are culturally sensitive and relevant, addressing the norms, attitudes, and beliefs of the target population. There are various types of programs with different approaches to pregnancy prevention, such as peer education, life options, working with parents, and working in schools and other settings.

Lessons Learned

Important lessons have been learned in the area of adolescent pregnancy prevention. For example, although some prevention efforts focus solely on the importance of **abstinence** from sexual intercourse, the bulk of current evidence indicates that this approach is not successful in delaying the onset of intercourse (Kirby, 1997). Furthermore, education alone is generally not sufficient to change risky behavior such as inconsistent contraceptive use (Howard & Mitchell, 1993). Multidisciplinary programs are needed that combine elements such as sexuality education, enhanced negotiation and communication skills, and access to services and contraceptives (AGI, 1994; Howard & Mitchell, 1993; Plouffe & White, 1996). Finally, although some have expressed concern that sexuality education and/or contraceptive distribution might encourage sexual activity among teens, recent research reviews have concluded that the opposite is actually true (Kirby, 1997; Kirby, Resnick, Downes, Kocher, Gunderson, Potthoff, Zelterman, & Blum, 1993).

TABLE 20-1   **CONSIDERATIONS FOR NURSING INTERVENTIONS**

ISSUE	CONSIDERATIONS
Adolescent father	Acknowledge the risk factors for adolescent fatherhood and encourage involvement in the prenatal and postnatal periods. In speaking with adolescent males, it is important for the nurse to identify and assess beliefs and diagnose problems that may be specific to the adolescent male. Personalize interventions to adolescent males, both in terms of preventing adolescent pregnancy through responsible sex and in terms of coping with the consequences of being a young father. Interventions that positively affect adolescent fathers may indirectly benefit their partners by enhancing partner support (Roye & Balk, 1996). Talking in a nonthreatening, engaging manner with the male adolescent will facilitate effective communication that will address risk factors and beliefs and promote healthy outcomes for the father, mother, their families, and their child (Roye & Balk, 1996; Sonenstein et al., 1997). Stress male responsibility in birth control. Increase his role in pregnancy and child care. Improve his parenting skills and support his lifestyle changes (completing school, job training, and working).
Developmental stage	Nurses who are knowledgeable about factors in adolescent development can better design developmentally appropriate primary interventions to prevent pregnancy, STDs, and HIV in their community. Recognize the developmental tasks and stages of adolescence in order to recognize the influence that those developmental factors have on adolescent sexual behavior. Consider the biophysical, cognitive, and psychosocial theories of development. Answer questions and educate the adolescent about physical development and sexual issues.
Culture/ethnicity	Assess and diagnose each adolescent client and family in order to develop culturally sensitive interventions that are tailored to address cultural factors that impact sexual behavior, contraception, and potential pregnancy.
Peer	Take advantage of the powerfully influential peer group to reach adolescents; trained **peer educators** may be used to deliver safer sex and abstinence messages.
Intrapersonal	Be aware that the adolescent is in a stage where she is developing self-identity and self-esteem and that the adolescent may use sexual activity and pregnancy to bolster her identity.
Attitudes	Explore nonjudgmentally the adolescent's attitudes about pregnancy.
Socioeconomic status	Assess the adolescent's economic situation and intervene to connect the adolescent and family with needed community resources.
Sexual abuse	Identify adolescents in potentially abusive situations and assess both the adolescent and the adolescent's family for abuse.
Positive health outcomes	Conduct home visits to adolescents during pregnancy and after birth to improve pregnancy outcomes and infant health status and to delay repeat pregnancies (Olds, 1992; Olds, Henderson, & Kitzman, 1994; Olds, Henderson, Tatelbaum, & Chamberlin, 1988).

Peer Education Approach

The **peer education** model shows great promise for use in adolescent pregnancy prevention (Minter, 1990) because the peer group is a common source for information about sex. In this model, peers are trained to lead prevention programs within their peer group. Community health nurses may serve as trainers and facilitators in these programs. Some of the advantages of peer education are that it provides positive role models, reinforces norms, empowers youth, and encourages personal responsibility (Coyle et al., 1996).

Life Option Approach

A promising approach that is worthy of additional study is programs that shift the focus to enriching an adolescent's life options across the board by addressing concerns such as academic performance, self-esteem, substance abuse, and long-term goal realization. These programs may include one-on-one mentoring and role modeling with successful adults, community service participation, remedial education, tutoring services, counseling by both professional and peer groups, self-worth enhancement techniques, and exposure to new experiences to expand life options (e.g., concerts, museums, travel). This approach attempts to expand an adolescent's future goals and expectations by improving educational and employment prospects. Because future-oriented, goal-directed adolescents are less likely to become pregnant, the expected result is a reduction in the rate of adolescent pregnancies. Although this approach does not directly address adolescent pregnancy, it targets many of the factors that contribute to an adolescent's risk for unintended pregnancy (Kirby, 1997; Loda, Speizer, Martin, Skatrud, & Bennett, 1997). Because the community health nurse is familiar with the community and its members, he or she may serve as a trusted mentor, educator, community liaison, and coordinator of such programs. In addition, for these programs to be effective, community health nurses must be aware of programs and resources that target adolescents in a broader sense, not only in terms of pregnancy prevention and contraception.

Working with Parents and Adults

Community health nurses may work with parents and other adults significant to the adolescent, such as adult relatives, teachers, coaches, and neighbors. This approach may be a promising avenue for prevention because parents and significant adults influence the behavior of adolescents, including sexual behavior, in their everyday interactions. Although there is no single way for parents to effectively communicate with their children, the nurse may suggest that parents follow the guidelines provided by the National Campaign to Prevent Teen Pregnancy outlined in Box 20-3.

School-Based Programs

A large number of pregnancy prevention programs target teens through school programs. Some of the programs in school may include sex education, family life education, and contraception education. Sex education is provided by some private schools and by public schools in approximately 70% of the states (Norr, 1991); however, most family life programs are offered at the junior or senior high school level as an elective course, which means they do not reach many adolescents and cannot target those at greatest risk. Also, most sex education teachers have little training in sex education, and it is not their primary focus. In school systems with school nurses, the nurse is involved in both sex and family life education. Nurses can also provide factual sex education to teenagers as they provide other health services. Nurses are effective sex educators because they are equipped to provide sexual content in a factual, nonjudgmental approach. They are also proficient at encouraging and guiding client discussion, characteristics helpful in addressing sex education with adolescents. These and other school-based programs receive limited funding, and access is limited for most students. However,

A CONVERSATION WITH...

This teenage mom was 17 when she had her first child. She married the father of the child, finished high school, and is pursuing a college education.

On learning I was pregnant, I was really sad. My world was coming to an end. Many changes took place. My boyfriend and I both wanted to finish high school. So we were married and moved in with my in-laws.

After the baby was born, we graduated and soon moved into a trailer. I was overwhelmed with the responsibility. I lost so much sleep I thought I would never feel rested again!

We made the choice to stay married and I chose to go on to college against all odds. Now that college graduation is only a little over a year away, and I've grown up a lot, my future has hope! It has taken us more than three years, but I can truthfully say the last four months have been happy for us as a family.

Two major factors that have helped me keep from giving up on education and my marriage were the support of my mother and the teen-mom support group leader who became a real friend to me. They gave me something to hang on to and hope for when the winds of strife seemed capable of blowing me over.

After almost four years, we are beginning to see ourselves as a family mostly because of two concepts learned in the support group. The first was that I realized decisions in life were mine to make. I was responsible for my life. The second concept was learning how to effectively communicate love to my husband and son. He and I are the two people in the world that will love our son more than anyone else. We are partners in our responsibility for his nurturance, guidance, and support. How different my life might have been if I had not involved myself with this community service.

—A Teen Mother
Source: A. McFarland. (1998, May 5).
"Family Matters." Fort Payne, AL:
The Times Journal, p. 4.

BOX 20-3 TEN TIPS FOR PARENTS TO HELP THEIR CHILDREN AVOID TEEN PREGNANCY

1. Be clear about your own sexual values and attitudes.
2. Talk with your children early and often about sex, and be specific.
3. Supervise and monitor your children's behaviors, setting rules, curfews, standards, and so on.
4. Know your children's friends and their families.
5. Discourage early, frequent, and steady dating.
6. Take a strong stand against your daughter dating a significantly older boy; do not allow your son to develop an intense relationship with a much younger girl.
7. Help your teenager to have options for the future that are more attractive than early parenthood.
8. Let your kids know that you value education highly.
9. Know that your kids are influenced by the media; pay attention to what they are watching, listening, and reading.
10. Develop strong, close relationships with your children at an early age.

Source: National Campaign to Prevent Teen Pregnancy, 1998.

school-based programs operate within a highly politicized environment. Decisions to include or exclude certain program elements within school-based programs may be made in an effort to minimize controversy rather than to maximize positive outcomes. As a result, community health nurses may need to broaden the focus of their prevention efforts beyond the domain of the school.

Working in Various Settings

Rather than limit the discussion of sexuality and pregnancy prevention to any one setting or a particular type of visit, community health nurses are uniquely positioned to seize opportunities to provide education and implement prevention in numerous settings. These settings, such as family planning clinics, primary health care clinics, school health clinics, and community-based health clinics, are all ideal settings for adolescent pregnancy prevention, even when the adolescent does not present for contraceptive services. Interventions targeting adolescents who use the services of family planning clinics appear to be particularly promising in that they can effectively reach a high-risk group, adolescent females (and potentially their partners) who come to the clinic for a pregnancy test (Zabin, Emerson, Ringers, & Sedivy, 1996). These clinics are logical sites because of the population that they serve: More than 60% of adolescents younger than 17 use family planning clinics (Zabin & Clark, 1981), and more than 82% of young African American adolescents use them (Mosher, 1990). In addition, they provide the opportunity to reach a population of vulnerable, high-risk adolescents at a timely moment.

Program Evaluation

Evaluation is an important part of the nursing process. Programs must be continually evaluated and modified by the community health nurse to ensure their effectiveness and appropriateness for preventing adolescent pregnancy. New prevention programs are constantly in the process of being designed; however, few programs are carefully and consistently developed and evaluated. Thus, efforts may be wasted on interventions that are not effective. One measure of a sound design is the incorporation of theory in the design. Community nurses should have a knowledge base that includes an understanding of various behavioral theories such as the health belief model (Becker, 1974), social cognitive theory (Bandura, 1986), and the theory of reasoned action (Azjen & Fishbein, 1980). These theories can be used to understand the factors that encourage or discourage health promotion behaviors and can guide both program design and evaluation. The lack of meaningful program evaluation is a major defect in the primary prevention of adolescent pregnancy. Evaluation by the community health nurse is critical not only to identify ineffective programs or program elements but also to identify effec-

tive interventions and provide the impetus for replication and reevaluation in a different population. An effective prevention intervention is one that makes positive behavioral changes in measurable outcomes such as decreased incidence of unprotected sex or decreased number of sexual partners.

Secondary and Tertiary Prevention

Prevention efforts may not reach all adolescents because the risk of pregnancy may not be associated with extremely negative outcomes (Stevens-Simon, Kelly, Singer, & Cox, 1996). Therefore, the community health nurse must implement secondary and **tertiary prevention** techniques. In secondary and tertiary prevention, the community health nurse focuses attention on the health care, prevention needs, and long-term development of pregnant adolescents and adolescents who are already young mothers or fathers (Table 20-2). Secondary prevention efforts are designed to promote healthier outcomes from adolescent pregnancy. Its efforts are aimed at improving participation in prenatal care, childbirth preparation, and parenting activities. Interventions may include early detection of pregnancy, options counseling, prenatal care, childbirth education, parenting education, and safer sex education.

Early Detection

A goal for the community health nurse is to identify pregnant adolescents early in their pregnancies, because many teens wait until they are visibly pregnant before they initiate prenatal care (Baker, 1996). Factors such as shame, denial, self-esteem issues, low value and knowledge of health, limited access to care, lack of future-oriented thinking, and lack of symptoms have all been linked to failure to receive early diagnosis and care (Baker, 1996; Lee & Grubbs, 1995; Thompson, Powell, Patterson, & Ellerbee,

TABLE 20-2	SECONDARY AND TERTIARY PREVENTION: NURSING INTERVENTION
ISSUE	**CONSIDERATIONS FOR NURSING INTERVENTIONS**
Early detection	Identify pregnant adolescents early in their pregnancies.
	Recognize factors linked to failure to receive early diagnosis and care.
Pregnancy options	Assess knowledge about pregnancy options.
	Be sensitive to the factors that impact her decision.
	Assess the support the adolescent receives throughout the pregnancy.
	Facilitate therapeutic relationships with the adolescent mother and father and their social support networks.
	Include the father of the baby. A comprehensive assessment should include identification of his attitudes, emotional reactions, plans for education, and plans for involvement with the pregnancy, his partner, and the child.
	Provide options counseling.

Continued

TABLE 20-2   SECONDARY AND TERTIARY PREVENTION: NURSING INTERVENTION—CONT'D

ISSUE	CONSIDERATIONS FOR NURSING INTERVENTIONS
Prenatal care	Encourage early and consistent prenatal care to reduce neonatal and maternal complications.
	Teach the adolescent and her partner about the special needs of pregnancy.
	Assess barriers to adolescent prenatal care.
	Provide health screening assessments, counseling, and education for pregnant clients.
The adolescent father	Encourage the father's participation in prenatal visits.
	Invite the father to prenatal classes, encourage questions and participation in prenatal visits, and acknowledge the father's role as a partner in the pregnancy.
	Encourage fathers to participate in the delivery.
Parenting education	Assess knowledge about parenting.
	Provide education about positioning and handling of infants, nutrition, hygiene, elimination, growth and development, immunization, and recognition of illnesses.
	When doing health teaching it is important to be sensitive to the ethnicity and culture of the client and integrate it into the care of the infant.
Postpartum care	Focus on the standard postpartum areas as well as on specific concerns of the adolescent, such as body image, weight loss, and fatigue.
	Assess the adolescent's adjustment to her new role and the emotional support systems available to her.
	Provide a health assessment of both the mother and infant, newborn care education and supervision, prenatal education on growth and development and parenting skills, review of role adjustment and available supports, and sex education and birth control information.
	Encourage the adolescent to continue developing as an individual (e.g., to continue her education, participate in some social activities, to explore relationships with peers) and at the same time increase her proficiency and confidence in parenting.
Support	Assess available physical and emotional support.
	Refer adolescents to other possible resources, such as parenting programs, cooperative day care, or programs that pair the new mother with an older adolescent mother with a successful experience.
Status of the newborn	Provide a newborn assessment/well-baby check.
	Assess for signs of adequate maternal-infant bonding.
	Provide information about child care.
Sexual activity and contraceptive use	Assess adolescents' plans for sexual activity and need for contraceptive methods.
	Initiate discussion about birth control while the adolescent is pregnant so that both partners have an opportunity to identify contraceptive and safer sex methods that they will use after the pregnancy.
	Provide instruction on condom use during pregnancy in your discussion of disease prevention in pregnancy.
	Help the adolescent explore the risks involved if they have sex without adequate protection.
	Help the adolescent select the most appropriate form of contraception from several alternatives
	If the adolescent has already used birth control, it is helpful to identify the method, how it was used, and the reason for discontinuance.
	Make sure that the adolescent is aware of community resources (family planning clinics) where she may be supplied with contraceptives.
	Encourage clinic attendance, promote access to contraception, and provide referrals to appropriate contraceptive services when counseling individuals or teaching sex education classes; emphasize the importance of contraceptive use by all sexually active adolescents.
	Monitor compliance and encourage cooperation with adolescents.

BOX 20-4 ADOLESCENTS AND ABORTION

Nearly 4 in 10 teen pregnancies (excluding miscarriages) end in abortion. There were about 289,000 abortions among teens in 1994.

Since 1980, abortion rates among sexually experienced teens have declined steadily because fewer teens are becoming pregnant, and in recent years fewer pregnant teens have chosen to have an abortion.

The reasons most often given by teens for choosing to have an abortion are concern about how having a baby would change their lives, feeling that they are not mature enough to have a child, and having financial problems.

Twenty-nine states currently have mandatory parental involvement laws in effect for a minor seeking an abortion: AL, AR, DE, GA, ID, IN, IO, KS, KY, LA, MD, MA, MI, MN, MS, MO, NE, NC, ND, OH, PA, RI, SC, SD, UT, VA, WV, WI, and WY.

Sixty-one percent of minors who have abortions do so with at least one parent's knowledge; 45% of parents know about their daughter's abortion. The great majority of parents support their daughter's decision to have an abortion.

Source: Alan Guttmacher Institute, 1998.

1995). Community health nurses can work to identify teens early in their pregnancies by using community outreach techniques such as advertisements for prenatal services in malls, schools, public transportation, and churches.

Options Counseling

In counseling the pregnant adolescent, the nurse must be aware that the adolescent's decisions about her pregnancy and subsequent pregnancy prevention will affect both the adolescent mother and her entire family. Once pregnancy is confirmed, the adolescent faces an important decision about her options, which include **abortion, adoption,** or keeping the baby (Box 20-4). The nurse has the responsibility to provide (or refer to someone who will provide) the adolescent with information about pregnancy options. Among adolescents, the most common outcome (55%) is a live birth. Only 1 in 20 pregnant adolescents chooses to place her infant for adoption, whereas 35% of adolescent pregnancies end in abortion (National Center for Health Statistics, 1990).

The community health nurse must recognize that many factors play a role in the decision the adolescent makes about the pregnancy. These factors may include cultural and religious up-

bringing, family attitude toward the pregnancy (perceived or real), partner attitude, and state law. Partner age plays an important role, as the data has shown that adolescent females with younger partners tend to terminate their pregnancies at a higher rate than adolescent females with adult partners (AGI, 1994).

Prenatal Care

Once an adolescent decides to continue the pregnancy, effort is directed toward ensuring a healthy outcome for the mother and infant. Early initiation and regular continuance of prenatal care significantly reduce the risk for both adolescents and their infants (ANA, 1987). The nurse should educate the adolescent and her partner about the special needs of pregnancy as they relate to adolescence, such as the following:

- *Special nutritional needs (Box 20-5)*
- *Physical changes and demands of pregnancy*
- *How pregnancy affects the female adolescent's growth and development*
- *Emotional changes during pregnancy for both parents*
- *What to expect during delivery*

BOX 20-5 ADOLESCENT PREGNANCY AND NUTRITION REQUIREMENTS

The nutritional needs of the pregnant adolescent are often different from those of adult women. Many adolescents are experiencing rapid physical growth and maturation during their teenage years. Pregnancy increases the nutritional requirements of the adolescent.

*The recommended nutritional goals of the adolescent depend on the **gynecological age** of the adolescent. (Gynecological age is the number of years between the chronological age and the age of menarche.) Adolescents with a gynecological age less than or equal to 2 years have increased nutritional needs because of their own physical growth requirements. When the gynecological age is less than 2 years, the pregnant teen may compete with the nutritional requirements of the fetus to meet those of the adolescent.*

Because adolescent diets are often high in salt, sugar, and fatty foods and low in protein, vitamins, and minerals, the nurse must be diligent about assessing and diagnosing deficits in the pregnant adolescent's diet.

- *Preterm labor*

- *Signs and symptoms of pregnancy complications*

Programs that address barriers to adolescent prenatal care have demonstrated positive outcomes, including reduced neonatal and maternal complications (Rogers, Peoples-Sheps, & Suchindran, 1996; Yoder & Young, 1997).

Prenatal care services that prove successful in getting teenagers to use and comply with the overall program of care are those that provide an accepting, caring atmosphere and work to reduce obstacles to beginning or continuing care. These results have been in comprehensive community-based programs with a heavy outreach and educational emphasis, using multidisciplinary health care teams, especially community health nurse involvement, and home visits. The community health nurse acts as the case manager of prenatal care and sees that clients are provided with needed services. The nurse is the team member who spends the most time with the adolescent, providing most of the health screening assessments, counseling, and education for pregnant clients.

Prenatal programs should also aim to improve the quality and duration of the father-child relationship. Community health nurses can assist in these efforts by encouraging the father's participation in prenatal visits. Most fathers are curious and interested in the process of gestation and delivery but are uncomfortable asking questions and hesitant in interacting with health care providers. The community health nurse can invite the father to prenatal classes, encourage questions and participation in prenatal visits, and acknowledge the father's role as a partner in the pregnancy. Fathers can be encouraged, but not forced, into participation in the baby's delivery.

Three types of programs offer prenatal care to adolescents: private medical services, clinic programs, and school-based prenatal programs. The choice of program depends on the accessibility and the financial circumstances of the adolescent and her family. Private medical services are provided by physicians in single or group practices or associated with health maintenance organizations. These services are available to people who have a medical insurance plan or can afford to pay. Clinic programs are for families without insurance or the financial resources to pay for prenatal care. School-based programs provide services in connection with other school-run clinic services or in separate schools designed for the exclusive use of pregnant adolescents (Olds, 1992). School-based prenatal services provide a comprehensive approach to care and are usually found in large school districts with high rates of adolescent pregnancy.

Parenting Education and Contraceptive Education

Adolescent parents typically need more structured education focusing on newborn care, parenting skills, and fostering developmentally appropriate interactions. Discussion about birth control should also be initiated while the adolescent is pregnant so that both partners have an opportunity to identify contraceptive methods that they will use after the pregnancy. The community

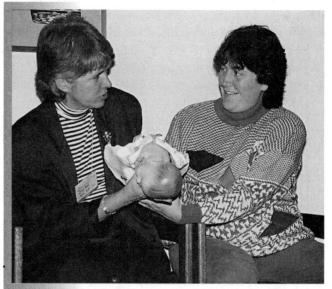

Nurse role modeling appropriate infant care with teen mother.

health nurse is in a unique position to provide these services at a group or individual level and promote continuity of care that focuses on the new family.

Transition from Prenatal to Postpartum Care

After delivery of the baby, the focus is on postpartum care, which varies widely in scope and duration of services. All prenatal programs provide a postpartum check for the mother. A well-baby check is included in most services, although a private obstetrical practice may rely on the mother to make her own arrangements for all infant care. The most extensive postpartum care is delivered in community programs that rely heavily on nurses. These programs usually include the following:

- *Health assessment of both the mother and infant*

- *Newborn care education and supervision*

- *Prenatal education on growth and development and parenting skills*

- *Review of role adjustment and available supports*

- *Sex education and birth control information*

One valuable component of these programs is the emphasis on regular contact with the new mothers, starting the first week after delivery. Studies show that regular nurse visits reduce anxiety and increase infant health as measured by fewer accidents and emergency department visits (Olds, 1992; Olds, Henderson, & Kitzman, 1994; Olds, Henderson, Tatelbaum, & Chamberlin, 1988). Mothers experience many concerns or problems before the first scheduled clinic or physician visit. Earlier contacts allow the adolescent and nurse to address these issues and reduce anxiety. Contact need not always be in person; some care can be provided by telephone monitoring of the new mother.

Health and Psychosocial Status of the Mother

At a minimum, the mother should have a 6-week postpartum examination. Some community health programs start home visits at about 2 weeks postpartum. The physical assessment should focus on the standard postpartum areas as well as on specific concerns of the adolescent, such as body image, weight loss, and fatigue. In addition, the nurses should assess the adolescent's adjustment to her new role and the emotional support systems available to her. Adjusting to the role of parent during adolescence is difficult. Conflict is not unusual. Family members may expect the adolescent to instantly become an adult and mother, or the opposite, to remain a child and allow her parents to assume all the responsibilities for the infant. Ideally, the adolescent should be encouraged to continue developing as an individual (e.g., to continue her education, participate in some social activities, to explore relationships with peers). The adolescent mother needs support in increasing her proficiency and confidence in parenting and integrating her new responsibilities into her daily routine. She may be juggling school, social activities, and infant care. Fatigue and stress are common.

The community health nurse can help the new mother look at the immediate family, other relatives, significant others, and the father of the infant and his family for support. The adolescent mother could also be referred to other possible resources, such as parenting programs, cooperative day-care programs, or programs that pair the new mother with an older adolescent mother with a successful experience. Even if support systems are adequate, the family may need some help in understanding and supporting the adolescent as a maturing individual. Adequate physical and emotional support, along with health teaching and realistic expecta-

tions for their children, successfully reduces the incidence of abuse and neglect from at-risk mothers (Marshall, Buckner, & Powell, 1991; Olds, 1992; Olds, Henderson, & Kitzman, 1994; Olds, Henderson, Tatelbaum, & Chamberlin, 1988).

Sexual Activity and Contraceptive Use

Ideally, the idea of future contraception should be introduced as part of the prenatal program. The adolescent must decide whether she will continue sexual activity after delivery and must be encouraged to be honest with the nurse about her decision. Sometimes, the mother is no longer involved with the father of the infant and announces that she does not intend to be sexually active or to have another child. In this case, the adolescent mother should be helped to explore the risks involved if she changes her mind without adequate protection. Once an adolescent has been pregnant, she risks repeating the situation (AGI, 1981; Brown, Saunders, & Dick, 1999).

Access to and regular use of birth control is the goal of contraceptive services for adolescents. Family planning clinics and private physicians are one source; school-based clinics are a more recent effort. Community health nurses can encourage clinic attendance, promote access to contraception, and provide referrals to appropriate contraceptive services when counseling individuals or teaching sex education classes. The nurse must emphasize the importance of contraceptive use by all sexually active adolescents (Kahn, Brindis, & Glei, 1999).

Health Status and Care of the Newborn

In addition to the usual newborn assessment, the community heath nurse should look for signs of adequate maternal-infant

CASE STUDY

You are a school nurse at Hilton High School. You have carefully followed several of your students who have become pregnant and helped them find resources for support both during and after their pregnancies. You have noticed, however, that several of your students have decided to discontinue breast-feeding. In speaking with Arlene Johnston, a 15-year-old sophomore with a 3-month-old son, Antonio, you find out that she too is reconsidering breast-feeding. She understands the benefits of breast-feeding and is able to discuss them with you. Both Arlene and her mom think that breast-feeding is good for Antonio. However, upon further questioning, you discover that her new partner, Sam, and her friends at school think that breast-feeding is "nasty." Arlene feels embarrassed that her friends know she breast-

feeds, and she is afraid that she will lose her friends and boyfriend.

1. What factors in Arlene's (and the other adolescents') cognitive development support her decision to discontinue breast-feeding?

2. How can you address this to continue to promote Arlene's breast-feeding Antonio?

You decide that one means to addressing attitudes toward breast-feeding is to address the attitudes of all students at Hilton High.

1. Consider different ways that you, as the school (community) health nurse, can address the students at Hilton High.

2. Think about what special considerations there are for such an intervention.

bonding. Evidence of attachment includes calling a child by its name, cuddling, talking to the infant, and demonstrating an interest in infant care and development. Adolescents sometimes demonstrate difficulty in bonding simply because they have had no previous experience with infants and are afraid to do anything. Sometimes, another person has assumed the role of caregiver and the adolescent becomes an observer rather than caregiver. Bonding can be assessed in clinic settings, but home visits by the community health nurse allow for a more accurate picture of the nature and scope of the mother-infant relationship. Considering the current trend of short postpartum length of stay, the community health nurse has the opportunity to observe the interaction among the infant, teenager, and other caregivers for a longer time than nurses in the clinical setting.

Tertiary Prevention

Tertiary prevention efforts may include prevention of additional adolescent pregnancies, support of positive parent-infant interaction, support groups for adolescent parents, and programs that support the adolescents while they pursue educational goals. The techniques discussed previously that are used in primary prevention may be used to prevent repeat pregnancies in adolescents. The nurse may work collaboratively with organizations that provide support such as child care and allowing adolescent parents to complete and pursue further education (Smith & Hanks, 1994). Other nursing interventions may include long-term child development education and parenting classes. Programs that foster maternal education, father involvement, and increased self-esteem show significant promise for better maternal and infant development (Diehl, 1997; Roye & Balk, 1996).

CONCLUSION

Despite the proliferation of prevention efforts, adolescent pregnancy is a significant and enduring community health problem. It has been linked to various problems such as increased poverty, decreased educational attainment, increased psychological stress, potential isolation from peers, and increased reliance on public funds. Multiple pregnancies among adolescents are not uncommon and are particularly disturbing because the negative effect of pregnancy increases dramatically.

Many factors contribute to adolescent pregnancy, and community health nurses must be aware of potential risk factors and understand the complex interaction of these factors. Without this awareness and understanding, the nurse will not be able to adequately perform the nursing process to de-velop and evaluate age-appropriate, culturally sensitive, convenient, comprehensive, and affordable interventions that will meet the special needs of adolescents. It is clear that unless community health nurses and other health professionals make an effort to provide information, few adolescents will actively seek out nurses or other professionals as resources. Nurses are well suited to address the issues of adolescent pregnancy. The professional roles in schools, clinics, screening programs, health departments, and community outreach centers provide access to at-risk populations. Community health nurses have the opportunity, sensitivity, and commitment to work to achieve positive outcomes for adolescents and their children.

CRITICAL THINKING ACTIVITIES

1. What are the social norms and cultural beliefs about adolescent pregnancy and sexuality in your community? How do you think that these beliefs affect adolescent behavior?

2. What strategies can the community health nurse implement to help the pregnant adolescent and her family cope with the changes in the family structure?

3. You are planning a pregnancy prevention intervention for adolescents in your community. Identify program characteristics that you might include in your intervention that have been shown to be effective in adolescent pregnancy prevention programs.

4. It is important for the community health nurse to be aware of community resources to appropriately refer clients. What resources are available in your community for pregnant adolescents? adolescents with children? adolescent fathers?

5. Does your school district provide child care for adolescents with children? Do you believe they should? Why?

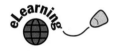

Explore Community Health Nursing on the web! To learn more about the topics in this chapter, access your exclusive web site:
http://communitynursing.jbpub.com

REFERENCES

Alan Guttmacher Institute (AGI). (1981). *Teenage pregnancy: The problem that hasn't gone away.* New York: Author.

Alan Guttmacher Institute (AGI). (1994). Sex and America's teenagers. New York: Author.

Alan Guttmacher Institute (AGI). (1998). *Facts in brief: Teens and pregnancy*: http://www.agi-usa.org/pubs/fb_teen_sex.html.

American Academy of Pediatrics, Committee on Adolescence. (1989). Adolescent pregnancy. *Pediatrics, 83*, 132–135.

American Nurses Association (ANA). (1987). *Access to prenatal care: Key to prevention of low-birth weight.* Kansas City, MO: Author.

Azjen, I., & Fishbein, M. (1980). *Understanding attitudes and predicting social behavior.* Englewood Cliffs, NJ: Prentice Hall.

Baker, T. J. (1996). Factors related to the initiation of prenatal care in the adolescent nullipara. *The Nurse Practitioner, 21*(2), 29–42.

Bandura, A. (1986). *Social learning theory.* Englewood Cliffs, NJ: Prentice Hall.

Becker, M. H. (1974). The health belief model and personal health behaviors. *Health Education Monographs, 2*, 324–508.

Blankson, M. L., Cliver, S. P., Goldenberg, R. L., Hickey, C. A., Jin, J., & Dubard, M. B. (1993). Health behavior and outcomes in sequential pregnancies of black and white adolescents. *Journal of the American Medical Association, 269*(11), 1401–1403.

Bowen, M. (1971). The use of family theory in clinical practice. In J. Haley (Ed.), *Changing families.* New York: Grune & Stratton.

Brown, H. N., Saunders, R. B., & Dick, M. J. (1999). Preventing secondary pregnancy in adolescents: A model program. *Health Care for Women International, 20*(1), 5–15.

Bulcholz, E. S., & Gol, B. (1986). More than playing house: A developmental perspective on the strengths in teenage motherhood. *Theory and Review*, 347–357.

Campaign for Our Children. (1996). *Fact sheet on adolescents who have babies*: http://www.cfoc.org/statsfactsheet.html.

Centers for Disease Control and Prevention (CDC). (1991). Premarital sexual experience among adolescent women—United States, 1970–1988. *Morbidity and Mortality Weekly Report, 39*, 929–932.

Cockey, C. D. (1997, June). Preventing teen pregnancy. It's time to stop kidding around. *Lifelines*, 32–40.

Coley, R. L., & Chase-Lansdale, P. L. (1998). Adolescent pregnancy and parenthood. Recent evidence and future directions. *American Psychologist, 53*(2), 152–166.

Coyle, K., Kirby, D., Parcel, G., Basen-Engquist, K., Banspach, S., Rugg, D., & Weil, M. (1996). Safer choices: A multicomponent school-based HIV/STD and pregnancy prevention program for adolescents. *Journal of School Health, 66*(3), 89–94.

Crowe, L. C., & George, W. H. (1989). Alcohol and human sexuality: Review and integration. *Psychological Bulletin, 102*, 374–386.

Darabi, K. F., Jones, J., Varga, P. L., & Hourse, M. (1982). Evaluation of sex education outreach. *Adolescence, 17*(65), 57–64.

Davis, K. A. (1980). *A theory of teenage pregnancy in the U.S. adolescent. Pregnancy and childbearing*. Washington, DC: Department of Health and Human Services.

Davis, S. M., & Harris, M. B. (1982). Sexual knowledge, sexual interests, and sources of sexual information of rural and urban adolescents from three cultures. *Adolescence, 18*(66), 471–492.

Davtyan, C. (2000). Contraception for adolescents. *Western Journal of Medicine, 172*(3), pp. 166–171.

Department of Health and Human Services (DHHS). (1990). *Healthy People 2000: National health objectives* (Publication No. 91-50213). Washington, DC: U.S. Government Printing Office.

Desmond, A. M. (1994). Adolescent pregnancy in the United States: Not a minority issue. *Health Care for Women International, 15*(4), 325–331.

Diehl, K. (1997). Adolescent mothers: What produces positive mother-infant interaction? *Maternal Child Nursing, 22*, 89–95.

DiIorio, C., Hockenbeery-Eaton, M., Maibach, E., Rivero, S., & Miller, K. (1996). The content of African American mothers' discussions with their adolescents about sex. *Journal of Family Nursing, 2*(4), 365–382.

Drake, P. (1996). Addressing the needs of pregnant adolescents. *Journal of Gynecological and Neonatal Nursing, 25*(6), 518–524.

DuPlessis, H. M., Bell, R., & Richards, T. (1997). Adolescent pregnancy: Understanding the impact of age and race on outcomes. *Journal of Adolescent Health, 20*, 187–197.

Fagot, B., Pears, K., Capaldi, D., Crosby, L., & Leve, C. (1998). Becoming an adolescent father: Precursors and parenting. *Developmental Psychology, 34*(6), 1209–1219.

Farber, N. (1994). Perception of pregnancy risk: A comparison by class and race. *American Journal of Orthopsychiatry, 64*(3), 479–484.

Fiscella, K., Kitzman, H. J., Cole, R. E., Sidora, K. J., & Olds, D. (1998). Does child abuse predict adolescent pregnancy? *Pediatrics, 101* (4 Pt. 1), 620–624.

Fisher, S. M. (1984). The psychodynamics of teenage pregnancy and motherhood. In M. Sugar (Ed.), *Adolescent parenthood*. Jamaica, NY: Spectrum Publications.

Flavell, J. H., Miller, P. H., & Miller, S. A. (1993). *Cognitive development* (3rd ed.). Englewood Cliffs, NJ: Prentice Hall.

Fortenberry, J. D., Orr, D. P., Katz, B. P., Brizendine, E. J., & Blythe, M. J. (1997). Sex under the influence. *Sexually Transmitted Diseases, 24*(6), 313–319.

Foster, H. W. (1997). The campaign to prevent teen pregnancy. *Journal of Pediatric Nursing, 12*(2), 120–121.

Geronimus, A. (1986). The effects of race, residence and prenatal care on the relationship of maternal age to neonatal mortality. *American Journal of Public Health, 76*(12), 1412–1421.

Grogger, J., & Bronars, S. (1993). The socioeconomic consequences of teenage childbearing: Findings from a natural experiment. *Family Planning Perspectives, 25*(4), 156–161, 174.

Hatcher, R. A., Trussell, J., Stewart, F., Stewart, G. K., Kowal, D., Guest, F., Cates, W., Jr., & Policar, M. S. (1994). *Contraceptive technology* (16th ed., rev.). New York: Irvington.

Howard, M., & McCabe, J. A. (1992). An information and skills approach for younger teens: Postponing sexual involvement program. In B. C. Miller, J. T. Card, R. L. Paifoff, & J. I. Peterson (Eds.), *Preventing adolescent pregnancy*. Newbury Park, CA: Sage Publications.

Howard, M., & Mitchell, M. E. (1993). Prevention of teenage pregnancy: Some questions to be answered and some answers to be questioned. *Pediatric Annals, 22*(2), 109–118.

Jemmott, L. S. (1993) AIDS risk among black male adolescents: Implications for nursing intervention. *Journal of Pediatric Health Care, 7*, 3–11.

Jemmott, L. S., & Jemmott, J. B., III. (1990). Sexual knowledge, attitudes, and risky sexual behavior among inner-city black male adolescents. *Journal of Adolescent Research, 5*, 346–369.

Jemmott, L. S. & Jemmott, J. B., III. (1992). Increasing condom-use intentions among sexually active inner city black adolescent women: Effects of an AIDS prevention program. *Nursing Research, 41*, 273–279.

Jemmott, J., Jemmott, L., & Fong, G. (1998). Abstinence and safer sex HIV risk-reduction interventions for African American adolescents: A randomized controlled trial. *Journal of the American Medical Association, 279*(19), 1529–1536.

Kahn, J. G., Brindis, C. D., & Glei, D. A. (1999). Pregnancies averted among U.S. teenagers by the use of contraceptives. *Family Planning Perspectives, 31*(1), 29–34.

Kenney, J. W., Reinholtz, C., & Angelini, P. J. (1997). Ethnic differences in childhood sexual abuse and teenage pregnancy. *Journal of Adolescent Health, 21*(1), 3–10.

Kirby, D. (1997). *No easy answers: Research findings on programs to reduce teen pregnancy* (Summary). Washington, DC: The National Campaign to Prevent Teen Pregnancy.

Kirby, D., Resnick, M. D., Downes, B., Kocher, T., Gunderson, P., Potthoff, S., Zelterman, D., & Blum, R. W. (1993). The effects of school-based health clinics in St. Paul on school-wide birthrates. *Family Planning Perspectives, 25*(1), 12–16.

Kokotailo, P. K., Langhough, R. E., Cox, N. S., Davidson, S. R., & Fleming, M. F. (1994). Cigarette, alcohol and other drug use among small city pregnant adolescents. *Journal of Adolescent Health, 15,* 366–373.

Landry, E., Bertrand, J., Cherry, F., & Rich, J. (1986). Teenage pregnancy in New Orleans: Factors that differentiate teens who deliver, abort, and successfully contracept. *Journal of Youth and Adolescence, 15,* 259–274.

Lee, S. H., & Grubbs, L. M. (1995). Pregnant teenagers' reasons for seeking or delaying prenatal care. *Clinical Nursing Research, 4*(1), 38–49.

Leppert, P. C., Namerow, P. B., & Barker, D. (1986). Pregnancy outcomes among adolescents and older women receiving comprehensive prenatal care. *Journal of Adolescent Health Care, 7,* 112–117.

Levy, S. R., Perhats, C., Nash-Johnson, M., & Welter, J. F. (1992). Reducing the risks in pregnant teens who are very young and those with mild mental retardation. *Mental Retardation, 30*(4), 195–203.

Lieberman, E. J. (1980). *The psychological consequences of adolescent pregnancy and abortion: Adolescent pregnancy and childbearing.* Washington, DC: Department of Health and Human Services.

Loda, F. A., Speizer, I. S., Martin, K. L., Skatrud, J. D., & Bennett, T. A. (1997). Programs and services to prevent pregnancy, childbearing, and poor birth outcomes among adolescents in rural areas of the Southeastern United States. *Journal of Adolescent Health, 21,* 157–166.

Males, M. (1993). School-age pregnancy: Why hasn't prevention worked? *Journal of School Health, 63*(10), 429–432.

Marshall, E., Buckner, E., & Powell, K. (1991). Evaluation of a teen parent program designed to reduce child abuse and neglect and to strengthen families. *Journal of Child Adolescent Psychiatric and Mental Health Nursing, 4*(3), 96–100.

McFarland, A. (1998, May 5). "Family Matters." Fort Payne, AL: *The Times Journal,* p. 4.

Minter, P. (1990). Teen talk: Peer groups addressing teen pregnancy. *American Journal of Public Health, 80,* 349–350.

Morrison, D. (1985). Adolescent contraceptive behavior: A review. *Psychological Bulletin, 98,* 538–568.

Mosher, W. D. (1990). *Use of family planning services in the United States: 1982 and 1988.* Hyattsville, MD: National Center for Health Statistics.

Mott, S. (1990). Adolescence. In S. Mott, S. James, & A. Sperhac (Eds.), *Care of children and families.* Redwood City, CA: Addison-Wesley.

National Campaign to Prevent Teen Pregnancy (1998). *Ten tips for parents to help their children avoid teen pregnancy.* Washington, DC: Author.

National Center for Health Statistics (NCHS). (1990). Advance report of final natality statistics, 1990. *Monthly Vital Statistics Report, 41*(9), Supplement.

Norr, K. (1991). Community-based primary prevention of adolescent pregnancy. *Birth Defects: Original Article Series, 27*(1), 175–199.

Olds, D. (1992). Home visitation for pregnant women and parents of young children. *American Journal of Diseases of Children, 146*(6), 704–708.

Olds, D., Henderson, C., & Kitzman, H. (1994). Does prenatal and infancy nurse home visitation have enduring effects on qualities of parental caregiving and child health at 25 to 50 months of life? *Pediatrics, 93*(1), 89–98.

Olds, D., Henderson, C., Tatelbaum, R., & Chamberlin, R. (1988). Improving the life-course development of socially disadvantaged mothers: A randomized trial of nurse home visitation. *American Journal of Public Health, 78*(11), 1436–1445.

Orshan, S. A. (1996). Acculturation, perceived social support, and self-esteem in primigravida Puerto Rican teenagers. *Western Journal of Nursing Research, 18*(4), 460–473.

Pittman, K., & Adams, G. (1988). *Teenage pregnancy: An advocate's guide to the numbers.* Washington, DC: Children's Defense Fund.

Plouffe, L., & White, E. W. (1996). Adolescent obstetrics and gynecology: Children having children—Can it be controlled? *Current Opinion in Obstetrics and Gynecology, 8*(5), 335–338.

Polaneczky, M. (1998). Adolescent contraception. *Current Opinion in Obstetrics & Gynecology, 10*(3), 213–219.

Pollack, A. E. (1992). Teen contraception in the 1990s. *Journal of School Health, 62*(7), 288–293.

Pratt, W., Mosher, W., Bachrach, C., & Horn, M. (1984). Understanding U.S. fertility: Findings from the National Survey of Family Growth, Cycle III. *Population Bulletin, 39,* 1–42.

Rew, L. (1998). The adolescent. In N. C. Frisch & L. E. Frisch (Eds.), *Psychiatric mental health nursing.* Albany, NY: Delmar Publishers.

Reynoso, T.C., Felice, M. E., & Shragg, G. P. (1993). Does American acculturation affect the outcome of Mexican-American teenage pregnancy? *Journal of Adolescent Health, 14,* 257–261.

Robinson, R. B., & Frank, D. L. (1994). The relation between self-esteem, sexual activity, and pregnancy. *Adolescence, 29*(113), 26–35.

Rogers, M. M., Peoples-Sheps, M. D., & Suchindran, C. (1996). Impact of a social support program on teenage prenatal care use and pregnancy outcomes. *Journal of Adolescent Health, 19*, 132–140.

Roye, C. F., & Balk, S. J. (1996). The relationship of partner support to outcomes for teenage mothers and their children: A review. *Journal of Adolescent Health, 19*, 86–93.

Smith, J. B., & Hanks, C. A. (1994). Reaching out to mothers at risk. *RN*, 42–46.

Sonenstein, F. L., Pleck, J. H., & Leighton, C. K. (1989). Sexual activity, condom use, and AIDS awareness among adolescent males. *Family Planning Perspectives, 21*, 152–158.

Sonenstein, F., Stewart, K., Lindberg, L., Pernas, M., & Williams, S. (1997). Practical advice and program philosophy. *Involving males in preventing teen pregnancy*

Sorenson, D. (1973). *Adolescent sexuality in contemporary America.* New York: World Press.

Spitz, A. M., Velebil, P., Koonin, L. M., Strauss, L. T., Goodman, K. A., Wingo, P., Wilson, J. B., Morris, L., & Marks, J. S. (1996). Pregnancy, abortion, and birth rates among US adolescents—1980, 1985, and 1990. *Journal of the American Medical Association, 275*(13), 989–994.

Stevens-Simon, C., Kelly, L., Singer, D., & Cox, A. (1996). Why pregnant adolescents say they did not use contraceptives prior to conception. *Journal of Adolescent Health, 19*, 48–53.

Taylor, H., Kagay, M., & Leichenko, S. (1986). *American teens speak: Sex myths, TV, and birth control.* New York: Planned Parenthood Federation of America.

Thompson, P. J., Powell, M. J., Patterson, R. J., & Ellerbee, S. M. (1995). Adolescent parenting: Outcomes and maternal perceptions. *Journal of Obstetrical, Gynecological and Neonatal Nursing, 24*(8), 713–717.

Toledo-Dreves, V., Zabin, L. S., & Emerson, M. (1995). Duration of adolescent sexual relationships before and after conception. *Journal of Adolescent Health, 17*, 163–172.

Trad, P. V. (1999). Assessing the patterns that prevent teenage pregnancy. *Adolescence, 34*(133), 221–240.

U.S. Public Health Service (USPHS). (1997). Put prevention into practice: Unintended pregnancy. *Journal of the American Academy of Nurse Practitioners, 9*(4), 193–198.

Widom, C. S., & Kuhns, J. B. (1996). Childhood victimization and subsequent risk for promiscuity, prostitution, and teenage pregnancy: A prospective study. *American Journal of Public Health, 86*(11), 1607–1612.

Yoder, B. A., & Young, M. K. (1997). Neonatal outcomes of teenage pregnancy in a military population. *Obstetrics & Gynecology, 90*(4), 500–506.

Zabin, L. S., Kantner, J., & Zelnik, M. (1979). The risk of adolescent pregnancy in the first months of intercourse. *Family Planning Perspectives, 11*, 215–226.

Zabin, L. S., & Clark, S. D. (1981). Why they delay: A study of teenage family planning clinic patients. *Family Planning Perspective, 13*, 205–217.

Zabin, L. S., Emerson, M. R., Ringers, P. A., & Sedivy, V. (1996). Adolescents with negative pregnancy test results: An accessible at-risk group. *Journal of the American Medical Association, 275*(2), 113–117.

Zelnik, M., & Kantner, J. F. (1979). Reasons for nonuse of contraception by sexually active women age 15–19. *Family Planning Perspectives, 11*(5), 289–296.

Zelnik, M., Kantner, J. F., & Ford, K. (1981). *Sex and pregnancy in adolescence*. Beverly Hills, CA: Sage Publications.

Zoccolillo, M., Meyers, J., & Assiter, S. (1997). Conduct disorder, substance dependence, and adolescent motherhood. *American Journal of Orthopsychiatry, 67*(1), 152–157.

Zuckerman, B. S., Walker, D. K., Frank, D. A., Chase, C., & Hamburg, B. (1984). Adolescent pregnancy: Biobehavioral determinants of outcome. *Journal of Pediatrics, 105*(6), 857–863.

Chapter 21
Children's Health

Harriet J. Kitzman, H. Lorrie Yoos,
and Anne C. Klijanowicz

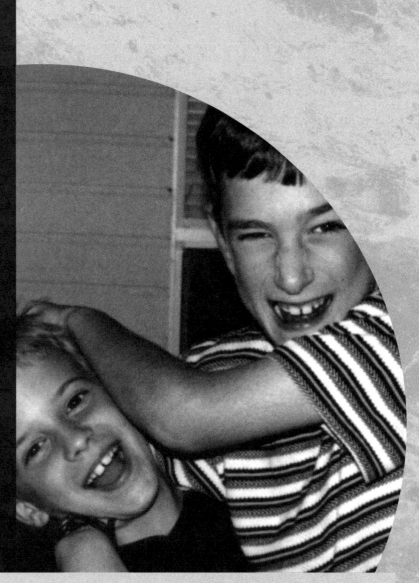

Ring-a-round o'roses
A pocket full of posies,
A-tishoo! A-tishoo!
We all fall down.

Old English children's rhyme which dates back to the Great Plagues
refers to the "rosy rash"; "posies" of herbs were kept in pockets as pro-
tection from the disease, and sneezing was often a final, fatal symp-
tom with resulting death and "falling down."
    The Oxford Dictionary of Nursery Rhymes

QUESTIONS TO CONSIDER

After reading this chapter, answer the following questions:
1. What is the significance of the infant mortality rate in the assessment of a community's health?
2. What are three common health problems of children?
3. How is chronic disease manifested in children?
4. How are risk-taking behaviors of adolescents related to health?
5. What are common behavioral problems that have health consequences during adolescence?
6. What is the scope of maltreatment of children in the United States?
7. What is the ecology of child health?
8. What is the United Nations Rights of the Child Convention?
9. What are delivery of care issues related to child health?
10. How does the role of the community health nurse in child health differ from the acute care setting?

KEY TERMS

Asthma
Attention-deficit
hyperactivity disorder
(ADHD)

Cancer
Cerebral palsy
Congenital malformations
Growth failure

Neonatal mortality
Preterm delivery and low
birth weight

Rights of children
Sudden infant death
syndrome (SIDS)

Children, our greatest national resource, are one of the nation's most vulnerable groups. Despite having the most expensive health care system in the world, the health status of children in the United States still lags behind many countries on important health indicators such as low birth weight, preterm delivery, and infant mortality. Data on the specific indicators of well-being of the nation's children and on the leading causes of death for specific age cohorts are available from the Federal Interagency Forum on Child and Family Statistics and the Centers for Disease Control and Prevention (CDC).

In addition to those who die, a significant number of U.S. children have compromised health. For example, 19% of children in 1996 were rated by their parents as having less than very good or excellent health, up only slightly from 1984 (Federal Interagency Forum on Child and Family Statistics, 1999).

Although parents and society want the best for children and youth, many infants begin their life compromised by low birth weight and/or prematurity and are often cared for by parents who are significantly stressed by overwhelming, competing demands resulting from young age, work, illness, disability, poverty, and isolation. They face day-to-day challenges as they attempt to nurture their children.

One of the most critical challenges of our times is to establish and maintain healthy physical and social environments for children. Communities are being challenged to support the nurturing role of parents. For generations, community health nurses have been central figures in the community's effort to protect the health of children and families (Deal, 1993; Kitzman, Cole, Yoos, & Olds, 1997). This chapter examines selected children's health problems, provides an ecological perspective of child health, explores societal responses to child needs in relation to community health nursing, and describes systems of care delivery that influence successful services in relation to children and their families.

• •

Children can infuse something special into our souls . . . it is a privilege to watch a child discover the world.
Arlene McFarland, RN, DNS, 1999

• •

Mothers and babies during the first half of the 20th century were at a greater risk for dying from acute infection.

Morbidity and Mortality Rates

One of the primary indicators of a nation's overall health status is its infant mortality rate. Despite the fact that the United States is one of the world's leaders in health care, its infant mortality rate, although improved between 1983 and 1994 (10.9 to 7.1 per 1,000 births), remains higher than many other industrial nations. Within the United States, infant mortality, like adult mortality, is related to socioeconomic status. The poor are more likely to die early than the more affluent.

• •

Remember the children behind the statistics. All over America, they are the small human tragedies who will determine the quality and safety and economic security of America's future, as much as your and my children will.
Marian Wright Edelman, *The Measure of Our Success: A Letter to My Children and Yours*, 1992

• •

Death rates for children ages 1 to 4 declined by almost half between 1980 and 1997 (64 to 36 per 100,000 children, respectively). Death rates for children ages 5 to 14 declined about a third (31 to 21 per 100,000), and those for adolescents ages 15 to 19 declined about 20% (89 to 79 per 100,000) (Federal Interagency Forum on Child and Family Statistics, 1999).

Depending on definition of terms, chronic illnesses and disabilities affect between 2% and 32% of the nation's children. Approximately 2% of children have conditions that lead to numerous limitations in daily activities and can be classified as severe, and approximately 9% of children experience conditions of moderate severity (Newacheck & Taylor, 1992). Among school-aged children 5 to 17 years old, approximately 12% have difficulty performing at least one daily activity, with learning being the most common difficulty (Federal Interagency Forum on Child and Family Statistics, 1999).

As treatment of childhood disease has improved over the past decades, so have survival rates, resulting in a population of children with severe chronic illness and disabilities who previously would not have survived to adulthood. Currently, 90% survive, and slow progress is expected for the future in further reducing the mortality rates in the chronically ill and disabled. Nevertheless, this leaves a significant population of children with complex, severe, and permanent impairments requiring specialized services.

Problems of Infancy, Childhood, and Adolescence

Preterm Delivery and Low Birth Weight

In industrialized countries where infectious and nutritional diseases have been largely eliminated, death in the first month of life (**neonatal mortality**) accounts for about three-fourths of all deaths occurring in those younger than 1 year of age. The most common causes of neonatal death are preterm delivery, low birth weight, and congenital malformations. About three-fourths of all neonatal deaths occur in infants weighing less than 2,500 g at birth, the World Health Organization's adopted definition of low birth weight. According to the 1999 National Center for Health Statistics report, the low birth weight rate in the United States (7.5% in 1997) differs by race and socioeconomic status. African Americans (13.1%) have rates that are more than double those for Caucasians (6.5%). Hispanic, Native American, and Asian American infants' birth weights are very close to those of Caucasians.

Preterm delivery is the primary cause of low birth weight. The cause of preterm delivery is thought to be multifaceted; however, it has eluded scientists. Although risk profiles for preterm delivery have been developed, the mechanism(s) by which risk factors affect preterm delivery has not been determined. Interventions, regardless of their nature, have been demonstrated to be of limited value (Goss, Lee, Koshar, Heilemann, & Stinson, 1997). Preterm delivery rates in the United States have not improved in the last 30 years; instead they have become worse. Similarly, low birth weight has remained largely unchanged during that time despite the fact that more than 85% of mothers currently receive care as early as the first trimester (Racine, Joyce, & Grossman, 1992).

The rates of multiple births increased 33% between 1980 and 1994 (currently 25.7 per 1,000 births), an increase believed to be a result of infertility treatments (National Center for Health Statistics, 1996). Twins and other multiples are more likely to be of low birth weight than singletons. Nevertheless, multiple births account for only a portion of low-birth-weight infants, and there remain significant opportunities for improvement in the low birth weight rate.

Limited progress was made toward meeting the *Healthy People 2000* objective for abstinence from tobacco and alcohol during pregnancy, despite their scientifically established detrimental effects on the fetus. Maternal smoking during pregnancy is associated with low birth weight. The rates of fetal alcohol syndrome are actually on the rise. *Healthy People 2010* has an objective related to smoking cessation during pregnancy. Although there are alcohol control objectives targeted to people of childbearing age, there are none that specifically address alcohol use and pregnancy (DHHS, 2000). Selected *Healthy People 2010* objectives appear in the box on p. 496.

Despite no improvement in the rates of low birth weight, the infant mortality rate has decreased dramatically over the past 30 years. This decrease is primarily due to improvements in technology and care available in neonatal intensive care units (Ahmann, 1996). Many more infants, particularly those of very low birth weight, are now surviving. The survivors are having a long-term impact on the demographics of the childhood population. Although infants weighing 500 to 1,000 g are now living, about 20% have serious handicaps, including cerebral palsy, mental retardation, deafness and blindness, and seizures. At least one-third have significant learning difficulties (Hack, Horbar, & Malloy, 1991), affecting the number of children requiring special education and other services. Those at highest risk for low birth weight (i.e., the poor and many African Americans) become increasingly vulnerable in childhood because of the combined impact of chronic disability and social disadvantage.

Until more is learned about the causes of **preterm delivery and low birth weight,** recommendations must follow what is known about factors associated with these conditions. Early and regular prenatal care and reduction in unhealthy habits such as cigarette smoking, drug and alcohol use, poor nutrition, and exposure to sexually transmitted diseases currently top the list of primary prevention strategy recommendations. Reduction in these unhealthy practices is among the goals of community health nursing practice with pregnant women; nurses working in homes and in the community are in an ideal position to give counsel about healthy practices to women who are planning to become or who are pregnant.

Injuries

Injuries kill more children than all diseases combined and are the leading cause of childhood morbidity and disability from year 1 through adolescence. Every year, approximately 25% of children in the United States have an injury for which they seek medical attention (Adams & Benson, 1993). Injuries in children generate more hospital days of care, cause a higher proportion of discharges to long-term care facilities, and result in a higher proportion who require home health care after hospital discharge than any disease.

Death rates for injury differ by age. Rates are high in infancy (26.7 per 100,000), gradually reducing to a low of 9.2 per 100,000 for those 5 to 9 years old and increasing to a high of 66.1 per 100,000 for those 15 to 19 years old. Although motor vehicle accidents and suffocation are the leading causes of death in infancy, motor vehicle accidents and firearms are the leading causes among adolescents. Death rates as a result of injuries also differ by race and socioeconomic status, with rates for African American children being nearly twice that for whites (Division of Injury Control, 1990).

As a society we have established multiple preventive strategies, with some strategies requiring more active participation than others. Legislation has made the environment safer, and less behavioral change in consumers is required to ensure children's protection. Product safety legislation has been effective. Legislation requiring safety caps on medication bottles, for example, has been instrumental in reducing poisoning. Legislation requiring seatbelt use, smoke detectors, and bike helmets have made specific preventive behaviors more difficult to avoid. Self-determined, preventive safety behaviors that are affected by beliefs and motivation, such as keeping household cleaners and irons out of reach, require more active decision making on the part of caregivers and are more difficult to change. Community health nurses, working in primary prevention of injuries, need to attend to the influence of health beliefs and social conditions of families when providing interventions (Russell, 1996). A nurse's recommendations need to take into consideration the parenting beliefs as well as the physical environment. The American Academy of Pediatrics (1997) recently published a comprehensive sourcebook on injury prevention and control for children and youth.

Although a safe environment is beneficial, caregiving activities that accommodate to the child's capacity are critical. Some children are more injury prone (e.g., those with hyperactivity and impulsivity) than are others and some mothers have greater capacity to respond to their children's supervision needs than do others. The community health nurse can assess the physical and social environment and the parent-child interaction and can work with the parent, helping the parent to understand the child's cognitive and physical capacities and to develop day-to-day practices that reduce risk of childhood injuries. See the following Research Brief for an example of an intervention.

RESEARCH BRIEF

Kitzman, H., Olds, D. L., Henderson, C. R., Hanks, C., Cole, R., Tatebaum, R., McConnochie, K. M., Sidora, K., Luckey, D. W., Shaver, D., Engelhardt, K., James, D., & Barnard, K. (1997). Effects of prenatal and infancy home visitation by nurses on pregnancy outcomes, childhood injuries and repeated childbearing. Journal of the American Medical Association, 278, 644-652.

A randomized trial of a program of home visiting by nurses found that children of low-income, first-time mothers visited by nurses had fewer health care encounters for injuries and poisonings than those who were not visited, concluding that nurses can be instrumental in helping parents protect their child from harm.

Inadequate Nutrition, Obesity, and Eating Disorders

As a society, we have worked to eliminate hunger in children. Food is provided to low-income pregnant and breast-feeding mothers and their children up to age 5 through the Women, Infants and Children (WIC) Program. Women enrolled in WIC receive other related services, including education about nutritional requirements, prenatal care, and other preventive services. Many low-income children qualify for school breakfast and lunch programs. According to the U.S. Bureau of the Census, in 1997, less than 5% of children lived in households where there was moderate or severe hunger as a result of food insecurity (less than 1% with severe hunger) (Federal Interagency Forum on Child and Family Statistics, 1999).

Despite the availability of WIC and other supplements, many children simply do not have adequate amounts of nutritious food (Yoos, Kitzman, & Cole, 1998). Even though food is expected to be available to every child, the food intake of many children does not match their metabolic maintenance and growth needs. Reports of a recent survey by the U.S. Department of Agriculture's Center for Nutrition Policy and Promotion showed that most children (76% of ages 2 to 5, 88% of age 6 to 12, and 94% of ages 13 to 18) had a diet that was either poor or needed improvement.

Grocery stores carry a wide range of foods, making adequate nutrition for children and youth at all ages possible at any time with limited work required for preparation. In most metropolitan areas, prepared food can be purchased 24 hours a day. Yet failure to thrive, undernourishment, and obesity continue to be problems for many young children.

The cause of **growth failure** is sometimes difficult to determine. In the past, failure to thrive was classified as organic or nonorganic. In recent years, there has been an increased appreciation of the multidimensional nature of the problem. Intense interventions with families in the home often are required as part of the diagnostic and treatment process. These interventions are aimed at providing adequate nutrition, understanding and enhancing the quality of parent-child interaction, and developing strategies whereby the methods of feeding match the biological, social, and emotional needs of the child. The community health nurse who visits in the home and has a therapeutic relationship with the parent is a critical member of the diagnostic and treatment team.

Many adolescents (rates range from 0.1% to 3%) are afflicted with anorexia nervosa, a disease associated with limited food intake and inadequate nutrition (Coupey, 1998). Anorexia nervosa is a disease that primarily afflicts middle and upper socioeconomic adolescent girls older than 14. Its cause remains unclear. Although often attributed to psychological and psychosocial factors, physiological origins continue to be investigated. Diagnostic criteria include refusal to maintain body weight, fear of gaining weight, amenorrhea, and disturbance in the way body weight and shape is experienced. There are two types of anorexia nervosa: restricting type and binge-eating/purging type. This is a serious, potentially life-threatening syndrome and may require extensive treatment.

Although failure to thrive and anorexia nervosa persist, obesity in childhood and adolescence is increasing, placing many children at risk for chronic illness in adulthood. The third National Health and Nutrition Examination Survey found 20% to 27% of children (depending on age group) meet the criteria for obesity. It is the most common nutritional disorder of youth. Many genetic and environmental factors influence the development of obesity. Of the environmental influences, unlimited access to unhealthy foods, facilitated by the lack of norms for specific mealtimes, and a sedentary lifestyle with limited exercise represent the primary factors. Although the relationship is not strong, obesity during the school-age years does appear to increase the child's risk for obesity in adulthood, with approximately 40% of obese children remaining obese as adults (The Third National Health and Nutritional Examination Survey 1988–1994, 2000).

The community health nurse can use multiple strategies in working with parents and children, beginning with counseling related to breast-feeding and infant feeding and continuing through the establishment of healthy food and feeding practices that are age appropriate. A comprehensive understanding of nutritional needs and growth and development challenges is required. The reader is referred to pediatric and growth and development texts for that information.

One of the most central assessment activities of the community health nurse is regularly and systematically plotting the child's weight and height on a growth chart. The graph of growth changes is an invaluable first screen in discovering problems and in assessing response to interventions. When the quality of the diet is evaluated, 1-day dietary recall and a diary of all food taken for each day of a week are very informative to both the community health nurse and the primary care team and often are enlightening to the parent. Nutritional counseling needs to start with an adequate assessment of current practices and cultural values related to food. Because foods are prepared in multiple ways in different cultures, care needs to be taken to evaluate the nutritional quality of the foods rather than the types of dishes being served.

•••••••••••••••••••••••••••••••

There is no finer investment for any country than putting milk into babies.

Winston Churchill

•••••••••••••••••••••••••••••••

Communicable Diseases

One of public health's most successful programs has been immunizations. Progress continues to be made in the development of vaccines for the more severe communicable diseases, sparing children from death and the ravaging effects of many of the complications of these diseases. For example, smallpox has been eliminated worldwide, and polio has been dramatically constrained.

Although immunization clinics were a common method of distributing vaccines in the past, today the responsibility for immunizing children is often assumed by the primary care provider. In 1997, 85% of children younger than 18 had health insurance coverage, making immunizations theoretically available to most children through health insurance. Schedules for immunizations are recommended with the first agents given in early infancy. For the child to be protected, it is important to give the appropriate number of doses. New immunizing agents are currently under development, making it vital for professionals to keep up to date on the most recent recommendations. Because recommendations for immunizing agents are undergoing change, the current recommendations are not included here. The CDC is an up-to-date source for recommended immunization schedules.

Immunization rates are considered an important indicator of the adequacy of health care for children and of the level of protection a community enjoys from preventable communicable diseases. Despite high rates of health insurance, in 1997, only 76% of children 19 to 35 months of age had received the key recommended vaccinations. Factors other than health care availability often stand in the way of universal vaccine coverage. The community health nurse is in a key position within the community to identify barriers to care, educate families regarding immunizations, and facilitate health care visits for immunization.

Viral gastrointestinal and respiratory infections remain common, particularly among infants and young children, resulting in frequent illness days and challenges for working parents who try to find quality care for sick children. Young children in organized child care tend to have greater exposure to these common infections, thus increasing the scope of the problem. Most of these infections are self-limiting in healthy children but may be serious in premature infants and children with chronic illness.

Sudden Infant Death Syndrome

Sudden, unexpected, and unexplained death during the first year of life is referred to as **sudden infant death syndrome (SIDS)**. It is the leading cause of infant death after the postneonatal period and most often occurs when the child is between 1 and 5 months of age. Although the cause is not known, male preterm and low-birth-weight infants, infants living in low socioeconomic households, and infants whose mothers smoke are more likely to die from SIDS.

A link between sleeping position and SIDS has been found: Infants who sleep in the prone position are more at risk for SIDS. A 1992 statement issued by the American Academy of Pediatrics (AAP) advised the supine position for sleeping and avoidance of soft materials such as pillows and quilts that might trap exhaled air and promote rebreathing. As for all children, a smoke-free environment is recommended.

There are undoubtedly numerous causes of SIDS. Abnormal control of heart rate or respirations is one of the factors associated with sudden death. Some infants with idiopathic apnea of infancy (AOI) who exhibit apnea during sleep, an episode of apnea while awake, or color change during sleep succumb to unexpected death. Thus, apnea episodes should be reported and evaluated. Home cardiorespiratory monitoring, medication, careful parent teaching of interventions for apnea events, and parent support may be required.

Parents of infants who die from SIDS have special needs, and community health nurses often are involved in their support during the grieving process. The National SIDS Resource Center has made important information available to parents and professionals alike.

Growth and Development in the Presence of Chronic Illness

Although the presence of a chronic illness does not imply developmental problems, the limitations imposed by chronic illness and disabilities place children at risk for a wide range of developmental lags as they confront their ever-expanding worlds. The goal of care for the chronically ill and disabled child is to minimize the biological manifestations of the illness or disability on health and development, avoid complications, and reduce further disease. Outcomes can be improved by careful periodic assessments and early, individualized treatment by a multidisciplinary team of which nurses are critical members. The family's responsiveness to the child as well as responsiveness of the broader environment contribute to the outcomes (McGrath & Sullivan, 1999); thus, they are among the factors that need to be considered in any assessment and plan.

Children with chronic illnesses and disabilities and their families have a broad range of health, education, and supportive service needs. Their primary and specialty health care needs often include a range of nutritional, physical, occupational, speech and hearing, respiratory, and other therapies. Because of the issues they face, including uncertain prognosis and ambiguity, families and children often benefit from a range of preventive mental health services. The costs of missed work and added expenses associated with frequent long-distance travel to obtain specialty services, and costs associated with day-to-day in-home care should not be underestimated.

Unlike common chronic illnesses of adulthood, with the exception of **asthma,** there are few common, severe disabling conditions in childhood. Most life-threatening and severe diseases are rare, leaving an insufficient client population base to develop extensive categorical services locally. Because families with a chronically ill or disabled child have needs in common, regardless of the diagnosis, community-based services that meet the generic needs of children and families have gradually been developed (Perrin, 1997).

Every domain of family life is affected when a child is chronically ill or disabled (Miles, Holditch-Davis, Burchenal, & Nelson, 1999). Health professionals increasingly appreciate the significant physical, psychological, social, and emotional burden that families experience. Significant improvements in child and family functioning have been demonstrated as a result of carefully crafted, innovative programs.

Families are very active partners of professionals in the treatment of their children with chronic illness and disability. Many have become important advocates for the services needed and active supporters of one another. Because many of the families are coping with rare diseases, feelings of isolation are common. Parents are reaching out to other parents of children with chronic illness and disability, providing information, understanding, and support. Community health nurses are helping them with this networking process. In addition, families who are sharing the same experiences are increasingly connecting through the Internet.

Asthma

In the United States, asthma is the major cause of morbidity in children. This chronic condition affects 5.8% of children in the United States and is responsible for 25% of days missed from school. There has been an increase in the prevalence and in the severity of asthma during the past 20 years, with hospitalizations for asthma on the rise. From 1980 to 1993, the death rate for children ages 5 to 14 years nearly doubled (CDC, 1996). Although medications and therapeutic regimens to control the disease have improved, this disease continues to have devastating effects on the lives of large numbers of children and their families. The prevalence and severity of the disease is greater in African American children living in poverty and in crowded conditions (Yoos & McMullen, 1998).

Viral respiratory infections as well as exposure to specific allergens, such as cigarette and other smoke, dust mites, molds, cockroaches, and pet dander, often provoke this disease. Asthma education programs have been developed that are aimed at increasing adherence to prescribed medical regimens and reducing exposure to allergens (Yoos, McMullen, Bezek, Hondors, Berry, Herendeen, MacMaster, & Schwartzberg, 1997). These programs have had varying degrees of success. One of the explanations for limited adherence to regimens is that the disease produces intermittent symptoms. It is difficult for families to maintain regular day-to-day prevention practices during asymptomatic times.

CASE STUDY

Ben is a 16-year-old, Hispanic male with severe asthma. Originally diagnosed at 6 months of age, Ben's asthma has escalated in severity over the past 3 years. He has experienced multiple emergency department visits and hospitalizations, often requiring intensive care.

Ben's parents are divorced. He lives with his father but often spends time at his mother's home or at his maternal grandmother's residence. Ben has experienced many school absences throughout this academic year as a result of the persistent nature of his symptoms and frequent need for hospitalization. He thinks his grades are suffering because of his absences. Ben's usual asthma triggers include dust, cigarette smoke, upper respiratory infection, and weather change.

Ben is currently being discharged after a 3-day hospitalization for an asthma exacerbation. One week before admission, Ben began to experience nasal congestion and cough. On the day of admission, he developed labored breathing and wheezing despite increased use of his albuterol inhaler. In the emergency department, Ben did not respond to continuous albuterol nebulizer treatments and was transferred to the pediatric intensive care unit. His condition gradually improved with supportive medical therapy. Because of Ben's anxiety associated with his asthma attacks, the psychiatry service was consulted and relaxation therapy was initiated.

At the time of discharge Ben was feeling well, with peak flow readings of 560 before and after albuterol treatments. Chest examination at discharge revealed an occasional expiratory wheeze but was otherwise clear to auscultation. His discharge medications included the following: prednisone 30 mg/day orally; fluticasone (Flovent) twice daily; nedocromil (Tilade) MDI 2 puffs twice daily; albuterol MDI 2 puffs every 6 hours, increasing to 2 puffs every 4 hours for cough or wheeze. A community health nursing referral was initiated.

1. What lifestyle changes might you recommend to Ben and his family for avoiding his asthma triggers? Be sensitive to his family situation and needs and consider cultural influences.

2. Education about asthma and its management is an essential part of your care. Develop a teaching plan for Ben and his family including learning objectives, content, and appropriate teaching strategies.

3. His father is very concerned about Ben's absences from school and the work that he has missed. What options might you consider for approaching this problem? How might you work with school personnel to help Ben remain in school?

4. Community-based, comprehensive service programs are needed to provide the full continuum of required services to asthmatic children and their families. Describe the role of the community health nurse in advocating for and developing such services. What resources are available in your community?

Because of the continued advancement of asthma therapy, like in other conditions, it is important for those providing care to be current in their understanding of the disease and its treatment. The community health nurse is in an ideal position to understand the day-to-day concerns of the family with a child with asthma and to facilitate their understanding of and adherence to the environmental and pharmacological regimen.

Cancer

The approximate overall incidence of malignancy in children younger than 15 years of age is 14 per 100,000 per year. Incidence for nearly all types varies worldwide. Among the common sites of childhood **cancer** are blood and bone marrow, bone, lymph nodes, brain, central nervous system, kidneys, and soft tissue. Although the disease may present itself as a mass or symp-

toms related to a mass, the symptoms are often nonspecific. Among the symptoms related directly to tumors are unexplained bleeding, bruising, or petechiae; headaches and vomiting; bony pain; limping; paleness; hematuria; and unexplained endocrine symptoms. There also may be signs of obstruction. Among the nonspecific symptoms are weight loss, failure to thrive, diarrhea, malaise, and low-grade fevers. Children with unexplained signs and symptoms should be referred promptly for an evaluation.

After diagnosis, state-of-the-art treatment can be provided in specialty cancer treatment centers where nurses are employed as members of multidisciplinary teams. The treatment is based on the type and extent of the cancer. Among the multiple treatments are surgery, chemotherapy and radiation therapy, and biological response modifiers. Bone marrow transplantation may also be used. The community health nurse may provide care to the child and family in consort with a long-distance, specialty cancer treatment center. Parents, of course, struggle with not only the illness of the child and the threats to the child's survival, but also the threat to long-term health and development caused by the toxic treatments provided. With new treatments, survival rates for children with cancer have improved, and the disease is considered a chronic illness.

Cerebral Palsy

Central nervous system damage or insult in the early periods of brain development (prenatally or within the first years of life) can result in nonprogressive disorders that cause abnormal movement and posture; these are referred to as **cerebral palsy**. The causes of cerebral palsy differ and include developmental anomalies, perinatal trauma, congenital infections, and perinatal period metabolic disorders. Cerebral palsy also has very different manifestations. Based on motor dysfunction, the four types of cerebral palsy are spastic, dyskinesia, ataxia, and mixed. The degree of dysfunction ranges from mild to severe.

In the United States, the incidence of cerebral palsy has remained relatively steady. Approximately 1.8 per 1,000 children younger than 18 are affected. Severe cases of cerebral palsy are usually diagnosed within the first 6 months of life, with parents often expressing concerns about lack of developmental progress. Often, moderate and mild spastic hemiplegia are not diagnosed until the second year. Delay in meeting developmental milestones as well as abnormal tone (either low or high) are among the presenting problems. Specific signs of neurological dysfunction that raise concerns include scissoring of the legs, abnormal crawling, and abnormal reflexes.

Maintaining mobility, maximizing joint range of motion, and developing optimal muscle control and balance are among the treatment goals for infants with cerebral palsy. Because of the variation in manifestations as well as the specific needs of families, treatment of the infant and toddler with cerebral palsy is individualized. It usually involves physical and occupational therapy. Diverse physical therapy programs have been developed for children with cerebral palsy, often requiring tremendous effort on the part of parents. The community health nurse practicing in homes and in child care and other community settings may be the first to listen to the parents' emerging concerns or observe signs of dysfunction. Support during diagnosis and treatment is important. It may be some time before the full extent of the disability will become evident. Care during the preschool and school-age period involves optimizing function.

Congenital Malformations

The community health nurse may encounter any of a large number of rare, **congenital malformations** and abnormality syndromes. The severity of these conditions ranges from very minor, circumscribed abnormalities to very severe, complex, multisystem malformations. Refer to current pediatric and pediatric nursing texts for more details.

Attention-Deficit Hyperactivity Disorder

A behavioral syndrome, **attention-deficit hyperactivity disorder (ADHD)** is thought to have its origins in biological variations in central nervous system development. Prevalence rates in elementary grades range from 3% to 10%, with the condition being more prevalent in males (Wender, 1998). Inattention, overactivity, and impulsiveness are among the behaviors exhibited. Although first appearing in childhood, symptom manifestation differs by age. Symptoms, however, persist through adolescence and adulthood. These behaviors, associated with lack of success in school, often are attributed to a learning disability.

Although some persons diagnosed with ADHD do indeed have a learning disability, it is not a symptom of the disease. Currently, it is thought that ADHD may be overdiagnosed. The use of methylphenidate (Ritalin), a common medication used to treat ADHD, increased nearly sixfold from 1990 to 1995 according to the U.S. Drug Enforcement Administration. ADHD is a complex disease requiring careful attention to accurate diagnosis, pharmacological treatment, environmental management, and counseling. Community health nurses working in schools, homes, and programs in the community are in ideal positions to assess children within the context of their day-to-day physical and social environments and to develop modifications in those environments that help align the environmental demands with the capacity of the child and family.

Behavioral Problems

Children develop a range of behaviors as they learn to accommodate to the demands of society. Many problematic behaviors have their origin in the impulsivity of young children, which makes it difficult for them to resist temptation, work toward distant goals, control emotions, and wait for their need to be fulfilled. As children work toward learning self-control, these behaviors are at times problematic. With the support of nurtur-

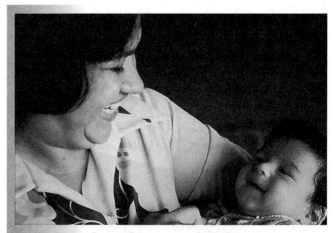

The health of an infant is greatly influenced by the ability of the mother to meet the infant's security needs.

ing parents, most of the common behavior problems of early childhood subside as the child develops self-control and self-regulating processes. In conjunction with those in the family's supportive network, health and social service professionals can help parents anticipate and respond to problematic but developmentally appropriate behaviors. As soon as problems such as aggression, sadness, and self-destructive behaviors are evident, however, a careful evaluation is warranted, because early intervention can reduce the risk of later parent-child interactional problems and more serious child psychological and antisocial behavioral problems.

Risk-Taking Behaviors of Adolescents

A variety of conflicts emerge with physical puberty, and adolescence is considered an age when many individuals become more vulnerable to risky behaviors and reckless deviance. There are multiple theories about the source of the conflicts that emerge during adolescence. One of the most noted is the "lack of fit between human organisms shaped by evolutionary forces that act very slowly and are difficult to change and opportunities for action determined by social conditions that change relatively quickly" (Csikszentmihalyi, 1998, p. 7). This theory suggests that as a society we are uncertain about the readiness of adolescents for contemporary adult roles. The desires that are genetically based in the adolescent do not match the opportunities provided by the culture. Anxiety that emerges in the adolescent is expressed in conflicts associated with taking responsibility, sexuality and intimacy, control and power, and interaction with adult role models (Csikszentmihalyi, 1998).

. . . .

I am not young enough to know everything.

Oscar Wilde

. . . .

The complexity of adolescent risk behaviors needs to be acknowledged because no single intervention is likely to be successful for all. Findings of recent research suggest that self-concept is important in the early stages of development of risky behaviors, as well as being the structure through which these behaviors continue and become enduring aspects of the self (Stein, Roeser, & Markus, 1998). These findings support the emphasis of recent adolescent programs on the development of self-esteem.

Regardless of origin, it is important to note that adolescents use a wide range of methods to manage their changing bodies and roles, some carrying more health risk than others. Nevertheless, experimentation with smoking, alcohol, illegal drugs, and other risk behaviors are serious matters. Communities are challenged to develop environments where youth can mature to adulthood without unnecessary risks. Community centers, sports programs, and volunteer programs are among the many approaches used.

Smoking

Despite extensive public health campaigns designed to reduce adolescent smoking, the rates remain high, placing yet another generation at risk for smoking-related chronic diseases in adulthood. Chemical dependency on nicotine is established easily. Approximately 50% of those who smoke half a pack of cigarettes a day in high school will have great difficulty stopping (MacKenzie & Kipke, 1998). Surveys in 1996 found that 22% of seniors smoked daily. Only 10% of adult smokers begin after age 20 and only 40% begin after age 14 (MacKenzie & Kipke, 1998). These statistics form the basis for the extensive public health efforts to cut the sale of cigarettes to minors and encourage adolescents not to smoke. In addition, for some cultural groups, cigarette use ushers in the subsequent use of alcohol and other drugs, making it particularly important to stop the introduction to smoking.

Substance Use

The United States leads the industrialized nations in its high teen alcohol and drug abuse rates. Alcohol remains the most popular drug, with 80% of adolescents having tried it by their 18th birthday and 51% of high school seniors having used it in the previous month (MacKenzie & Kipke, 1998). White males have higher rates of use than do African American males and higher rates than their female counterparts.

Although the use of other drugs is lower, drug use continues to place adolescents at risk. For example, prevalence rates of marijuana use by high school seniors in 1996 was 36%; cocaine use was 7%; and amphetamines and other stimulants use was 15% (MacKenzie & Kipke, 1998). Although rates were somewhat lower in 1998, use of illicit drugs remains a significant problem.

Sexual Activity

Unintended pregnancy, sexually transmitted disease, and pregnancy compromised by sexually transmitted disease are among the problems encountered by adolescents who engage in unprotected sex (Institute of Medicine, 1995). Recent surveys indicate that approximately half of all high school students have had sexual intercourse at some time. An estimated 12% of all adolescent females 15 to 19 years of age become pregnant each year, with half of these pregnancies carried to term (Gold & Gladstein, 1998). It is difficult to determine the number of pregnancies that are welcomed versus the number that are intended because many adolescents do not have intercourse with the intent of becoming pregnant but know that it could happen, do nothing to prevent it, and welcome it when it occurs. The intention of having a child in adolescence differs by culture and socioeconomic status, with some groups accepting parenthood earlier than others.

The risk of contracting a sexually transmitted disease increases with each additional sexual partner and with the addition of their partners' partners, over a lifetime of sexual activity. Many adolescents do not feel vulnerable, expecting any sexually transmitted disease to be treated successfully if they become infected. Nevertheless, some infections, if undetected and left untreated, and others for which there is no cure, result in chronic infection, infertility, and pregnancies compromised by preterm labor or neonatal infection. Strains of at least one sexually transmitted disease, human papillomavirus (HPV), have been associated with cervical dysplasia. Human immunodeficiency virus (HIV) infection and acquired immunodeficiency syndrome (AIDS) increasingly involve adolescents who engage in unprotected sex. Because there may be as much as a 10-year latency period between development of the HIV infection and development of AIDS, many people become infected during adolescence but are not aware of their infection.

Public health campaigns have been developed to encourage delaying the introduction of sexual intercourse in adolescence, to encourage the use of condoms for protection from disease and pregnancy, and to encourage the use of other forms of birth control. Nevertheless, evidence suggests that many adolescents have significant deficits and inaccuracies in knowledge related to sexual risk and its prevention. In addition, knowledge of contraception and condom use does not ensure their actual use because behavior does not always follow information. This makes it important to understand the motivation of the adolescent when providing preventive service. Communities and health care providers continue to struggle to find effective prevention strategies.

Violence

A major source of morbidity and mortality in the United States today is adolescent peer violence. Peer violence may be considered an epidemic and most often involves people who know one another. Complex factors contribute to peer violence. Inflicted injury most commonly occurs as a result of a fight among classmates and peers. A number of intervention programs have been developed, including those that teach conflict resolution.

Homicide is the second leading cause of death for older adolescents and young adults, leading to debate about society's responsibility in regulating exposure to violence and accessibility of handguns. Recent outbreaks of violence in schools and other public places that have resulted in deaths have raised the level of concern for violence and increased government awareness that violence is an important public health problem.

Primary prevention strategies for violence are recommended to begin at birth and continue throughout childhood. Avoidance of guns, television violence, and exposure to neighborhood and family violence is appropriate for all ages. In addition, there are recommended strategies that are age specific. Prevention for children from birth to 4 years old involves helping parents establish effective parenting practice with behavioral management skills that do not involve corporal punishment. Children 5 to 12 years old risk exposure to bullying and fighting in school. Because bullies and their victims are both at risk for poor performance and long-term relationships, identification of these prac-

tices as important is recommended. Although this behavior has often been overlooked in the past, it is now taken seriously. Henry J. Kaiser Family Foundation and Children Now (a nonpartisan, independent advocacy group for children) recently published information and tips for talking with children about violence.

Adolescents who are not in school, are using drugs, and are involved in fights are at particularly high risk for violence. Adolescents who are trying to use nonviolent techniques should be supported to continue and those engaged in combative behavior should be encouraged to become involved in a conflict resolution program.

The potential negative impact of domestic violence among adults in the household on children of all ages needs to be an ongoing concern. Not only do children risk injury themselves, but they also risk the emotional trauma associated with seeing the abuse (Eisenstat & Bancroft, 1999). Because more than 90% of domestic violence includes women being abused by men, children often see the abuse of their mother. Clinical issues related to domestic violence are complex and not easily resolved. The community health nurse needs to be open to the possibility and willing to address the problem as it emerges.

Delinquency

The number of youth ages 12 to 17 who have been identified as perpetrators of serious violent crimes had decreased from 52 crimes per 1,000 in 1993 to 31 crimes per 1,000 in 1997. Similarly, youth have been less likely to be the victims of crime (rates were 44 per 1,000 in 1993 versus 27 per 1,000 in 1993) (Federal Interagency Forum on Child and Family Statistics, 1999). The reason for the decrease is not known.

Although federal, state, and local governments have funded numerous primary prevention programs that target youth groups, the degree to which they are efficacious is not known. From a community health perspective, statistics suggest that there may be duplication and overlap of services to prevent delinquency on one hand and services that are too limited in scope to be effective on the other. Services that are broad-based, responding to the psychological needs of individual youth while simultaneously creating a positive environment within which youth can thrive, appear to be more effective than services that speak to only the youth or the environment.

Suicide

Suicide rates for males increased more than fivefold between 1950 and 1990. The rate in 1990 for males 15 to 19 was 18.8 per 100,000 and for females 3.7 per 100,000 persons (National Center for Health Statistics, 1996). When there is a handgun in the house, the teen is six times more likely to commit suicide, perhaps because it facilitates one to act impulsively. Community health nurses who work with children and youth need to be continuously conscious of suicide potential and able to detect early signs of problems for which suicide is the end outcome. A public health and educational campaign of the Educational Fund to End Handgun Violence has developed a program, Hands Without Guns, for youth.

Child Maltreatment

It is estimated that nearly 1 in 20 children is a victim of physical abuse. Of those who die from maltreatment (estimated at more than 2,000 children in the United States annually), 48% are a result of abuse, 37% of neglect, and the remainder from the combination (Lung & Daro, 1996). Of the injury-related deaths to infants in 1995, 761 were deemed unintentional, 311 were homicide, and 57 were undetermined (National Center for Health Statistics, 1996). The number of children identified as experiencing harm from neglect, physical abuse, emotional abuse, and sexual abuse continues to increase (Sedlak & Proadhurst, 1996). Because of the increasing awareness of the phenomenon and mandated reporting, it is unclear whether the real extent of child maltreatment has increased or whether our methods to identify it have improved. Nevertheless, the number of reports has increased each year since the Child Protective Service (CPS) was established.

Children younger than 3 years of age are more likely than older children to be identified as abused or neglected. Parents at increased risk to maltreat their children include those who are living in stressful situations, have poor parenting skills, are substance abusing, and have been maltreated themselves as children.

It has been hard to determine rates of maltreatment in children with disabilities because of the difficulty many children have in communicating their experience (Reichert & Krugman, 1997). Children with mild and moderate disabilities do appear to be at greater risk for physical and sexual abuse. Their needs and their behaviors often make parenting particularly challenging. In addition, it is often difficult to know what can be expected of the child with mild or moderate disabilities and parents at times expect behaviors that do not match the child's abilities. When children are severely disabled and expectations are clearer, it is believed that parents tend to accommodate and the children do not appear to be at greater risk for maltreatment.

It has been estimated that as many as 1 in 10 children before age 18 have been exposed to some form of sexual abuse, probably the most underdiagnosed of all types of maltreatment. The child knows the offender in approximately 90% of the cases, and offenders are predominantly male. Family risk factors for sexual abuse include poor relationships between parents and with the child, the presence of a nonbiologically related male in the house, and parental alcohol and drug abuse.

Impact of Maltreatment

The physical, emotional, and psychological damage to the child from maltreatment is determined by multiple factors, including developmental stage at time of maltreatment, the severity and duration of the abuse, and the relationship of the perpetrator to the victim. Child maltreatment occurs across social, ethnic, geographic, cultural, and economic boundaries; however, because it often occurs in the context of poverty, substance abuse, and family stress, it is difficult to determine the independent impact of the maltreatment on the negative outcomes in the child. For children with chronic illness or disability, it is particularly difficult to determine the added contribution of maltreatment to their behavioral and physical functioning over and above the disability. Nevertheless, there is substantial evidence of a relationship between maltreatment and such outcomes as later school failure, relationship disorders, substance abuse, and arrests.

Government Involvement

The extent of government involvement in the lives of families where children are maltreated is controversial. Although there is general agreement that there should be involvement when there is high risk of immediate serious injuries or death, there is less agreement about involvement with emotional and physical neglect, even when these may have significant long-term consequences. In the United States, cases of suspected child abuse and neglect are reported to governmental child protective agencies.

There is an ongoing need for a system that is both balanced and flexible in its protection of children. Individual child tragedies, with the associated media attention, far too often have driven case decisions and reform, upsetting the balance between protecting the child and maintaining the family on behalf of the child (Larner, Stevenson, & Behrman, 1998). Removing a child from home and parents is a serious act with significant long-term consequences for the child and the family.

A very important role for the community health nurse in child maltreatment is in primary prevention. By providing information, guidance, and support, the nurse helps parents develop the competencies necessary to care for their children. The nurse also helps parents define and identify methods to meet their own needs, whether they are for socioemotional or cognitive fulfillment or for material resources. Because parents are helped to meet their own needs, they are more able to provide care to their children.

Nurses who care for families with children also are responsible for early detection of child maltreatment. They, as well as other professionals, are required by law to report to the appropriate state agency any case of suspected abuse and neglect. Thus, they need to be well prepared to identify signs and symptoms of all kinds of maltreatment and to act as an advocate for the child as well as for the parent. It needs to be recognized that, regardless of the sensitivity exhibited by officials investigating a report of suspected child abuse and neglect, the experience is stressful for the parents and ultimately the family.

Children need to be protected from abuse while abusive parents or caregivers obtain the services necessary to meet their needs (these include parenting skills; financial, job, and housing support; and psychiatric services). Thus, when situations of immediate risk come to the attention of authorities, children are removed from the home until the family situation can be stabilized. Very often, it is the community health nurse who supports the family, provides many if not all of the necessary educational and counseling services, and acts as a case manager as families work to prepare themselves for the retention of, or return to, custody of their children.

A voluntary program of home visiting for families at risk for maltreatment (Wallach & Lister, 1995) has been recommended as a primary prevention strategy by the U.S. Advisory Board on Child Abuse and Neglect. There is now evidence that some home visiting programs are effective in reducing the incidence of maltreatment (Olds & Kitzman, 1993). As secondary prevention strategies, intensive family preservation programs have been developed for those facing serious and immediate threats, with the short-term goal of keeping the child in the home or returning him to the home soon. These intensive programs have low caseloads (two to six families), 24-hour availability, and intensive contact.

• •

The undeniable fact is that our children's future is shaped both by the values of their parents and the policies of our nation.
Putting Children and Families First: A Challenge for our Church, Nation, and World. National Conference of Catholic Bishops—Pastoral Letter, November, 1991

• •

The Ecology of Child Health

Children reside in multiple contexts, and their health is affected by each of these settings. The theory of human ecology emphasizes the importance of social contexts on child development (Bronfenbrenner, 1979). The structural characteristics and interrelations of families, social networks, schools, neighborhoods, communities, and culture affect the day-to-day life experiences of the child. Although families are the closest to and have the greatest impact on young children, the nurturing that families can provide depends on their social and physical environmental context.

Poverty

Although the overall poverty rate for children younger than 6 years of age decreased more than 10% between 1993 and 1996, poverty still places a significant proportion of our children at risk for poor health and developmental outcomes (Aber, Bennett, Conley, & Li, 1997; National Center for Children in Poverty, 1998). The most recent drop in rate can be attributed to improvements in rates of full-time employment. The Earned Income Tax Credit has also been effective in helping move some families out of poverty. There are important differences in poverty rates by states, with the rates for some states (e.g., Louisiana, Mississippi) being more than three times higher than for other states (e.g., Utah, New Hampshire).

In 1996, among children younger than 6 years of age, 11% were living in extreme poverty, an additional 12% were living in less severe poverty, and an additional 20% were living near

> ## A Conversation With...
>
> *Too many young people—of all colors, and all walks of life—are growing up today unable to handle life in hard places, without hope, without adequate attention, and without steady internal compasses to navigate the morally polluted seas they must face on the journey to adulthood.*
>
> *As a result, we are on the verge of losing two generations of Black children and youths to drugs, violence, too-early parenthood, poor health and education, unemployment, family disintegration— and to the spiritual and physical poverty that both breeds and is bred by them. Millions of Latino, Native American, and other minority children face similar threats. And millions of white children of all classes, like too many minority children, are drowning in the meaninglessness of a culture that rewards greed and guile and tells them life is about getting rather than giving.*
>
> **—Marian Wright Edelman**
> Source: Edelman, 1992.

poverty (defined as combined family income between 100% and 185% of the federal poverty line). In 1997, African American and Hispanic children younger than 6 years of age were much more likely than white children to be living in poverty (37% and 36%, respectively, versus 11%) (Federal Interagency Forum on Child and Family Statistics, 1999).

The risks of being poor increases with single parenthood, low educational attainment, part-time employment or unemployment, and low wages (National Center for Children in Poverty, 1998). In mother-only families, 55% of children younger than 6 years of age lived in poverty, in contrast to 12% of two-parent families. The educational level of parents was a strong predictor of family income. The poverty rate was 62% among children younger than 6 when neither parent had a high school education.

Effects of Poverty on Children

Poverty increases the barriers to a healthy environment. The negative influences of poverty on child health and development have been well established. Neonatal and postneonatal mortality rates are higher in children living in poverty. Poor children also are at greater risk for accidents, maltreatment, developmental delays, and some diseases.

Poverty varies in severity and in duration. For some children, poverty is transitory and sporadic, whereas for others, it is persistent. The relative impact of the severity and duration of poverty on child outcomes has not been determined. Persistent poverty may have greater negative consequences on the child's expectations for the future than intense poverty of short duration.

Although children are at higher risk for adverse outcomes when they are persistently very poor, there is no consensus about how the experiences of poverty work to negatively influence child health and development. Income poverty directly affects the resources of the family and in many ways defines the social context into which the child is born and lives. Social context affects the risk of low birth weight and gestational age of infants, which in turn makes the children more vulnerable to cognitive, physical, and mental health problems. It also affects children's social environment, the quality of their physical environment, the physical care they receive, the quality of their interaction with caregivers (including their stimulation), discipline and expectations, and the social and educational resources available to them in the community (Aber, Brooks-Gunn, & Maynard, 1995).

The social context in which youth develop affects their risk for developing maladaptive behaviors. Teens living in poverty are three times more likely than those not living in poverty to drop out of school. High school dropout rates continue to be high, particularly among ethnic minorities, with 27% of Hispanics dropping out of school in 1993. Youth who drop out of school are more likely to be unemployed and subsequently be in trouble with the law.

It is important to note that many children who live in poverty succeed and even excel in education, employment, and family and community life. These children are often referred to as *resilient*. Community health nurses, as well as other important people in their lives, can help create the environment within which children can develop the psychological resources necessary for future health.

Environmental Hazards

Playgrounds
The availability and quality of playgrounds and recreational areas for children of all ages differs by location, with some neighborhoods having much better developed and safer facilities than others. Developmental capacity, as well as presence or absence of disability, is important when developing a safe playground. Nurses often provide consultation to community groups in the development of play areas.

Environmental Smoke
More than 40% of children are exposed to environmental tobacco smoke or secondhand smoke. This environmental pollutant places a large proportion of our children at increased risk for impairment in lung growth, middle ear infection, higher incidence of respiratory infections, and exacerbation of symptoms of asthma. The recent attempts to eliminate smoking in many closed public places have been helpful in reducing unwanted exposure. Community health nurses can provide information to parents about the risks of secondhand smoke to children and can support parents as they participate in programs to stop smoking.

Toxins
Although the toxicity of some hazards, such as lead, diazinon, and mercury, is now well accepted, the long-term risks to development associated with other chemicals is not well known. For example, the impact of chemicals used on lawns in children's playgrounds and to clean and disinfect the home often is not fully known. The most common form of birth defect is cognitive development deficits. The causes of many are unknown, but scientists have speculated that many birth defects may be associated with environmental toxicants during the prenatal period (Dietrich, 1999).

An important exposure to toxins occurs during the preconception and intrauterine periods. Among the well-established toxins are lead, alcohol, drugs, and tobacco. There now is significant evidence that these substances can have a profound effect on the neurodevelopmental integrity of the infant and child. Public health warnings urging women to avoid these substances during pregnancy are backed by a substantial body of research.

Infants and children have different kinds of exposure to environmental toxins than do adults. They tend to be in the same room for longer periods and to be in different parts of the room than adults. For example, infants spend the majority of the time in a crib and toddlers/preschoolers spend nearly half their time in their bedroom. Also, because small particles in the air may be distributed in layers, air near the floor where the infants and young toddlers play may be more toxic than air at the level of the room where adults inhale. Similarly, chemicals and pesticides on treated carpets are more accessible to creeping infants and exploring toddlers than they are for adults. Some children spend considerable time using potentially toxic art and craft supplies.

In addition to differential exposure, the internal biological mechanisms of young children make them more vulnerable to toxins. Because of developmental differences, infants and children breathe or ingest, process, and excrete toxic substances from the air, water, and food differently than do adults. The growth and maturation of the organs make them more susceptible to harmful substances. For example, a 2-year-old child will absorb about five times as much of the ingested lead as will an adult (Rout & Holmes, 1991), making occupational limits that are set for adults many times higher than are safe for children.

Lead is an environmental toxin that has been attacked through public health measures after empirical research found the deleterious impact of lead poisoning on the long-term intellectual capacity of children. Significant legislation to reduce this environmental hazard has been enacted. Aggressive legislation has been effective in reducing lead in gasoline and paint and in elimination of lead in older homes, thus reducing the incidence of lead in the environment. Although lead poisoning in children has been reduced dramatically, some children continue to be at risk. At the level of the individual child, health care providers currently incorporate risk assessment and early detection as tools against this devastating disease that has reduced the intellectual potential of many children. Health care providers can complete risk assessments, however, only when children seek service. Therefore, it is

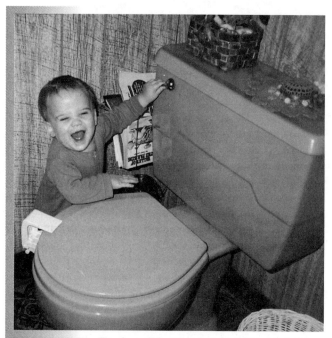

Creating a healthy environment is critical to raising a healthy child. This toilet has a safety latch to prevent accidents.

important that the community health nurse recognize conditions that place the child at risk and ensure that the child seeks care and is tested and treated if necessary. Some families need to be moved to different housing while their house is being deleaded.

Overall, environmental hazards produce unique risks for children because of their developmental demands. Thus, constant vigilance is required. Continued research is needed to understand the potential toxicity of old and new environmental agents. With evidence of their toxicity, policy makers supported by health care providers, teachers, community members, and families can support laws and regulations necessary to reduce environmental risks. There remains, however, significant responsibility on the part of parents and caregivers to continuously monitor and avoid environments that may be harmful to children.

One of the most critical challenges of our times is to establish and maintain healthy physical and social environments for children. Because community health nurses work within the community, they often are the first to be aware of a hazard and the first to make the hazard known to others. They may act as advocates for the families and problem solvers with community planners and community service providers.

Social Responses to the Needs of Children

Rights of Children
Children are the most vulnerable group in society. They do not have the political power that other potentially vulnerable groups

have (e.g., disabled, seniors, ethnic minorities). To ensure that children do not suffer unduly, adults must assume responsibility. The United Nations Convention of the Rights of the Child has provided some guidance about **rights of children** through its convention report (Box 21-1).

As a society, we have placed the primary responsibility for assuring that the rights of individual children are respected with parents. The community, however, is increasingly held responsible for creating an environment that supports parents as they care for their children and for acting as a safety net for children whose parents are unable to meet their children's basic needs.

There is increasing consensus among those advocating for children that as a society we should strive for children to be conceived by parents who have established their physical and emotional readiness to protect the fetus during pregnancy and to provide care for their child after birth.

Respecting the rights of children is a societal responsibility and is shared by all. The need for a broad community approach to the development of optimal nurturing of our youngest children is found in the following statement by David Hamburg (1994), President of the Carnegie Corporation. (The assumptions underlying this quote are the same for all children and youth.)

> If some traditional sources of stability and support have become weakened by enormous historical changes, then how can young children's development best be nurtured? The pivotal institutions are the family, the health care system, the emerging child care system, religious institutions, community organizations, and the media.

Family Context
Human infants grow and develop in a social environment where they are protected and cared for by others. Increasingly, grandparents and extended family live at distances and are unable to provide help to parents. It is useful for parents, with the help of

communities, to have established supportive informal (friends and relatives) and formal (service providers) social networks as they face the challenges of parenthood. Community health nurses hold important responsibilities in helping communities and families create a context where these social networks can thrive.

In addition to information that comes from direct contact with others, there are many sources of information for parents, including books, television, and the Internet. The support obtained from discussing this information with peers, as well as professionals, however, should not be underestimated.

Home visiting programs are an important source of support for families, particularly those with children at high risk because of physical or social condition (Kang, Barnard, Hammond, Oshio, Spencer, Thibodeaux, & Williams, 1995). Most of the primary prevention home visiting programs begin during pregnancy or early infancy and continue until the child is between 1 and 3 years of age. More than half a million children currently are enrolled in home visiting programs. The goals of the programs include the promotion of effective parenting practices, the prevention of child maltreatment, the promotion of healthy child development, and the improvement in the mothers' lives (Gomby, Culross, & Behrman, 1999). Because of the positive impact of some of these programs, there is renewed interest in home visiting as a support to young families, and new funding streams are increasingly becoming available.

Child Care

There has been a dramatic, steady increase in the number of women working. This trend is expected to continue with welfare to work initiatives. The demand for child-care vouchers is growing as welfare loads decline (National Center for Children in Poverty, 1999). The proportion of married women with children younger than 6 years of age in the United States who work has increased from approximately 10% in 1948 and 30% in 1970 to 60% in 1994. Day care is rapidly becoming the norm for children, and securing a quality child-care arrangement is an important challenge for parents (Hofferth, 1996).

Who cares for children when their mothers work? For children younger than 5 years of age whose mothers were in the workforce in 1993, parents or relatives cared for 47%, center-based programs cared for 30%, family child care cared for 17%, and in-home sitters cared for 5% (West, Wright, & Hausken, 1995). Children increasingly are entering formal, center-based day care and at earlier ages.

There are five major challenges facing dual-earner parents and single-parent families related to the care of their children. First, the time available to share activities with children is constrained. Second, the energy necessary to be emotionally involved with the children may be limited. Third, monitoring and supervision of children's activities is difficult. Fourth, in an attempt to meet the children's need, the parent's own needs for friendships, diversion, recreation, and relaxation may be difficult to meet, leaving them more vulnerable to the first three chal-

lenges. Fifth, the challenge may leave questions about competency that in turn threatens the maternal self-concept. It is argued by many, however, that low-income women face the same challenges as do middle-income women but also have the added burden of meeting the challenges with fewer resources, for example, less reliable transportation, and more chronic illness.

Each age group of children provides a new set of challenges to working parents who use child care and a new set of potential risks to the child. Because of the developmental needs for attachment, particular attention has been given to children younger than 1 year of age (Broom, 1998). Yet in 1994, more than half of all infants were cared for by someone other than their parents on a regular basis.

The consequences for children of poor mothers entering the workforce are not known. There is fear by some that the children's basic needs for food, shelter, and protection will not be met. If adequate, nurturing child care is not available, women, already stressed by social conditions, may need to leave their children in conditions that do not support optimal development. There is also concern than children will be denied access to health care because they will not be eligible for Medicaid (Larner,

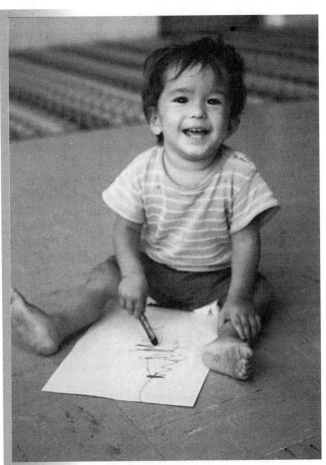

As children grow, they need a stimulating environment for optimal development.

Terman, & Behrman, 1997). The developmental consequences for infants and young children are unclear. Among mothers who have been receiving welfare, research to date suggests that maternal employment may influence positive child development and not be harmful in school-age children (Larner, Terman, & Behrman, 1997).

Choice of child care is one of the most important decisions parents make. Community health nurses involved with children need to become familiar with the resources available in the community and the financing of child care. In addition to providing information about characteristics of quality child care, nurses direct parents to resources and assist them in problem solving as they make their decisions about child care. Community health nurses are also an important resource for child care providers who struggle with developing a safe and nurturing environment, particularly when children become ill.

Child-care financing has fluctuated widely in the United States because there has not been a broad-based purpose or approach. Funding has been provided to meet immediate crises but has not been sustained, resulting in a collection of funding streams rather than a coherent system (Cohen, 1995). In some situations, child-care services have been considered custodial care, while at others they are considered educational services. Increased public support for direct child-care service subsidies has emerged with subsequent changes in the tax code and entitlements (Cohen, 1995). There is increased recognition by industry of the importance of family life to employees and some companies are offering daycare for children as a support to employees.

Systems of Care for Children and Families

Financial Support: Welfare to Work Programs

Although Americans have valued the protection of children, the Aid to Families with Dependent Children (AFDC) program increasingly has been seen as a system that simply does not work and also is inconsistent with American values that stress individual work and self-sufficiency (Payne, 1998). Originally passed in 1935, the AFDC program guaranteed cash assistance for poor single-parent families and enabled mothers to remain at home with their children. In recent years, many social scientists have charged that the AFDC program traps families in dependency and poverty and results in families being negatively stereotyped. With the passage of the Personal Responsibility and Work Opportunity Reconciliation Act in 1996, welfare was reconstructed in an attempt to discourage out-of-wedlock parenting and encourage mothers to work. It is not known how the stress imposed on poor women with limited social resources will affect the quality of their parenting. Although many experts believe that the negative impact of family stress associated with the mother working out of the home will be more than offset by the advantages gained in the self-worth

that comes from self-sufficiency, others are less certain. Experience to date is too limited to draw conclusions

Primary Health Care

One of the primary goals in health care is consistent health care providers who work in partnership with parents on behalf of the health of the child. The health care provider would know the child and family and have a comprehensive record of health assets, problems, and current therapeutic regimen. Ideally, primary care services are proactive and anticipatory. Preventive strategies, such as immunizations and safety counseling, necessary for the child's optimal growth, development, and protection, should be included. The services also need to be reactive to health problems, based on the needs identified through health supervision and those expressed by the family. Services extend, through referral and consultation, to other specialty and supportive services. The community health nurse is an active partner of the primary care provider in the care of many children who are at risk because of physical, developmental, or social conditions. There is increasing recognition that for many families, needs extend beyond a traditional primary care system. A more integrated system of health and social services is emerging. Managed care provides new opportunities for health care systems and communities together to develop a more comprehensive approach to the health needs of children. The approaches to managed care differ, and it is important for the community health nurse to understand how services are integrated in the community being served.

School Health Services and School-Based Primary Care

There was early recognition in the United States that the health of children affects their ability to attend school and to be ready to learn. School health services were built on that understanding. By the early 1900s, health and social services had become important components of the educational experience for children. The 1994 Joint Statement on School Health, presented by the secretaries of the Department of Education and the Department of Health and Human Services, provided a renewed focus on the interactive nature of health and education (Riley & Shalala, 1994). (See Chapter 12.)

While school health in the early part of the 20th century focused primarily on communicable disease control, health education, emergency services, and screening, some primary care services began to be introduced into the schools by 1960. School nurse practitioners joined the schools in Denver in 1969 and began providing primary care services. Since the 1980s, health clinics have been established in many schools, introduced primarily to make it easy for youth to receive primary health care services. School-based clinics provide a range of diagnostic and treatment services, primarily to adolescents. Funding for school-based clinics have ranged from private foundations to public funds. For more information on the role of the community health nurse in the school, see Chapter 12.

Home Care

With the survival of more children with complex diseases and disabilities, greater demands have been placed on the health care system to meet basic nursing needs, needs that more appropriately are met in the home than in the hospital. Home care has replaced hospitalization for care of many children with complex care needs. Nurses in the community often direct or provide around-the-clock care to children on ventilators and other life-saving technologies. They rapidly become partners with parents as they plan to meet the needs of the children.

Services for Children: Early Intervention

The basis for health is formed in the early years. Early intervention recognizes that education in infancy and early childhood can enhance the functioning of some children with disabilities and developmental delays. This position has evolved over a period of years following extensive research that has demonstrated the impact of environments on subsequent functioning of children at risk for developmental delays. In the late 1970s, children with disabilities between the ages of 6 and 18 had a right to education as a result of the Education for All Handicapped Children Act of 1975. The 1986 amendments to that act, often referred to as *Early Intervention,* mandated services for children 3, 4, and 5 years of age with disabilities. It also established a system of services that would benefit children with disabilities from birth to age 3 and their families. It is designed to provide a coordinated payment system, facilitating and enabling states to develop statewide, comprehensive, coordinated, multidisciplinary, interagency programs of early intervention services for infants and toddlers with disabilities and their families (Ruppert, 1997).

In 1991, through grants to states to plan and deliver services, the Individuals with Disabilities Act made coordinated intervention services available to infants and toddlers with disabilities who are or are at risk of becoming developmentally delayed. Services include "(1) early identification, screening, and assessment services, (2) medical services only for diagnostic or evaluation purposes, (3) health services necessary to enable the infant or toddler to benefit from the other early intervention services, (4) family training, counseling, and home visits, (5) special instruction, (6) speech pathology and audiology, (7) occupational and physical therapy, (8) psychological services, and (9) case management" (Ruppert, 1997). Early intervention in its ideal form also includes education for family life, pre-conception counseling, education and support for healthy behaviors during pregnancy, and identification and treatment of infants at risk for developmental delays. Participation of parents is considered central, with some services being provided in the home and others being center based.

Services for Children with Special Health Care Needs

Originally established in 1935, Title V of the Social Security Act was designed as a means for states to develop public health programs that serve children with special health care needs. Originally referred to as the *State Crippled Children's Services Program,* several legislation amendments have resulted in the current State Programs for Children with Special Health Care Needs. Its current mission includes: "1) the provision and promotion of family-centered, community-based, coordinated care for children with special health care needs; 2) the development of community-based systems of services for these children and their families; and 3) the provision of rehabilitation services for blind and disabled children who meet certain eligibility requirements" (Wallace & Gittler, 1998).

In the past, many services have been organized around specific diseases. Professionals, expert in the diagnosis and treatment of single or closely related conditions, have produced important condition-specific therapies. As special services have developed, eligibility for coverage has been determined by diagnostic labels. These diagnostic labels also determined eligibility for other benefits, including Social Security Supplemental Security Income, which provides supplements to poor and low-income blind and disabled children. A recent decision by the U.S. Supreme Court has resulted in a change by requiring children's functioning, as well as severity of specific diagnosis, to be considered in determining eligibility for services and benefits. The future of generic and specialized health and supportive services for children with chronic illnesses and disabilities and their families will depend on the future financing of health and social services.

Many children have chronic illnesses and disabilities, such as ADHD, that can interfere with progress in education. Public Law No. 94-142 (Education for All Handicapped Children; later referred to as the Individuals with Disabilities Act [IDEA]), passed in 1975, mandated all states to provide a free, appropriate public education to all students with disabilities. IDEA includes protections regarding special education eligibility, parental rights, a requirement for least restrictive environment for the child, the provision of related services, and individualized education programs.

When regular education is unable to accommodate the educational needs of the child because of persistent and substantial individual differences, the student is considered "disabled" from an educational perspective. Special needs may be physical, cognitive, behavioral, or a combination thereof. More than 10% of children are found to have a disability, and learning disabilities account for about half of all disabilities.

Children often have co-morbidities as well as different strengths and weaknesses, making their educational needs different. Recommendations for a specific set of services by disability category have been judged to be inappropriate. Therefore, individual plans appropriate to the child's needs are considered optimal. School administrators and teachers look to the nurse for consultation and support in their daily work with students and with the establishment of individual plans for the child. This is particularly important for children with multiple physical and behavioral disabilities.

As children with chronic illnesses and disabilities have been mainstreamed into regular classrooms for the child to be in the least restrictive environment, they have brought with them a host of special needs, including gastrostomy tube feedings, catheterizations, special medications, and related therapies. Although supervision of these procedures generally has been considered the province of the school nurse, staffing often leads to procedures being carried out by teachers or teacher's aides with limited supervision.

Transitioning Children to Adult Services

Many children with severe diseases, such as cystic fibrosis and sickle cell anemia, are now surviving into adulthood, leaving professionals and society in general with questions relating to their intimate relationships, employment, independence in living, and health services. Many medical care and supportive services have eligibility requirements that are age-based, leaving those reaching adulthood abruptly uncovered. Public Law No. 94-142 and IDEA do address the need for preparation for adult services, including planning with interagency links for supported employment, independent living, and so on, based on the needs of the client. The community health nurse often is the professional who identifies the gaps in services for individuals no longer eligible for children's services but who have extensive

prevention as well as health promotional needs as they strive for adult independence.

A Look to the Future of Children's Health

When comparing the mortality and morbidity rates for infants and children in the United States with those of other industrialized countries, it is apparent that there is considerable opportunity for improvement in the United States. If, as a society, we are to succeed in lowering these rates, ongoing consideration needs to be given to programs and policies that have the potential to support parents in providing care to their children. The direct health and human services that are offered to families with children, whether those children be healthy or with significant chronic illness and/or disability, need to be sufficiently coordinated to ensure that families receive the needed services. The number of children with complex chronic illness calls for continued effort on the part of health and human services to integrate services in a way that will respond to their needs. The ultimate goal is to support every parent and child so that the child can achieve his or her potential and unnecessary future costs associated with preventable health and behavioral problems can be avoided.

HEALTHY PEOPLE 2010

OBJECTIVES RELATED TO CHILDREN'S HEALTH

Immunization and Infectious Diseases

Vaccination Coverage and Strategies

14.22   Achieve and maintain effective vaccination coverage levels for universally recommended vaccines among young children.

Injury and Violence Prevention

Unintentional Injury Prevention

15.20   Increase use of child restraints.

Violence and Abuse Prevention

15.33   Reduce maltreatment and maltreatment fatalities of children.

Maternal, Infant, and Child Health
Fetal, Infant, and Child Death

16.1   Reduce the rate of child death.

Mental Health and Mental Disorders
Treatment Expansion

18.7   Increase the proportion of children with mental health problems who receive treatment.

Vision and Hearing
Vision

28.2   Increase the proportion of preschool children aged 5 years and younger who receive vision screening.

Hearing

28.12   Reduce otitis media in children and adults.

Source: DHHS, 2000.

CONCLUSION

Nurses working in the community have a unique opportunity to visit families in their homes and community and observe as parents go about their day-to-day activities, struggling to do the best for their children, often in the face of tremendous adversity. Because of their perspectives and the information they have available to them, nurses become critical members of community effort of planning for services for children and families. Finally, in providing direct care, nurses can individualize services to the needs of the family being cared for and the health and human resources available in the community.

CRITICAL THINKING ACTIVITIES

1. Is it necessary for prospective parents to be prepared for pregnancy and parenthood?

2. The United Nations Convention on the Rights of the Child suggests that a woman planning on becoming pregnant should be in a state of optimal health. She should schedule a pre-conception health examination (including a review of nutritional status); have a plan for regular prenatal care with early detection and treatment of complication and have a plan for managing day-to-day demands during pregnancy; be free from infections and chemical agents that may affect the sperm, ovum, and fetus; be emotionally, psychologically, and economically committed to being a parent; be socially connected with a supportive network and living in a community that values the rights of children.

   - Are these suggested conditions feasible?

   - What are the social implications of these recommendations?

   - Do these recommendations conflict with the rights of individuals as they have been operationalized?

   - What is the role of the community health nurse in education and advocacy regarding the bases for these recommended conditions?

   - What role should nurses play when working with families who do not meet these conditions?

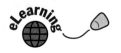

Explore Community Health Nursing on the web! To learn more about the topics in this chapter, access your exclusive web site:
http://communitynursing.jbpub.com

REFERENCES

Aber, J. L., Bennett, N. G., Conley, D. C., & Li, J. (1997). The effects of poverty on child health and development. *Annual Review of Public Health, 8,* 463–483.

Aber, J. L, Brooks-Gunn, J., & Maynard, R. A. (1995). Effects of welfare reform on teenage parents and their children. *The Future of Children, 5,* 53–71.

Adams, P., & Benson, V. (1993). *Vital health stat 10, 1991.* Hyattsville, MD: National Center for Health Statistics.

Ahmann, E. (1996). Profile of the high-risk premature infant. In E. Ahmann (Ed.), *Home care for the high-risk infant* (pp. 1–16). Gaithersburg, MD: Aspen Publishers.

American Academy of Pediatrics. (1997). *Injury prevention and control for children and youth.* Elk Grove Village, IL: Author.

Bronfenbrenner, U. (1979). *The ecology of human development: Experiments by nature and design.* Cambridge, MA: Harvard University Press.

Broom, B. L. (1998). Parental sensitivity to infants and toddlers in dual-earner and single-earner families. *Nursing Research, 47*(3), 162–170.

Centers for Disease Control and Prevention (CDC). (1994). Program for the prevention of suicide among adolescents and young adults. *Morbidity and Mortality Weekly Report, 43* (RR6), 1–7.

Centers for Disease Control and Prevention (CDC). (1996). Asthma mortality and hospitalization among children and young adults—United States, 1980–1993. *Journal of the American Medical Association, 275,* 1535–1536.

Children Now. (1998). *Right time, right place: Managed care & early childhood development.* Oakland, CA: Author.

Children's Defense Fund. (1994). *The state of America's children yearbook.* Washington, DC: Author.

Cohen, A. (1995). A brief history of federal financing for child care in the United States. *The Future of Children, 6,* 26–40.

Coupey, S. (1998). Anorexia nervosa. In S. Friedman, M. Fisher, S. Schonberg, & E. Alderman (Eds.), *Comprehensive adolescent health care* (pp. 247–262). St. Louis: Mosby.

Csikszentmihalyi, M. (1998). Evolution of adolescent behavior. In S. Friedman, M. Fisher, S. Schonberg, & E. Alderman (Eds.), *Comprehensive adolescent health care.* St. Louis: Mosby.

Deal, L. W. (1993). The effectiveness of community health nursing interventions: A literature review. *Public Health Nursing, 11,* 315–323.

Dietrich, K. (1999). Environmental toxicants and child development. In H. Tager-Flusberg (Ed.), *Neurodevelopmental disorders.* Cambridge, MA: The MIT Press.

Division of Injury Control, Centers for Disease Control and Prevention. (1990). Childhood injuries in the United States. *American Journal of Diseases of Children, 144,* 627–649.

Edelman, M. W. (1992). *The measure of our success: A letter to my children and yours.* Boston: Beacon Press.

Eisenstat, S., & Bancroft, L. (1999). Domestic violence. *The New England Journal of Medicine, 341,* 886–892.

Federal Interagency Forum on Child and Family Statistics. (1999). America's children: Key national indicators of well-being. Washington, DC: U.S. Government Printing Office.

Freeman, M. (1996). *Children's rights: A comparative perspective.* Brookfield, VT: Dartmouth.

Freeman, M. (1996b). Introduction: Children as persons. In M. Freeman (Ed.), *Children's rights: A comparative perspective.* Brookfield, VT: Dartmouth.

GAO report to congressional requesters. At-risk and delinquent youth. (GAO/HEHS-96-34). Washington, DC: U.S. Government Printing Office.

Gold, M. A., & Gladstein, J. (1998). Epidemiology of mortalities and morbidities in adolescents. In S. Friedman, M. Fisher, S. Schonberg, & E. Alderman (Eds.), *Comprehensive adolescent health care.* St Louis: Mosby.

Gomby, D., Culross, P., & Behrman, R. (1999). Home visiting: Recent program evaluations—Analysis and recommendations. *The Future of Children, 9,* 4–26.

Goss, G. L., Lee, K., Koshar, J., Heilemann, M. S., & Stinson, J. (1997). More does not mean better: Prenatal visits and pregnancy outcome in the Hispanic population. *Public Health Nursing, 14,* 183–188.

Hack, M., Horbar, J. D., & Malloy, M. H., et al. (1991). Very low birth weight outcomes of the National Institutes of Child Health Neonatal Network. *Pediatrics, 87,* 587–597.

Hamburg, D. (1994). *Starting points: Meeting the needs of our youngest children.* New York: Carnegie Corporation of New York.

Hofferth, S. (1996). Child care in the United States today. *The Future of Children, 6,* 41–61.

Institute of Medicine. (1995). *The best intentions: Unintended pregnancy and the well-being of children and families.* Washington, DC: National Academic Press.

Kang, R., Barnard, K., Hammond, M., Oshio, S., Spencer, C., Thibodeaux, B., & Williams, J. (1995). Preterm infant follow-up project: A multi-site field experiment of hospital and home intervention programs for mothers and preterm infants. *Public Health Nursing, 22,* 171–180.

Kitzman, H., Olds, D. L., Henderson, C. R., Hanks, C., Cole, R., Tatebaum, R., McConnochie, K. M., Sidora, K., Luckey, D. W., Shaver, D., Engelhardt, K., James, D., & Barnard, K. (1997). Effects of prenatal and infancy home visitation by nurses on pregnancy outcomes, childhood injuries and repeated childbearing. *Journal of the American Medical Association, 278,* 644-652.

Kitzman H., Cole, R., Yoos, H. L., & Olds, D. (1997). Challenges experienced by home visitors: A qualitative study of program implementation. *Journal of Community Psychology, 25,* 95-109.

Larner, M., Stevenson, J., & Behrman, R. (1998). Protecting children from abuse and neglect: Analysis and recommendations. *The Future of Children, 8,* 4–22.

Larner, M., Terman, D., & Behrman, R. (1997). Welfare to work: Analysis and recommendations. *The Future of Children, 7,* 4–19.

Lung, C. T., & Daro, D. (1996, April). *Current trends in child abuse reporting and fatalities: The results of the 1995 annual fifty states survey* (Working Paper No. 808). Chicago, IL: National Committee to Prevent Child Abuse.

MacKenzie, R., & Kipke, M. (1998). Substance use and abuse. In S. Friedman, M. Fisher, S. Schonberg, & E. Aderman (Eds.), *Comprehensive adolescent health care.* St Louis: Mosby.

McGrath, M. M., & Sullivan, M. C. (1999). Medical and ecological factors in estimating motor outcomes of preschool children. *Research in Nursing and Health, 22*(2), 155–167.

Miles, M., Holditch-Davis, D., Burchenal, P., & Nelson, D. (1999). Distress and growth outcomes in mothers of medically fragile infants. *Nursing Research, 48,* 129–140.

National Center for Children in Poverty. (1998). *Young child poverty in the States—Wide variation and significant change* (Research Brief 1). New York: Columbia School of Public Health.

National Center for Children in Poverty. (1999). Demand for child care vouchers grows as welfare loads decline. *News and Issues, 9,* 5.

National Center for Health Statistics. (1996). *Epidemiology and health promotion from data compiled by the Division of Vital Statistics. U.S. Bureau of Census population file RESD9795.* Washington, DC: U.S. Government Printing Office.

Newacheck, P., & Taylor, W. (1992). Childhood chronic illness: Prevalence, severity, and impact. *American Journal of Public Health, 3,* 364–371.

Olds, D. L., & Kitzman, H. (1993) Review of research on home visiting for pregnant women and parents of young children. *The Future of Children, 3,* 53–92.

Payne, J. (1998). *Overcoming welfare.* New York: Basic Books.

Perrin, J. (1997). Systems of care for children and adolescents with chronic illness. In H. Wallace, R. Biehl, J. MacQueen, & J. Blackman (Eds.), *Children with disabilities and chronic illness* (pp. 156–161). St. Louis: Mosby.

Racine, A. D., Joyce, T. J., & Grossman, M. (1992). Effectiveness of health care services for pregnant women and infants. *The Future of Children, 2,* 40–57.

Reichert, S., & Krugman, R. D. (1997). Child abuse, neglect, and disabled children. In H. Wallace, R. Biehl, J. MacQueen, & J. Blackman (Eds.), *Children with disabilities and chronic illness* (pp. 137–143). St. Louis: Mosby.

Riley, R. W., & Shalala, D. E. (1994). *Joint statement on school health.* Washington, DC, U.S. Departments of Education and Health and Human Services.

Rout, U. K., & Holmes, R. S. (1991). Postnatal development of mouse alcohol dehydrogenases: Agarose isoelectric focusing analysis of the liver, kidney, stomach, and ocular isozymes. *Biology of the Neonate, 59,* 93–97.

Ruppert, E. (1997). Early intervention. In H. Wallace, R. Biehl, J. MacQueen, & J. Blackman (Eds.), *Children with disabilities and chronic illness* (pp. 338–345). St. Louis: Mosby.

Russell, K. M. (1996). Health beliefs and social influence in home safety practices of mothers with preschool children. *Image: The Journal of Nursing Scholarship, 28,* 59–64.

Sedlak, A. J., & Proadhurst, D. D. (1996). *The third national study of child abuse and neglect.* Washington, DC: Department of Health and Human Services.

Stein, K., Roeser, R., & Markus, H. (1998). Self-schemas and possible selves as predictors and outcomes of risky behaviors in adolescents. *Nursing Research, 47,* 97–106.

Wallace, H., & Gittler, J. (1998). Federal legislation for children with special health care needs and their families: Past, present, and future. In H. Wallace, R. Biehl, J. MacQueen, & J. Blackman (Eds.), *Children with disabilities and chronic illness.* St. Louis: Mosby.

Wallach, V. A., & Lister, L. (1995). Stages in the delivery of home-based services to parents at risk of child abuse: A healthy start experience. *Scholarly Inquiry for Nursing Practice: An International Journal, 9,* 159–173.

Wegman, M. E. (1993) Annual summary of vital statistics—1992. *Pediatrics, 92,* 743–54.

Wender, E. (1998). Attention-deficit hyperactivity disorder. In S. Friedman, M. Fisher, S. Schonberg, & E. Alderman (Eds.), *Comprehensive adolescent health care* (pp. 967–972). St. Louis: Mosby.

Vital Statistics of the United States. (1997). *Mortality Detail, 1994.* Washington, DC: National Center for Health Statistics.

West, J., Wright, D., & Hausken, E. G. (1995). *Child care and early education program participation of infants, toddlers, and preschoolers.* Washington, DC: U.S. Department of Education.

Yoos, H. L., Kitzman, H., & Cole, R. (1998). Family routines and the feeding process. In D. Kessler & P. Dawson (Eds.), *Failure to thrive and pediatric undernutrition: A transdisciplinary approach* (pp. 377–387). Baltimore: Paul H. Brookes Publisher.

Yoos, H. L., & McMullen, A. (1996). Illness narratives of children with asthma. *Pediatric Nursing, 22,* 285–290.

Yoos, H. L., & McMullen, A. (1998). Risk factors for asthma. Unpublished, University of Rochester.

Yoos, H. L., McMullen, A., Bezek, S., Hondors, C., Berry, S., Herendeen, N., MacMaster, K., & Schwartzberg, M. (1997). An asthma management program for urban minority children. *Journal of Pediatric Health Care, 11,* 66–74.

Chapter 22
Elder Health
Virginia Lee Cora

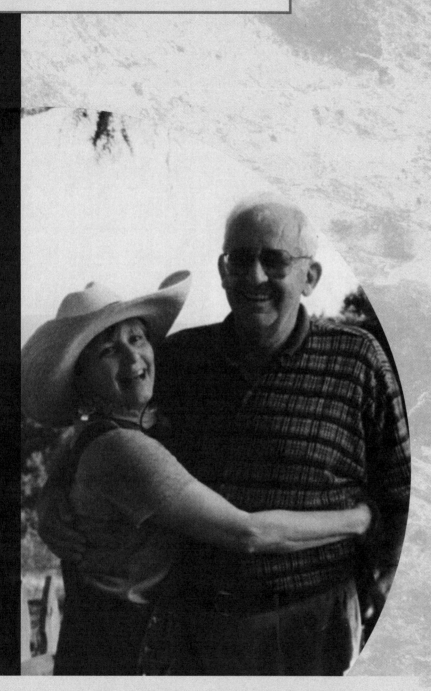

As community health nurses stand at the dawn of a new century, more than one-third of our nation's citizens are elderly. How can we prepare for the future of a generation of more than 76 million whose numbers, demands, expectations, and diversity have no precedent?

QUESTIONS TO CONSIDER

After reading this chapter, answer the following questions:

1. What are the various meanings of *aging*?
2. What is gerontological nursing?
3. What are the major health concerns of the aging population?
4. How are ideas and misconceptions about aging related to the care of elders?
5. What are the major preventive health issues of the elderly?
6. What are specific intervention strategies for the community health nurse in promoting the health of elders?
7. What are special health considerations that the community health nurse should be aware of in caring for the elder?
8. What ethical issues are involved when working with the elderly?

KEY TERMS

Ageism
Aging
Activity of daily living
  (ADL)
Advance directives
Alzheimer's disease
Cohort
Confusion

Delirium
Dementia
Depression
Elder abuse
Geriatrics
Gerontology
Instrumental activity of
  daily living (IADL)

Life expectancy
Life review
Life span
Longevity
Orthostatic
  hypotension
Osteoporosis

Presbycusis
Presbyopia
Primary aging
Polypharmacy
Respite care
Secondary aging
Senescence

In caring for elders, we cannot look to the past for direction, for never have so many people lived this long and in such good health. We cannot expect our current ways of thinking about aging and models of caring for the elderly population to provide us with much guidance. Such ways of thinking are outdated in our quest for more progressive attitudes about aging and health. As nurses work with ever increasing numbers of elderly persons in a variety of settings, we must develop improved ways of promoting independence, dignity, and self-care among our older clients. Most of our investments in health care for elders have been in institution-based secondary and tertiary prevention strategies, with little attention to preventive, holistic "aging-in-place" centered care. In the future, home- and community-based alternatives will become the norm for health care of elders, and nurses will provide the leadership to promote maximum levels of independence and the highest possible quality of life for elders and their families.

• •

Grow old along with me. The best is yet to be!

Rabbi Ben Ezra

• •

Aging

Elders differ from middle and young adults in many ways. Persons 80 years old obviously are not the same as persons 20 or 50 years old. Aging is the sum of all the changes that normally occur in a person with the passage of time; life and aging begin at conception and end at death. Aging is a natural, lifelong, and total process that varies among individuals and within various domains and organ systems of each individual. Aging is *universal*—it occurs at different rates and degrees; *progressive*—it interferes with lifestyle; *decremental*—it has a general gradual decline; and *intrinsic*—it is unmodifiable.

Primary aging is "a biologic process whose first cause apparently is rooted in heredity" (Busse & Blazer, 1980, p. 4). Secondary aging is "the defects and disability whose first cause comes from hostile factors in the environment, particularly trauma and disease" (Busse & Blazer, 1980, p. 4). Although health care providers may have little impact on *primary aging*, they can have a significant impact on *secondary aging* by altering risk factors associated with lifestyle, safety, and the like. Nurses can identify genetic predispositions in family health histories, use data from screening tests, and teach appropriate lifestyle changes (e.g., healthy diet, regular exercise, weight management, pollution reduction). For example, for an elder with heart disease in both parents and a sibling, total cholesterol levels greater than 240, and low-density lipoprotein (LDL) levels greater than 160, the nurse can encourage a low-fat diet and exercise; the primary care provider may prescribe hypolipidemic agents.

• •

I'm not afraid of growing old, because I am. That's just a fact of life. I'm not out to "arrest" life, the way some people do. I'm living with it, and that's a part of your journey, that's part of who you are. You carry it with you.

Robert Redford, actor, age 60,
May 1998

• •

Aging Terminology

In working with elderly populations, community health nurses must differentiate among several age-related terms: age, life span, life expectancy, longevity, senescence, and cohort. Age, of course, is the length of time a person has existed. **Life span** is the maximum potential for survival of a particular species. The maximum duration of existence for a human being is 115 to 120 years. **Life expectancy** ("expected life") is the average observed years of life of a species from birth to death or at any stated age. For example, the life expectancy of a child born today is 75 years; the life expectancy of an 85-year-old is 6 more years. Living most of the potential human life span is a relatively contemporary phenomenon. The life expectancy during the Stone Age was 15 years; in the time of Hippocrates (460-377 BC), it was about 18 years; in the time of George Washington (1732-1799), it was 30 years; in the time of Florence Nightingale (1820-1910), it was 50 years; in 2000, it was 75 years. **Longevity** ("long life") usually is the expected length of an individual's life, based on the lives of their immediate family members. **Senescence** ("grown old") is the last stage of a lifelong process of aging. This period culminates in changes in behavior with decreased powers of survival and adjustment (Comfort, 1990). In the United States, old age, or senescence, was designated by the 1935 Social Security act as being over age 65. **Cohort,** a term derived from the Roman military unit, is a group of people who share a particular age, historical moment, or geographical area (e.g., born between 1900 and 1920, Depression era, or urban ghetto). Cohorts tend to develop similar attitudes and values because they share experiences of a certain period (e.g., frugalness may be seen in many elders who survived the Great Depression).

Language used to designate elderly persons is more poorly differentiated than it is for children. It is inexact to lump together all individuals ages 65 to 120 years simply as old. Elders usually are persons age 65 years or older. They often are referred to as pre-old, ages 55 to 64 years; young-old, ages 65 to 74 years; middle-old, ages 75 to 84 years; and old-old, ages 85 and older.

Geriatrics (*geras,* "old age," *iatros,* "physician") is a medical term for the branch of health science concerned with the diseases and problems of old age. **Gerontology** (*geron,* "old man," *logos,* "word") is a sociological term for the study of old age and aging. It is a multidisciplinary, applied science that can be examined from several perspectives: myths and folk wisdom, efforts to prolong life, demographics, and scientific inquiry (Ebersole & Hess,

1998). Gerontology has no core, unifying theory of aging. Instead, there are biological theories at the molecular, cellular, and system levels; psychological theories of the life span; and sociological theories of elders as social beings (see appendix A).

• •

To learn from the old, we must love them, not just in the abstract, but in the flesh, beside us in our homes, businesses, churches and schools. We must work together as a people to build the kinds of rituals, communities, institutions, and language that allow us to love and care for one another.

Mary Pipher, 1999

• •

FYI

As a result of 30 years of study, the *Baltimore Longitudinal Study of Aging*, sponsored by the National Institutes of Health, has reached two critical conclusions:

1. Aging is not a disease.
2. There is no single, simple pattern of aging.

Source: The Baltimore Longitudinal Study of Aging, National Institute on Aging, National Institutes of Health, Department of Health and Human Services, Older and Wiser, 1989.

Gerontological Nursing

Although elderly populations in poorhouses and rural settings were the focus of nurses in the 1800s and early 1900s (Burnside, 1988), the evolution of a nursing specialty concerned with older people is a recent phenomenon (Box 22-1). Gerontological nursing, the nursing of the aged, began evolving as an area of practice in the early 1960s. The standards and scope of gerontological nursing practice are well defined by the American Nurses Association (see appendix B). *Gerontic nursing* also is a nursing term coined by Gunter and Estes (1979) to define "a health service for the aged." Because most elders live in the community, especially in rural settings, as opposed to being in institutions, the needs of elders have been a focus of community health nurses throughout their history.

Aging and Health

With this country's many advantages, Americans are able to live long enough to grow old. As community health nurses we must examine our own attitudes and values about aging and elderly people to gain holistic, realistic views and provide age-appropriate care for this elderly population.

Aging does not equal health. The changes associated with normal aging are differentiated from the changes associated with health problems. For example, a 65-year-old may be confined to bed with end-stage rheumatoid arthritis while an 85-year-old may run a 26-mile marathon.

Aging changes are both relative and absolute. For example, the individual who has poor eye-hand coordination as a young adult will have poorer eye-hand coordination as an elder than his or her peers, a *relative* change. A person with a 10% reduction in vital capacity of the lungs has an *absolute* change. The principal of individual variation is that the best predictor of a person's current performance is that person's previous performance. Elders should not be judged by the average age-related decline seen in cross-sectional studies (Kane, Ouslander, & Abrass, 1999).

Aging is a comprehensive process. It is not only a series of biological changes; it also is a complex series of psychosocial, socioeconomic, and spiritual changes that influence and are influenced by the elders, their families, communities, and society. Any changes that affect one domain simultaneously affect all other domains.

Old age is a time of continued growth, development, and fulfillment (i.e., achieving self-actualization or ego integrity). This culmination of the life cycle is a balance of both gains and losses

---

BOX 22-1 EVOLUTION OF GERONTOLOGICAL NURSING

THE AMERICAN NURSES ASSOCIATION (ANA)

1966	Established a Division of Geriatric Nursing Practice
1968	Developed the first standards of geriatric nursing practice
1973	Established certification in geriatric nursing as generalists (1974), nurse practitioners (1976), and clinical nurse specialists (1989)
1981	Developed the first statement of the scope of gerontological nursing practice
1983	Creation of The National Conference of Gerontological Nurse Practitioners (NCGNP)
1984	Creation of the National Gerontological Nursing Association (NGNA)
1985	Creation of Canadian Gerontological Nursing Association (CGNA)
1986	Creation of the National Association of Directors of Nursing administration in Long-Term Care (NADONA/LTC)

of the processes of change. As with other transitional periods of life, old age is a time of holding on and letting go. Some performance may be enhanced with aging. For example, with greater wisdom, perspective, and problem-solving skills, cognitive function may improve.

The elderly population is heterogeneous and diverse. Human beings tend to be more homogeneous (similar) at birth and become quite heterogeneous (different) in old age. As with other age or ethnic groups, we must avoid simplistic generalizations and neither romanticize elders nor stereotype or stigmatize them. Rather, we must balance their positive aspects with their negatives to accept them as they are with specific health problems countered by many real strengths.

Elders are tough. Very few elders are frail; a great majority are hardy, vigorous, and active through the very end of their lives. They are not *victims* of aging processes, but rather *survivors* of life's experiences as part of family systems within their environment. They usually appreciate direct, factual information rather than ambiguous indirect statements.

. . . .

You don't get old from calendar years. You get old from inactivity.
Jack LaLanne

. . . .

Nursing of Elders

The "age wave" is coming, and society will need well-educated and experienced nurses to meet the challenge of providing care for this ever-increasing, complex segment of the population. To provide holistic care, community health nurses will need to consider these elders within the context of their community, their family, and themselves.

Elders in the Community

The status and roles of elderly people in the community are influenced by the values placed on aging by society. In some cultures, elders and their collective wisdom are held in very high esteem; in other cultures, old age exemplifies loss of productivity with subsequent loss of status and stigmatization. **Ageism** is the systematic stereotyping of and discrimination against people because they are old (Butler & Lewis, 1998). Learned at an early age, these prejudices may surface in younger people's negative beliefs about older people, as well as from the elders' beliefs about themselves. These views can influence the outcomes of health care. For example, elders may be viewed as too old for surgical interventions when most tolerate surgery well. Demented elders may be seen as not needing analgesics or comfort measures when

in pain. Nurses need to listen for ageism in themselves and others, then confront it as they would racism or sexism in any age group through the education about the realities of old age, both positive and negative.

Demography of Elders

The aging population is growing by both absolute and relative numbers (U.S. Bureau of the Census, 1991). In 1900, persons 65 and older numbered 3 million, or 3% of the American population. With a 10-fold rise, they currently make up 32 million, or 12% of the total population, the "graying of America." In 2010, the "age wave" will hit as the first of the Boomers turns 65 years of age. In 2050, they will be 20% of the population and number 80 million. Elders are 6% of the world population. The old-old, age 85 and older, are the fastest growing segment of the population, projected to grow from 50,000 now to 1 million in 2050. Most older men (74%) are married, and many older women (40%) are not. The elderly population in this country is becoming more racially, ethnically, and culturally diverse than ever before: 87% are Caucasian, 7.7% are African American, 3.4% are Hispanic, 1.4% are Asian/Pacific Islanders, and 0.4% are Native American. By 2050, African American elders will increase to 12%, Hispanics will grow eightfold, and Asian and Native American groups will increase significantly. Cultural and ethnic differences in aging and health are reflected in the life expectancy of men and women. For example, the life expectancies of white men and women are 73 and 80 years, respectively; life expectancies of black men and women are 65 and 74 years, respectively. Elders of various cultural groups may have different responses to health problems, modifiable risk factors, and health promotion activities like education. Community health nurses need to determine the values of elderly populations within their local area and how these cultural differences affect health care. For example, elderly family members may be immigrants to this country. They may not understand or speak English; they may not be literate in any language. These individuals may delay seeking health care because of fear of the system.

The distribution of the elderly population is four to one in rural settings compared with urban settings. Rural elders are the oldest old, are poorer, and have more chronic illness, compounded by greater problems with access, transportation, and inadequate health care facilities. In 1990, nine states had more than 1 million elders: California, Florida, New York, Pennsylvania, Texas, Illinois, Ohio, Michigan, and New Jersey. The largest percentage of the oldest old are clustered in five farm states: Iowa, South Dakota, Nebraska, North Dakota, and Kansas.

Currently, the median annual income of elderly men is approximately $15,000; for elderly women, it is approximately $8,500. Only 11% are below the poverty line, but 27% are near poor. Women make up 74% of poor elders; African Americans account for 24% of these poor. The major source of income for elders is the federal Social Security program; more than half have pensions and 19% have private pensions. Eight percent receive public assistance, 6% receive food stamps, and 12% have Medicaid. The education of elders is improving from a median level of 9 years in 1970 to 12 years in 1990, but currently, only 55% have a high school education and 13% have completed college. As many as 50% to 80% of elders have inadequate *functional health literacy;* that is, they are unable to read prescription bottle labels, comprehend health literature and appointment slips, complete health insurance forms, follow diagnostic test instructions, and so on (Williams, Parker, Baker, Parikh, Pitkin, Coates, Nurss, 1995).

Twenty-one million households are headed by elders, 78% are owners and 22% are renters. Approximately 15% of elderly men and 79% of elderly women live alone, primarily because women tend to live longer than men. Because of their economic status, disabilities, or social needs, many elders resort to a wide variety of living arrangements, including senior housing units, home sharing, home equity conversion, group homes, "granny flats," and others. Although only about 5% of elders age 65 years live in nursing homes, about 20% of elders age 85 years are in these facilities, with many more women and Caucasians comprising this population than men or other ethnic groups. A growing number and variety of alternative housing arrangements for frail and/or demented elders are emerging. These newer services include adult day-care centers, personal care homes, and assisted living facilities.

With regard to health care access, the elderly population accounts for 36% of America's health care expenditures: $72 billion from Medicare, $20 billion from Medicaid, and $10 billion from other sources. Health care consumes up to 20% of the income of elders, an average of $1,500 out-of-pocket expenses annually. Although only 12% of the total population, older adults account for 37% of hospital stays and 47% of hospital days. Most of these hospital expenditures are made in the last 6 months of life. Individual, family, cultural, and health provider beliefs and values all may influence choices for health care during this period. For example, family members may refuse to "give up" on an elder and want every medical intervention to be done for a terminal illness, whereas the elder may believe "the only cure for old age is death" and resist further care, even pain management.

Healthy People 2010 *for Older Adults*

For the elderly population, *Healthy People 2010* goals are to maintain their health and functional independence and compress morbidity and dependence into the shortest possible time. Objectives related to improvements in nutrition, reductions in tobacco use, weight control, physical activity, immunizations, and health care visits are focused on all age groups. Community health nurses can help address the need for more health educa-

tion and programs for older adults. For example, only 30% of elders participate in moderate physical activity (e.g., walking, gardening), and less than 10% in vigorous physical activity; only 10% have had the pneumococcal vaccine, and less than 20% get an annual influenza vaccine. All these problems can be addressed during clinic and home visits or other contacts with elders. Selected objectives for older adults are summarized in the *Healthy People 2010* box on p. 506. Some of the programs and organizations concerned with improving the health and living situation of elders are suggested in Box 22-2.

Elders in the Family

As the basic social unit mediating between the individual person and the whole of society, the family is the focus of intervention for elders in the community. One definition of family is that a family is "a social system of multiple, interdependent generations of persons who identify each other as being related by birth, marriage, adoption, or mutual consent, as being committed to one another over time, and as having common properties, rights, and responsibilities" (Cora, 1985). By helping families maintain positive attitudes toward aging, nurses can assist elders to look forward to and take advantage of their long and active lives. Elders can give their children one final gift: a positive model of old age.

Aging Families

Aging families are assessed according to their structure, functions, or development, or as systems that encompass all of these attributes. No matter the setting, elders should be approached as members of multigenerational families.

The structural approach to aging families is demonstrated by the family genogram, including at least three generations. Even when elders live alone, their families influence their needs, behaviors, and health care. When assessing elders' families, community health nurses need to develop brief genograms of immediate, distant, and extended family members to help explain their behaviors and understand their meanings as well as to establish support systems for frail or demented elders. Nurses may need to help contact these family members or create surrogate families to assist with care.

The functional approach to aging families describes activities to meet the sexual, economic, reproductive, and educational needs of aging family members and provides a convenient checklist for identifying functional and dysfunctional family relationships (see Duvall in Box 22-3). However, in modern societies, the state has assumed many responsibilities for functions that previously were within the family. Care of elders may be added to the list of services performed by the state in the form of elder care centers, residential centers, and nursing homes. Examining the functional tasks of aging families is helpful for nurses when assessing their patterns of control and levels of involvement with their elders. For example, when helping adult children adjust to

HEALTHY PEOPLE 2010

OBJECTIVES RELATED TO OLDER ADULTS

Cancer

3.13   Increase the proportion of women aged 40 years and older who have received a mammogram within the preceding 2 years.

Heart Disease and Stroke

Heart Disease

12.6   Reduce hospitalization of older adults with heart failure as the principal diagnosis.

Immunization and Infectious Diseases

14.29   Increase the proportion of adults who are vaccinated annually against influenza and ever vaccinated against pneumococcal disease.

Injury and Violence Prevention

Unintentional Injury Prevention

15.27   Reduce deaths from falls.

15.28   Reduce hip fractures among older adults.

Medical Product Safety

17.3   Increase the proportion of primary care providers, pharmacists, and other health care professionals who routinely review with their patients aged 65 and older and patients with chronic illnesses or disabilities all new prescribed and over-the-counter medicines.

Vision and Hearing

Vision

28.6   Reduce visual impairment due to glaucoma.

28.7   Reduce visual impairment due to cataract.

Hearing

28.14   Increase the proportion of persons who have had a hearing examination on schedule.

28.15   Increase the number of persons who are referred by their primary care physician for hearing evaluation and treatment.

Source: DHHS, 2000.

---

familial roles and responsibilities as caregivers, knowledge of family tasks may assist nurses to support family members and prevent burnout from overtaxing the system.

The developmental approach emphasizes the synchronization of several dimensions of time: individual time, family time, and historical time (Erikson, 1963). Individual time is the chronological movement of a person over a lifetime. Family time is the timing of epoch events in the family that involve birth, death, and transitions of persons from one role to another. Historical time is the chronology of a society over an extended period, such as decades or centuries. Elders nearing the end of their individual time are experiencing role changes that involve the transition of power from themselves to younger family members. These changes become important events in the evolving of family time, but also must be interpreted in the context of the historical moment of the society of which they are a part (Erikson, 1963). (See Carter and McGoldrick in Box 22-3.)

Family Caregivers

As part of the intergenerational family life process, family members accept familial responsibility in times of crisis. More than 23% of American households include at least one caregiver, of whom more than 76% are caring for a relative or friend who is at least 50 years old (AARP, 1997). The average age of caregivers is 46 years. These individuals often represent the "sandwich generation," adults who may be both raising children and caring for elders—often while working outside the home; however, 12% of caregivers are elders age 65 and older. More than 73% of the caregivers are female; two-thirds are working. The average Amer-

BOX 22-2 LEGISLATION, PROGRAMS, AND ORGANIZATIONS CONCERNED WITH OLDER ADULTS

FEDERAL PROGRAMS

- Social Security Act of 1935: Social Security Administration (SSA), Old Age, Survivors, and Disability Insurance (OASDI), Social Security (SS), Supplemental Security Income (SSI)

- Older Americans Act (OAA) of 1965: Administered by Department of Health and Human Services (DHHS) Administration on Aging (AOA)

- State and area agencies on aging, multipurpose senior centers (social, recreational, educational, and nutritional services for senior citizens), senior employment and volunteer programs (ACTION: Foster Grandparents, RSVP, Senior Companions), senior nutrition programs, health education and prevention activities, senior transportation services, in-home health care. National Aging Information Center (202-619-7501). Eldercare Locator (800-677-1116).

- Research on Aging Act of 1974: Created the National Institute on Aging (NIA) within National Institutes of Health. Publishes a resource guide for older Americans (Age Pages)

- Health Care Financing Administration (HCFA): Administers Medicare and Medicaid insurance programs

- Department of Agriculture: Offers food and nutrition programs including food stamps

- Department of Veterans Affairs: Provides services and benefits to veterans

- Department of Housing and Urban Development: Offers low-cost public housing for elders

- Department of Treasury Internal Revenue Service (IRS): Offers assistance with income tax problems and filing

- Department of Interior: Access to federal park system, Gold age Passports (free), Golden Eagle Passports (low-cost)

NATIONAL PRIVATE AND VOLUNTARY NONPROFIT ORGANIZATIONS

- National Council on Aging (NCOA): Established in 1950 as a national resource for information, consultation; sponsors publications, special programs, advocacy activities, research, training, Health Promotion Institute

- American Association of Retired Persons (AARP): Founded in 1958 by Dr. Ethel Percy Andrus (also National Retired Teachers association); 30 million members; 4,000 local chapters; largest nonprofit, nonpartisan membership organization in the world; purpose is to enhance quality of life for older persons; promote independence, dignity, and purpose for older persons; provide leadership in determining the role of older persons in society; and improve the image of aging. Members 50+. *Modern Maturity* magazine, AARP News Bulletin. Tax assistance, health insurance, mail order drugs, information.

- National Eldercare Institute on Health Promotion

- Andrus Foundation on gerontological research

- American Society on Aging (ASA): Enhance knowledge and skills of those working with older adults and their families

- Gerontological Society of America (GSA): Multidisciplinary professional and scientific organization for those working in the field of gerontology.

- Gray Panthers: Founded in 1970 by Maggie Kuhn (1905-1995) as an intergenerational activist group dedicated to social change. "Speak your mind. Even if your voice shakes, well-aimed slingshots can topple giants. . . . The best age to be is the age you are."

---

ican woman will spend 16 years caring for children and 17 years caring for elderly relatives. A majority of the care recipients are female relatives. Twenty-one percent of caregivers live in the same household as the recipient and 94% live within 2 hours' commuting distance. The average time of care provided is 18 hours per week, but 57% provide 40 or more hours of weekly care. While the average outlay for caregiving expenditures is $171 per month, the average for high-intensity caregivers is $357 a month. Most caregivers provide assistance with at least one **instrumental activity of daily living (IADL)** (e.g., telephon-ing, shopping, transportation, medications, money, food preparation, housekeeping, and laundry), about half assist with one **activity of daily living (ADL)** (e.g., bathing, dressing, toileting, transfer, continence, and feeding), and a third help with at least three ADLs. Most view caregiving as having some impact on family life, leisure time, work life, and personal finances. They also see caregiving as an overall positive experience (AARP, 1997).

Community health nurses need to assess caregivers for their *competence* (i.e., caregiving knowledge, skills, confidence, and

BOX 22-3 CHECKLISTS OF AGING FAMILY TASKS AND PROCESSES

Duvall's (1977) family developmental tasks for elderly family members:

- Do the elders have satisfactory living arrangements for their current situation?
- Have the elders established comfortable routines for their old age?
- Are the elders adjusting to their retirement income?
- Is the family helping safeguard the elders' physical and mental health?
- Are the elderly couple maintaining love, sex, and marital relations?
- Are the elders remaining in touch with other family members?
- Are the elders keeping active and involved with family and community?
- Are the elders and family finding meaning in the elders' life?
- Are the elders and family finding meaning in the elders' death?

Carter and McGoldrick's (1980) family life cycle of aging families:

Primary emotional transition:

- Are the elders and family members accepting their shifting generational roles?

Second-order changes in family status required to proceed developmentally:

- Are the elders maintaining their own and/or the couple's functioning and interests in face of physiological decline? Are they exploring new familial and social role options?
- Are the elders providing support for a more central role for the middle generation?
- Is the family making room in the system for the wisdom and experience of the elders, supporting the older generation without over functioning for them?
- Are the elders dealing with loss of spouse, siblings, and other peers and preparation for own death? Is there life review of elders and integration of the family?

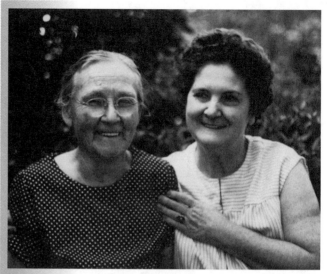

More women than men survive, and the very old are often cared for by their elder children.

objectivity), *burden* (number of hours of caregiving per day/week, nature of tasks to be completed), and *burnout* (psychological stress related to the nature of the illness and the necessary care and support system). Because many caregivers are elderly themselves, their own health issues need to be addressed, especially if they too are frail. When problems are identified, caregivers may need to expand their support systems through family, friends, or community agencies (e.g., home health social services, area agencies on aging, religious groups). Caregivers may need assistance to manage financial and legal concerns, or they may benefit from participation in caregiver groups for their educational and social support. They usually need to increase their access to resources and may need respite services for relief of stress.

A respite ("look back") is an interval of rest; **respite care** provides family members temporary relief of caregiving responsibilities for elders. The availability of these services varies widely in rural and urban areas and different regions of the country. They may be offered in the home by other family members, religious organizations, or federal or state programs; they may be offered in institutional settings by adult day-care centers, assisted living facilities, or nursing homes. Social workers may be helpful in locating respite services in various communities, or the community health nurse may need to help create opportunities for respite for overburdened caregivers.

Elder Abuse, Exploitation, and Neglect

With most caregiving for elders occurring in homes, community health nurses must be aware of the potential for abusive, dysfunctional family relationships. More than 1 million elderly women are victims of abuse each year. They often fail to report maltreatment because of shame, fear of retaliation, or previous unsatisfactory experiences with police, district attorneys, or social workers who lacked sensitivity to the concerns and needs of older people. As a form of domestic violence, **elder abuse** or maltreatment is defined as the willful infliction of physical pain, injury, or debilitating mental anguish, unreasonable confinement, or willful deprivation by a caregiver of services that are necessary to maintain physical and mental health (O'Malley, 1987). *Elder neglect* refers to elderly persons who are either living alone and not able to provide for themselves the services that are necessary to maintain physical and mental health or are not receiving necessary services from responsible caretakers (O'Malley, 1987). Types of elder maltreatment are described in Table 22-1. Maltreatment occurs with 5% to 10% of elders, typically by family members. The most frequently abused, exploited, and neglected elders are those with functional disabilities who are frail, confused, and dependent; are older than 70, female, and of minority status; and have poor social networks. The abuse often is invisible—it is repeated, not reported. Adult protective service laws require mandatory (46 states) or voluntary (4 states) reporting of suspected abuse or neglect.

Nurses who encounter elders in the community have opportunities to assist with both primary prevention and secondary prevention of elder maltreatment. The goals of primary prevention are to support caregivers and reduce the potential for abuse. The goals of secondary prevention are early case finding of abuse and crisis intervention, referral, and follow-up with the elders and family caregivers. Techniques for interventions in the maltreatment of elders are summarized in Box 22-4.

Elders as Individuals

The goals of health care for individual elders are to maximize independence and to minimize dependence. For nurses working directly with elders in the community, the focus of intervention is on health promotion and primary prevention to maintain autonomy of the elders as members of family systems within their environment. Health care providers need to focus on the elders' abilities, what's left to build on, rather than disabilities, what's lost. The ability to function depends on individual characteristics and the setting/environment. The health care providers' role is to enhance coping ability by careful clinical assessment and management of remediable problems and facilitating changes in the environment to maximize function in the face of those problems that remain (Kane, Ouslander, & Abrass, 1999).

Elders usually exhibit multiple health problems with complex interactions. Health care interventions often require multidisciplinary approaches. Nurses work in collaboration with primary care providers (e.g., physicians, nurse practitioners, physician assistants), therapists (e.g., physical, occupational, speech therapists), pharmacists, social workers, psychologists, and many others. Health care for these elders must consider the issues of access, quality, and cost.

In the community, providers of health care become integral to the elder's environment. Nurses may be viewed as friendly visitors or surrogate family members rather than as health care providers. We must be aware of factors that foster dependency, including our own attitudes and behaviors. The aversion to risk of health care providers, families, and the elders themselves can bias thinking toward conservative interventions without consideration of quality of life issues (Kane, Ouslander, & Abrass, 1999). For example, fear of falling in an elder may suggest using a wheelchair with further deconditioning rather than emphasizing walking to strengthen muscles and improve balance and gait. Nurses can help keep elders as active and healthy as possible, encourage their independence, and support their health decisions.

Chronic Illness

The cost of surviving the acute illnesses and injuries of young and middle ages are the chronic illnesses of old age. Approximately 85% of elders have at least one chronic disease; 30% of the aged have three or more chronic conditions (Reuben, Yoshikawa, & Besdine, 1996). There is an increase in functional disabilities with 20% of elders being dependent in at least one ADL. The causes of morbidity and mortality in elders are summarized in Table 22-2. With the focus of nursing for health promotion being on self-care, a universal prescription for every age, including elders, is reduction of health risks. In the United States, there is ample evidence that at the start of the 21st century, we are living better, as well as longer. The disability rate,

TABLE 22-1	TYPES OF ELDER MALTREATMENT

TYPES	BEHAVIORS OF ABUSERS AND/OR ELDERS
ABUSE	
Physical or sexual	Slapping, pushing, restraining, molesting
Psychological	Threats, intimidation
Exploitation	Misappropriation of funds or property
Medical	Withholding necessary medications, treatments, or assistive devices
NEGLECT	
Passive	Unintentional lack of caregiving because of lack of knowledge and/or skills
Active	Abandonment or intentional failure to provide caregiving
Self-neglect	Intentional or unintentional lack of attention to self-care

FYI

Elders Have Their Own Dreams

John Glenn, Osceola McCarty, and Lillian Carter are well-known public figures who pursued their dreams throughout their lives. Each took different paths toward realizing their dreams as they grew older.

John Glenn took his first ride in space in 1962, becoming the first man to orbit the earth. Thirty-six years later, he became the oldest person in space when at the age of 77, he returned as part of the crew of the Discovery. When Glenn went into space in 1962 as a young man, the thought of sending a 77-year-old into orbit seemed unthinkable; today it is not only possible but expected. Glenn states, "Just because we grow older, doesn't mean we give up our dreams."

Ms. Osceola McCarty never set out to get attention. McCarty, a tiny 87-year-old woman, washed clothes all her life. She lived a simple life, never married, and never had children, yet amazingly she was able to amass a small fortune of $250,000. When she donated $150,000 to the University of Southern Mississippi to fund scholarships for African American students, she was surprised at the reaction. Her generosity so touched people the world over that she became a cultural heroine: She shared the spotlight with Oprah Winfrey and Jesse Jackson and received the Presidential Citizen's Medal from President Bill Clinton. She simply said, "If you can help somebody, help them." She dreamed of a future in nursing but was forced to drop out of school in the sixth grade. The USM College of Nursing made her an honorary graduate of its nursing program in 1996.

Lillian Carter, mother of President Jimmy Carter, was a retired RN at the age of 68 when she joined the Peace Corps and served as a nurse in Bombay, India, for 2 years.

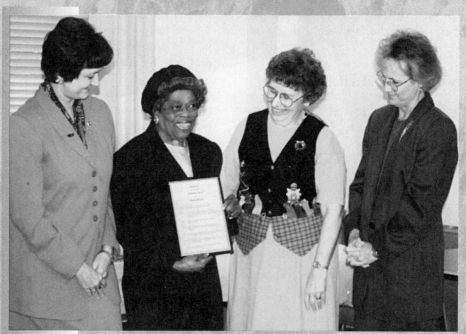

Ms. Osceola McCarty with her "honorary nurse" certificate from the Mississippi Nurses Association.

Contributed by Karen Saucier Lundy.

Continued

FYI—CONT'D

Miss Lillian Sees Leprosy for the First Time

When I nursed in a clinic near Bombay,
A small girl, shielding all her leprous sores,
Crept inside the door. I moved away,
But then the doctor called, "You take this case!"
First I found a mask, and put it on,
Quickly gave the child a shot and then,
Not well, I slipped away to be alone
and scrubbed my entire body red and raw.
I faced her treatment every week with dread
and loathing—of the chore, not the child.
As time passed, I was less afraid,
and managed not to turn my face away.
Her spirit bloomed as sores began to fade.
She'd raise her anxious, searching eyes to mine
To show she trusted me. We'd smile and say
a few Marathi words, then reach and hold
Each other's hands. and then love grew between
Us, so that, later, when I kissed her lips
I didn't feel unclean.

By Jimmy Carter
Source: Carter, 1995.
Used with permission.

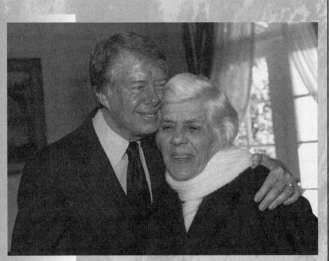

Mrs. Lillian Carter greets her son, President Jimmy Carter, in 1977, upon her return from India, where she spent 2 years working as a nurse in the Peace Corps.

BOX 22-4 TECHNIQUES FOR INTERVENTION IN THE MALTREATMENT OF ELDERS

PRIMARY PREVENTION

- Be aware of the risk factors for potentially abusive situations—in both elders and caregivers (e.g., frailty, confusion, dependence, functional disabilities, age 70+ years, female, minority status, poor social networks).
- Provide anticipatory guidance to help families plan for future needs of frail and/or demented elders.
- Broaden support systems for families with dependent elders by involving other family and friends in caregiving activities.
- Teach families stress management techniques and provide information about caregiving and local resources (e.g., caregiver classes, support groups, respite and day care, financial aid, counseling).

SECONDARY PREVENTION

- Observe for physical injuries (e.g., bruises, lacerations, burns, fractures, pressure sores, malnutrition, poor hygiene, dehydration, recurring injuries) and/or psychological damage (e.g., unusual fears, caregiver not letting elder be alone with providers).
- Ask direct questions while alone with the elder: "Has anyone tried to hurt you or make you do things you didn't want to do?"
- Do a complete physical examination, including the skin, head, neck, breasts, abdomen, genitals, and rectum.
- Document findings with the elder's own words, detailed descriptions, and, if possible, photographs of injuries.
- Assess the severity and frequency of the abuse and the safety of the elder. Report findings to adult protective services. If potentially lethal, make immediate referrals (call the police).
- Provide follow up with the elder and family, because many abusive situations are repetitive.

TABLE 22-2   MORBIDITY AND MORTALITY IN ELDERS

MORBIDITY: INCIDENCE OF *CHRONIC DISEASES* OF PERSONS AGED 65+ YEARS

Arthritis	47%	Orthopedic impairments	17%
Hypertension	37%	Sinusitis	15%
Heart disease	32%	Diabetes	10%
Hearing impairments	29%	Visual impairments	10%

MORTALITY: CAUSES OF *DEATH* IN PERSONS AGED 65+ YEARS

CAUSE	RATE*	RISK FACTORS	RISK REDUCTION
Heart disease	217.3	Smoking, hypertension, hypercholesterolemia	Take aspirin, estrogen, low-fat diet, exercise
Cancer	104.7	Tobacco use, radiation	Screen breast, colon, skin, prostate, uterus, mouth
Stroke	46.4	Hypertension, tobacco	Aspirin, smoking cessation
Lung disease (COPD, pneumonia/influenza)	20.6	Tobacco use, allergies	Immunization, smoking cessation
Diabetes	9.6		Screen, diet, exercise
Accidents/falls	8.7	Weakness, imbalance, polypharmacy	Exercise, drug review, home and community safety
Kidney disease	6.1	Hypertension, diabetes	Treat infections
Liver disease	3.4	Avoid toxic substances	ETOH; immunization

Rate per 10,000 population.

Adapted from Kane, Ouslander, & Abrass, 1999.

although high for elders, has been falling steadily since the early 1980s. There is a shrinking percentage of elders older than 65 who have hypertension, arteriosclerosis, and dementia. All of this is most likely the result of improved treatment of disease and the acceleration of studies in the science of aging. A growing body of knowledge confirms that chronic illness and disability are not an inevitable consequence of aging as we have been led to believe. Those individuals who suffer the most and the longest from disabilities are often the victims of unhealthy lifestyle choices, such as smoking, obesity, sedentary lifestyle, or poor adaptation to stress. There is convincing evidence that the way we age is more dependent on how we live than who our parents are.

Assessment of Elders

Nurses in community health emphasize wellness with the goal of maintaining optimal function, physically, mentally, socially, and spiritually so as to be as independent as possible for as long as possible. The four primary domains of geriatric assessment to accomplish this goal are functional ability, physical health, mental health, and socioenvironmental factors.

Functional assessment

As a measure of physical and mental abilities to manage ADLs, functional assessment is an important parameter for determining an elder's ability for self-care at home. (See appendix C.) In addition to self-reports by the elder and family members, the ability to perform the ADLs also needs to be observed by the nurse by having the elder perform as many of these activities as possible (e.g., putting on a button shirt, getting on the toilet, picking up a penny). (See appendix D.)

Physical assessment

In the physical assessment of elders, emphasis is placed on areas that most impact functional ability (e.g., vision, hearing, strength). The health history for older adults must include frequent inquiries about exercise, nutrition, medications, substance use (tobacco, alcohol, caffeine), incontinence, memory and depression, social activities, and isolation. In addition to the usual height, weight, and vital signs, blood pressure needs to be checked sitting, lying, and standing for **orthostatic hypotension**, a common problem in elders. Along with the usual adult physical examination, vision and hearing, mouth, skin, breasts (women), prostate (men), and feet need to be checked regularly in elders. Diagnostic screening tests performed by primary care providers for asymptomatic, low-risk older adults usually include cholesterol every 5 years, clinical breast examination and mammography every 1 to 2 years, sigmoidoscopy every 3 to 5 years, and digital rectal examination and fecal occult blood testing (FOBT) annually. Complete blood count, urinalysis, thyroid

FYI

Clinical Pearls for the Community Health Nurse

- *Ten pennies make one dime.* Loss of independence in elders may be the result of many subtle changes accumulated over time rather than sudden, dramatic events. Look for multiple simple interventions (the pennies) to support existing strengths and maximize function (the dime). For example, correcting poor vision, losing a few pounds of excess weight, and strengthening deconditioned extremities through a walking program may enable elders threatened with impending relocation to become more mobile and remain in their own homes living independently.

- *Never ask an elder's age.* Rather than ask elders their ages, ask when they were born to identify their cohort and the rich information this fact provides about the physical, psychological, and social factors that have influenced their lives. For example, to know a man is 91 identifies him as old-old; to know he was born in 1909 places him at the depth of the Great Depression during his early adulthood while trying to establish work and family roles.

- *Listen to be heard.* Community health nurses usually are younger than their elderly clients. There is a tendency for nurses to "preach" about health care and for elders to "turn off" these young "know-it-alls." After all, they are the survivors of many hardships in their life experience. If you are talking more than 50% of the time, you are not listening. To avoid this common pitfall, each nurse needs to center the self to focus on the elder; ask clarifying questions, then listen to the elder's answers; reinforce positive aspects of the situa-

tion and support the elder's control, then listen to the elder's concerns; verify understandings, then listen to the elder's responses; reinforce outcomes and enable maximum autonomy, and, yes, *LISTEN* to the elder! Then you just may hear each other.

- *To hydrate elders, encourage them to drink fluids in small, frequent amounts:* a 4- to 6-oz. glass of juice offered every 1 to 2 hours, or a 1-pint, covered plastic mug sipped frequently between breakfast and lunch, refilled, and consumed again between lunch and supper. Avoid fluids after the evening meal to reduce nocturia.

- *Be realistic about weight management goals for elders.* Rather than using ideal body weight (IBW), ask about the usual body weight (UBW) at about age 30 to 50 to establish more individualized goals for gaining or losing weight.

- *For health teaching with elders, remember the four S's:* Start small and stay simple. Take more time, break content into smaller units, present one idea at a time, be concrete (not abstract), increase repetitions (three to seven times), and use more than one modality (visual, verbal, and written).

- *Be aware of bowel function.* Any time an elder presents with anorexia, nausea and vomiting, constipation, abdominal pain, loose stool, fecal incontinence, urinary retention or incontinence, delirium, fever, arrhythmia, or tachypnea, inquire about the last bowel movement and check for a fecal impaction.

- *Teach elders to use it or lose it.* "The right amount of exercise in old age is 'more than yesterday.' If you don't do it today, you can't do it tomorrow" (Ham & Sloane, 1997).

---

screen are done periodically depending on the situation. Pap smears usually are not indicated after age 70 or after a hysterectomy. The normal values on diagnostic laboratory tests and other physical findings may differ between younger and older adults. For example, uric acid and alkaline phosphatase increase slightly with age; the erythrocyte sedimentation rate (ESR) and C-reactive protein increase significantly with age.

Mental assessment

The assessment of mental health in elders is focused on memory and mood. The Folstein, Folstein, and McHugh (1975) Mini-Mental State Examination (MMSE) is an 11-item instrument designed to screen five areas of cognitive functioning: orienta-

tion, registration, attention and calculation, recall, and language and praxis. Scores may be adjusted for educational and visual deficits, but generally a score of 24 to 30 indicates no cognitive impairment, 18 to 23 is *mild impairment*, and 0 to 17 is severe impairment (see appendix E).

The 30-item Yesavage and Brink (1983) Geriatric Depression Scale is used to screen for depression in elders with intact cognition or only mild cognitive impairment (see appendix F). The 15-item short form is used for initial screening, and if depression is indicated by missing 5 or more items, the remaining 15 items are administered. Depression is suspected if the elder misses 11 or more items on the full instrument (sensitivity, 84%; specificity, 95%). Elders with significant mental/emotional impairments are referred to their primary care provider for further evaluation and treatment.

Socioenvironmental assessment

Socioenvironmental factors are assessed to identify family and living situations, social support systems, financial status, and environmental hazards. A home safety checklist may be administered on the initial visit and periodically thereafter to monitor for the hazards contributing to accidents, falls, and injuries in elders (see appendix G). A community assessment can be completed as described elsewhere in this text.

Interpreting assessment data

In analyzing the findings of geriatric assessments, nurses must remember that the effects of normal aging are being redefined continuously. The presentation of signs and symptoms of illnesses in older adults may be atypical. They may underreport or overreport symptoms of illnesses or have multiple, nonspecific complaints that require explication. Older adults may have a lessened tolerance for stress, yet have difficulty communicating their health needs. The focus of this chapter is on maintaining abilities for a vigorous old age through health promotion and environmental management and preventing disabilities through disease prevention in elders.

Preventive Health Care

In providing preventive health care for elders in the community, nurses can use 16 verbs that represent basic functions. These eight verb sets are easily understood by elders and their families. How well does the elder:

- *see* and *hear*
- *think* and *feel*
- *eat* and *sleep*
- *work* and *play*
- eliminate *bladder* and *bowel*
- *heat/cool* and *touch/feel*
- *walk* and *talk*
- *hurt* and *believe?*

Sensory Integrity

The elderly person depends on accurate perception of environmental information from all of the senses to maintain independence. Interventions to maximize perception are essential for successful living alone or with the family. In addition to regular assessment of vision and hearing, the community health nurse needs to be aware of the potential for sensory overload or sensory isolation in elders.

Vision

Normal aging is associated with increasing impairment of vision, most commonly a progressive farsightedness called **presbyopia**.

In addition, four major ocular diseases are commonly seen in elders ages 75 to 85: cataracts (46%), macular degeneration (28%), glaucoma (7%), and diabetic retinopathy (7%) (Kane, Ouslander, & Abrass, 1999). Approximately 92% of elders older than 65 wear eyeglasses; however, the vision of only 65% of those older than 85 are corrected well enough to be able to recognize a friend across the street or read newsprint. Yellowing of the lens reduces color clarity, so reds, oranges, and yellows are seen more clearly than greens, blues, and purples. Decreased lens elasticity and pupil size (miosis) decrease accommodation and contribute to central ("tunnel") vision, and night blindness. Diminished lacrimation may cause xerophthalmia ("dry eyes"). Loss of skin elasticity may result in entropion (inversion) or ectropion (eversion) of the eyelids, which are associated with conjunctivitis and blindness.

Visual acuity should be assessed annually. Individuals with scores greater than 20/40 are referred to an ophthalmologist. Correction typically involves magnification with bifocal glasses. Other interventions to improve function in visually impaired elders are summarized in Box 22-5.

Auditory

Because of its implications for social interactions and safety, hearing is an essential component of sensory integrity. Hearing

---

BOX 22-5 TECHNIQUES FOR VISUALLY IMPAIRED ELDERS

- Increase background color contrast; use warm tones.
- Increase light intensity, but avoid or reduce glare by using blinds, unwaxed floors, and so on.
- Check corrective glasses daily for cleanliness and fit; use magnifying lenses.
- Simplify and unclutter the environment; check for safety hazards (e.g., throw rugs).
- Caution about altered perception when using uneven surfaces (e.g., stairs, escalators, ramps).
- Avoid night driving; assess driving ability every year.
- Increase print size, use large print books.
- Consult the local library for the Library of Congress directory of publishers of large type books, talking books, and catalogues of visual aids, appliances, and computer training.
- Check radio reading services that offer the weather, news, sports, and readings of interest.
- Have annual visual acuity screening; refer to an ophthalmologist as indicated.

impairment is the most common sensory problem experienced by elders. It occurs in 25% to 30% of people older than 60, especially males. It is the most poorly recognized and undercorrected sensory deficit. Only 25% of those who might benefit from a hearing aid actually use one (Reuben, Yoshikawa, & Besdine, 1996). The most common impairment of aging is **presbycusis,** a gradual, progressive bilateral sensorineural hearing loss of predominately higher frequencies and impairment of speech discrimination (especially the consonants *f, s, th, h,* and *sh*). Hearing sensitivity may be assessed with the simple whisper test: Whisper random numbers about 12 inches from each ear while covering the opposite ear. Those with hearing deficits require referral to a audiologist for amplification with a hearing aid or assistive listening device such as the "pocketalker." Techniques to improve communication with hearing impaired elders are summarized in Box 22-6.

Because of the increased viscosity of cerumen and coarseness of hairs lining the auditory canal, another common problem that can affect hearing in elders is cerumen impaction. A simple intervention is to soften the ear wax daily for 3 to 4 days with a ceruminolytic agent (e.g., Cerumenex, Debrox), then irrigate with warm water until the wax is removed (see package instructions). The client should be referred to a primary care provider if the impaction is not resolved.

Nutrition and Sleep

In every culture, meals have great social significance as well as nutritional value. Changes in appetite and weight may be the first indicators of altered health status. A balance of activity and rest are important for feelings of well-being. Therefore, nutrition and sleep are functions to be assessed thoroughly and often in elderly individuals.

Nutrition

Of community dwelling elders, 15% to 50% are believed to have poor nutrition or be malnourished. Because of this major health problem, the Nutrition Screening Initiative (1992), a coalition of the American Academy of Family Physicians, the American Dietetic Association, and the National Council on Aging, was developed to identify nutritional problems, improve nutrition, and improve delivery of nutrition programs. Common factors associated with malnutrition in community-dwelling elders include physical illness, medications, lack of hydration, social isolation, oral health problems, limited mobility, lack of transportation, limited vision, poverty, dementia, depression, and alcoholism.

The nutritional needs of elders change significantly with advanced age. For example, calorie requirements progressively decrease, about one-third from a lowered metabolic rate and two-thirds from reduced physical activity. There is a decrease in the acuity and differentiation of taste (dysgeusia) and smell (anosmia), which contributes to anorexia and malnutrition. With loss of salty and sweet tastes, foods taste more bitter and sour. Less volume and acidity of salivation contributes to xerostomia ("dry mouth"), dysphagia ("difficult swallowing"), and difficulty digesting starches. Loss of gingiva and wearing down of teeth contributes to gingivitis, loss of teeth, ill-fitting dentures, and potential mouth ulcers. Thinning of the esophageal wall and relaxed cardiac sphincter contribute to early satiety (feeling of fullness) and dyspepsia (acid indigestion/heartburn), as does less mucin, decreased gastric juices (HCl, enzymes), and slower peristalsis in the stomach. Thinning of the intestinal wall and slower peristalsis in the colon contributes to increased flatulence, polyps, and diverticula. As with other age groups, the nutritional requirements for elders differ in some categories (Table 22-3). The health problems and associated nutritional deficits of elders are summarized in Table 22-4.

Changes in weight may be early indicators of multiple health problems in older adults (e.g., depression, congestive heart failure, diabetes). Height and weight should be measured

---

BOX 22-6 TECHNIQUES FOR HEARING IMPAIRED ELDERS

- Minimize background noise (e.g., turn off or down the television or radio).
- Stand within 2 to 3 feet of the person.
- Speak face-to-face, on the same level, and toward the best ear.
- Speak at a normal level or slightly louder volume—do *not* shout (it distorts sound).
- Speak a little more slowly in a clear, slightly lower pitched voice.
- Get the person's attention; call his or her name first.
- Use short, simple sentences; pause at the end of each sentence (e.g., "Ms. Smith, here is a glass of water").
- Repeat by paraphrasing the message in a different way.
- Provide extra time for responses and give visual clues or transitional sentences to preface a message (e.g., pointing to the door, "It's time for lunch"); avoid appearing frustrated.
- Write down key words if the person can read.
- Have the person repeat to be certain the message was understood.
- Be sure hearing aids are worn, functioning (check batteries), and fit properly.
- Inspect ears at least every 3 months for impacted cerumen.

TABLE 22-3   NUTRITIONAL REQUIREMENTS OF ELDERS

MACRONUTRIENTS

Protein	1.0-1.25 g/kg/day
Calories	1,800-2,100 kcal/day
Water	2 L/day; 30 ml/kg/day
Sodium	Minimum, 0.5 g/day; maximum, 2.4 g/day
Sodium chloride	Minimum, 1.3 g/day; maximum, 6.0 g/day
Dietary fiber	Typical 8-17 g/day; ideal 20-35 g/day

MICRONUTRIENTS

Vitamins	
Water-soluble (B and C)	Become deficient over weeks to months
Fat-soluble (A, D, E, and K)	Become deficient over many months to years
Minerals	
Calcium	1,200-1,500 mg/day
Zinc	12-15 mg/day

Source: Adapted from Reuben, Yoshikawa, & Besdine, 1996, pp. 145-148.

BOX 22-7   FORMULAS FOR CALCULATING THE NUTRITIONAL STATUS OF ELDERS

World Health Organization calorie estimates for adults over age 60 years:

Women $(10.5) \times$ (weight in kilograms) $+ 596$

Men $(13.5) \times$ (weight in kilograms) $+ 487$

Harris-Benedict equations for estimating resting calorie requirements:

Women $= 655 + (9.6)$(Weight in kg) $+ (1.7)$(Height in cm) $- (4.7)$(Age in yr)

Men $= 66 + (13.7)$(Weight in kg) $+ (5.0)$(Height in cm) $- (6.8)$(Age in yr)

where kg = Weight in pounds $\times$ 0.45
cm = Height in inches $\times$ 0.39

$$\text{Body mass index} = \frac{\text{Weight in kilograms}}{(\text{Height in meters}) 2} \quad \text{OR}$$

$$\frac{\text{Weight in pounds}}{(\text{Height in inches}) 2} \times 703.1$$

M = Height in inches $\times$ 0.025

Percentage of weight change =

$$\frac{\text{Usual/previous weight} - \text{Actual/current weight}}{\text{Usual/previous weight}} \times 100$$

Importance of weight change:

Time Interval	Significant	Severe
1 week	1%-2%	>2%
1 month	5%	>5%
3 months	7.5%	>7.5%
6 months	10%	>10%

and the body mass index (BMI; 24 to 25 is ideal in elders) should be calculated with the initial assessment of the elder's nutritional status, then, on every visit, the client's weight should be rechecked and the percentage of change calculated. The client should be referred to the primary care provider if the percentage of change is significant or severe. The formulas for calculating the caloric needs and BMI and the standards for estimating the significance of weight change over time are in Box 22-7.

The community health nurse can begin the nutritional assessment with a 3-day diet recall and calorie count. Consider *financial* (fixed income, buying habits), *physical* (transportation, limited mobility, poor vision), and *personal barriers* (food prepa-

TABLE 22-4   HEALTH PROBLEMS AND NUTRITIONAL DEFICITS OF ELDERS

HEALTH PROBLEM	NUTRITIONAL DEFICIENCY
Resistance to infection	Protein, calories
Poor wound healing and skin friability	Vitamins A, B_6, D, E; selenium; zinc; copper, iron
Osteopenia	Protein, zinc, vitamins C and E
Anemia	Calcium, vitamins D and K, estrogen
Cardiovascular diseases	Iron, folate, vitamin B_{12}
Cataracts, age-associated macular degeneration	Folate, Vitamins E, B_{12}; excess fat
Constipation	Zinc; selenium; vitamins A, C, E
	Water, dietary fiber

Source: Adapted from Reuben, Yoshikawa, & Besdine, 1996. p. 145.

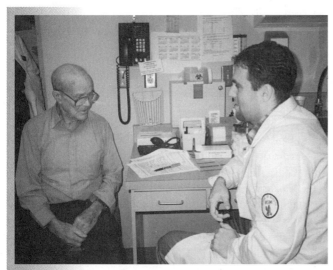

Elders are living longer than in generations past and are healthier than their predecessors.

ration, preferences, eating problems, medications). Oral assessment includes checking for ill-fitting dentures, lost teeth, periodontal disease, and the last dental visit.

The goals for nutrition are to assist elders to plan and provide a well-balanced diet with a variety of foods from each food group and maintain a desirable weight. They need to be encouraged to eat low-fat, high-fiber foods and avoid fried, fatty, concentrated sweet, and salty foods.

Nutritional services may start with shopping assistance, which can be provided by family, friends, religious groups, senior centers, and local homemaker services. Grocery stores may offer senior parking and electric shopping carts. Community services include aggregate meal sites in senior centers, Meals on Wheels, area agencies on aging, and county extension services.

For elders with limited income, stretching money to purchase both food and medications can be a challenge. They may buy easy-to-prepare "empty calorie" foods (concentrated sweets or salty snacks) rather than foods for a balanced diet. The nurse can suggest a variety of foods that will not break the budget, including dried legumes, beans, whole cereal grains, poultry, fish, dried fortified milk, less expensive cuts of meat, low-fat cheeses, yogurt, and dried instant breakfast.

The goal of weight management is to help elders approach an ideal body weight (IBW) for their age, sex, and body frame. These individuals may be involuntarily gaining or losing weight and need to stabilize their weight, or they may have a long history of being seriously overweight or underweight and now are experiencing health problems. Techniques for maintaining or improving the nutritional status of elders are suggested in Box 22-8.

Underweight

For elders who are malnourished or underweight (BMI less than 20 or more than 10% *below* IBW), the goal is to increase the calorie

intake, including daily multivitamin with mineral supplementation. Loss of smell affects taste and enjoyment; loss of appetite may be from loneliness and depression. The nurse calculates the caloric needs based on the desired weight for these elders. For example, if an 83-year-old frail man's current weight is 130 pounds; his height is 5 feet, 11 inches; and his usual body weight is 160 pounds, his caloric needs are between 1,460 (World Health Organization [WHO] formula) and 2,160 calories (estimated formula) per day.

Overweight

For elders who are obese or overweight (BMI greater than 29 or more than 20% *above* IBW), the weight management goals are to decrease calories and increase activity levels. Diets to promote weight loss generally limit intake to 1,500 to 1,800 calories per day (including daily multivitamin with mineral supplementation) with adjustments for age, sex, and body frame. The lifestyle adjustments required for weight loss are difficult to accomplish and maintain at any age, and no less so in elders. In addition to reducing amounts or eliminating certain types of foods, elders must incorporate exercise into daily routines to compensate for their reduced metabolism and achieve their weight loss goals. They are especially prone to fads and gimmicks rather than adjustment of eating and exercise patterns. Appetite suppressants should be avoided because they generally are ineffective and may have serious side effects in elders. To assist with weight loss, many nutritionally sound, holistic commercial weight loss programs (e.g., Weight Watchers) are available. Public television may offer low-impact exercise programs, such as chair aerobics. Community and religious groups also may offer weight loss and exercise programs, or the nurse can facilitate the formation of a neighborhood weight loss group. Whatever the approach, overweight elders often need weight loss programs that are relatively inexpensive, easily accessible, age appropriate, and socially supportive. Obese persons on weight loss diets also need to be weighed weekly.

Hydration

Often overlooked as part of nutrition, adequate hydration is a key factor to prevent dehydration, soften stools, increase salivation and expectoration, maintain skin and renal function, and aid in absorption of medications and high-fiber foods. Elders usually require at least 12 quarts or 1,500 ml of fluids per day, especially water. For diabetic or overweight elders or those who dislike the taste of water, sugar-free liquids (e.g., Crystal Light, Sugar Free Kool-Aid) can be encouraged.

As with infants, elders are particularly vulnerable to variations in fluid volume (overhydration or underhydration) because of their decreased cardiovascular and renal reserves. Signs of dehydration include weight loss; concentrated urine, decreased output; elevated temperature; sunken eyeballs; dry, parched, coated tongue; pallor, poor skin turgor, and dry mucous membranes. A weight loss of 2% to 4% is mild, 5% to 9% is moderate, and 10% or more is severe dehydration with danger of circulatory collapse and death. These individuals require immediate referral to their primary care provider for careful rehydration.

Sleep

Adequate periods of sleep and rest are essential for the restoration of energy in all living beings. Elderly persons commonly experience changes in both sleep pattern and sleep structure. These changes can result in initial insomnia (disturbances, difficulty falling asleep), interim insomnia (frequent awakenings), and terminal insomnia (earlier morning awakenings), or hypersomnolence (excessive sleep).

Community health nurses can prevent or intervene in many of these problems by thorough assessments of patterns of activity and rest. Consider the nature of the sleep problem by determining its onset and duration (i.e., acute, transient, or chronic [>3 weeks]). A sleep history can be obtained by having the el-

der keep a "sleep log" for several days and nights; then the log can be analyzed for patterns of wakefulness and sleep: total sleep time, total time in bed, sleep problems, day problems that interfere with sleep. The nurse should inquire about recent changes in behavior or performance and evaluate the use of caffeine (e.g., coffee, tea, cola), xanthine (e.g., chocolate), nicotine, alcohol, and medications that interfere with sleep (prescription and over-the-counter [OTC] drugs). The nurse should consider health problems that may interfere with sleep, especially pain (e.g., arthritis, heart failure, chronic obstructive pulmonary disease [COPD], gastroesophageal reflux disease [GERD], diabetes, anxiety, depression, dementia, nocturnal myoclonus, sleep apnea). Finally, the nurse should teach the client good sleep hygiene (Box 22-9).

....

I still climb Mount Everest just as often as I used to. I play polo just as often as I used to. But to walk down to the hardware store I find a little bit more difficult.

From an interview with Theodor S. Geisel, "Dr. Seuss," in the *New York Times Book Review.* Cited in *Seuss-isms: Wise and Witty Prescriptions for Living from the Good Doctor,* New York: Random House, 1997

....

Elimination

Problems with elimination can have devastating consequences for elders. Fear of "accidents" may contribute to social withdrawal and isolation. An inability to control the bladder or the bowels is a major precipitant to institutionalization. Therefore, nurses must take every opportunity to maintain elimination patterns in older adults.

Urinary Elimination

Although aging alone does not cause urinary incontinence, several age-related changes and health problems can contribute to its development (e.g., childbirth, menopause, prostate surgery, stroke). Urinary incontinence is the involuntary loss of urine severe enough to have social or hygienic consequences. The prevalence is 15% to 30% in elderly community-dwelling men and women, respectively (Reuben, Yoshikawa, & Besdine, 1996). Stress, urge, and overflow incontinence are caused by failure to store urine or empty the bladder. Functional incontinence is caused by an inability to toilet efficiently. A neurogenic bladder usually is associated with urinary retention; it often requires an indwelling catheter or intermittent catheterizations and is managed on an individual basis. As much as 80% of incontinence can be eliminated with bladder rehabilitation programs.

To assess the nature of urinary incontinence, the nurse must determine previous patterns of urination and daily activities. The nurse should ask the elder to record fluid intake and voiding patterns for at least 3 days to establish the current schedule of urination. In collaboration with the primary care provider, the nurse should determine cause, duration, and degree of incontinence. Common factors associated with this problem include medications, caffeine, and fecal impactions. For frail or confused elders, it is especially helpful to observe the level of function for toileting activities (e.g., walking, dressing, transfers, hygiene). When establishing realistic goals for urinary continence, the nurse should consider the anticipated cooperation of the elder

---

BOX 22-9 TECHNIQUES FOR SLEEP HYGIENE

- Standardize bedtime and rising time. Go to bed at the same time each night and get out of bed at the same time each morning regardless of sleep during the night. Avoid drastic shifts in sleep-wake cycle.

- Minimize daytime napping to 30 to 60 minutes in early afternoon.

- Encourage daily exercise and both daytime and evening activities with adequate exposure to bright light during the day.

- Avoid large meals and fluids within 4 hours of bedtime. Eliminate or limit caffeine, xanthines, nicotine, and alcohol, especially within 4 hours of bedtime. Avoid diuretics within 8 hours of bedtime.

- Engage in bedtime rituals (e.g., personal hygiene, toileting, relaxation activities, prayer, meditation).

- If in pain, provide comfort measures (e.g., acetaminophen 500 mg, one to two tablets HS if indicated).

- If hungry, have a light bedtime snack with milk (contains tryptophan).

- Wear comfortable sleep clothes and keep bedroom cool, clean, and quiet, with only a night light if desired. Use the bedroom only for sleep and sex (not for reading, watching television, eating, or working).

- If unable to sleep within 30 minutes, go to another room and engage in restful activities (reading, soft music, hobbies); avoid active television. Return to bed only when sleepy.

- Avoid over-the-counter drugs for sleep (especially diphenhydramine [Benadryl], which interrupts the sleep cycle, can be cumulative, and may cause delirium in elders). Avoid regular use of hypnotics (they cause interruption of sleep cycle, tolerance, and habituation); limit to three times per week.

- Consult with primary care provider concerning health problems and medications that interfere with sleep.

---

and family for bladder rehabilitation activities (e.g., total continence, daytime continence with nighttime padding).

Treatments for urinary incontinence include pelvic muscle rehabilitation (Kegel exercises, biofeedback, vaginal weight training, pelvic floor electrical stimulation), behavioral therapies (bladder training, toileting assistance), medications (oxybutynin, estrogen), and surgeries (AHCPR, 1996). Techniques for urinary incontinence in elders are summarized in Box 22-10. By working on bladder rehabilitation with these elders, their caregivers, and primary care providers, community health nurses often can prevent or minimize this condition with significant impact on overall functioning and quality of life.

Fecal Elimination

Bowel elimination has significant implications for elders' comfort and quality of life. Bowel regularity and fecal continence take on enormous significance for some elders. Common problems include diarrhea, fecal incontinence, and constipation.

Diarrhea

For diarrhea in elders, the criterion is the volume of stool per day, rather than the number or consistency of stools, which may be altered with changes in food or fluid intake but still may be within normal limits. Diarrhea can be infectious or noninfectious and is a significant cause of morbidity and mortality among those elders who are frail and more susceptible to fluid and electrolyte imbalances. This condition is prevented by scrupulous food preparation and storage, frequent handwashing, and avoidance of fecal contamination and polypharmacy. Initial assessments include onset, volume, number, consistency of stools; duration (acute versus chronic); the presence of bright red blood in the stool (hematochezia) or black, tarry stool (melena); the presence of other symptoms (e.g., abdominal cramping or distension, lassitude, thirst, nausea, vomiting, fever, malaise); diet; and medications. The nurse should evaluate the elder's general appearance, vital signs, and weight and perform an abdominal examination for pain or tenderness.

Although common diarrhea often is treated in the home (Box 22-11), any condition lasting more than 24 hours in elders should be referred to their primary care provider for evaluation and possible rehydration. The protocol for chronic diarrhea, often a part of an irritable bowel syndrome, is developed in collaboration with the primary care provider and usually includes a high-fiber diet, possibly with a bulking agent (e.g., methylcellulose or psyllium hydrophilic mucilloid [Citrucel or Metamucil]) or loperamide (Imodium A-D).

Constipation

For elders, the most common bowel problem is constipation, a difficulty in passing stools or incomplete or infrequent passage of hard stools (usually less than three per week). The usual causes of small, hard, or infrequent stools are poor bowel habits, including a lack of dietary fiber, poor fluid intake, inadequate exercise, psychological factors, and medications, often with inappropriate use

BOX 22-10 TECHNIQUES FOR BLADDER REHABILITATION IN ELDERS WITH URINARY INCONTINENCE

- Explain the nature of urinary incontinence and establish mutual goals to encourage participation and cooperation in bladder rehabilitation activities.

- Provide adequate fluid intake, at least 1,500 ml/day, to dilute urine and minimize bladder and skin irritation and odor.

- Check for medications that precipitate incontinence (e.g., diuretics) and give them early in the day. Check caffeine use (e.g., coffee, tea, colas) and reduce or eliminate (switch to decaffeinated beverages).

- When usual voiding times have been established, prompt the elder to toilet 2 hours before these times, usually hourly at first, then every 2 hours, and finally every 3 hours if tolerated. Encourage the elder to void before meals, after naps, before bed, and before any special activities, such as walks or outings. Advance times only when the elder is successful during shorter periods of continence for several days.

- Encourage the elder to empty the bladder completely at each voiding by leaning forward and gently pushing down with abdominal muscles (Crede maneuver).

- Observe the amounts of urine voided (i.e., bladder capacity). If the quantity is very large, schedule more frequent visits to the toilet; or if it is very small, schedule less frequent voiding.

- For women with stress incontinence, teach Kegel exercises to help recondition pelvic muscle and improve sphincter control. With the woman on the toilet, instruct her to stop the flow of urine for a few seconds; repeat several times. When she has learned to interrupt her flow of urine, have her execute the same contractions while sitting in a chair, starting with 5 repetitions and advancing to 10 repetitions held for 5 seconds, with each set done four or more times a day. An alternate activity is to contract and relax successively the urethral, vaginal, and rectal sphincter muscles in the same manner described above.

- For urge incontinence, once on the commode, teach elders to hold back the urine as long as possible by tightening the pelvic musculature.

- If elders are confused, demented, or demonstrate anxious behavior, check them frequently for the need to void. During activities, place elders nearest the bathroom and remove barriers in their path.

- Encourage the elder and family to use incontinence pads (not diapers!), such as Attends or Depends, to promote dryness until continence is reestablished. These products are not much more bulky than regular underwear and can be worn with confidence under everyday clothing. If skin breakdown is a problem, coat the perineum with a thin layer of petroleum or zinc oxide ointment (e.g., Vaseline, A&D Ointment, or Desitin).

- Monitor rehabilitation activities daily and evaluate them at least weekly until a voiding pattern is established. Check for dryness and odor, use of toilet for voiding, skin integrity, and self-concept. Encourage the elder frequently, praise successes, reinforce teaching frequently, and do not permit discouragement when accidents occur. Reconditioning of the bladder may require several weeks, but with patience and persistence it usually is successful.

BOX 22-11 TECHNIQUES FOR COMMON DIARRHEA IN ELDERS

- Place the bowel at rest for 36 to 72 hours. Give clear liquids for the first 12 to 24 hours, full liquids or soft diet for next 24 to 48 hours, then regular diet as tolerated. Maintain adequate hydration (1,500 to 2,000 ml/day).

- Give an over-the-counter antidiarrheal agent:
  - Absorbent agents (Kaopectate) 15 to 30 ml every 4 to 6 hours prn loose stool × 24 hr OR
  - Bismuth subsalicylate (Pepto-Bismol) 15 to 30 ml every 4 to 6 hours prn loose stool × 24 hr OR
  - Opioid (Imodium AD) two 2-mg tables initially, then one tablet prn loose stool × 24 hr (maximum, 16 mg/day).

- Teach elder to avoid irritating foods.

- If not improved in 24 hours, refer to primary care provider for prompt evaluation.

of laxatives. Common complications are fecal impaction and fecal incontinence.

To assess the nature of constipation, the nurse must determine previous patterns of previous bowel habits and daily activity patterns. The nurse should ask the elder to record food and fluid intake (noting dietary fiber and free water) and bowel movements (frequency, timing, difficulty) for at least 3 days. The elder's general physical and mental condition should be evaluated, and if the client is frail or confused, the nurse should observe the level of function for toileting activities (e.g., walking, dressing, transfers, hygiene). The nurse must consider possible associated factors (e.g., medications, fecal impactions, illnesses) and make referral to primary care provider if indicated. When setting goals for bowel elimination, the nurse should consider anticipated cooperation of the elder and family for bowel rehabilitation activities. By working with these elders, their caregivers, and primary care providers, community health nurses often can prevent and intervene with a bowel rehabilitation including a high-fiber diet, adequate fluids, daily exercise, and elimination of laxatives (Box 22-12).

BOX 22-12 TECHNIQUES FOR BOWEL REHABILITATION IN ELDERS WITH CONSTIPATION

- Explain the nature of constipation and establish mutual goals to encourage participation and cooperation in bowel rehabilitation activities.

- Encourage a high-fiber diet that adds bulk to stool. This diet usually starts with high-fiber cereals (i.e., more than 10 gm of dietary fiber per serving, such as All Bran, Bran Buds, 100% Bran, or Fiber One), and/or supplemental wheat bran (miller's bran) 1 to 4 tablespoons per day added to moist foods (e.g., cereals, grits, oatmeal, cream of wheat, applesauce, soup, cottage cheese, ice cream). Vegetables and fruits also add bulk to stools (e.g., at least 5 servings per day of green leafy vegetables, raw fruits, vegetables).

- Provide adequate fluids to make the stool softer and easier to pass. Include at least $1/2$ to 2 quarts (1,500 to 2,000 ml) of fluids per day, unless contraindicated (see Hydration, p. 518).

- Encourage exercise daily to promote circulation to the bowel and stimulate evacuation. For example, walk at least 1 mile per day, ride a stationary bicycle or swim for at least 30 minutes per day, unless contraindicated (see Critical Thinking Activities).

- Establish a regular evacuation time to correspond with daily activities or family lifestyle patterns. Defecation is a learned, conditioned response that generally occurs at the same time each day. Most elders prefer an early morning time for bowel evacuation, but if scheduling of family activities in the morning precludes sufficient time for bowel hygiene, an evening bowel program is recommended (i.e., after supper and before bathing).

- Start the bowel program with a clean bowel (i.e., give a laxative or enema if necessary). For 3 consecutive days, insert a bisacodyl (Dulcolax) suppository into the rectum approximately 30 minutes before the established evacuation time. Wait 30 minutes, then assist the elder to the toilet with a book or magazine to promote relaxation. Another approach is to use 1 to 3 tablespoons of an osmotic agent (lactulose or sorbitol) daily for 3 to 5 days to get a bowel pattern established. Stool softeners (e.g., docusate [Colace, Dialose]) generally are ineffective for constipation in elders.

- Absolutely avoid laxatives, especially the long-term use of stimulant laxatives with phenolphthalein (i.e., Correctol, Ex-Lax, Feen-a-Ment) because of their blunting of natural evacuation and purging of the bowel. A daily bowel movement is not necessary, but avoid going for more than 3 days without defecation. If no BM occurs in 2 days, use a bisacodyl (Dulcolax) suppository. If no BM occurs in 3 days, use a phosphate (Fleets) enema. If the enema is not successful, use 1 ounce (30 ml) of Milk of Magnesia to get the bowels restarted. Daily osmotic agents may be needed; consult primary caregiver

- Observe the consistency of stools (i.e., normal, soft, hard, or watery). If stools are hard or painful, increase the water intake. If stools are small or scant, increase the bulk with dietary fiber. Recommend a stool softener, such as docusate (e.g., Colase, Dialose) only if needed because of hemorrhoids or other rectal problems.

- Monitor rehabilitation activities daily and evaluate them at least weekly until a bowel pattern is established. Check for constipation, use of the toilet for defecation, fecal impaction, skin integrity, and self-concept. If relapses occur, restart the program with suppositories for 3 days. Encourage the elder frequently, praise successes, reinforce teaching frequently, and do not permit discouragement when accidents occur. Reconditioning of the bowel may require several weeks to overcome years of poor bowel habits, but with patience and persistence it usually is successful.

Mobility and Communication

The ability to move about the environment is crucial for independent living. The ability to communicate one's thoughts and feelings to others is essential for well-being. Therefore, nurses must take an active role in maintenance of mobility and communication in elderly individuals striving to remain in the community.

Mobility

Adequate mobility is critical for elders to maintain their functional independence. Even brief periods of immobility can lead to rapid deconditioning and loss of flexibility and strength in elders increasing the risk of falls and injury. Conversely, daily exercise helps the elder to prevent diseases (e.g., osteoporosis, arterial/venous insufficiency, gastrointestinal stasis, musculoskeletal stiffness, coronary heart disease, obesity, stroke, depression, anxiety, dementia); improve sleep, mobility, strength, flexibility, and mood; increase life expectancy; and improve quality of life. Community health nurses can encourage elders to exercise individually, with families, or in groups.

BOX 22-13 TECHNIQUES FOR EXERCISE AND MOBILITY IN ELDERS

- Explain to the elder and family the benefits of an exercise program, and set mutual, realistic goals to encourage participation and cooperation in physical rehabilitation activities. It is important to emphasize functional independence rather than an arbitrary physical goal (e.g., the ability to walk to the bathroom unassisted rather than to walk 100 feet).

- Maximize visual and hearing functions by referral to an ophthalmologist and/or otologist and wearing corrective glasses and/or hearing aids (see Sensory Integrity, p. 514).

- In collaboration with the primary care provider, evaluate medication regime for drugs that alter cardiovascular function, impair central nervous system function, interact, and polypharmacy, and simplify the drug regime by eliminating all nonessential drugs.

- Check footwear for proper fit and condition. Athletic shoes with shock absorbent soles and good support are ideal for an exercise program; shoes with Velcro closures are more easily managed by elders with hand problems. Check clothing for comfort and fit. Athletic apparel (e.g., cotton fleece or windbreakers) is designed for maximum movement, comfort, and convenience, if acceptable to the elder.

- In collaboration with the primary care provider, refer to a physical therapist or rehabilitation facility for correction of major physical decrements (i.e., stroke, arthritis).

- Provide for gait retraining through a program of physical exercise, basically walking outside or at a covered mall for at least 30 to 60 minutes per day for at least 5 to 6 days per week. *Start low, go slow* with regular, low impact, unstressed, but progressive exercise. Begin with a distance the elder can manage (e.g., 100 feet or $1/4$ mile); increase the distance at weekly intervals until the elder is walking 1 to 2 miles, then gradually increase the speed until a comfortable cadence is achieved (i.e., mild perspiration, increased respiratory and pulse rate). Alternatively, use stationary exercise machines, bicycling, swimming, or low impact aerobic, strengthening, flexibility programs (Tai Chi, YMCA/YWCA, fitness centers, community parks, senior programs, senior Olympics). Exercise is better maintained if done with a partner (spouse, friend) at the same time every day.

- Use assistive devices (e.g., straight cane, four-pronged cane, or walker) for balance and support, and/or support stockings for venous return. Check these devices for proper fit and safety, including nonskid tips on canes and walkers.

- Use mild analgesics for relief of soreness, aches, and pains. Acetaminophen, one or two 500-mg tablets for up to four times a day, is recommend over aspirin or ibuprofen, which have increased side effects in elders. Taking analgesics 30 minutes before exercise may minimize discomforts from deconditioning.

- Encourage the use of adaptive behaviors (e.g., rising slowly, using rails or furniture for balance) to minimize the risk of falls and, when appropriate, teach techniques for falling and getting up after a fall to minimize complications.

- Avoid physical restraints that actually increase, rather than decrease, falls and injuries, and compound immobility.

- Monitor the exercise program daily and evaluate at least weekly for improvement in muscle strength, flexibility, and gait stability. Check for orthostatic hypotension, falls, pain, motivation, and self-concept. Encourage elders frequently, praise successes, reinforce teaching frequently, and do not permit discouragement when problems occur. Reconditioning of muscles may require several weeks or months, but with patience and persistence some progress will be made.

Impaired mobility in elders usually involves multiple factors, including an initial physical deficit (i.e., fractured hip or degenerative joint disease), compounded by a sedentary lifestyle, deconditioning, inadequate daily exercise patterns, sensory impairment (i.e., vision and hearing), confusion, inappropriate medications, improper assistive devices, and/or environmental hazards. To assess the mobility of elders, the nurse must determine previous types and levels of exercise and daily activity patterns, any history of activity-related injuries and falls, and possible associated factors influencing mobility (e.g., medications, confusion, illnesses). The nurse should then evaluate the elder's general physical and mental condition, food and fluid intake, environmental safety, and availability of assistive devices, and observe the level of function for physical activities (e.g., posture, gait, balance, strength, endurance). When establishing a program for exercise or physical rehabilitation, the nurse should consider the anticipated cooperation of the elder and family for physical activities and address the physical deficits as well as contributing factors (Box 22-13).

Falls

Accidents are the fifth leading cause of death among elders, and falls account for two-thirds of these deaths. Seventy percent of fall injuries are in persons older than 75; 50% of those hospitalized do not survive for 1 year. Fear of falling further inhibits many elders from performing activities that would prevent falls (e.g., exercise) and contributes to functional decline, depression, helplessness, and social isolation. Falls result from environmental hazards, deconditioning, sensory deficits, and impaired central processing. The best prevention for falls is a combination of rehabilitative, environmental, and behavioral strategies. For example, correcting vision, using assistive devices, installing bathroom grab bars, and initiating a progressive exercise program that emphasizes conditioning of the lower extremities all help reduce the occurrence of falls.

Osteoporosis

A multifactorial disease of increased skeletal fragility, **osteoporosis** places elders at risk of fractures during activities of daily living. Postmenopausal women are affected initially, but men also are subject to senile bone loss. With a bone mineral density more than 2.5 standard deviations below young normals, the vertebral bodies, proximal femur, and distal radius are common fracture sites. In collaboration with primary care providers, community health nurses can assist with preventive strategies for osteoporosis (Box 22-14).

Communication

Other than slower speech, verbal communication usually is unaffected by aging. The most common causes of language disorders in elders are strokes and dementia resulting in some form of aphasia. Strategies for improving communication are summarized in Box 22-15.

BOX 22-14 PREVENTION OF OSTEOPOROSIS IN ELDERS

- Establish a daily exercise program.
- Encourage dietary intake of calcium (1,200 to 1,500 mg/day) with dairy products (milk, cheese, yogurt) and/or calcium supplementation 500 mg tid with meals (e.g., Tums 500, Oscal).
- Encourage dietary intake of vitamin D (400 to 800 IU/day) and/or supplementation with multivitamin with minerals once or twice daily.
- In collaboration with primary care provider, consider estrogen replacement therapy, selective estrogen receptor modulators, or bone density enhancers.
- On sunny days, try to sit outside for 2 to 3 hours (avoiding 11 AM to 2 PM) to enhance vitamin D intake.

Cognition and Affect

Because people are sentient beings, attention, memory, and emotion are integral with personal identity, environmental adaptation, and quality of life. Changes in cognitive abilities may be stereotyped as "senility" and either minimized or maximized by elders and family members. Altered mood and emotional responses may further confound the situation. Impaired cognition and affect may exhaust family resources and precipitate relocation from the home to a long-term care facility. Therefore, nurses can assist elders to remain independent in their own environments by being sensitive to cognitive and affective changes.

BOX 22-15 TECHNIQUES FOR SPEECH IMPAIRED ELDERS

- Reduce environmental distractions (radios, television) before engaging the elder in conversation.
- Gain the elder's attention and maintain eye contact.
- Speak slowly and use a simple vocabulary with short sentences; ask simple yes/no questions.
- If the elder does not respond, repeat the question with the same wording.
- Encourage the elder to say one word at a time; if unable to say a word, substitute another word.
- Praise successes. If unable to complete a thought, avoid appearing frustrated; take a break, then try again.

Cognition

Cognitive functioning changes very little with normal aging. Intelligence is unchanged, and with the wisdom gathered from life experience, problem solving often is improved. Memory involves pattern recognition and is declarative (factual, "what") and procedural (process, "how"). With diminished attention and immediate recall, elders may have some declarative memory loss (forgetfulness), but procedural memory usually is not affected. Learning, which depends on memory, also is undisturbed but is slower. Performance may be slower but often is more precise.

Confusion is a common problem in some elders and may result from alterations in sensory or central processing. The most common causes of confusion are delirium, dementia, and depression.

Delirium

Acute confusional state (**delirium**) is a physiological state that usually is reversible and is characterized as an altered level of consciousness, disorganized thinking (incoherent speech, repetitive speech and behavior), with a rapid onset and fluctuating course; it is often worse at night and has an underlying medical cause (e.g., pneumonia, urinary tract infection, fecal impaction, septicemia). Prevention involves adequate oxygenation, hydration, nutrition, elimination, sensory stimulation, exercise, and avoidance of certain medications.

Dementia

Age-associated memory impairment is the mild, gradual deterioration in memory performance, speed of cognitive processing, and executive functions that accompanies normal aging and does not interfere with activities or relationships. **Dementia** is "a syndrome of progressive decline that relentlessly erodes intellectual abilities, causing cognitive function deterioration leading to impairment of social and occupational functioning" (AHCPR, 1996, p. 1). Dementia occurs in 5% of persons age 65, a rate that doubles every 5 years after age 65, and affects almost 50% of persons 85 or older. This cognitive impairment is irreversible, has an insidious onset, and is stable over time, with progressive amnesia (loss of memory), aphasia (loss of language), agnosia (loss of object recognition), apraxia (loss of motor function), and loss of executive function (abstract thinking and complex behavior). **Alzheimer's disease** is a cortical degeneration that accounts for 80% of dementia. Most elders with mild or moderate dementia live at home and are cared for by family members. Community health nurses can assist with early case finding and referral to a primary care provider or specialist (geriatrician, neuropsychologist, or psychiatrist). Assessment includes elimination of reversible causes (e.g., drugs, depression, delirium, thyroid dysfunction, vitamin B_{12} deficiency). Cognitive functioning is screened with mental status examinations, which test orientation, memory, attention, language, and praxis.

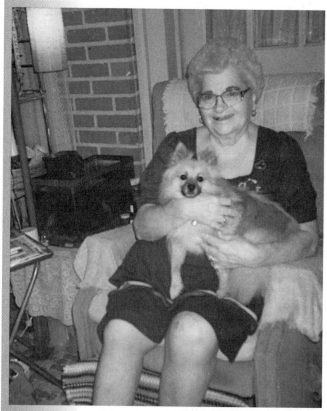

Pets are often very important to elders who live alone.

The basic principles for working with elders who have cognitive deficits are to *simplify the environment*, *provide structure* for daily activities, *minimize changes* in that structure, and when changes are necessary, *prepare for changes* well in advance. The goals of cognitive behavioral programs are to help elders maintain their highest level of function, enable them to continue living at home, and offer support to caregivers. These programs are based on strengths, areas of deficit, and realistic goals for their living situations. Strategies for the management of dementia are summarized in Box 22-16.

Affect

Self-concept evolves from what persons think and feel about themselves, what they think and feel about others, and what they think and feel others think and feel about them (Satir, 1964). Assurance of personal worth is based on feeling valued, useful, and competent. Old age is accompanied by many epoch events—retirement, altered health, relocation of home, deaths of family and friends, and finally one's own transition from life to death. With the frequent, multiple losses associated with old age, elders may experience feelings of powerlessness, hopelessness, and spiritual distress. These feelings may result in anxiety, fear, and anger or depression.

BOX 22-16 STRATEGIES FOR MANAGEMENT OF DEMENTIA IN ELDERS

- Structure time/place. Use daily and weekly schedules that provide consistency, predictability, and repetition. Structure and simplify activities of daily living, family activities, specific tasks, and the environment to maximize ability with less clutter, complexity, and hurry. For example, activities are done in the same order and at the same times and places each day (e.g., arise at 7:00, breakfast at 7:30); certain activities are done on the same days of the week every week (e.g., bathe on Tuesday and Saturday, laundry on Monday).

- Anticipate change. Known events, such as holidays and family gatherings, are anticipated several weeks in advance, mentioning every day the names of people who will be involved and using photos, stories, or other aids to familiarize the elder with the anticipated situation. Persons with cognitive deficits can learn, but the key is repetition—as many as 7×7 times!

- Modify the environment. Reorganize the elder's living situation to compensate for sensory and functional impairments. Use memory aids (e.g., clocks, calendars, simple written cues) for orientation and identification of items and places. Keep the environment as simple and uncluttered as possible. Avoid situations that stress intellectual capabilities. For those with early dementia, newspapers, television, telephone calls, and e-mail may be helpful. For those with severe dementia, security devices and electronic monitoring may be indicated. Recommend identification jewelry, photo ID, and current photos; suggest Medialert or the Alzheimer's Association Safe Return Program (800-272-3900).

- Manage problem behaviors. Analyze each behavioral problem in three parts:
  - **A** Antecedents (what happens before to trigger or cause the behavior)
  - **B** Behavior (what specific actions can be seen and described)
  - **C** Consequences (what happens after or because of the behavior)

- Develop a plan to either avoid or prevent problem behaviors by changing either the antecedents or the consequences of the behavior. Avoid catastrophic reactions by minimizing the common antecedents (too much too fast, fatigue).

- Support caregivers. Because persons with dementia may not be able to change as a result of their illness, the caregivers have to be the ones to change. Altering problem behaviors is not easy, and not every attempt will be successful. If the plan isn't working, look at the situation again and try another approach. Be flexible and willing to try new approaches as the elder changes over time. Reward successes, no matter how small. Remember to laugh.

- Provide information and referral: Contact the Alzheimer's Association (919 North Michigan Ave., Suite 1000, Chicago, IL 60611; 800-272-3900), Alzheimer's Disease Education and Referral (ADEAR), area Agency on Aging, community mental health centers, and/or Internet groups.

- Community-based care: adult day centers, home health agencies.

- Caregiver burden: caregivers classes, support groups, respite care.

- Long-term care: personal care/assisted living homes, skilled care nursing homes.

Depression

The most common disturbance of mood experienced by elders is **depression**. Prevalence varies by setting: 5% to 20% in community-dwelling elders, 25% in hospitalized elders, and 40% in nursing home residents (AHCPR, 1993). Its presentation may differ from younger populations, with somatic complaints being more likely in elders than emotional statements about guilt, anger, or depressed mood. The cause may be exogenous (situational), resulting from poor finances, disability, bereavement, loneliness, or social isolation; or endogenous (biochemical), resulting from physical illnesses, pain, or medications; or both. Among community-dwelling elders, depression can be clinical (1%) or subsyndromal (15%) (Reuben, Yoshikwa, & Besdine, 1996).

The assessment of depression in elders requires information from the elder and family members. New physical complaints or exacerbations of previous pain, gastrointestinal symptoms, cardiovascular symptoms, preoccupation with poor health or physical limitations, diminished interest in pleasurable activities, sleep disturbances, fatigue, poor concentration, patchy memory loss, and expressions of negativism should be noted. The Geriatric Depression Scale should be administered and the elder referred to a primary care provider as indicated by assessments. In collaboration with the primary care provider, the nurse should

BOX 22-17 STRATEGIES FOR MANAGEMENT OF DEPRESSION IN ELDERS

- Offer unconditional positive regard for the changes of aging and altered function.

- Emphasize with the elder and family that depression is very manageable and reversible; offer hope.

- Encourage the elder to maintain control over self and the situation by offering choices for simple decision making.

- Assist the elder to identify positive aspects of the situation and opportunities for gains as well as losses.

- In collaboration with primary care provider, encourage the use of medications, psychotherapy, and exercise to treat the depression.

BOX 22-18 STRATEGIES FOR PREVENTION OF SUICIDE IN ELDERS AT RISK

- Reduce the immediate danger of self-harm by removing hazardous articles.

- Refer any potentially suicidal elder promptly to their primary care provider (same day). Provide a constant companion (family, friend) in route.

- Extract a promise from the elder not to attempt suicide before the agreed intervention (e.g., clinic visit, your next visit).

- Mobilize resources by restoring a sense of control, reconnecting the elder with significant others, and developing lifelines of support systems and community resources.

- Follow up with regular calls on the elder and maintenance of support systems.

check for physical problems and medications that cause depression. Interventions for depression are summarized in Box 22-17.

Suicide among elders

With the prevalence of depression among elders, it is not surprising that they have the highest suicide rate of any demographic group. Suicides among elders are characterized by physical illnesses and functional losses rather than the problems with employment, finances, and family relations that are more common among younger adults. Completed suicides more often are by men (60%); attempted suicides more often are by women (75%). The methods include guns, hanging, drug overdose, and cutting or slashing. Threats are real, and first attempts usually are successful. Half to two-thirds of victims see primary care providers in the month before the suicide; 10% to 40% have seen providers within 1 week of their death (Reuben, Yoshikawa, & Besdine, 1996). These visits represent a cry for help and provide a window of opportunity to intervene. More insidious sui-

CASE STUDY

Martha Miller is a 72-year-old widow who has lived alone for 12 years. She has four grown children, two who live in a nearby town and two who live in a distant state. Mrs. Miller has a history of coronary artery disease and hypertension that is controlled with medication. She is unemployed and living on social security and a small pension from her deceased husband. Two weeks ago, Mrs. Miller was involved in a collision while making a left turn at an intersection near her home. She was not injured except for some bruising of her right arm and shoulder. She was evaluated by her family physician immediately after the accident and sent home with instructions to rest and take Tylenol for any discomfort. However, her car, which she had recently purchased, was sent to the garage for exten-

sive repairs. Since the accident, Mrs. Miller has not left the house and calls one of her children every day crying. She is not eating or sleeping well and says she is not able to live alone any longer. One of her children calls the agency where you work to ask for assistance and you are sent to assess Mrs. Miller in home and make a recommendation for action.

1. What kind of information are you seeking regarding Mrs. Miller's condition?

2. What kind of assessment data would you collect?

3. Can you think of any specific assessment tools that might be appropriate to use in this situation?

4. Just from the information you have received before your visit, what do you think might be some issues Mrs. Miller is dealing with?

cide activities used by elders include a refusal to eat, take medications, or follow simple safety procedures and the overuse of alcohol and drugs.

Nurses must consider the potential for suicide in any elders who are depressed or exhibit negativism and hopelessness. Elders fear loneliness, abandonment, loss of control, and pain, but they do not always fear death. Incidence of suicide is higher among elders who are white, male, Protestant, or widowed; they often live alone, have financial problems, have a history of alcoholism, and have poor health, especially a recent diagnosis of terminal illness. The nurse must not hesitate to inquire about suicidal fantasies and ideation. Such questions do not increase the likelihood of suicidal behavior. If these thoughts are present, the nurse should ask directly about plans, method, and means. Behavioral clues such as getting personal affairs in order, giving away possessions, making wills and funeral arrangements, self-neglect, erratic behavior, suspiciousness, hoarding of pills, and personality changes must be attended. Community health nurses have unique opportunities for suicide prevention through early case finding and enrichment of resources and support systems (Box 22-18).

Employment and Retirement

Approximately 12% of older adults are employed or actively seeking employment, 7% men and 5% women, with an increasing trend toward women working in their later years. Of these working elders, more than 50% work part-time (often without benefits) and 24% are self-employed (U.S. Bureau of the Census, 1991). With a life expectancy of 20 years at age 65, transition from work into retirement, a 20th century phenomenon, is the major normative event of the second half of life. Issues for retirement planning include financial security; role restructuring; location; new or part-time careers; educational, recreational, and leisure activities; and relationships with family and friends. With the loss of a formal work role and more leisure time, many elders enjoy volunteering with community agencies or programs such as the Retired Senior Volunteer Program (RSVP) through the local area agency on aging. They also pursue lifelong learning through community education programs through schools (including high school equivalency programs), colleges, and universities, and Elderhostel programs throughout the world. Travel around the country or abroad also may be an option.

By being aware of the meanings of *work* and *play* for elders, community health nurses can be alert for the problems that may arise during these transition periods. For those who are able to redefine themselves with meaningful activities, the latter stages of life can be times for achieving ego integrity (Erikson, 1963) and self-actualization (Maslow, 1968) through lifelong learning and creativity. For those who are unable to make these transitions, old age may become a time of loneliness, hopelessness, and boredom. Quality of life rather than quantity of life becomes the issue. Mastery of the past is the basis for adaptation to the present and hope for the future. Family, friends, and faith are integral with self-concept and spirituality.

Nurses can help alert elders to the characteristics and normality of aging and the **life review** process to find purpose in life (Ebersole & Hess, 1998). Interventions to facilitate these transitions are summarized in Box 22-19. For frail and/or demented elders, programs are needed to combat the plagues of loneliness, boredom, and helplessness in nursing homes by using companionship, variety, and helpfulness. The integration of resident animals, abundant plants, children, and community activities into this environment makes it a more human habitat. For example, a nursing home may adopt suitable dogs and cats from animal shelters, sponsor a scout troop, offer their meeting rooms for local gardener groups, and provide summer day camps for children.

Sexuality

Aging is no deterrent to the need for love and belongingness. The desire for intimacy usually is with one's own generation (spouse, partner, friend), rather than with previous generations (parents) or subsequent generations (children). Elders in any community

---

BOX 22-19 STRATEGIES FOR LATE LIFE TRANSITIONS

- Encourage spontaneous reminiscence and life review that provide opportunities for elders and their families to recapture events in their lives, for elders to create material and/or symbolic legacies, and for families to develop their family and cultural heritage.

- Facilitate connections between past hopes, present events, and future expectations. Support the elder's spiritual belief system. Confront conflicts and anxiety regarding death, guilt, and dependency; instill a sense of hope.

- Use an eclectic approach with counseling, coaching, and listening based on individual situations. Be a dependable confidant, and be aware that life review may be carried out sporadically over several months or years.

- Recommend motivation and remotivation, purpose in life, or validation therapies for frail and/or demented elders.

- Avoid stereotyping and premature closures by elders, families, and caregivers, including nurses.

- Suggest age-appropriate social, recreational, and diversional activities with family and peers to establish support systems and prevent social isolation (e.g., volunteerism, educational programs, 50 Plus, RSVP, civic and religious groups, senior citizens centers).

BOX 22-20 SAFETY PRECAUTIONS FOR ELDERS

- Check to see that stairs are well lighted, free of clutter, and have nonskid surfaces and handrails.
- Check bathrooms for handrails, nonslip adhesive surfaces in tubs/showers, nonslip flooring.
- Provide rooms with adequate, nonglare lighting; eliminate clutter and throw rugs, casters on chairs, dangling cords, waxed floors. Avoid sedation with narcotics and sedatives. Use carbon monoxide and smoke detectors.
- Provide for easy access to the local emergency system, including telephone numbers. If frail and/or homebound, suggest "Friendly Caller" or lifeline services.
- Encourage defensive driving; suggest the local AARP mature/defensive driving program.
- Recommend identification jewelry (i.e., bracelet or necklace) and current photo identification.
- When accidents occur, investigate for specific information on location, time, environmental factors, and intervene to prevent their recurrence.

setting need social interactions with their peers. Their sexual expressions may take a variety of forms, including touching, holding, kissing, fondling, petting, and intercourse, and as with other age groups, these expressions may be heterosexual or homosexual. For older adults living with children or in institutions, nurses may need to facilitate their needs for privacy and intimacy. For those with no spouse or partner, masturbation or fantasy may be alternatives. As with any age group, sexually active elders are at risk for sexually transmitted diseases (STDs), including human immunodeficiency virus (HIV) and acquired immunodeficiency syndrome (AIDS). The PLISSIT model (Permission, Limited Information, Specific Suggestions, Intensive Therapy) is helpful for assessing and intervening in sexual problems with elders (Annon, 1976). For example, nurses can support the sexuality of elders indirectly by saying gently that romance does not end at a certain age and wonder if the person has any questions or concerns in this area (get permission to discuss sexuality). If men indicate a problem, the nurse should ask them more directly, but tactfully, if they are having problems with erections or intercourse; if women indicate a problem, the nurse should ask about lubrication; both should be asked about satisfaction and what they want to do about it. The nurse should provide limited information and make specific suggestions for simple problems (e.g., mild analgesia and alternate positions for painful joints), then make referrals to a primary care provider for intensive therapy as indicated.

Safety and Security

As an aspect of work and play, safety for elders is concerned with accidental injuries in the home and community, especially from falls, fires, and motor vehicle accidents. Older adults with generalized weakness, slow reaction time, unstable gait, visual changes, hearing loss, and multiple medications are at greater risk for accidents and crime. Unfortunately, their vulnerability makes them frequent targets of purse snatchings, pickpocketing, fraud (e.g., fraudulent claims, confidence games, medical quackery), theft, vandalism, and harassment. Community health nurses need to assess home safety to eliminate hazards (see appendix G), teach elders and caregivers basic safety measures, and advocate for greater safety in the community. Safety precautions for elders are summarized in Box 22-20.

Thermal Regulation and Skin Integrity

With less efficient thermal regulation, elders are at higher risk for health problems during temperature extremes. As the largest organ in the body, the skin of elderly people undergoes many age-related changes and is subject to serious complications. Nurses are at the forefront of preventive health care for both thermal regulation and skin integrity.

Thermal Regulation

Internal body temperature is a balance of cellular metabolism, muscle activity, and heat loss by radiation, convection, and evaporation through the skin (Ebersole & Hess, 1998). The ability to feel heat and cold is impaired in elders, and their return to core body temperature in response to heating or cooling is twice as long as in their youth. Drugs such as sedative-hypnotics, phenothiazines, and alcohol may further impair thermoregulatory mechanisms (Reuben, Yoshikawa, & Besdine, 1996). Fear of costly utility bills may decrease their use of air conditioning or heating systems during extreme temperatures. These factors place community-dwelling elders at high risk for hypothermia and hyperthermia during very hot and cold weather. Community health nurses can help prevent life-threatening emergencies by encouraging elders and families to check homes for insulation and caulking to maintain heat and cool. Assistance with fuel costs, which is available in most states, also may be needed. Nurses can help establish "buddy" systems among family, friends, and neighbors for daily checks on elders during weather extremes. A low threshold of suspicion should be used for referrals of at-risk elders to primary care providers or emergency care centers.

Hypothermia

Elders produce less heat per kilogram of body weight. They usually have decreased muscle mass and subcutaneous fat, reduced muscle activity, and less efficient shivering. Their vasoconstriction response of the skin arterioles to cooling is diminished, so heat within the body is not conserved. They are less able to discriminate temperature differences and may have delayed perception of being cold. These age-related changes contribute to an increased risk of hypothermia in elders when indoor temperatures are below 65°F. Symptoms of hypothermia include a body temperature of 95°F (96°F rectal) or below, cold to touch, absent shivering and piloerection, slow capillary refill, pallor or cyanosis, bradypnea, arrhythmia and bradycardia, hypotension, slurred speech, and lethargy. Treatment requires slow warming and may require hospitalization for metabolic imbalances if cooling is prolonged or extreme. See Box 22-21 for techniques to prevent hypothermia.

Hyperthermia

The vasodilation response of the arterioles to heating is diminished in elders so that heat is not delivered to the skin for dissipation. A greater threshold temperature is needed to initiate perspiration and less sweat is produced in response to heating. Elders also are less sensitive to thirst. Individuals with cardiovascular and peripheral vascular diseases, diabetes, and infections, as well as those taking certain medications (e.g., anticholinergics, antihistamines, diuretics, β-blockers, antidepressants, antiparkinsonian drugs), are at risk for hyperthermia. The three types of hyperthermic emergencies are heat syncope, heat exhaustion, and heat stroke. Symptoms include increased body temperature (especially 105°F and above), flushed skin, tachypnea, tachycardia, headache, weakness, and seizures. Suggested techniques to prevent hyperthermia in elders are listed in Box 22-21.

Skin Integrity

With increased elasticity and decreased surface acidity, dryness of the epidermis (xerosis), thinning of the dermis, and loss of subcutaneous fat, skin integrity is an ever-present potential problem in this age group. Skin also has strong symbolic significance and influence on self-esteem. Some elders feel "untouchable" as they experience the wrinkling associated with aging. Gentle touch on the hand, arm, or shoulder helps establish contact with many elders. Nurses need to inspect the skin during any clinical encounter or procedure to check for the many skin disorders of elders (e.g., pruritus [itching], urticaria, intertrigo, seborrheic dermatitis and keratosis, rosacea, psoriasis); several skin cancers are common in elders (e.g., actinic keratoses [precancerous], basal cell and squamous cell carcinomas, melanomas). The nurse should check skin lesions for the ABCD of cancers: Asymmetry, irregular Boarder, multiple Colors, Diameter greater than 1 cm; positive findings should be reported to the primary care provider. Lacerations (especially skin tears), abrasions, and pressure ulcers also are common. Maintenance of skin integrity can be accomplished by limiting bathing (i.e., two to three times a week in warm weather, once or twice a week in cold weather), liberally using emollients (e.g., Eucerin lotion, Vaseline ointment), and avoiding direct sun exposure (i.e., wearing protective clothing or sunscreens). Bath oils should be avoided because they may exacerbate skin problems and increase the risk of falls; water softeners and perineal wipes often are too harsh for the thin skin of elders and should be avoided.

Pressure ulcers

Maintenance of skin integrity and prevention of pressure ulcers requires ever-present vigilance of elders, family caregivers, and nurses in the community. As with other age groups, skin problems are prevented with adequate nutrition and avoidance of pressure, friction, shear, and moisture (AHCPR, 1992). Individuals most at risk are immobile, incontinent, malnourished, frail, or confused. With elders who are confined to bed or wheelchairs, the most common sites of pressure ulcers are the ischium (24%), sacrum (23%), trochanters (15%), heels (35%), and malleolus (7%). Community health nurses can help prevent these painful, costly, and life-threatening complications by being systematic, comprehensive, and routine about skin care. Two instruments often used for assessment of risk factors are the Braden Scale for predicting pressure sore risk and the Norton Risk Assessment

BOX 22-22 TECHNIQUES TO PREVENT PRESSURE ULCERS IN ELDERS

- Teach elders and family members to inspect the skin daily, especially the sacrum, hips, and heels. Use a hand mirror for pressure sites not easily seen. Nurses directly observe the skin of vulnerable elders on *every* visit.

- Improve skin tolerance to pressure by cleansing vulnerable areas with mild soap; avoid hot water and excessive friction. Treat dry skin with moisturizers or emollients. Avoid massage over bony prominences.

- Minimize exposure to moisture. Check persons with incontinence at least every 2 hours, clean the skin, and change clothing or pads immediately. Use topical moisture barriers if necessary.

- While in bed, absolutely reposition the elder every 2 hours (post a schedule); use positioning devices (i.e., pillows, foam wedges) at no more than 30 degrees lateral inclined position; avoid trochanters. Use pressure-reducing devices such as 4-inch dense foam mattresses. Use the lowest degree of head elevation (30 degrees maximum) and limit time of head elevation. Keep the heels off the bed —*no doughnuts.*

- While in a chair or wheelchair, absolutely reposition every hour. Consider postural alignment, weight distribution, balance, and stability. Use pressure-reducing devices, such as a 4-inch dense foam cushion—*not a doughnut.*

- Use lifting devices (i.e., trapeze, bed linens) to avoid friction and shear.

Scale. Techniques to prevent pressure ulcers in elders are listed in Box 22-22.

Comfort and Spirituality

Elders may not complain of discomfort or pain; health care providers may treat it inadequately; and poorly managed pain may aggravate other health problems. With all the age, health, and lifestyle changes experienced by elders, an intact spiritual belief system is essential. Comfort and spirituality conclude this section on preventive health care.

Comfort

Altered proprioception is more common in elders with increased light touch and pain thresholds. Maintaining comfort and managing pain, both acute and chronic, are essential to keep elders mobile and fully involved in their daily activities. Community health nurses need to assess comfort levels frequently using standard pain

scales for persistent problems. Gentle massage, warm (*not* hot) baths, and fragrances are just a few of the techniques that may be helpful for common discomforts. In collaboration with the primary care provider, regular use of analgesics may be helpful to raise the pain threshold and improve comfort and mobility (e.g., acetaminophen 500 mg one to two tablets four times daily as needed for discomfort). Nurses must be vigilant for overuse of OTC nonsteroidal antiinflammatory drugs (NSAIDs, e.g., aspirin, ibuprofen, naproxen), which can lead to gastrointestinal bleeding in elders, and they must be cautious with narcotic and sedative drugs, which can contribute to delirium and falls in this age group.

Spirituality

With the experiences of aging and changes in health status, many elders and families are faced with the need to discover a continuing purpose in the elder's life, find new meanings in their existence, and prepare for their transcendence from life to death. As they approach the end of their lives, elders may contemplate their movement from the concrete reality of their physical existence toward more abstract, metaphorical conceptualizations of their oneness with God, a divine being, or a higher power. Spirituality, the essence of the soul, may be integral with elders' beliefs, hope, energy, creativity, acceptance of life and death, and transcendence (Ebersole & Hess, 1998). As with other age groups, nurses assess the spiritual health of elders by inquiring discretely about their spiritual perspectives and religious commitments. Observations include their ability to discover continuing meaning and purpose in life, give and receive love, have hope, be creative, and share humor. The goals of spiritual care are to preserve the elders' unique beliefs and values and support their religious practices. Nurses may need to help elders make contact with religious advisors (e.g., minister, priest, rabbi, shaman) and use religious articles (e.g., Bible, Koran, crucifix, medals, prayer shawls, incense). They may need to have privacy for prayer and meditation or may want to sing hymns, read or write poetry, or offer other forms of self-expression. Elders may ask the nurse to share in these practices, as is appropriate for the situation. Other spiritual issues, life review, and advance directives are discussed elsewhere in this chapter. However elders express their spirituality, it is important that nurses recognize these needs and assist with their being met.

Special Elder Health Issues

Community health nurses must consider special issues in the elderly population. Comprehensive health care for elders includes immunizations, medication review, chemical abuse, and ethical dilemmas.

Immunizations

Pneumonia and influenza combined are a leading cause of death in the United States. Elders with chronic illnesses are at the highest risk for these respiratory illnesses. In the elderly population, immunizations usually are limited to three vaccines: influenza, pneumococcal, and tetanus/diphtheria. For elders who travel to foreign countries, other immunizations may be indicated. Elders should be referred to their local health department immunization clinic for information about the requirements for specific countries.

Medications

Elders purchase 40% of all prescription drugs (most commonly cardiovascular, anti-infective, antipsychotic, antidepressant, and diuretic agents) and 40% of OTC medicines (mostly analgesics, laxatives, and antacids). An average of five prescription drugs and three OTC drugs are taken by 90% of elders (Ebersole & Hess, 1998). Because aging changes affect the absorption, distribution, metabolism, and elimination of pharmacological agents, elders are more prone to drug interactions, adverse reactions, and toxicities.

Polypharmacy (many drugs) is a multifactorial problem that results from a "pill-oriented" society, elders' beliefs about

health care and their various acute and chronic health problems, the prescribing practices of primary care providers, and the use of multiple primary and specialty providers. Problems of adherence to drug regimes occur with 25% to 50% of medications, including underuse, overuse, and misuse; many of these errors contribute to unnecessary hospitalizations (Ebersole & Hess, 1998). Medicare does not fund prescription drugs; Medicaid limits recipients to five prescriptions per month; some insurance plans may offer assistance with drugs. Because of their expense, elders may not fill prescriptions or may discontinue medications or decrease dosages and/or frequencies to stretch their medicines.

Community health nurses must be attentive for errors of omission (e.g., unfilled prescriptions, skipped doses, discontinuing medicines) and errors of commission (e.g., self-medication by increasing or decreasing dosages, changing times, using another person's drugs, taking OTC drugs). Nursing interventions for drug therapies are summarized in Box 22-23.

BOX 22-23 STRATEGIES TO IMPROVE MEDICATION USE BY ELDERS

- Obtain a medication history and consider the ability of elders to manage their medications, including financial status (purchase), environmental situation (storage), educational level (literacy), cognitive status (memory), visual acuity (reading labels), functional status (opening containers), and drug allergies.

- Remind elders to bring their medicines to each clinic visit; do a drug review ("brown bag check") for correct medications, dosages, instructions, refills, and their drug knowledge.

- Check medications frequently during home visits, including their storage and the disposition of old medications.

- In collaboration with primary care providers, simplify drug regimes and eliminate all unnecessary drugs, both prescribed and over-the-counter. Use once or twice daily dosing whenever possible.

- Teach elders and family members about all medications and prepare a written schedule, including each drug name and strength, size/color, frequency (specific times), purpose, and important side effects.

- Encourage elders to purchase all medications through the same pharmacy to check for drug allergies and interactions.

- Encourage elders to take medications at the same times and place every day with 4 to 6 ounces of water. Use memory aids to assist with adherence to drug regimes (e.g., written lists, medication calendars, pill boxes).

- Store all medicines together in a safe dry place, in their original containers, and out of the reach of small children.

- Remind elders to take a sufficient supply of all medicines when traveling away from home.

- If elders have memory problems, functional impairments, or complicated drug regimes, suggest the use of medication boxes pre-filled by the elder or caregiver either daily or weekly.

- If elders have arthritic problems, suggest easy-opening containers; if they have visual problems, use large print for labels; if they have swallowing problems, use liquid forms. Caution against crushing tablets or emptying capsules into food or fluid before checking with a pharmacist.

- Monitor elders continually for efficacy and side effects of medications. Use the abnormal involuntary movement scale (AIMS) to monitor drugs (especially antipsychotics) with extrapyramidal side effects such as tremors, akinesia, akathisia, and rigidity (tardive dyskinesia).

Chemical Abuse

Among elders, chemical abuse include all of the psychoactive chemicals used by younger populations, with alcohol being the substance that is most commonly abused. Alcoholism is estimated to affect 10% to 15% of community-dwelling elders. With their decreased tolerance to alcohol combined with normal aging changes and use of multiple prescription and OTC drugs, elders are at higher risk for falls, accidents, and burns. Nurses in the community can help identify these individuals by noting changes in behavior (e.g., anxiety, memory loss, depression, blackouts, confusion), health status (e.g., weight loss), hygiene, falls, and injuries. Elders can be screened with the TWEACK test (Reuben, Yoshikawa, & Besdine, 1996):

Tolerance	How many drinks before you feel effects of alcohol?
Worry	Have you ever felt worried by criticism of your drinking?
Eye opener	Have you ever taken a morning eye opener?
Amnesia	Are there times after drinking when you can't remember what you did?
Cut down	Have you ever felt the need to cut down on drinking?
Drin**K**ing	How many drinks before you fall asleep or pass out?

Those elders and families found to have alcohol problems are referred to their primary care providers, community mental health centers, Alcoholics Anonymous, or other local agencies for treatment of chemical abuse. Because denial of alcohol abuse is so prevalent and the necessary lifestyle changes are so difficult to maintain, recovery often is a long, irregular process. Nurses need to persist in their support, referral, and follow-up for these individuals and their families.

Other substances abused by elders include nicotine, caffeine, prescription and OTC drugs, illicit street drugs, and food. Assessments and interventions for these chemicals are similar to those for younger populations.

All We Need To Know

All we need to know is that we're needed.
All we have to feel is we're worthwhile.
It's not very difficult; indeed, it's
Something you can do with just your smile.

All we ask from you is some attention.
Notice us! We're special. If you please,
Pardon us, if now and then we mention
We would like a tender loving squeeze.

Old and gray, we wait. And don't forget that
Inside us, the child is waiting, too.
Help us feel important.
You can bet that
Then we'll want to be our best for you!

Ellen Johnston-Hale, age 83

Ethical Dilemmas

Because community health nurses become so involved with elderly people in their own environment, they often encounter ethical dilemmas and end-of-life issues. All too often there is no simple, easy, "right" answer to these complex situations—if there were, the dilemma would not exist. Usually, the choice is between two or more "bad" options. Beware of simple solutions for these usually ignore the complex nature of dilemmas. For example, when a frail, demented elder is anorexic, losing weight, and at risk for complications, one option is to insert an enteral feeding tube—which may improve nutrition, but also may prolong the person's suffering and dying and may be against his or her wishes for end-of-life care.

In American society, critical values in most ethical dilemmas concern autonomy (freedom of choice), nonmaleficence or beneficence (do no harm/do good), and distributive justice (use of resources). Because elders consume large amounts of health care resources, ethical conflicts occur around the issues of old versus young and quantity of life (adding years to live) versus quality of life (adding life to years). For many elders, the finality of death must be weighed against dependence, pain, abandon-

RESEARCH BRIEF

Gloth, F. M., Tobin, J. D., Sherman, S. S., & Hollis, B. W. (1991). Is the recommended daily allowance for vitamin D too low for the homebound elderly? Journal of the American Geriatrics Society, 39, 137–141.

The recommended daily allowance (RDA) for vitamin D is 200 IU for adults. Although there is inadequate research on the specific requirements for elders older than 65, there is evidence that homebound and institution-bound elders are at special risk for vitamin D deficiency. Symptoms of vitamin D deficiency include weakness, pain, and bone loss, which can lead to osteoporosis and spontaneous fractures, all devastating conditions for elders. These symptoms compound the hardships already suffered by many older persons whose health is already impaired. The body's main source of vitamin D is direct exposure to the sun's ultraviolet rays. Approximately 5% of the U.S. population age 65 and older is in nursing homes. In addition, many older people in poor health at home tend to stay indoors and therefore are not exposed to sunlight. Recommendations of the study include encouraging all elders to sit outside on sunny days for 2 to 3 hours to enhance their vitamin D intake.

ment, and loneliness. Clarification of beliefs and values of the elder, the family, and the health care providers may offer insights into these perspectives and facilitate satisfactory resolution of these conflicts.

Advance directives can help clarify elders' desire for health care interventions in the event of life-threatening situations. Nurses can encourage elders and families to discuss end-of-life issues (e.g., cardiopulmonary resuscitation, hospitalization, antibiotics, intravenous and enteral feedings) while elders are relatively young, healthy, and competent to express their wishes. The elder can complete a living will and/or durable power of attorney for health care in accordance with state statutes to assist family members to implement these wishes. In elders, intellectual competence for informed consent can be determined with the FMMSE (see appendix E).

For elders who have no advance directives and are very frail or demented, nurses can anticipate the occurrence of end-of-life issues. Nurses should take the initiative to approach families about these decisions *early*, encourage them to talk with extended family members as appropriate, and consider what the elders would prefer if they were able to express their wishes. Consider criteria for decision making (e.g., reversibility or irreversibility of the condition), communicate with the primary care provider, and document decisions appropriately. If elders are able to participate in these decisions, the nurse should encourage them to do so. Supporting the spiritual integrity of all concerned helps sort out the issues and maintain positive attitudes and behaviors.

• •

The Long Walk
We have walked a long way—the old woman said.
I no longer know the way—The trees are so tall—they all look the same. Are we near to the end?

We are close—You see – right there—the cleared meadow on the top of the next hill—we have just one more hill to climb. We are very close to the end my dear—the old man said.

I am growing tired—is it much further—she asked.

See my dear we are close. Just beyond the next hill—see how the trees part—just one more hill to climb.

Are you sure this is the way? We have walked for such a long time and climbed so many hills.

We are close now my dear—you can almost see the stream. Listen we are very close—just behind that hill—see how the valley opens.

It's growing late—have we reached the end?
My legs are tired and I would like to rest.

See the top of the hill –see how the trees are black picture cuts against the sky—you can almost see it now.

Look where the sun is setting—home is just beyond that bend—we can almost smell the evening fire—my dear.

The shadows are growing long and I would like to rest.
Are we near home?

Just one more hill to climb—then we can rest.

It is so dark and my eyes are not so good—do you see the end of our journey?

Dr. Ann Thedford Lanier

• •

CONCLUSION

With the "graying of America," elders are integral with the delivery of community health care. These older adults were socialized in a reactive health care system that focused on illness. Until recently, they have not been especially proactive or focused wellness or prevention. Community health nurses in 21st century can help elders by the three A's: awareness, assessment, and advocacy. Nurses can help elders practice health promotion and primary disease prevention through good nutrition, regular exercise, family and community involvement, stress management, anticipatory guidance, and safety checks. Secondary prevention requires self-monitoring activities (e.g., breast or testicular self-examinations), periodic screening, regular physical and oral health examinations, and adherence to therapeutic regimens. By working collaboratively with primary care providers, nurses can improve the health and quality of life of older adults—and help celebrate the joy of aging.

CRITICAL THINKING ACTIVITIES

1. After reading the following, what are some ways that community health nurses can help "reconnect" elders with other clients in the health care delivery system? Identify settings where health promotion interventions might be created to meet this need.

On the need to reconnect with elders . . .

A great deal of America's social sickness comes from age segregation . . . . We segregate the old for many reasons: prejudice, ignorance and a lack of good alternatives . . . If we aren't around dying people, we don't have to think about dying . . . and, the more involved we are with the old, the more pain we feel at their suffering . . . The old often save the young. And the young save the old . . . If 10 people ages 2 to 80 are grouped together, they will fall into a natural hierarchy that nurtures and teaches them all . . . the incredible calculus of old age—that as more is taken, there is more love for what remains.

Mary Pipher (1999, March 19-21). The new generation gap: For the nations health, we need to reconnect young and old. *USA Weekend,* p. 12.

2. Using photographs, assist an elderly client with visualizing independence in his or her life today. How can photographs throughout our lives assist in maximizing our ability to care for ourselves and promote our autonomy? Think of times in your own life when you were dependent and had limitations. What kinds of images helped improve your confidence in becoming self-sufficient again?

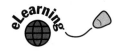

Explore Community Health Nursing on the web! To learn more about the topics in this chapter, access your exclusive web site: http://communitynursing.jbpub.com

REFERENCES

Agency for Health Care Policy and Research (AHCPR). (1992). *Pressure ulcers in adults: Prediction and prevention*. Rockville, MD: U.S. Government Printing Office.

Agency for Health Care Policy and Research (AHCPR). (1993). *Depression in primary care*. Rockville, MD: U.S. Government Printing Office.

Agency for Health Care Policy and Research (AHCPR). (1996a). *Recognition and initial treatment of Alzheimer's disease and related dementias*. Rockville, MD: U.S. Government Printing Office.

Agency for Health Care Policy and Research (AHCPR). (1996b). *Managing acute and chronic urinary incontinence*. Rockville, MD: U.S. Government Printing Office.

American Association for World Health. (1999). *Healthy aging, healthy living—Start now! Resource booklet*. Washington, DC: Author.

American Association of Retired Persons (AARP) and National Alliance for Caregiving. (1997). *Family caregiving in the U.S.: Findings from a national survey*. D16474 Washington, DC: AARP.

American College of Physicians. (1994). *Guide for adult immunization* (3rd ed.). Philadelphia: Author.

Anderson, K., & Anderson, L. (1994). *Mosby's pocket dictionary of medicine, nursing, & allied health* (2nd ed.). St. Louis: Mosby.

Annon, J. (1976). The PLISSIT model: A proposed conceptual scheme for behavioral treatment of sexual problems. *Journal of Sex Education and Therapy*, January, pp. 18–20.

Bellack, P., & Edlund, B. (1992). *Nursing assessment and diagnosis* (2nd ed.). Boston: Jones and Bartlett.

Burnside, I. (1988). *Nursing and the aged: A self-care approach* (2nd ed.). New York: McGraw-Hill.

Burnside, I., & Haight, B. (1994). Reminiscence and life review: Therapeutic interventions for older people. *Nurse Practitioner*, *19*(4), 55-61.

Butler, R., & Lewis, M. (1998). *Aging and mental health* (5th ed.) Boston: Allyn & Bacon.

Busse, E., & Blazer, D. (1980). *Geriatric psychiatry*. Washington, DC: American Psychiatric Press.

Carter, E., & McGoldrick, M. (1980). *The family life cycle: A framework for family therapy* (pp. 3-20). New York: Gardner.

Carter, Jimmy. (1995). *Always a reckoning*. New York: Random House.

Cora, V. L. (1985). *Family life process of intergenerational families with functionally dependent elders*. Dissertation. University of Alabama at Birmingham.

Comfort, A. (1990). *Say yes to old age: Developing a positive attitude toward aging*. New York: Crown.

Duvall, E. M. (1977). *Marriage and family development*. Philadelphia: J. B. Lippincott.

Ebersole, P., & Hess, P. (1998). *Toward healthy aging: Human needs and nursing response* (5th ed.). St. Louis: Mosby.

Erikson, E. (1963). *Childhood and society*. New York: Norton.

Folstein, M., Folstein, S., & McHugh, P. (1975). Mini-mental state: A practical method for grading the cognitive state of patients for the clinician. *Journal of Psychiatric Research*, *12*, 189-198.

Gunter, L., & Estes, C. (1979). *Education for gerontic nursing*. New York: Springer.

Ham, R., & Sloane, P. (1997). *Primary care geriatrics: A case-based approach* (2nd ed.) St. Louis: Mosby.

Healthy People 2000: The nation's health. (pp. 23-26, 588-591).

Kane, R., Ouslander, J., & Abrass, I. (1999). *Essentials of clinical geriatrics* (4th ed.). New York: McGraw-Hill.

Katz, S., Ford, A., Moskowitz, R., et al. (1963). Studies of illness in the aged. The index of ADL. *Journal of the American Medical Association*, *185*, 914.

Lawton, M., & Brody, E. (1969). Assessment of older people: Self maintaining and instrumental activities of daily living. *Gerontologist*, *9*, 179–186.

Lueckenotte, A. G. (1996). *Gerontologic nursing*. St. Louis: Mosby.

Maslow, A. (1968). *Toward a psychology of being* (2nd ed.). Princeton, NJ: Van Nostrand.

National Center for Health Statistics, Centers for Disease Control and Prevention. (1994). *Health United States, 1993* (U.S. Public Health Service, DHHS Publication No. 94-1232). Washington, DC: U.S. Government Printing Office.

Nutrition Screening Initiative. (1992). *Consensus conference.* Washington, DC.

O'Malley, R. (1987). *Inadequate care of the elderly: A health care perspective on abuse and neglect.* New York: Springer.

Reuben, D., Yoshikawa, T., & Besdine, R. (1996). *Geriatrics review syllabus: A core curriculum in geriatric medicine* (3rd ed.). Dubuque, IA: Kendall/Hunt.

Satir, V. (1964). *Conjunct family therapy: A guide to theory and technique.* Palo Alto, CA: Science & Behavioral Books.

Staab, A., & Lyles, M. (1990). *Manual of geriatric nursing.* Glenview, IL: Scott, Foresman/Little, Brown.

U.S. Bureau of the Census. (1991). *Statistical abstract of the United States: 1993* (112th ed.). Washington, DC: U.S. Government Printing Office.

United States Public Health Service (USPHS). (1994). *Clinician's handbook of preventive services: Put prevention into practice.* Washington, DC: Department of Health and Human Services.

Williams, M., Parker, R., Baker, D., Parikh, N. S., Pitkin, K., Coates, W. C., & Nurss, J. R. (1995). Inadequate functional health literacy among patients at two public hospitals. *JAMA, 274,* 1677-1720.

Yesavage, J., & Brink, T. (1983). Development and validation of a geriatric depression screening scale: A preliminary report. *Journal of Psychiatric Research, 17,* 37-49.

APPENDIX A

SELECTED THEORIES OF AGING

BIOLOGIC THEORIES

Molecular Theories

Gene: Selected genes become active in later life, causing the organism to fail to survive

Error, error catastrophe:
  Somatic mutation
  Transcription

Programmed, programmed senescence

Run-out-of-program

System Level Theories

Neuroendocrine control (pacemakers)
Immunological/autoimmune

Cellular Theories

Free radical, antioxidants
Cross-link/connective tissue
Clinker
Wear-and-tear

PSYCHOLOGICAL THEORIES

Maslow's hierarchy of human needs
Jung's individualism
Course of human life
Erikson's (1963) eight stages of life:
  Sense of ego integrity versus sense of despair
Peck (1968):
  Ego differentiation versus work-role preoccupation
  Body transcendence versus body preoccupation
  Ego transcendence versus ego preoccupation
Feil (1982): resolution of the past versus vegetation
Butler's (1963) life review
Levinson's (1977) Seasons of Life
Lowenthal's (1973) life transitions
Havighurst's (1974) developmental tasks:
  Establishing satisfactory living arrangements
  Adjusting to retirement and reduced income
  Adjusting to decreasing physical strength and health

Establishing an explicit affiliation with one's age group
Meeting civic and social obligations
Adjusting to death of spouse
Psychosocial theories of aging:
Interpersonal, disengagement, continuity, activity (life review, reminiscence)

SOCIOLOGICAL THEORIES

Cummings & Henry (1961): Disengagement
Lemon (1972): Activity
Havighurst (1963): Continuity
Age stratification
Person-environment fit
Sociological aging life course, life transitions, status and role changes, social supports

APPENDIX B

ANA STANDARDS OF GERONTOLOGICAL NURSING PRACTICE

STANDARDS OF CLINICAL GERONTOLOGICAL NURSING CARE

Standard I. Assessment

The gerontological nurse collects client health data.

Information obtained from the aging person, significant others, and the interdisciplinary team and nursing judgment based on knowledge of gerontological nursing are used to develop the comprehensive care plan. Interviewing, functional assessment, environmental assessment, physical assessment, and review of health records enhance the nurse's ability to make sound clinical judgments. Assessment is culturally and ethnically appropriate.

Standard II. Diagnosis

The gerontological nurse analyzes the assessment data in determining diagnosis.

The gerontological nurse evaluates health assessment data to identify the aging person's state of health and well-being, and treatment of and responses to illness, aging, and reduced activity. Each person responds to aging in a unique way. Nursing diagnoses form the basis for nursing interventions.

Standard III. Outcome Identification

The gerontological nurse identifies expected outcomes individualized to the client.

The ultimate goals of providing gerontological nursing care are to influence health outcomes and improve the aging person's health status. Outcomes often focus on maximizing the aging person's state of well-being, functional status, and quality of life.

Standard IV. Planning

The gerontological nurse develops a plan of care that prescribes interventions to attain expected outcomes.

A plan of care is used to structure and guide therapeutic interventions and achieve expected outcomes. It is developed in conjunction with the aging person and significant others.

Standard V. Implementation

The gerontological nurse implements the interventions identified in the care plan.

The gerontological nurse implements a care plan in collaboration with the aging person, significant others, and the interdisciplinary team. The gerontological nurse provides culturally competent direct and indirect care, using concepts of health promotion, illness prevention, health maintenance, rehabilitation, restoration, and palliation. The nurse educates and counsels the aging person and significant others involved in that person's care. In addition, the gerontological nurse supervises and evaluates both formal and informal caregivers to ensure that their care is supportive and ethical and demonstrates respect for the aging person's dignity. Gerontological nurses select interventions according to their level of practice.

Standard VI. Evaluation

The gerontological nurse evaluates the aging person's progress toward attainment of expected outcomes.

Nursing practice is a dynamic process. The gerontological nurse continually evaluates the aging person's responses to therapeutic interventions. Collection of new data, revision of the database, alteration of nursing diagnoses, and modification of the care plan are often required. The effectiveness of nursing care depends on ongoing evaluation.

STANDARDS OF PROFESSIONAL GERONTOLOGICAL NURSING PERFORMANCE

Standard I. Quality of Care

The gerontological nurse systematically evaluates the quality of care and effectiveness of nursing practice.

The dynamic nature of geriatric care and the growing body of gerontological nursing knowledge and research provide both the impetus and the means for gerontological nurses to improve the quality of client care.

Standard II. Performance Appraisal

The gerontological nurse evaluates his or her own nursing practice in relation to professional practice standards and relevant statutes and regulations.

The gerontological nurse is accountable to the public for providing competent clinical care and has an inherent responsibility to practice according to standards established by the profession and by regulatory bodies.

Standard III. Education

The gerontological nurse acquires and maintains current knowledge in nursing practice.

Scientific, cultural, societal, and political changes require a continuing commitment from the gerontological nurse to pursue knowledge, to enhance nursing expertise, and advance the profession. Formal education, continuing education, certification, and experiential learning are some of the means for professional growth.

Standard IV. Collegiality

The gerontological nurse contributes to the professional development of peers, colleagues, and others.

The gerontological nurse is responsible for sharing knowledge, research, and clinical information with colleagues and others through formal and informal teaching methods and collaborative educational programs.

Standard V. Ethics

The gerontological nurse's decisions and actions on behalf of clients are determined in an ethical manner.

The gerontological nurse is responsible for providing nursing services and health care that are responsive to the public's trust and client's rights. Co-workers and other formal and informal care providers must also be prepared to provide the care needed and desired by the aging person and to render services in an appropriate setting. Special ethical concerns in gerontological nursing care include informed consent; emergency interventions; nutrition and hydration of the terminally ill; pain management; need for self-determination by the aging person; treatment termination; quality-of-life issues; confidentiality; surrogate decision making; nontraditional treatment modalities; fair distribution of scarce resources; and economic decision making.

Standard VI. Collaboration

The gerontological nurse collaborates with the aging person, significant others, and health care providers in providing client care.

The complex nature of comprehensive care for aging persons and their significant others requires expertise from a number of different health care providers. Collaboration between consumers and providers is optimal for planning, implementing, and evaluation care. Meetings of the interdisciplinary team provide a forum to evaluate the effectiveness of the care plan and make necessary adjustments.

Standard VII. Research

The gerontological nurse uses research findings in practice.

Gerontological nurses are responsible for improving nursing practice and the future health care for aging persons by participating in research. At the basic level of practice, the gerontological nurse uses research findings to improve clinical care and identifies clinical problems for study.

Standard VIII. Resource Utilization

The gerontological nurse considers factors related to safety, effectiveness, and cost in planning and delivering client care.

The aging person is entitled to health care that is safe, effective, and affordable. Treatment decisions must maximize resources and maintain quality of care.

Source: American Nurses Association (ANA). (1995). Scope and standards of gerontological nursing practice. *Washington DC: Author.*

APPENDIX C

ACTIVITIES OF DAILY LIVING AND INSTRUMENTAL ACTIVITIES OF DAILY LIVING

	INDEPENDENT	ASSISTED	DEPENDENT		INDEPENDENT	ASSISTED	DEPENDENT
Bathing	0	1	2	Telephoning	0	1	2
Dressing	0	1	2	Shopping	0	1	2
Toileting	0	1	2	Transporting	0	1	2
Transfer	0	1	2	Medicating	0	1	2
Continence	0	1	2	Handling money	0	1	2
Feeding	0	1	2	*Preparing food	0	1	2
				*Housekeeping	0	1	2
				*Laundry	0	1	2

ADL Score (0-12) _____   IADL Score (0-16)_____   Total Score (0-28)_____

0	Independent	0	Independent	0	Independent
1-6	Assisted	1-8	Assisted	1-14	Assisted
7-12	Dependent	7-16	Dependent	15-28	Dependent

Source: Adapted from Katz, 1963, and Lawton & Brody, 1969 (alternate scoring).

APPENDIX D

TINETTI FALL ASSESSMENT SCALE

BALANCE:	(SEATED IN HARD, ARMLESS CHAIR)	SCORING
Sitting balance	leans or slides in chair	5 0
	steady, safe	5 1 _____
Arises	unable without help	5 0
	able, uses arms to help	5 1
	able without using arms	5 2 _____

Attempts to rise	unable without help	5 0
	able, requires 1 attempt	5 1
	able to rise, 1 attempt	5 2 _____
Immediate standing	balance (1st 5 sec)	
	unsteady (staggers, moves feet, trunk sway)	5 0
	steady but uses walker or other support	5 1
	narrow stance without other support	5 2 _____

Standing balance	unsteady	5 0
	steady but wide stance and uses other support	5 1
	narrow stance without support	5 2 _____
Nudged	begins to fall	5 0
	staggers, grabs, catches self	5 1
	steady	5 2 _____
Eyes closed	unsteady	5 0
	steady	5 1 _____
Turning 360°	discontinuous steps	5 0
	continuous steps	5 1
	unsteady (grabs, staggers)	5 0
	steady	5 1 _____
Sitting down	unsafe (misjudged distance, falls into chair)	5 0
	uses arms or not a smooth motion	5 1
	safe, smooth motion	5 2 _____
Balance Score:		_____ /16

Gait:	(stands, walks about 10 ft at usual pace, then back at rapid, but safe pace with aids)	Scoring
Initiation of gate	any hesitancy or multiple attempts to start	5 0
	no hesitancy	5 1 _____

Step length and height

right swing foot	does not pass left stance foot with step	5 0
	passes left stance foot	5 1
	right foot does not clear floor completely	5 0
	right foot completely clears floor	5 1

left swing foot	does not pass right stance foot with step	5 0
	passes right stance foot	5 1
	left foot doesn't clear floor completely	5 0
	left foot completely clears floor	5 1 _____
Step symmetry	right & left step length not equal (estimate)	5 0
	right & left step appear equal	5 1 _____
Step continuity	stopping or discontinuity between steps	5 0
	steps appear continuous	5 1 _____
Path	marked deviation	5 0
	mild/moderate deviation or uses walking aid	5 1
	straight without walking aid	5 2 _____
Trunk	marked sway or uses walking aid	5 0
	no sway but flexion of knees or back or spread arms out while walking	5 1
	no sway, no flexion, no use of arms, and no use of walking aid	5 2 _____
Walking time	heels apart	5 0
	heels almost touching while walking	5 1 _____

Gait Score: _____ /12

Balance and Gait Score: Score _____ /28

Key to Risk for Falls:	Score
low	25-28
moderate	19-24
high	0-18

APPENDIX E

MINI-MENTAL STATE EXAM

FOLSTEIN MINI-MENTAL STATE EXAM

Highest school grade completed _____

Maximum	Score	Orientation
5	_____	What is the (year), (season), (date), (day), (month)?
5	_____	Where are we: (state), (city), (county), (facility), (floor)?

Registration

3	_____	Name 3 objects: 1 second to say each; ask person all three objects after they are said. Give 1 point for each correct answer. Then repeat objects until all three are learned. Count trials and record: _____

Attention and Calculation

5 _____ Serial 7s. One point for each correct. Stop after 5 answers. 93 86 79 72 65. Alternatively, spell "world" backwards: D L R O W

Recall

3 _____ Ask for three objects repeated above. Give 1 point for each correct answer.

Language and Praxis

2 _____ Name a pencil and a watch.

1 _____ Repeat the following phrase: "No ifs, ands, or butts."

3 _____ Follow a 3-stage command: "Take this paper in your right hand, fold it in half, and put it on the table."

1 _____ Read and obey the following command: **CLOSE YOUR EYES**

1 _____ Write a sentence:

1 _____ Copy this design:

___

30

Key to FMMSE Scores

no cognitive impairment	24-30
mild cognitive impairment	18-23
severe cognitive impairment	0-17

Source: Folstein, Folstein, & McHugh, 1975.

APPENDIX F

GERIATRIC DEPRESSION SCALE

Mood Scale

1.	ARE YOU BASICALLY SATISFIED WITH YOUR LIFE?	yes	NO
2.	HAVE YOU DROPPED MANY OF YOUR ACTIVITIES AND INTERESTS?	YES	no
3.	DO YOU FEEL THAT YOUR LIFE IS EMPTY?	YES	no
4.	DO YOU OFTEN GET BORED?	YES	no
5.	Are you hopeful about the future?	yes	NO
6.	Are you bothered by thoughts that you just can't get out of your head?	YES	no
7.	ARE YOU IN GOOD SPIRITS MOST OF THE TIME?	yes	NO
8.	ARE YOU AFRAID THAT SOMETHING BAD IS GOING TO HAPPEN TO YOU?	YES	no
9.	DO YOU FEEL HAPPY MOST OF THE TIME?	yes	NO
10.	DO YOU OFTEN FEEL HELPLESS?	YES	no
11.	Do you often get restless and fidgety?	YES	no
12.	Do you prefer to stay home at night rather than go out and do new things?	YES	no
13.	Do you frequently worry about the future?	YES	no
14.	DO YOU FEEL THAT YOU HAVE MORE PROBLEMS WITH MEMORY THAN MOST?	YES	no
15.	DO YOU THINK IT IS WONDERFUL TO BE ALIVE NOW?	yes	NO
16.	Do you often feel downhearted and blue?	YES	no
17.	DO YOU FEEL PRETTY WORTHLESS THE WAY YOU ARE NOW?	YES	no
18.	Do you worry a lot about the past?	YES	no
19.	Do you find life very exciting?	yes	NO
20.	Is it hard for you to get started on new projects?	YES	no

21.	DO YOU FEEL FULL OF ENERGY?	yes	NO
22.	DO YOU FEEL THAT YOUR SITUATION IS HOPELESS?	YES	no
23.	DO YOU THINK THAT MOST PERSONS YOUR AGE ARE BETTER OFF THAN YOU ARE?	YES	no
24.	Do you frequently get upset over little things?	YES	no
25.	Do you frequently feel like crying?	YES	no
26.	Do you have trouble concentrating?	YES	no
27.	Do you enjoy getting up in the morning?	yes	NO
28.	Do you prefer to avoid social gatherings?	YES	no
29.	Is it easy for you to make decisions?	yes	NO
30.	Is your mind as clear as it used to be?	yes	NO

Score   Circled capitalized answers   _____

Crossed out lowercase answers   _____

Total   15 or 30

Key to Scoring   **GDS**

No depression   0–4 capitalized on 15-item screen

Mild depression   5–10 capitalized on 30-item scale

Severe depression 11–30 capitalized on 30 item scale

Directions for Scoring: This scale is intended to be administered orally to the elderly person in a quiet, private setting. Circle the capitalized *answer* if the elder answers the question with the capitalized response. Draw a line through the lower case *answer* if the elder answers with the lower case response.

Score 1 point for each circled capitalized answer.

Score 0 for each lower case answer.

For screening purposes, use the 15 short-form *questions* which are capitalized. If the elder scores more than 5 points, administer the full 30-item scale.

Interpretation: A score of 5 or more capitalized responses on the 15-item screen is suggestive of depression and indicates the need to administer the full scale. a score of 0-10 is in the Normal range; a score of 11 or more capitalized responses on the 30-item scale is positive for depression.

According to Yersavage and Brink (1983), a cut-off score of 11 has a sensitivity of 84% and a specificity of 95%. A cut-off score of 14 has a sensitivity of 80% and a specificity of 100%.

Source: Yesavage & Brink, 1983.

APPENDIX G

HOME SAFETY CHECKLIST

HOME INTERIOR

Floors: clean, clutter-free, rugs anchored and in good repair (no scatter rugs), surface smooth and nonskid wax;

Electrical appliances: cords in good repair and out of traffic lanes

Lighting: adequate not-glare lighting; stairs illuminated; night lights where needed

Temperature: range 70-75°F; adequate heating, cooling, and ventilation; insulation; fireplace/heaters with protective screens

Furniture: sturdy, good repair

Stairs: sturdy railings; nonskid steps; uncluttered

Organization: uncluttered, navigable traffic lanes

COMMUNICATION

Lock/unlock door; reach light switches

Emergency telephone numbers posted, legible (fire, ambulance, doctor, family)

If no telephone, life line, neighbor, "buddy," or other means to summon help

Smoke alarms available with working batteries

KITCHEN

Food: adequate supply, fresh

Stove: free of grease and flammables, baking soda or fire extinguisher

Refrigerator: cooling effectively, food available and fresh

Sink: draining properly, hot (check temperature) and cold water; dishes washed

Cleaning supplies: stored separately and clearly marked

Garbage: taken out; regular pick up

Ladder or step stool: sturdy with handle

BATHROOM

Handrails for tub and toilet

Skid-proof mats for tub and/or shower

Nonskid rug on floor

Electrical outlets safe distance from tub

MEDICATIONS

Stored safely; current; disposal of old medicines

Current list with times, dosage, description, purpose

OUTSIDE

Walks, driveways, and stairs: smooth surfaces in good repair (no raised or uneven places); edges painted or clearly visible; handrails secure

Doors and windows: panes and screens in good repair

Fire escape or alternate exit from house

Source: Adapted from Burnside, 1988.

Chapter 23
Community Mental Health
Sarah Steen Lauterbach

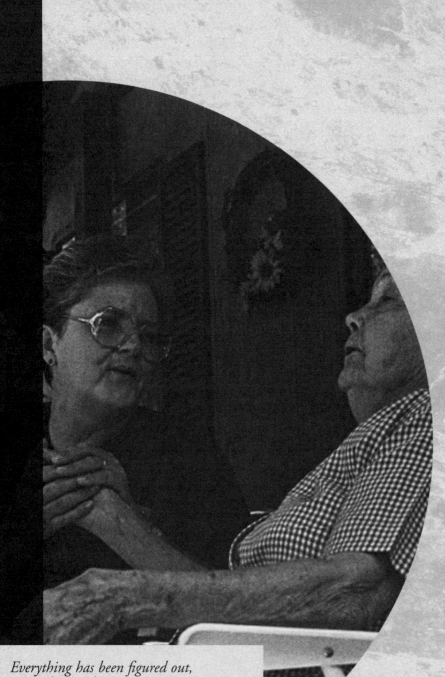

*Everything has been figured out,
except how to live.*

Jean Paul Satre

CHAPTER FOCUS

Definitions of Mental Health

History of Community Mental Health
   Early Humanitarian Reform
   Community Mental Health Reform

The Art and Science of Mental Health Nursing
   History of Psychiatric-Mental Health Nursing

Current Assessment of Mental Health Status
   Pattern of Use of Psychiatric-Mental Health Services
   Individuals and Groups Needing Psychiatric-Mental Health
      Services
   Ethics of Psychiatric-Mental Health Services

Psychiatric-Mental Health Nursing's Roles and
Phenomena of Concern

Models for Psychiatric-Mental Health Nursing Practice
   Public Health Model
   Primary Care Model
   Primary Mental Health Care Model
   Person-Focused Model of Practice and Nursing's
      Therapeutic Use of Self

The Future of Psychiatric-Mental Health Nursing
Practice

Healthy People 2010: Objectives Related to Mental
Health and Mental Disorders

QUESTIONS TO CONSIDER

After reading this chapter, answer the following questions:
   1. What is the definition of *mental health in the community*?
   2. What is the history of community mental health nursing?
   3. What is the current mental health status of Americans?
   4. What are some of the models for psychiatric-mental health nursing practice?
   5. What will psychiatric-mental health nursing practice be like in the future?

KEY TERMS

Advocacy
Community Mental Health
   Centers (CMHCs)

Phenomena of
   concern
Prevention

Psychiatric-mental
   health nursing
Seriously mentally ill

Universal human
   experiences

....

No temper could be more cheerful than hers, or possess, to a greater degree, that sanguine expectation of happiness which is happiness itself.

Jane Austen, 1775–1817

....

Definitions of Mental Health

Definitions of mental health in literature range from a focus on the absence of disease to the attainment of one's potential. The definition provided by *Healthy People 2000* "refers to an individual's ability to negotiate the daily challenges and social interactions of life, without experiencing undue emotional or behavioral incapacity" (DHHS, 1990). Missing in this definition is the human expectation and experience of living happily, as well as functionally, mentally healthy.

Concepts of mental health and illness have changed drastically over the last few centuries. In the 15th century the mentally ill were thought to be witches "possessed" by demons. Some cultures historically regard persons with psychiatric conditions as worthy of great respect, as having uncanny abilities and visionaries. At one time, mental illness was thought to be caused by a lesion or physical injury to the brain. If no objective injury or lesion was found, mental illness was thought to be a defect in morality and character.

....

Everything has been figured out, except how to live.

Jean Paul Sartre, 1905–1980

....

Since the early 1900s, identifying the mentally ill has been the focus of psychiatry. Great efforts were made toward the diagnosis and treatment of specific mental disorders and conditions. The development of the *Diagnostic and Statistical Manuals* (DSM) by the American Psychiatric Association (APA) since the 1950s (APA, 1980, 1987, 1992) has contributed to differentiation and research. Designated as "the decade of the brain," the focus of research in the 1990s has contributed to a fuller understanding of biological determinants of behavior (Hedaya, 1996). The major psychiatric milestones of the 20th century included the development of the diagnostic manual and assessment procedures; psychotherapy, including psychoanalysis; developmental theories; behavioral, cognitive, and psychological foci for psychotherapy, including crisis intervention, short-term, group, family, and long-term therapy; psychopharmacology; and knowledge concerning the biological determinants of behavior.

The definition of *mental health* is still in need of our attention and continued thinking in nursing. Many believe that the focus on biology has obscured, once again, the understanding of mental illness or mental health. The view of mental health in this chapter encompasses the notion that *mental health* involves connection of body, mind, and spirit, mental and physical wholesomeness. The concept of "balance" is common in holistic literature. Mental health is further viewed as involving a process through which a holistic balance between mind, body, and spirit (of individuals, families, and groups) is pursued through meaningful life activities. The mentally healthy person seeks experiences that promote well-being, productivity, and happiness as fully as possible given the particular situational contexts and limitations.

Nursing has historically embraced a role with caring that has focused on maximizing human potential. A focus on maintaining harmony and balance is needed in many areas of human endeavor and experience: in meaningful work, occupation or pursuit; in relationships with loved ones, significant others, and in social relationships, friendships, and work relationships; in meaningful relaxation, leisure, balanced nutrition, and fitness activities; and in having a respect and responsibility for the planet and world.

Mental illness or dysfunction, although it exists more in vulnerable population groups, is not wholly a respecter of vulnerability. There have been and currently are many gifted as well as ordinary people who have periodic mental health issues and conditions. The arts and sciences are filled with examples of brilliant and revolutionary contributions from people who had mental health problems. For example, the symbolist artist Edvard Munch, born in 1863, was an alcoholic and experienced depression throughout his life. His work focuses on themes of life and death and his experience with mental illness. The lithograph *The Scream* is one of his most important and popularized pieces. Of particular interest are three other works, *Anxiety, The Sick Child,* and *Death in the Sick Room.* As a young child, Munch experienced the death of his mother, and when he was 14, his sister died. *Death in the Sickroom* depicts the family scene years earlier. The following quote by Munch illustrates this anguish:

> I was born dying . . . Sickness, insanity, and death were the malevolent angels that guarded my cradle and have followed me through my life ever since.

History of Community Mental Health

In the United States today, the community mental health program is the primary model of care for people with serious mental illness. Begun in 1963, President John Kennedy raised awareness and attention to mental health with the Community Mental Health Centers Act. Federal funds were committed for the construction and staffing of **community mental health centers**

BOX 23-1 MENTAL HEALTH LEGISLATION AND ITS INFLUENCE ON MENTAL HEALTH SERVICES

1935	**Social Security Act**
	Shifted care for ill people from state to federal government.
1943	**National Institute for Mental Health**
	Established as one of the Institutes of Health, where funds for research and development were committed to mental health.
1955	**Mental Health Study**
	Established Joint Commission on Mental Illness & Health.
	Led to the transformation of state hospitals to establishment of CMHCs.
1963	**Community Mental Health Centers Act**
	Marked beginning of CMHCs and deinstitutionalization of large psychiatric hospitals.
1960s	Funds were committed from federal government for grants for education for mental health disciplines, including nursing; stipends were made available for traineeships for undergraduate and graduate nursing students; gradually these were less frequent and finally were no longer available.
1975	**Developmental Disabilities Act**
	Addressed rights of developmental disabilities and provided for similar actions for individuals with mental disorders.
1977	**President's Commission on Mental Health**
	Reinforced importance of community-based services, protection of human rights, and national health insurance for mentally ill persons.
1978	**Omnibus Reconciliation Act**
	Rescinded much of the 1977 commission's provisions and shifted funds for all health programs from federal to state governments in the form of block grants.
1986	**Protection and Advocacy for Mentally Ill Individuals Act**
	Legislated advocacy programs for mentally ill persons.
1990	**Americans with Disabilities Act**
	Prohibited discrimination and promoted employment opportunities for people with disabilities, including mental disorders.

Source: Adapted from Stanhope & Lancaster, 1996.

(CMHCs), using the catchment area concept, which distributed mental health services throughout states all over the country. Today these programs provide access to a range of services that before this legislation were nonexistent.

Community mental health development has been closely associated with legislation. Box 23-1 describes the major mental health legislative efforts and its influence on the development of mental health services.

....

Mental illness is the last great stigma of the 20th century. Most people treat someone with a mental illness as if it's their fault or as if they can just snap out of it.

Tipper Gore, June 18, 1999

....

Early Humanitarian Reform

Early treatment for people with mental illness was both cruel and inhumane. In 1843, Dorothea Dix, a school teacher, started the reform movement for the treatment of criminals, the mentally ill, and later, victims of the Civil War. Her work led to the establishment of asylums dedicated to humane treatment for the mentally ill. States built institutions for housing and treating persons with severe mental disorders. Intended as a humane movement, the large numbers of patients, combined with little knowledge and information about either cause or cure of mental illness, the establishment of asylums was, in retrospect, anything but humane. Within a few years, these large state institutions provided the only mental health treatment and grew to be overcrowded. Patients were not discharged to families in communities that had no treatment services. Psychiatric treatment was limited to somatic therapies and did very little to handle difficult symptoms. The asylum population continued to grow as new people were admitted and the long-term residential population grew. It was not uncommon for these patients to have stays of 20 to 40 years.

Community Mental Health Reform

From the mid-nineteenth century reform efforts of Dorothea Dix to the reforms of the latter half of the twentieth century, there has been much progress made in mental health science and treatment. The development of psychopharmacology was a milestone in treatment reform. Previously untreatable conditions were opened to the possibility of treatment. Since the early 1900s, psychotherapy had also been the focus of scholarship from several disciplines, including psychiatry, psychology, social work, and nursing. Psychotherapies that developed included long- and short-term and crisis intervention with individuals, groups, and families.

Currently, large numbers of clients discharged from the state institutions and those who would have required institutional care in years past are residing in communities. A large number of the homeless population in urban centers are chronically mentally ill. They continue to have exacerbating mental conditions and experience environmental stresses, including the stress of meeting basic needs. This group of homeless, chronically mentally ill is especially vulnerable.

As individuals were discharged from state mental institutions, private fee-for-service psychiatric services sprang up quickly in communities all over the country. Although care and a full range of treatment services are now more easily accessible within the community, there is inequity in access as a result of economic issues. Often, the families of the **seriously mentally ill** are unable to do what is necessary to ensure continuity of care or to get any care.

The goals and dreams of young mental health professionals of the community mental health movement showed great promise but have never been realized fully. The inequity in access and economics of mental health care and physical care continues to dominate the environment of mental health care. Within most communities, supportive services have been developed, primarily by the consumer movement, to meet particular support needs of clients. Box 23-2 identifies vulnerable groups who are in need of preventive, health promotion, and specialized treatment. Box 23-3 provides a listing of support services and groups available in many communities.

Beginning with the consumer movement of the 1970s, the groups focusing on support and psychoeducational issues with particular conditions have grown. These groups are available to the public, are listed in the telephone directories, and are advertised in varying community bulletin boards.

There is a growing need for identifying areas in need of care and attention, such as recent experiences of community loss, stress, and crisis experienced in the destruction of the World Trade Center in New York City in 2001. The high school shootings in Colorado at Columbine High (1999) and in Mississippi at Pearl High

BOX 23-2 VULNERABLE GROUPS

- Children and elders
- Adolescents
- Those experiencing work and vocational problems and transitions in work settings
- The unemployed
- The very old, older than 85
- Those living in poverty
- Single parents
- Adolescent parents
- Grandparents in parenting roles
- The uneducated
- The isolated and marginalized
- Those with learning and attention deficits
- Minority populations
- Depressed individuals
- Angry individuals
- Acutely or chronically ill individuals
- The incarcerated
- Victims of human and environmental abuse
- Victims of oppressive political systems
- Immigrants seeking asylum
- Those experiencing stress, crisis, change, and trauma

(1998) demonstrate that there is a growing need for both crisis and preventive intervention with adolescents and in schools. There is also need for more humanitarian reform involving economics and equity of mental health care. Increasingly, community programs are being called to provide consultation to schools and communities in dealing with sensitive issues needing professional mental health attention.

Mental health programs offer many services to the seriously mentally ill population. Box 23-4 provides a listing of examples of mental health services available in a community mental health center in Mississippi.

Inpatient services for the severely mentally ill are still provided by state hospital systems. Clients experiencing acute problems or acute exacerbations of chronic conditions are usually housed within jails in holding facilities, which usually have consultative psychiatric services. Despite attempts to build in continuity and access to care, there are needed reforms in all systems that use holding rather than inpatient treatment facilities. Inpatient services for the private system exist within relative geographic access in most communities. However, as cost containment measures have been instituted, inpatient care is often too brief. Insurance and economics are currently

BOX 23-3 SUPPORT GROUPS

- Compassionate Friends: focus on death, bereavement and loss (spouses, sudden infant death syndrome, perinatal, sibling)
- Cancer Support: focuses on variety of cancers, including breast cancer and ostomy
- Caregivers Support Group: for caregivers of elderly, cancer, mentally ill
- Infertility Support: for couples experiencing infertility
- Parents without Partners
- Suicide Survivors
- Addictions Anonymous: for alcohol, gambling, exercise, shopping, food
- Smoking Cessation: including smokeless tobacco
- Families of Murdered Victims
- Families of Seriously Mentally Ill
- Medication follow-up and education: for clients and families
- Parenting Groups: for parents of adolescents, learning disabilities, autism, incarcerated
- Grandparenting
- Homeless Mothers
- Diabetes Education
- Alzheimer's Family Support: including Parkinson's
- Fibromyalgia Support
- Cardiac: Mended Hearts
- Organ Donor Group Support: families of donors and recipients of organs
- Physical Disabilities Support

BOX 23-4 COMMUNITY MENTAL HEALTH SERVICES

SERVICES

- Seriously mentally ill day treatment
- Acute partial hospitalization for seriously mentally ill
- Children's services
- Adult day care
- Day Treatment Club House: for those with chronic conditions who live in the community
- Alcohol and chemical addictions programs
- Outpatient follow-up
- Group living

POSSIBLE TREATMENT MODALITIES AVAILABLE IN THESE PROGRAMS

- Resocialization, remotivation, and life skills assistance
- Social services
- Psychological services, including testing
- Medical services management and referral
- Psychopharmacological management
- Occupational therapy
- Recreational therapy
- Group, family therapy, and individual therapy
- Outreach and home visiting
- 12-step program
- Vocational rehabilitation
- Psychotherapy, long and short term

the greatest barriers to access to comprehensive, appropriate, and timely care in both the private and public systems.

The Art and Science of Mental Health Nursing

History of Psychiatric-Mental Health Nursing

As a nurse, I try to do for them what they would do for themselves if they had the strength, the will, and the knowledge that a nurse has. And I try to do it in such a way that I don't make them dependent on me, any more than is necessary.
            Interview with Virginia Henderson in Baer, 1990

The role of nursing, defined by Henderson, is relevant to the role of nursing in mental health. Box 23-5 identifies important events in the history of psychiatric nursing. Hildegard Peplau (1952), considered the founder of psychiatric nursing, further proposed that the context and development of the nurse-client relationship underpinned the professional nursing role. The early nursing leaders were involved with social reform movements and human rights and advocated for the poor and politically powerless. In addition, they knew the critical importance of social support. Nurses must learn to care for each other and the profession or else caring for others will continue to suffer (Lauterbach & Becker, 1996).

BOX 23-5 IMPORTANT EVENTS IN PSYCHIATRIC NURSING HISTORY, 1773–1955

1773	*First mental hospital in the United States established in Williamsburg, Virginia*
1846	*First use of the term psychiatry by physicians attempting to upgrade the status of their work with the mentally ill*
1882	*First school for psychiatric nurses (or mental nurses) established at the McLean Asylum in Somerville, Massachusetts*
1913	*Johns Hopkins Hospital included psychiatric nursing in the course of study for general nurses*
1920	*Publication of the first psychiatric nursing textbook, Nursing Mental Diseases, by Harriet Bailey*
1946	*Passage of the National Mental Health Act, which established the National Institutes of Mental Health (NIMH)*
1948	*Publication of the Brown Report, which recommended that psychiatric nursing be included in general nursing education*
1952	*Publication of Interpersonal Relations in Nursing by nurse theorist Hildegard Peplau*
1955	*National League for Nursing made psychiatric nursing a requirement for accreditation of basic nursing programs*

Source: Adapted from Frisch & Frisch, 1998.

BOX 23-6 PSYCHIATRIC MENTAL HEALTH NURSING: AREAS OF PRACTICE

BASIC-LEVEL FUNCTIONS

- Health promotion and health maintenance
- Intake screening and evaluation
- Case management
- Milieu management and therapy
- Self-care activities
- Psychobiological interventions
- Health teaching
- Crisis intervention
- Counseling and therapeutic relationships
- Home visiting
- Community action
- Advocacy

Source: Adapted from ANA, 1994.

and services be integrated *within* the health care system. Ideally, the role encompasses routine as well as specialty and advanced care, alongside a full range of primary, secondary, and tertiary care. There is potential for nursing to be involved in all levels of prevention and promotion of mental health, especially in advocacy for the inclusion of mental health care in community health care and mental health promotion and education. Box 23-6 identifies basic practice for psychiatric-mental health nursing. These are discussed later as the role of the nurse is fully articulated.

There is a particular need for psychiatric-mental health nursing to promote personal and professional health and well-being. The idea that caring for self before caring for others is the central thesis in Lauterbach and Becker's work (1996) on caring for self.

Current Assessment of Mental Health Status

In 1978, President Carter's commission on mental health estimated that nearly 15% of the U.S. population needed some type of mental health services at any given time. More recent epidemiological data show that approximately 32% of the U.S. population report symptoms meeting criteria for one or more psychiatric disorders during their lifetime (Tsuang, Tohen, and Zahner, 1995).

The community mental health (CMH) movement of the 1960s provided nursing an opportunity for **advocacy** and social reform. Concurrent with the Civil Rights movement, the movement heightened awareness and articulated rights of persons suffering with mental illness. Furthermore, at the 100th International Congress for Nursing in London (July 1999), human abuse was discussed as a global concern in the etiology of mental illness.

To address the current state of the art, science, and spirit of psychiatric-mental health nursing, particular attention will be given to nursing within the community context. The potential role of psychiatric-mental health nursing mandates that mental health care

Pattern of Use of Psychiatric-Mental Health Services

According to Tsuang, Tohen, and Zahner (1995, p. 202), mental health services data show that the burden of mental disorders in the population is large. Even with only 1 in 5 individuals with a diagnosable disorder using services in 1 year, the cost of treatment is large. The human costs are exorbitant when the ability to have a quality, meaningful, and productive life is considered.

Mental health services comprise a very large portion of the health care budget. It was estimated that in 1988, the total costs to society (including costs relating to accidents, crime, and other problems associated with mental disorders) were $273.3 billion. Insurance plans typically require the covered individual seeking mental health services to pay a larger co-payment and perhaps a higher deductible than for physical health services. Many people with mental disorders are among those with little or no health insurance coverage.

....

We are more alike, my friends,
than we are unalike.

Maya Angelou

....

HEALTHY PEOPLE 2010

OBJECTIVES RELATED TO MENTAL HEALTH AND MENTAL DISORDERS

Mental Health Status Improvement

18.1 Reduce the suicide rate.

18.2 Reduce the rate of suicide attempts by adolescents.

18.3 Reduce the proportion of homeless adults who have serious mental illness (SMI).

18.4 Increase the proportion of persons with serious mental illnesses who are employed.

18.5 Reduce the relapse rates for persons with eating disorders, including anorexia nervosa and bulimia nervosa.

Treatment Expansion

18.6 Increase the number of persons seen in primary health care who receive mental health screening and assessment.

18.7 Increase the proportion of children with mental health problems who receive treatment.

18.8 Increase the proportion of juvenile justice facilities that screen new admissions for mental health problems.

18.9 Increase the proportion of adults with mental disorders who receive treatment.

18.10 Increase the proportion of persons with co-occurring substance abuse and mental disorders who receive treatment for both disorders.

18.11 Increase the proportion of local governments with community-based jail diversion programs for adults with serious mental illnesses.

State Activities

18.12 Increase the number of states and the District of Columbia that track consumers' satisfaction with the mental health services they receive.

18.13 Increase the number of states, territories, and the District of Columbia with an operational mental health plan that addresses cultural competence.

18.14 Increase the number of states, territories, and the District of Columbia with an operational mental health plan that addresses mental health crisis interventions, ongoing screening, and treatment services for elderly persons.

Source: DHHS, 2000.

RESEARCH BRIEF

Beck, C. (1998). The effects of postpartum depression on child development; a meta-analysis. Archives of Psychiatric Nursing, 12(1), 12–20.

The adverse, short-term effects of postpartum depression on maternal-infant interaction has been documented, but are there long-term sequelae for children of these women? This meta-analysis was to determine the magnitude of cognitive and emotional development of children older than 1 year of age. Nine studies were examined and indicated that postpartum depression had a small but significant effect. The strength of the effect seems to have weakened as the child grew older. An earlier meta-analysis by the same researcher found that postpartum depression displayed a moderate to large adverse effect on infants' behavior. Implications for future research as well as the cautioned use of meta-analyses of research using linear thinking, was discussed.

BOX 23-7 COMMON HUMAN EXPERIENCES

- Loss, death, separation
- Crisis
- Relationships with significant others—family, friends, work, society
- Anxiety
- Sadness, depression, and mood conditions
- Developmental eras and transitions—individual, family, group, societal
- Illness—acute and chronic
- Stress and coping
- Coping with change

RESEARCH BRIEF

Co-Occuring Addictive and Mental Disorders

El-Mallakh (1998) examined national co-morbidity surveys of epidemiological research, which indicate that 51% of individuals with a serious psychiatric disorder are also dependent on or addicted to illicit drugs. However, only 50% of these clients received treatment for both co-occurring conditions. El-Mallakh's article provides a historical overview of treatment philosophies and approaches to treatment. It also describes current models and outcome data regarding efficacy of treatment. Recommendations were made to include effective treatment models into nursing practices.

Individuals and Groups Needing Psychiatric-Mental Health Services

Healthy People 2010 identifies mental health problems and populations in need. Parents with young teens are aware of the growing population of youth who are encountering very serious substance use, including cigarettes, smokeless tobacco, an incredible variety of inhalants, abuse of prescription "pills," and daily and large quantities of marijuana use, coupled with alcohol. In addition, the epidemics of rape, violence, legal entanglements, and pregnancy among junior and senior high school students is, from the perspective of the youth, much greater than statistics demonstrate. The pattern of misuse and abuse that is reflected in the aforementioned behaviors, along with a recognition that problems with anxiety, depression, and attention to school and learning warrant careful investigation, research, and concurrent social action. Many of the behaviors are seen by professionals as attempts to self-medicate. However, research is needed to identify factors that are associated with and contribute to "using" behaviors. We need to understand more about these human **phenomena**.

There are a growing number of individuals and groups at risk in need of primary mental health nursing as well as specialized psychiatric-mental health care. This reflects the growing consumer and public recognition that specialized support is needed to cope with particular human phenomena and experiences. Box 23-7 lists common, **universal human experiences** that are often in need of special support and crisis or continuing care. The potential direction and roles for psychiatric-mental health nursing will focus on assisting persons and groups in handling living through difficult human experience.

Changes in the American family warrant particular attention. A growing number of children grow up in single-parent homes, usually with the father absent. There are changes in the structure and function of families. Single parents and working women are growing in number. This combined with poverty serves to compound vulnerability.

The growing elderly population with cognitive impairments, institutionalized elders, and those with Alzheimer's and

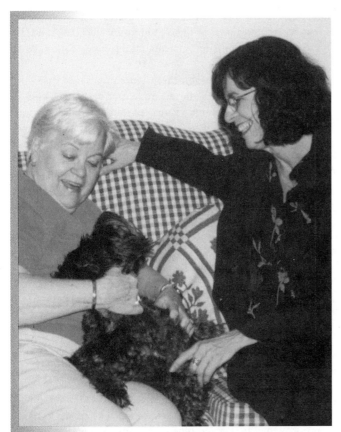

Dr. Sarah Steen Lauterbach, chapter author, in encounter with client.

ment is a human rights issue. While mental health is much improved today, there is still great need for equity and mainstreaming of mental health services into the health care system of services.

Mental health problems, in contrast to physical health problems, are often very complex, involving an interaction of many factors, including heredity, culture, social class, living conditions, lifestyle, family relationships, occupation, and economics and politics. There are often unrecognized mental health issues surrounding and involved with physical health and illness conditions that, if treated along with the physical illness, would promote a healthier adjustment. The separation of mental health services from other health services creates problems of access to treatment. Problems occur both for those with major or chronic and debilitating mental health conditions and for those who have symptoms that, if treated appropriately at the time, would contribute to the recovery, health, and well-being of the person.

their families further reflect the concept of compounding vulnerability. More work, more research, and more preventive efforts are needed for serious mental health conditions and diagnoses, such as schizophrenia, which involve exacerbations of acute symptoms of distress and disturbance. This population represents a large number of persons and families who experience periods of acute exacerbation of chronic illness. Other chronic illnesses, such as diabetes, have patterns involving crisis and management and need psychiatric-mental health nursing attention.

Ethics of Psychiatric-Mental Health Services

Inequity that exists around mental health care impoverishes a group of people who are already at risk. Furthermore, cost of services is a factor in access and serves to compound risk in an already vulnerable population. This is in direct conflict with prevention concepts and health promotion, which require delicate timing and appropriate intervention within the least restrictive environment. The right to fair and equal mental health treat-

Psychiatric-Mental Health Nursing's Roles and Phenomena of Concern

The American Nurses Association (ANA, 1994a) identified a list of actual or potential mental health problems presented in Box 23-8 that comprise phenomena of psychiatric-mental health nursing's concern. These include phenomena presented earlier as universal human experiences in need of attention, care, and research. Basic-level functions of psychiatric-mental health nursing presented previously are inclusive of both prevention and promotion activities as well as treatment and intervention activities.

The psychiatric-mental health nursing role includes health promotion, health maintenance, health teaching, community action, and advocacy; however, this area comprises one of the greatest needs in community mental health program development. Currently, nurses in practice within community programs function primarily as managers of care, overseeing care, administering medication, and maintaining records. Community action and advocacy activities are often limited. Some nurses are involved in developing and maintaining the therapeutic milieu, but staffing issues are prevalent throughout the private and public programs.

Missing from the list of functions is the nurse's key role in providing continuity of care. The nurse's unique role and position with persons and groups over time provide opportunities for support and intervention that others on the treatment team simply do not have. In addition, the commitment to using strengths of people and active involvement of those cared for place nursing in a key position.

BOX 23-8 PSYCHIATRIC-MENTAL HEALTH NURSING'S PHENOMENA OF CONCERN

Actual or potential mental health problems of clients pertaining to the following:

- The maintenance of optimal health and well-being and the prevention of psychobiological illness
- Self-care limitations or impaired functioning related to mental and emotional distress
- Deficits in the functioning of significant biological, emotional, and cognitive systems
- Emotional stress or crisis components of illness, pain, and disability
- Self-concept changes, developmental issues, and life process changes
- Problems related to emotions such as anxiety, anger, sadness, loneliness, and grief
- Physical symptoms that occur along with altered psychological functioning
- Alterations in thinking, perceiving, symbolizing, communicating, and decision making
- Difficulties in relating to others
- Behaviors and mental states that indicate the client is a danger to self or others or has a severe disability
- Interpersonal, systemic, sociocultural, spiritual, or environmental circumstances or events that affect the mental and emotional well-being of the individual, family, or community
- Symptom management, side effects/toxicities associated with psychopharmacological intervention and other aspects of the treatment regimen

Source: ANA, 1994.

Since the beginning of modern nursing, the concept of *prevention as intervention* has been a key concept of health care. The unique vantage provided by the nursing perspective, nursing presence, and the temporality of this role is often underused in therapeutic relationships with individuals, groups, and communities. This is an area in need of attention in both public and private programs.

The psychiatric-mental health nurse of the 21st century has assumed more coordinating, collaborative, and case management activities than ever before. At the same time, the role encompasses direct service and therapeutic interventions with individual and groups within services and programs that are located at a variety of locations, within community agencies, and the home. The role of nursing in mental health needs continued assessment and evaluation.

In primary mental health care environments, the basic-level psychiatric-mental health nurses are key professionals who are ideally positioned to assume a variety of roles in multiple settings ranging from acute inpatient to community settings. They are often the only member of the health care team who has the knowledge to monitor general health as well as mental health needs and care. They are prepared in early identification of problems, including preventive intervention, primary prevention, and health promotion. They possess skills in assessment, social intervention, and psychoeducational processes connected with understanding illness and experience of mental illness, and also have knowledge of symptom management, pharmacology, and rehabilitation.

Models for Psychiatric–Mental Health Nursing Practice

Public Health Model

The traditional public health model includes all levels of prevention: primary, secondary, and tertiary. It has been a viable model for psychiatric-mental health nursing practice. Central to this model is the critical role of public education. This model uses concepts of mental health and illness, epidemiology, and statistics in assessing mental health needs as well as risks.

Currently, the major thrust of American mental health care is toward secondary prevention efforts, providing treatment and minimizing disability. There is a need for research and funding in all areas of prevention, but particularly within primary prevention. The following primary prevention activities are in need of public policy inquiry and research: mental health promotion and dysfunction prevention; holistic, meaningful, mind-body wellness activities; personal and community education; acquisition of effective coping skills; wholesome early attachments and healthy lifelong relationships; facilitating environments conducive to meaningful work and mental and physical health; and finally, self-empowerment. There is need for large-scale community studies of stress, crisis, and post-trauma, especially in the United States following the catastrophic events of September 11, 2001.

Secondary prevention activities are the major thrust of care and include early diagnosis and intervention, accessible services, and timely, appropriate treatment. One of the most important contributions of the community mental health movement of the 1960s to the present has been the development of crisis intervention services. This, combined with the consumer movement of the 1970s, has made a significant contribution to support services for individuals and communities. Still, major primary prevention work is needed to address the conditions and environments that create and perpetuate interpersonal crises. Situational crises, which are superimposed on predicted developmental crises, further create risk, but with proper attention, they can be addressed. Consumer involvement has been helpful in the development of suicide prevention programs, services for rape crisis and victim recovery, and other phenomena needing support and therapeutic intervention. However, more research into crisis prevention, intervention, and impact of crises on life is needed. Human abuse and violence needs to be researched and better understood. Where treatment usually is focused on the victim, more work is needed in addressing the treatment and rehabilitation of the perpetrator, facilitating a violence-free environment. Phenomena need to be reconceptualized and investigated as a community and social phenomenon as well as an individual phenomenon.

Tertiary care has been the focus of community mental health programs and currently provides most of the care for the seriously mentally ill public, including state hospitalization. The community mental health care system includes a range of community-based services addressing a full range of needs and particular groups needing care. These programs address ongoing and acute exacerbations of conditions and chronic care. Activities aimed at rehabilitation and reducing the discomfort and suffering associated with particular mental health problems need research.

Primary Care Model

Since the beginning of modern nursing, nursing has offered two different perspectives for the focus of care: caring for the individual and caring for the needs of communities. There is often tension between these two different perspectives. This is especially true for psychiatric-mental health nursing, where the individual often is seen as the identified client but in reality reflects dysfunction within a family, community, or larger social system. Taking the example of the state of the mental health care system in the United States, there are stigma and economic differences within systems providing physical care and mental health care. Privatization of mental health care, reimbursement differences between physical and mental care, and the current contrast with public mental health care's focus on tertiary care are reflective of sentiment and thinking in a society that values economics and physical care over mental health.

Nursing has traditionally been able to provide care to both individuals and groups, using both paradigms for providing care: the public health model and person-focused or family-centered model. Nurses have seen the need for the current "illness care" system to be transformed into a "health care" system.

Primary health care is increasingly being viewed as synonymous with provision of health care (Haber, 1995). If this concept is to be fully actualized, then primary care will necessarily have to include mental health care. Nursing needs to take a position for advocating planned change and the right for each citizen to have responsive, quality mental health care as a component of quality health care.

FYI

Primary Mental Health Care: A Model for Psychiatric-Mental Health Nursing

Haber and Billings (1995) state that primary care is increasingly becoming synonymous with the provision of health care. In addition to discussing roles of basic and advanced level nursing practice in primary mental health care, these authors state that anxiety disorders, depression, and substance abuse are among the most commonly misdiagnosed categories in primary health care practice. In addition, they propose that the boundaries of mental health care delivery must be redefined and expanded from a specialty focus to a primary mental health care model. Furthermore, they state that nurses are beginning to find their niche in nontraditional settings.

Primary Mental Health Care Model

Increasingly, the discussion of a primary mental health care model is being proposed as a model for delivering community-based, comprehensive psychiatric-mental health nursing (Haber, 1995). It has the potential to integrate the two traditional models of care and puts nursing in a key role meeting needs of both individuals and communities. There is need for continued dialog between psychiatric nurses themselves, represented by the Coalition of Psychiatric Nursing Organizations (COPNO), including the ANA Council on Psychiatric Mental Health Nursing, the American Psychiatric Nursing Association (APNA), the Association of Child and Adolescent Psychiatric Nurses, and the Society for the Education and Research in Psychiatric Nursing (SERPN). Even though many nurses belong to more than one organization, there is need for uniting as a body, a process that has been under way.

Primary care roles need to be conceptualized to include providing psychiatric-mental health care within front-line health care and should include more than case management of psychiatric clients receiving tertiary and chronic psychiatric-mental health care.

I always said that mental health got what was left over after everybody else in the health field got what they wanted.

Rosalyn Carter, who as first lady served as co-chair of the President's Commission on Mental Health and championed the rights of those with mental illness

We do not see things as they are, we see them as we are.

Talmud

The Future of Psychiatric-Mental Health Nursing Practice

Current psychiatric-mental health nursing practice operates within the managed care, cost containment drive behind health care. A growing number of persons, groups, and communities are not receiving care, do not have basic needs met, and are being lost between services and programs. Preventive care is still in need of development. Psychiatric-mental health nurses need to be in integrated into primary health care environments and in community-based programs, such as in schools, day-care programs, parenting programs, and self-help and support programs. Most importantly, there is need for psychiatric-mental health advocacy in the area of health policy and health care planning. Increasingly, communities are experiencing acts of violence. Grandparents are parenting their dysfunctional adult children's children. The future looks bleak as the future grandparents are today's dysfunctional adults. Within this day of information and technology, the growing Third World vulnerable populations, within the larger affluent American society, are cause for concern. Unless we support and care for all our population's needs, health and human rights, including shelter, nutrition, and meaningful life, the health and happiness of the public is threatened. Caring comprehensively for a multicultural population and world is key.

CONCLUSION

Isolation and stigma that surround mental health has in the past surrounded other conditions. Cancer was in years past such a dreaded and stigmatized disease. Education and knowledge along with progress in making scientific advances and successful treatment contribute to increased awareness and understanding.

It was not until the 1950s, with the advent of psychopharmacology, that symptoms were treated successfully. The reliance on somatic therapies, such as hydrotherapy, insulin shock, and physical restraints before the psychopharmacological agents, further produced fear and stigma. The newer developments with antipsychotics and antidepressive agents have greatly enhanced treatment of serious episodes and acute exacerbations of chronic conditions. With knowledge has come greater openness and acceptance. Although we have come a long way, we still have a long way to go in meeting the public's mental health needs. Psychiatric-mental health nursing must continue a commitment to social reform. Of all specialties, we offer to guide the world in becoming more aware of meanings of human experiences. Through our interventions in the planning and policy arena and in our daily interactions with clients, families, communities, and colleagues, we hope to enable all people to live as fully as possible—in the words of one young man, "to live life out" as meaningfully, productively, healthfully, and happily as possible.

CRITICAL THINKING ACTIVITIES

1. Consider what is it like to experience the following:
   - Serious mental illness, such as schizophrenia, mania, or depression
   - Paranoid feelings, to the degree that you know that if you do not take medication, you will get sicker and sicker
   - Feeling that the medication dulls your attention, which helps you stay vigilant; feeling that something bad will happen if you let down your guard

2. What is it like to experience the following?
   - Having no one who you feel understands you and likes you just the way you are
   - Having no friends
   - Experiencing your little brother's death after he was sick so long with leukemia
   - Watching your dad begin to drink heavily in the evenings
   - Feeling fat, even though you only ate lettuce today, weigh 105 and are 5 feet, 7 inches tall
   - Wanting and feeling very independent but still being told by your parents what time you must come in

3. What is it like to experience the following?
   - Wanting your parents to stop fighting
   - Wanting your parents to get back together even though you remember how awful it was before they separated
   - Being devastated when your dad moved out
   - Living with your mom, who works too hard and still does not have enough money even though she gets some child support
   - Visiting your dad, who has forgotten what it is like to have anyone, much less a child, around

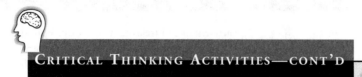

CRITICAL THINKING ACTIVITIES—CONT'D

4. What is it like to experience the following?
   - Being so depressed that you simply are too tired to get out of bed
   - Feeling that you have nothing to live for
   - Feeling that the world and your family would be better off if you just died
   - Being 17 and suddenly discovering that you had lost all your dreams and goals

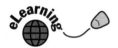

Explore Community Health Nursing on the web! To learn more about the topics in this chapter, access your exclusive web site:
http://communitynursing.jbpub.com

REFERENCES

American Nurses Association (ANA). (1994a). *A statement on psychiatric-mental health clinical nursing practice and standards of psychiatric-mental health clinical nursing practice*. Washington, DC: American Nurses Publishing.

American Nurses Association (ANA). (1994b). *Scope and standards of advanced practice registered nursing*. Washington, DC: American Nurses Publishing.

American Nurses Association (ANA). (1994c). *Psychiatric mental health nursing psychopharmacology project*. Washington, DC: American Nurses Publishing.

American Psychiatric Association (APA). (1980). *Diagnostic and statistical manual of mental disorders* (3rd ed.). Washington, DC: Author.

American Psychiatric Association (APA). (1987). *Diagnostic and statistical manual of mental disorders (3rd ed.,* rev.) Washington, DC: Author.

American Psychiatric Association (APA). (1992). *Diagnostic and statistical manual of mental disorders* (4th ed.) Washington, DC: Author.

Angelou, M. (1971). *Just give me a cool drink of water 'fore i die: The poetry of Maya Angelou*. New York: Random House.

Angelou, M. (1993). *Wouldn't take nothing for my journey now*. New York: Random House.

Baer, E. (1990). *Editor's notes. Nursing in America: A history of social reform, a video documentary*. New York: National League for Nursing Press.

Beck, C. (1998). The effects of postpartum depression on child development; a meta-analysis. *Archives of Psychiatric Nursing, 12*(1), 12–20.

Caplan, G. (1964). *Principles of preventive psychiatry*. New York: Basic Books.

Department of Health and Human Services (DHHS). (2000). *Healthy People 2000: Conference edition*. Washington, DC: U.S. Government Printing Office.

Department of Health and Human Services (DHHS). (1978). *Women's Worlds: NIMH supported research on women*. Washington, DC: U.S. Government Printing Office.

Department of Health, Education, & Welfare. (1978). *Women's worlds: NIMH supported research on women*. Washington, DC: U.S. Government Printing Office.

Donahue, M. (1989). *Nursing: The finest art*. St. Louis: Mosby.

El-Mallakh, P. (1998). Treatment models for clients with co-occurring addictive and mental disorders. *Archives of Psychiatric Nursing, 12*(2), 71–80.

Frisch, H., & Frisch, L. (1998). *Psychiatric mental health nursing*. Albany, NY: Delmar.

Haber, J., & Billings, C. (1995). Primary mental health care: A model for psychiatric-mental health nursing. *Journal of the American Psychiatric Nurses Association, 1*(5), 154–163.

Hedaya, R. (1996). *Understanding biological psychiatry*. New York: W. W. Norton & Company.

Henderson, V. (1966a). *The nature of nursing*. New York: Macmillan.

Henderson, V. (1966b). *The nature of nursing: Reflections after 25 Years*. New York: National League for Nursing Press.

Lauterbach, S., & Becker, P. (1996). Caring for self: Becoming a self-reflective nurse. *Holistic Nursing Practice, 10*(2), 57–68.

Leighton, A. (1982). *Caring for mentally ill people: Psychological and social barriers in historical context*. Cambridge, UK: Cambridge University Press.

May, R. (1961). *Existential psychology*. New York: Random House.

Nightingale, F. (1859). *Notes on nursing: What it is and what it is not*. New York: Dover Publications.

Peplau, H. (1952). *Interpersonal relations in nursing*. New York: G. P. Putnam's Sons.

President's Commission on Mental Health. (1978). *Report to the President from the President's Commission on Mental Health*. Stock # 040-000-00390, Vol. 1. Washington, DC: US Government Printing Office.

Stanhope, M., & Lancaster, J. (1996). *Community health nursing*. St. Louis: Mosby.

Todd, M., & Higginson, T. (1982). *Collected poems of Emily Dickinson*. New York: Random House. (Originally published in 1890.)

Tsuang, M., Tohen, M., & Zahner, G. (1995). *Textbook in psychiatric epidemiology*. New York: John Wiley and Sons.

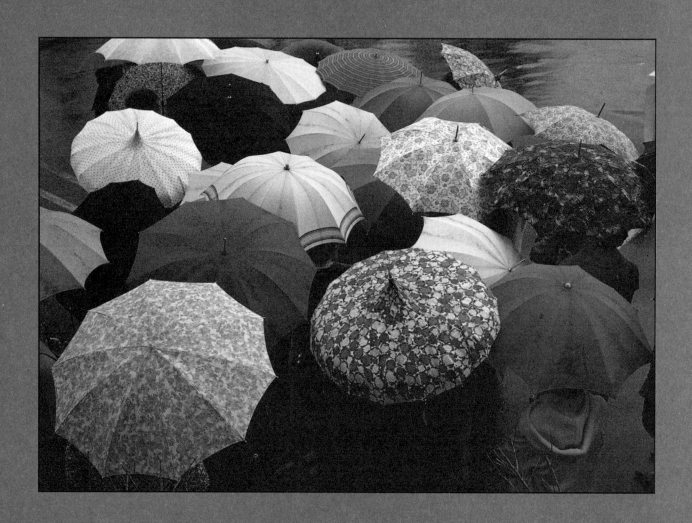

Appendix

Healthy People in Healthy Communities

A Systematic Approach to Health Improvement

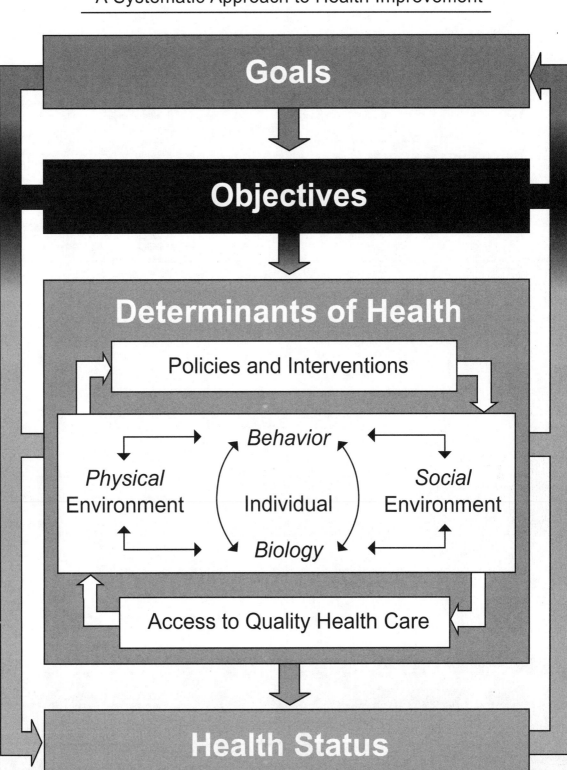

Index